D1483476

Clinical Manual of Contact Lenses

THIRD EDITION

Clinical Manual of Contact Lenses

THIRD EDITION

Edward S. Bennett, OD, MSEd
Associate Professor of Optometry
Co-Chief, Contact Lens Service
Director of Student Services
College of Optometry
University of Missouri-St. Louis
St. Louis, Missouri

Vinita Allee Henry, OD
Clinical Professor of Optometry
Co-Chief, Contact Lens Service
Director of Residency Programs
College of Optometry
University of Missouri-St. Louis
St. Louis, Missouri

Wolters Kluwer | Lippincott Williams & Wilkins
Health

Philadelphia · Baltimore · New York · London
Buenos Aires · Hong Kong · Sydney · Tokyo

Executive Editor: Jonathan W. Pine, Jr.
Senior Managing Editor: Anne E. Jacobs
Project Manager: Alicia Jackson
Senior Manufacturing Manager: Benjamin Rivera
Marketing Manager: Lisa Parry
Designer: Terry Mallon
Cover Designer: Joseph DePinho
Production Service: Maryland Composition

© 2009 by LIPPINCOTT WILLIAMS & WILKINS, a WOLTERS KLUWER business

530 Walnut Street
Philadelphia, PA 19106 USA
LWW.com

First Edition: Lippincott Williams & Wilkins, 1994, Second Edition: Lippincott Williams & Wilkins, 2000.

All rights reserved. This book is protected by copyright. No part of this book may be reproduced in any form by any means, including photocopying, or utilized by any information storage and retrieval system without written permission from the copyright owner, except for brief quotations embodied in critical articles and reviews. Materials appearing in this book prepared by individuals as part of their official duties as U.S. government employees are not covered by the above-mentioned copyright.

Printed in China

Library of Congress Cataloging-in-Publication Data

978-0-7817-7829-9
0-7817-7829-8
Clinical manual of contact lenses / [edited by] Edward S. Bennett, Vinita Allee Henry.—3rd ed.
    p. ; cm.
  Includes bibliographical references and index.
  ISBN 978-0-7817-7829-9
  1. Contact lenses—Handbooks, manuals, etc. I. Bennett, Edward S. II. Henry, Vinita Allee.
  [DNLM: 1. Contact Lenses. WW 355 C641 2008]
  RE977.C6C525 2008
  617.7′523—dc22

2008021814

Care has been taken to confirm the accuracy of the information presented and to describe generally accepted practices. However, the authors, editors, and publisher are not responsible for errors or omissions or for any consequences from application of the information in this book and make no warranty, expressed or implied, with respect to the currency, completeness, or accuracy of the contents of the publication. Application of the information in a particular situation remains the professional responsibility of the practitioner.

The authors, editors, and publisher have exerted every effort to ensure that drug selection and dosage set forth in this text are in accordance with current recommendations and practice at the time of publication. However, in view of ongoing research, changes in government regulations, and the constant flow of information relating to drug therapy and drug reactions, the reader is urged to check the package insert for each drug for any change in indications and dosage and for added warnings and precautions. This is particularly important when the recommended agent is a new or infrequently employed drug.

Some drugs and medical devices presented in the publication have Food and Drug Administration (FDA) clearance for limited use in restricted research settings. It is the responsibility of the health care provider to ascertain the FDA status of each drug or device planned for use in their clinical practice.

To purchase additional copies of this book, call our customer service department at (800) 638-3030 or fax orders to (301) 223-2320. International customers should call (301) 223-2300.

Visit Lippincott Williams & Wilkins on the Internet: at LWW.com. Lippincott Williams & Wilkins customer service representatives are available from 8:30 am to 6 pm, EST.

10 9 8 7 6 5 4 3 2 1

CCS1108

To our families for their devotion and encouragement

Jean, Matthew, Josh, Emily, and my mother, Mary Edith Snider

ESB

Sam, Amanda, Emily, Elizabeth, and my parents,
Vincel and Anita Allee

VAH

Contributing Authors

Joseph T. Barr, OD, MS
Professor of Optometry Emeritus
College of Optometry
The Ohio State University
Columbus, Ohio
Vice President Global Clinical and Medical
    Affairs and Professional Services Vision
    Care
Private Practice
Rochester, New York

P. Douglas Becherer, OD, FAAO
Adjunct Professor of Optometry
College of Optometry
University of Missouri–St. Louis
Private Practice
St. Louis, Missouri

Carolyn G. Begley, OD, MS
Professor
School of Optometry
Indiana University
Bloomington, Indiana

William J. Benjamin, OD, PhD
Professor of Optometry and Vision Science
School of Optometry
The University of Alabama at Birmingham
Birmingham, Alabama

Edward S. Bennett, OD, MSEd
Associate Professor of Optometry
Co-Chief, Contact Lens Service
Director of Student Services
College of Optometry
University of Missouri-St. Louis
St. Louis, Missouri

John de Brabander, PhD, FAAO
Senior Researcher/Research Coordinator
Eye Research Institute
Department of Ophthalmology
Maastricht University
Academic Hospital
Maastricht, The Netherlands

Dennis Burger, OD
Clinical Professor of Optometry
Department of Optometry
University of California
Berkley, California

J. Bart Campbell, OD
Professor of Optometry
The Eye Center
Southern College of Optometry
Memphis, Tennessee

Carmen Castellano, PhD, FAAO
Private Practice
St. Louis, Missouri

Walter Choate, OD
Private Practice
Madison, Tennessee

Larry J. Davis, OD
Associate Professor and Dean
College of Optometry
University of Missouri-St. Louis
St. Louis, Missouri

Michael DePaolis, OD, FAAO
Clinical Associate in Ophthalmology
University of Rochester
Private Practice
Rochester, New York

Kathy Dumbleton, BSc (Hons), MSc, MCOptom, FAAO (DipCL), FBCLA
Senior Clinical Scientist
Centre for Contact Lens Research, School of
    Optometry
University of Waterloo
Waterloo, Ontario, Canada

Stephanie Erker
Department of Optometry
College of Optometry
University of Missouri–St. Louis
St. Louis, Missouri

N. Rex Ghormley, OD, FAAO
Assistant Professor of Optometry
College of Optometry
University of Missouri–St. Louis
Private Practice
St. Louis, Missouri

Jeff Harter
Department of Optometry
College of Optometry
University of Missouri–St. Louis
St. Louis, Missouri

Vinita Allee Henry, OD
Clinical Professor of Optometry
Co-Chief, Contact Lens Service
Director of Residency Programs
College of Optometry
University of Missouri-St. Louis
St. Louis, Missouri

John Mark Jackson, OD
Associate Professor of Optometry
Southern College of Optometry
Memphis, Tennessee

Lyndon Jones, PhD, FCOptom, FAAO
Professor of Optometry
School of Optometry
University of Waterloo
Waterloo, Ontario, Canada

Frans Jongsma, PhD
Senior Researcher
Eye Research Institute
Department of Ophthalmology
Maastricht University
Academic Hospital
Maastricht, The Netherlands

Janice M. Jurkus, OD, MBA
Professor of Optometry
Illinois College of Optometry
Chicago, Illinois

Kimberly A. Layfield, OD
Private Practice
Winfield, Missouri

John W. Marohn, OD
Private Practice
St. Joseph, Michigan

Ron Melton, OD, FAAO
Private Practice
Concord, North Carolina

Julie Ott DeKinder, OD, FAAO
Assistant Clinical Professor of Optometry
College of Optometry
University of Missouri–St. Louis
St. Louis, Missouri

Keith Parker, NCLEC
President
Advanced Vision Technologies
Golden, Colorado

Marjorie Rah, OD, PhD
Assistant Professor of Optometry
The New England College of Optometry
Boston, Massachusetts

Jack Schaeffer, OD
Private Practice
Schaeffer Eye Center
Birmingham, Alabama

Terry Scheid, OD, FAAO
Diplomate AAO Cornea and Contact Lenses
Associate Clinical Professor of Optometry
SUNY College of Optometry
New York, New York

Peter G. Shaw-McMinn, OD
Assistant Professor of Optometry
Southern California College of Optometry
Private Practice
Sun City, California

Joseph Shovlin, OD, FAAO
Adjunct Faculty
Pennsylvania College of Optometry
Director of Contact Lens Service
Northeastern Eye Institute
Scranton, Pennsylvania

Christine Sindt, OD
Clinical Associate Professor
Department of Ophthalmology
University Hospitals and Clinics
Iowa City, Iowa

**Luigina Sorbara, OD, MSc, FAAO,
   Dipl C&CL**
Associate Professor
School of Optometry
University of Waterloo
Waterloo, Ontario, Canada

Loretta Szczotka-Flynn, OD, FAAO
Associate Professor of Ophthalmology
Department of Ophthalmology
Case Western Reserve University
Cleveland, Ohio

Randall Thomas, OD, MPH, FAAO
Private Practice
Concord, North Carolina

Eef van der Worp, BOptom, FAAO, FIACLE
Researcher/Lecturer
Eye Research Institute
Department of Opthalmology
Maastricht University
Academic Hospital
Maastricht, The Netherlands

Heidi Wagner, OD, MPH
Associate Professor
College of Optometry
Division of Health Professions
Nova Southeastern University
Fort Lauderdale, Florida

Ronald K. Watanabe, OD
Associate Professor of Optometry
Department of Specialty and Advanced Care
The New England College of Optometry
Boston, Massachusetts

Walter West, OD, FAAO
Private Practice
Brentwood, Tennesse

Brad Williams, OD, FAAO
Private Practice
Lincoln, Nebraska

Preface

In this Third Edition of the *Clinical Manual of Contact Lenses*, we have sought to not only update and revise this manual, but also to introduce new chapters on expanded areas in the field of contact lenses. New soft extended wear options, multifocal designs, orthokeratology and post-surgical fitting are areas that are increasing in popularity and can represent a challenge to contact lens practitioners. More emphasis has been given in this text to keratoconus, which impacts more patients than previously believed.

This book addresses a wide variety of clinical topics, including rigid gas permeable (GP) lens design and fitting, soft lens problem-solving, astigmatic management and bifocal correction. It is written so the practitioner can easily locate a topic and information about that topic without having to read an entire chapter. Each chapter concludes with sample cases that reinforce and demonstrate the practical nature of the chapter's topic. Nomograms and proficiency checklists also summarize and emphasize the important points in the chapters.

The purpose of Clinical Manual of Contact Lenses is to help students and practitioners fit, evaluate, and troubleshoot contact lenses, especially specialty contact lens designs. We hope this strictly clinical text will aid in everyday fitting situations and be an easy reference source to answer questions that might arise during the evaluation of a contact lens patient. It is written generically to be current for many years.

Edward S. Bennett, OD, MSEd
Vinita Allee Henry, OD

Acknowledgments

It is not possible to author a clinical text without it being a collaborative effort. We would like to first acknowledge our contributors, without whom this text would not have been possible. They include: Joe Barr, Doug Becherer, Carolyn Begley, Denny Burger, Joe Benjamin, Bart Campbell, Carmen Castellano, Walter Choate, Larry Davis, Julie DeKinder, Mike DePaolis, Kathy Dumbleton, Stephanie Erker, Rex Ghormley, Jeff Harter, John Mark Jackson, Lyndon Jones, Jan Jurkus, Kim Layfield, John Marohn, Ron Melton, Keith Parker, Marjie Rah, Jack Schaeffer, Terry Scheid, Peter Shaw-McMinn, Joe Shovlin, Christine Sindt, Luigina Sorbara, Loretta Szczotka-Flynn, Randall Thomas, Eef van der Worp, Heidi Wagner, Ron Watanabe, Walt West, and Brad Williams.

We appreciate the assistance of our graphical artist, Janice White for her contributions to this text. We would also like to acknowledge Drew Biondo, Sally Dillehay, Kylie Divine, and Amy Langford for their contributions. The support of Lippincott Williams & Wilkins—in particular, Senior Executive Editor Jonathan Pine—is greatly appreciated.

The support of our families and especially our spouses, Jean and Sam, made it possible for us to devote the time necessary to make this text as timely and clinically applicable as humanly possible.

This year marks the 25th year of our working together. It has been a privilege and a blessing to work as a team. Only the most fortunate have the opportunity to have a professor become a mentor, a colleague, and a close friend. This book is a celebration of that friendship.

Finally, we would like to acknowledge all practitioners who believe that contact lenses and, in particular, specialty lens designs, have an important application in their respective practices. We hope this text serves as a beneficial guide in helping you build your contact lens practice and our students who will be the future of our profession.

Contents

Clinical Manual of Contact Lenses

THIRD EDITION

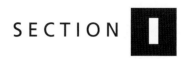

Introduction

CHAPTER 1

Preliminary Evaluation

Edward S. Bennett, Ronald K. Watanabe, and Carolyn G. Begley

▓ PURPOSE

A comprehensive preliminary evaluation is the essential first step in the contact lens fitting process. It is extremely important for the practitioner to evaluate every potential contact lens wearer to determine whether the patient is suitable for contact lens wear. This will minimize the risk of future failures or problems because of poor patient selection. If the patient is deemed a good candidate, the information obtained during the prefitting examination will help determine the most appropriate lens material, lens design, wearing time, and care regimen. It also serves as baseline data with which changes caused by contact lens wear can be compared.

▓ HISTORY

A good history includes the patient's reasons for wanting to wear contact lenses, ocular and medical histories, and any previous contact lens history. The history should guide the clinician in determining which tests to perform and the expected results for those tests. It should also contribute to the fitter's recommendations on contact lens types, care regimens, and wearing schedules.

Reasons for Contact Lens Wear

1. Cosmesis. Many patients do not like their appearance in glasses.
2. Inconvenience of glasses. They may be uncomfortable, get misplaced or broken, and have to be cleaned.
3. Improved vision. Patients with high ametropias, high astigmatism, keratoconus, corneal trauma, corneal distortion, and poor refractive surgery outcomes benefit visually from contact lenses.
4. Sports and recreation. Most athletes, both professional and recreational, benefit from the wider field of vision provided by contact lenses.
5. Occupation. In addition to athletes, individuals in the performing arts benefit greatly from contact lens wear. Celebrities, politicians, and others in the public eye may prefer their cosmetic appearance in contact lenses. However, contact lenses are contraindicated for patients who work in dusty, dirty environments (e.g., coal miners, sanitation workers) where debris and particulate matter may become trapped under the lens. In addition, individuals such as laboratory workers and hairdressers who work around noxious fumes are borderline contact lens candidates because of the possibility of a chemical keratitis and lens surface contamination. Some workers such as plumbers and automobile mechanics may experience difficulty cleaning all of the dirt and oils off their hands and therefore may be poor candidates. Other individuals, such as pilots, flight attendants, and video display terminal operators, may work in low-humidity environments and perform tasks during which blinking is inhibited. These individuals are not contraindicated for contact lens wear but should be managed as potential dry-eye patients.

Ocular History

1. Previous correction. Glasses or contact lenses?
2. Strabismus and amblyopia. Significantly reduced acuity? Diplopia? Past treatment?
3. Vision therapy. Binocular vision problems or symptoms?
4. Eye trauma.
5. Eye surgery.

Medical History

The following symptoms and conditions may contraindicate or restrict contact lens wear:

1. Itching, burning, or tearing.
2. Seasonal or chronic allergies.
3. Recurrent ocular infection or inflammation.
4. Sinusitis.
5. Dryness of mouth, eyes, or mucous membranes.
6. Nocturnal lagophthalmos.
7. Convulsions, epilepsy, and/or fainting spells. Such an individual should be identified as a contact lens wearer.
8. Diabetes. Type 1 diabetics, in particular, may have varying degrees of corneal anesthesia, poor corneal epithelial healing, and the potential to develop neurotrophic keratitis.
9. Collagen vascular disorders. Patients with rheumatoid arthritis and related collagen vascular disorders may have Sjögren's syndrome with keratoconjunctivitis sicca and associated tear film abnormalities. In addition, handling difficulties may be present.
10. Pregnancy. During pregnancy, particularly the third trimester, the tear film and corneal curvature may change significantly. This usually stabilizes shortly after childbirth.
11. Psychiatric treatment. Patients on medications to control anxiety, depression, or manic-depressive states should be screened but not necessarily discouraged from contact lens wear, especially if contact lenses would benefit them visually.
12. Thyroid imbalance. Hyperthyroidism, for example, may result in exophthalmos and lack of blinking, which can make contact lens wear difficult because of insufficient tear flow to the cornea.
13. Systemic medications. Certain medications can affect contact lens wear by reducing production of the aqueous phase of the tear film. Patients currently taking any of these medications should either be contraindicated as a contact lens wearer until the medication is discontinued or placed on a limited wearing schedule and carefully monitored. These medications include antihistamines, anticholinergics, some β-adrenergic blockers, tricyclic antidepressants, and oral contraceptives.[1]
14. Topical ocular medications. Patients using topical ocular medications may have restricted wearing times during contact lens wear. Soft lenses absorb the medication and alter drug delivery to the cornea, while gas-permeable (GP) lenses may block access to the cornea or increase contact time for any medication that collects under the lens.[2] In general, topical medications should be instilled 15 to 20 minutes before application of contact lenses or after they are removed.

Contact Lens History

If the patient is currently wearing lenses or has worn them in the past, it is important to determine why the person desires a refit, since this will likely affect what lens material and design will be used. The following questions should be asked:

1. What type of contact lens does (or did) the patient wear? Satisfaction? Symptoms?
2. What is (are) the reason(s) for discontinuing wear or desiring a change?

3. What is the patient's current wearing and lens replacement schedule?
4. What is the patient's care regimen (if appropriate)? Satisfaction? Symptoms?
5. Is there a history of a contact lens-related problems or complications in the past?
6. Is there a frequent history of changing lens materials (i.e., "shopper")?

■ ANATOMIC MEASUREMENTS

Ocular and eyelid dimensions influence the selection of lens type, initial lens parameters, and fitting technique to be used (i.e., lid attachment vs. interpalpebral).

Horizontal Visible Iris Diameter

1. Horizontal visible iris diameter (HVID) provides an approximation of the corneal diameter and ranges from 10 to 13 mm.
2. HVID is measured with a pupil diameter (PD) ruler tilted inward and read using the horizontal scale (Fig. 1.1).
3. This measurement will help determine overall diameter of the contact lens.

Pupil Diameter

1. Measurement of pupil diameter is similar to that for HVID (Fig. 1.2).
2. Perform this measurement under both normal and dim illumination. The latter will help in determining the optical zone diameter of a GP lens, which should be 1 to 2 mm larger than the pupil to minimize flare with vertical blink movement and pupil dilation in dim lighting conditions (e.g., driving at night).
3. Pupil sizes (dim illumination) are categorized as follows:
   Small pupil: <5 mm.
   Medium pupil: 5 to 7 mm.
   Large pupil: >7 mm.
4. For large pupil sizes, select a large optical zone (e.g., >8 mm) or a soft lens with a large optical zone. (Do not assume all soft lenses have large optical zones!)

Palpebral Aperture Height/Lid Position

1. Palpebral aperture height is equal to the vertical measurement of the opening between the upper and lower lids, with the patient gazing straight ahead.

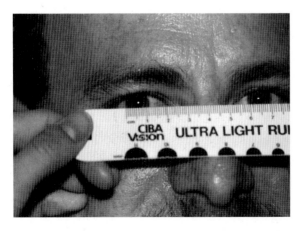

■ **FIGURE 1.1** Proper measurement of corneal diameter.

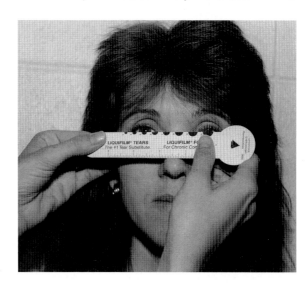

■ **FIGURE 1.2** Measurement of pupil diameter.

2. Perform this measurement with the patient relaxed and looking straight ahead (Fig. 1.3); also note and record the lid-to-cornea relationship.
3. This procedure will help determine type of lens and lens diameter for optimum patient comfort. A patient with an abnormally large palpebral fissure (e.g., ≥12 mm) will need a large-diameter lens for stability and comfort; likewise, a patient with an abnormally small palpebral fissure (e.g., ≤9 mm) will require a small-diameter lens.
4. Similarly, the position of the lower and upper lid to the limbus should be determined. A patient with a low upper lid that overlaps a large portion of the superior cornea is more likely to have a superior lid attachment. Likewise, a patient with a high upper lid that does not overlap much of the superior cornea is more likely to have an inferior lens position.[3]

Lid Tension

1. Lid tension is determined by lid eversion. Grasping the upper lid between the thumb and forefinger and gently pulling outward will give the practitioner an estimation of the lid tension over the globe.
2. Tight lids will pull a lens upward or may squeeze it downward (watermelon seed effect). Loose (heavy, fatty) lids will displace a lens downward.

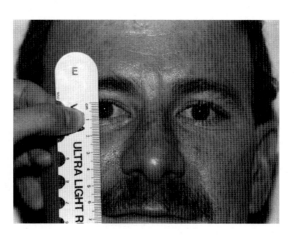

■ **FIGURE 1.3** Measurement of palpebral aperture height.

Blink Rate

1. A normal blink rate is 10 to 15 per minute.
2. Blink rate should be measured without the patient's knowledge; note the amplitude, length, and completeness of a typical blink.
3. If the patient presents with only 10% to 50% completeness of the blink, GP lenses are contraindicated unless a lid attachment or superior fitting relationship exists after the blink.[4] If the patient is a very infrequent blinker, soft lenses for social/occasional wear are recommended. On follow-up of patients with incomplete blinks, interpalpebral corneal and conjunctival desiccation should be monitored.

▮ REFRACTIVE INFORMATION

An evaluation of corneal topography and refractive status, with subsequent determination of predicted residual astigmatism, is imperative for proper contact lens design and parameter selection so that the likelihood of future success is maximized.

Corneal Topography

An evaluation of the patient's corneal topography is important in determining the appropriate lens parameters to be diagnostically fit. The base curve radius (BCR) and diameter for both GP and soft lens materials are selected based on corneal curvature measurements.

Corneal Contour

The cornea is an aspheric surface with greatest curvature at the apex and progressively flatter curvature toward the periphery. It is classically visualized as consisting of an essentially spherical central corneal cap (apical zone/apical cap) and a surrounding peripheral zone that gradually flattens. The corneal cap is defined as the area within which the corneal power does not change more than 1 D and is approximately 4 mm in diameter. A more accurate description of the corneal contour is an ellipsoid centrally with progressively increasing radius of curvature and eccentricity toward the periphery.[5] It is important to understand this corneal shape so that a contact lens can be optimally fit. For example, two patients having identical central corneal curvatures but different peripheral corneal curvatures and eccentricities are likely to be optimally fit with different contact lens parameters.

Evaluation

Methods for evaluating corneal topography include keratometry, autokeratometry, photokeratoscopy, and videokeratography (computer-assisted corneal topographic modeling).

Keratometer: The most common instrument for measuring corneal topography, the keratometer averages the curvature values of a few points on the cornea separated by approximately 3 mm in both the vertical and horizontal meridians. This instrument has the advantages of both ease of use and low cost. However, there are disadvantages:

- Only the central 3 mm of the cornea (approximately 8% of the corneal area) is evaluated.
- The apex is not directly measured.
- The central 3 mm of the cornea is assumed to be spherical, which may not be true. The magnitude of error is related to the rate of peripheral corneal flattening.
- A decentered corneal apex may cause inaccuracy.
- Examiner error is possible.
- Keratometric change may not correspond with refractive change.

Despite its drawbacks, most practitioners still use keratometry for the initial selection of lens parameters because of its accessibility and ease of use. In fact, for initial base curve selection and prediction of residual cylinder, it has proven to be quite reliable. However, fluorescein pattern evaluation is still the most important assessment in GP contact lens fitting, while centration and lens lag are most important for soft lens fit assessments.

Autokeratometer: Currently available automated keratometers provide accurate and consistent measurements of the central corneal curvature. The Humphrey Autokeratometer also assesses a larger area of the cornea (6.4 mm in the vertical meridian; 2.6 mm in the horizontal meridian), calculates the corneal curvature at the apex, provides the location of the apex, and calculates the shape factor. The disadvantages of automated keratometers include a much higher cost to the practitioner and a limited area of evaluation.

Photokeratoscope: A photokeratoscope presents a hemispherical, lighted Placido disk image to the cornea. The observer focuses on a virtual image (plus sign) reflected from the corneal apex. A Polaroid photo is taken and analyzed to determine corneal curvature. Since the camera magnification is fixed and known, the amount of separation between rings can be used to determine curvature.[6] The advantages of these instruments are their ability to provide a topographic analysis of at least 55% of the corneal surface, their ability to detect subtle topographic shifts, and the availability of data. The disadvantages include the more complicated data analysis and presentation, the limited availability of the instrument (it is no longer in production), and the expense.

Videokeratograph: The videokeratograph (computer-assisted corneal topography system) is a state-of-the-art instrument that measures and analyzes thousands of points on the corneal surface to provide information on corneal curvature and contour. It produces a color-coded corneal topographic map that provides the examiner with an easy-to-read representation of the curvature of virtually the entire corneal surface. Most systems use a combination of computer technology and a photokeratoscopic (Placido disk) image (Fig. 1.4) to produce a comprehensive topographic map of the cornea. Alternative methods utilizing projected grids (raster photogrammetry),[7] pachymetry,[8] and Fourier analysis of sine waves[9] have also been developed.

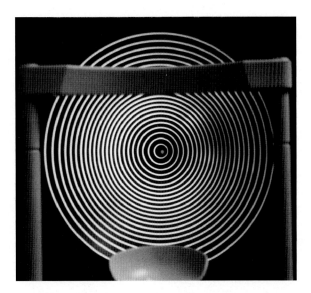

■ FIGURE 1.4 Photokeratoscopic cone used in Placido disk-based videokeratographers.

In addition to calculating corneal curvature, videokeratography software is able to determine corneal eccentricity, surface regularity, and elevation. With this information, the practitioner can detect corneal irregularities that may be causing reduced visual acuity and more effectively manage corneal distortion induced by contact lens wear, trauma, or surgery. Also, all videokeratographers have software that can design GP contact lenses based on the topographic information it has obtained. These software programs can design GP contact lenses successfully, but for most normal corneas, it may still be more efficient and just as accurate for the practitioner to use keratometry values for initial lens selection.[10,11] For irregular corneas, videokeratography more extensively describes the corneal contour, which may allow the practitioner to make contact lens-fitting decisions with greater confidence.[12]

The advantages of videokeratography include the availability of significantly more information, ease of use and analysis, and the most accurate method of monitoring topographic changes over time. The primary disadvantage is cost, although most systems are becoming very affordable for most practitioners.

Final Analysis

Despite the vast amount of information that videokeratography provides, most still consider keratometry the method of choice for diagnostic lens selection; however, it is important to remember that it represents only a starting point. As more accurate and accessible contact lens-fitting software becomes available for videokeratography, it may replace keratometry. Currently, it is more valuable for qualitative evaluations of the overall shape of the cornea, particularly for distorted and highly astigmatic corneas, for which both initial fitting and long-term management are enhanced.

Refraction

It is important to perform a careful binocular refraction to help calculate the contact lens power and expected residual astigmatism. Residual astigmatism for spherical soft lenses is simply equal to the refractive astigmatism. For GP contact lenses, calculated residual astigmatism is determined by the following formula:

$$\text{CRA (calculated residual astigmatism)} = \text{Refractive astigmatism} - \text{Keratometric astigmatism}$$

Example: Keratometry = 42.00 @ 180; 42.25 @ 090

Refraction = −2.00 − 1.00 × 180

CRA = (−1.00 × 180) − (−0.25 × 180) = −0.75 × 180

Typically, if the actual residual astigmatism (ARA) measured by refracting over a GP contact lens is >0.75 D, a spherical GP lens is not recommended because of reduced vision. Depending on the amount of keratometric (corneal) astigmatism, either a soft or GP toric lens would be a better option. In the above case, if the ARA equals the CRA, the best option may be a soft toric lens since the ARA with a spherical soft lens will equal the refractive astigmatism, or −1.00 D.

■ BINOCULAR VISION STATUS

Contact lenses may alter the binocular status of patients with high refractive errors or significant binocular anomalies. It is therefore important to test binocular function prior to lens fitting and make the necessary recommendations for lens wear.

Accommodation and Convergence

Pre-presbyopic moderate to high myopes may experience accommodative problems when switching from spectacles to contact lenses. In addition, they should be advised that a bifocal correction will probably be required at an earlier age. Convergence is similarly affected. A spectacle-corrected myope has a base-in prism effect when viewing at near, while a spectacle-corrected hyperope has a base-out prism effect. When contact lenses are worn, the myope loses the base-in prism effect at near and must converge more. Likewise, the contact lens-corrected hyperope loses the base-out prism effect at near and must converge less. Exophoric myopes and esophoric hyperopes may therefore experience more nearpoint symptoms with contact lenses than with spectacles.

Prismatic Correction

If base-in or base-out prism is necessary to provide binocularity and relieve asthenopic stress, it must be prescribed in spectacles. Although contact lenses can be worn together with spectacles, most patients would not appreciate the benefits of contact lens wear if glasses must be worn also. A small amount of base-down prism can be corrected in a contact lens, but base-up prism must be placed in spectacles.

▥ SLIT-LAMP EVALUATION

A comprehensive slit-lamp examination plays a vital role in determining whether the patient is a good contact lens candidate. The following should be evaluated on all prospective contact lens wearers:

External Observation

It is important to evaluate the eyelashes and external eyelids for the following conditions:

Blepharitis

Swollen inflamed lid margins reduce prognosis for successful contact lens wear. Debris from the lids may act as an irritant, and abnormal meibomian gland secretions will create an oily film on the lens surface. Staphylococcal blepharitis is also a potential cause of corneal infiltrates and may predispose the wearer to peripheral corneal ulcers. Acute and chronic forms of blepharitis should be treated before the patient is fit with contact lenses.

Entropion/Trichiasis

In-turned or disorganized lash patterns are not a contraindication for contact lens wear. In fact, a soft lens would protect the cornea from irritation caused by in-turned lashes.

Conjunctiva

The bulbar and tarsal conjunctiva should be evaluated biomicroscopically with white light. Rose bengal and lissamine green dye can be used to stain damaged or dead conjunctival cells, thus visualizing defects. Upper eyelid eversion is also required.

Bulbar Conjunctiva

Moderate injection of the bulbar conjunctiva, especially if persistent, may be caused by infection, dry eye, blepharitis, an allergic reaction, or other inflammatory process, and may contraindicate contact lens wear. Interpalpebral conjunctival staining is also suggestive of dry eye and should be investigated further with a tear film evaluation prior to contact lens fitting. Dense or coalesced rose bengal or lissamine green staining of the interpalpebral conjunctiva is often associated with the symptoms of dry eye. The presence of a pinguecula could necessitate GP lens wear if the edge of a soft lens irritates this condition. The presence of a pterygium should contraindicate contact lens wear; however, if only a small region of the peripheral cornea is affected, contact lenses can be considered.

Tarsal Conjunctiva

After upper eyelid eversion, the superior tarsal conjunctiva should be evaluated with and without fluorescein using the following scale[13]:

0 = satin. No papillae are observable.
1 = mildly elevated papillae, 0.1 to 0.2 mm in diameter, with uniform distribution (several papillae per millimeter of lid area).
2 = papillae are 0.5 to 1.0 mm in diameter, with nonuniform distribution.
3 = papillae 1 mm in diameter or greater are present on all regions of the upper lid.

Seasonal allergies result in mild papillary hypertrophy of the upper lid, usually of grade 1. A patient with giant papillary conjunctivitis (GPC, also known as contact lens papillary conjunctivitis [CLPC]) will exhibit large, irregularly sized papillae of grade 2 or 3 on the superior tarsal plate, which may be flattened and scarred if the condition is chronic (Fig. 1.5). GPC improves when a new contact lens is worn or with cessation of contact lenses. Thus, a new patient with GPC may be fitted in a daily disposable soft lens or a 2-week disposable lens, in combination with a decreased lens wearing time until the condition resolves. A mast cell inhibitor and/or corticosteroid may be used initially to decrease the inflammation.

Cornea

It is critical to carefully evaluate all aspects of the cornea prior to fitting. The presence of any significant corneal defect or disease process contraindicates contact lens wear until the condition has resolved. Many corneal defects are best visualized using the technique of indirect illumination. Chronic conditions, such as corneal dystrophies, may alter the type of contact lens, wearing schedule, and care regimen prescribed.

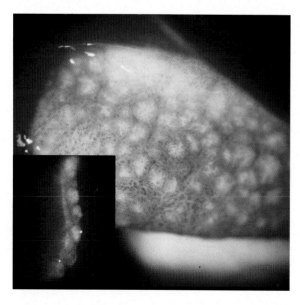

■ FIGURE 1.5 An everted upper lid from a patient with giant papillary conjunctivitis (GPC), showing grade 3 papillae on the upper tarsal plate

Limbal Vasculature

A 360-degree evaluation of the limbal vessels should be performed. Documentation of limbal vessel encroachment onto the cornea should be made. It is important to differentiate normal limbal vasculature from contact lens-induced vascularization. Encroachment of 1 to 2 mm suggests chronic hypoxia and may indicate the need for refitting with a silicone hydrogel, even on a daily wear basis, or refitting with GP lenses. Encroachment of >2 mm requires refitting to increase oxygen to the cornea, a decreased wearing time, and careful monitoring to prevent further advance of the neovascularization.

Epithelial Staining

Fluorescein application using a fluorescein strip moistened with preservative-free saline is essential when evaluating a new patient. Any areas of punctate epithelial staining should be noted. Sequential staining with liquid fluorescein is also recommended.[14] The presence of dense, coalesced staining may contraindicate fitting at that time and require treatment. It is important to always perform this procedure even if it is likely that the patient desires soft lenses. The eye can be thoroughly irrigated to rinse out the dye before lens application. Tear breakup time (TBUT) can be performed at this time as well.

Edema

The presence of deep stromal striae or folds, epithelial microcysts and vacuoles, or epithelial and stromal clouding indicate corneal edema and may contraindicate contact lens wear. The cause of the edema should be determined and treated, if possible. Occasionally, corneal dystrophies may cause edema; contact lenses are sometimes used in the management of these conditions. Epithelial microcysts are commonly found in extended-wear patients, and indicate that a period of oxygen deprivation has occurred.

Opacities: Scars versus Infiltrates

Carefully scan the cornea to differentiate an active from an inactive condition. Any active corneal infection or inflammation (e.g., corneal infiltrates, microbial keratitis) contraindicates contact lens wear at that time and requires the appropriate treatment.[15] Corneal scars and other inactive opacities are not contraindications to contact lens wear.

Endothelium

Evaluate the endothelial layer for the presence of guttata and polymegethism. The presence of an endothelial dystrophy may contraindicate contact lens wear.

■ TEAR FILM EVALUATION

The preocular tear film plays an important role in contact lens wear. It maintains hydration of soft contact lenses, determines lens surface wettability, acts as the primary anterior refracting surface, and deposits protein, lipids, and mucin onto the lens surface. Poor tear quality or quantity will reduce the patient's prognosis for successful contact lens wear. There are several tear evaluations that should be performed to determine whether a patient is a good contact lens candidate.

Tear Meniscus Evaluation

The height and quality of the lower tear prism (lacrimal lake) are evaluated during the slit-lamp examination. This is a good test for detecting the borderline dry-eye patient. If the tear prism is not sufficient, an aqueous deficiency is present. The anterior border of the tear meniscus is just behind the meibomian gland orifices. Where the meniscus meets the cornea, a black line exists that represents localized thinning. To evaluate the tear meniscus, fluorescein should be applied over the inferior bulbar conjunctiva about 1 to 2 minutes before evaluation[4] and then observed with cobalt blue and Wratten no. 12 filters. When the meniscus is so thin that it appears as a fine line, it is a significantly insufficient tear meniscus (Fig. 1.6).

Tear Breakup Time

TBUT is the most widely used test of tear film quality and a good predictor of contact lens success. It is equal to the postblink time for dry spots to form in the tear film and it is theoretically caused by contamination of the mucin layer by lipids. Fluorescein is instilled, and the cornea is evaluated with a wide slit-lamp beam (i.e., 2 to 4 mm) under low magnification (i.e., $10\times$ to $20\times$) with the cobalt blue filter. When wetting the fluorescein strip with saline, it is important to use unpreserved saline and shake excess moisture from the strip to avoid artificially destabilizing the tear film. The number of seconds until a dry spot forms is recorded. These dry spots appear as dark regions in the green-dyed tear film (Fig. 1.7). The patient is instructed to refrain from blinking during this period. An average normal value is 15 to 20 seconds. Less than 10 seconds indicates the patient may have dry eye, although many asymptomatic patients show tear breakup times in this range.[16] However, a low tear breakup time indicates that the patient is best suited for daily wear, may suffer from end-of-the-day dryness,

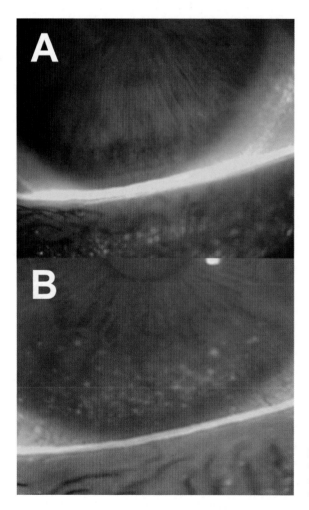

■ FIGURE 1.6 The inferior meniscus of a normal **(A)** and a dry-eye patient **(B)**. Note the inferior corneal staining in the dry-eye patient. (Courtesy of Wendy Harrison.)

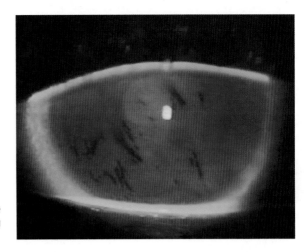

■ **FIGURE 1.7** The formation of dry spots in the precorneal tear film observed when measuring tear breakup time (TBUT).

and may not be able to obtain a comfortable all-day wearing schedule. Several important considerations could affect results:

- Do not manipulate the lids immediately prior to testing.
- It is best to use unpreserved saline to wet the fluorescein strip.
- No applanation tonometry should be performed before the test.
- Repeat the test several times, especially if low values are being obtained.
- Fluorescence of the tear film is enhanced if a Wratten no. 12 or similar yellow filter is placed over the observation system.
- Do not perform this test immediately after contact lens removal. Wearing contact lenses decreases tear breakup time, possibly for several hours after lens removal.

Two noninvasive breakup time (NIBUT) tests have been developed to minimize any disruption to the tear film.[17] In one technique a grid pattern is projected onto the anterior ocular surface, which is observed using a biomicroscope under low magnification.[18] When the grid pattern is disrupted, the tear film is breaking up. A second NIBUT technique involves using the keratometer mire image to observe tear film rupture.[19] In both techniques, a value of 8 to 10 is the cutoff for dry eye.

Interference Phenomena Evaluation

The lipid layer can be evaluated by specular reflection or interferometry of the tear film. Clinically, the slit lamp can be used, but the viewable area is very limited. The Keeler Tearscope is a commercially available instrument that provides a larger area of specular reflection, which allows the majority of the precorneal tear lipid layer to be visualized at once. With either technique, colored interference patterns of the lipid layer will be observed. A good lipid layer will have an amorphous pattern that appears gray to brown in color. Thinner lipid layers have a marblelike pattern, and if the lipid layer is absent, no interference patterns will be observed.[20,21]

Schirmer Tear Test

The Schirmer tear test evaluates basal tear secretion and part of the reflex secretion and has been used to screen contact lens candidates for suitability for lens wear. Although this is a simple test to administer, it has several problems including discomfort, inconsistency, and unreliability.[22–24] Nevertheless, it can be useful in detecting the aqueous-deficient dry-eye patient.

With the patient viewing superiorly, place a Schirmer test strip over the lower lid such that the 5-mm notched portion of the strip is approximately one-third of the way from the outer

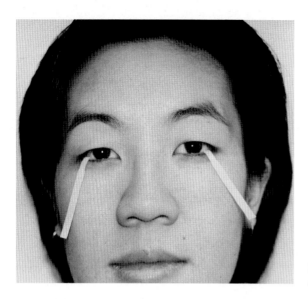

■ **FIGURE 1.8** Proper Schirmer strip placement at the outer one-third of the lower eyelids.

canthus. Several techniques are used to perform the test. In one technique the patient continuously looks upward with the room illumination lowered to reduce reflex tearing from light sensitivity (Fig. 1.8). After 5 minutes, the strip is removed, and the amount of wetting is measured in millimeters. Another technique is to ask the patient to keep the eyes closed after placement of the strip. A cutoff value of 5 mm in 5 minutes is considered normal.[25] The Schirmer tear test is most useful when a very low volume of tears is detected. A very high volume of tears, noted by the wetting of the complete strip or most of the strip, may not be repeatable, whereas an extremely low volume, noted by a very small area of strip coverage (0 to 4 mm), usually indicates aqueous deficiency. This test can be performed with or without anesthetic. If anesthetic is used, it is best to do the test several minutes after the anesthetic is instilled. However, performing the test without anesthetic is more useful for evaluating the success of contact lens wear because it demonstrates the more natural response of the ocular surface response to irritation. If the patient's tear volume is low and little or no tearing results from instillation of the irritating Schirmer strip, then the volume of tears is likely to remain low with contact lens wear. Thus, a low Schirmer value indicates that the patient will be likely to suffer from dry-eye symptoms with contact lens wear.

Important considerations when performing the Schirmer tear test include the following:

• Use low room illumination.
• The strip should rest in a slightly temporal position so that when the lower lid kicks inward during blinking, contact with the cornea, which may cause excess ocular irritation and reflex tearing, is avoided.

Phenol Red Thread Test

The phenol red thread test, developed by Hamano et al.[26] consists of a high-quality 70-mm cotton thread soaked in phenol red dye. It is performed similar to the Schirmer test: the end of the thread is inserted over the lower lid onto the temporal palpebral conjunctiva while the patient views superiorly. The test is performed for 15 seconds, and the amount of the test strip that has turned to a red color is measured (Fig. 1.9). The average value in the United States has been found to be 24.3 mm.[27] A value <9 mm has been diagnostic of dry eye. The benefits of this test include the following:

1. No anesthesia necessary; minimal discomfort.
2. A 15-second test time.

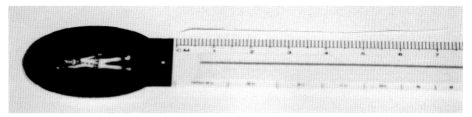

■ **FIGURE 1.9** The phenol red thread test.

3. Little reflex secretion.
4. More valid than the Schirmer tear test.[28]
5. Minimal environmental effects such as humidity because of the short testing time.

Criticisms of this test include the following:

1. Relatively low absorption capacity; individuals may secrete tears at a higher rate than can be absorbed by the thread.[29]
2. This test may only measure residual tears in the cul-de-sac, not tear volume.

Rose Bengal

Rose bengal stains damaged ocular surface cells that are not protected by an intact mucin layer. Therefore, the dye stains cells on the ocular surface of dry-eye patients, whose conjunctival cells become keratinized and lose their mucins.[30–32] For that reason, it has traditionally been used as a conjunctival stain for the dry-eye patient, although it is noticeably painful for those patients because it shows cellular toxicity if the mucin layer is breached.[33] A drop of 1% rose bengal (or use of an impregnated strip moistened with unpreserved saline) is instilled into the conjunctival sac; this is followed by irrigation of the external eye with an isotonic saline solution. The amount and location of the red stain will dictate the severity of the condition. Typically in keratoconjunctivitis sicca, the inferior cornea and conjunctiva will exhibit a large amount of staining. It particularly stains dead cells an intense red color, while it stains cells that are devitalized a weaker color. In marginally dry eyes, the conjunctival surface may stain in a discrete punctate fashion (Fig. 1.10), whereas in pathologic dry eye it is more coalesced. Typically, the adjacent triangular sections of the exposed bulbar conjunctiva, both nasally and temporally, will stain. After the patient has blinked three to six times and the excess dye has

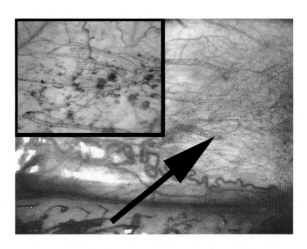

■ **FIGURE 1.10** Rose bengal staining of the conjunctiva in a dry-eye patient (*arrow*). Staining is magnified in the inset showing the typical punctate pattern.

been washed away by the tears, the eye is examined with white light. The following grading sequence has been recommended for evaluating this condition[34]:

0 = absence of staining.
1 = staining of <1/3 of the cornea.
2 = staining of between 1/3 and 2/3 of the cornea.
3 = staining of between 2/3 and the entire cornea.
4 = staining over the entire cornea.
5 = inferior conjunctival staining.

Lissamine Green

Lissamine green is a dye that provides information similar to the more traditional rose bengal dye, but without pain or discomfort for the patient. It works by diffusing into damaged or keratinized cells,[35,36] similar to sodium fluorescein. One drop of 1% lissamine green is instilled in the lower cul-de-sac, and the ocular surface is then examined with the slit lamp in white light. It has been shown that this dye yields staining scores that are not significantly different from rose bengal. In addition, lissamine green produces noticeably less irritation than rose bengal, and the irritation is of shorter duration.[36] Therefore, lissamine green can be used interchangeably with rose bengal when evaluating the eye for keratitis sicca. The grading scale is the same as for rose bengal.

Dry-Eye Questionnaire

The use of a dry-eye questionnaire can be beneficial in determining if the patient has some dryness characteristics or is in an environment that could be prone to inducing dryness. One such questionnaire, adapted from McMonnies et al.[28,37] is given in Appendix A. It can also be useful to ask about end-of-the-day dryness because that is a common complaint among contact lens wearers.[38]

What Series of Tests Should Be Used?

1. TBUT reveals tear quality and should be performed on all prospective contact lens wearers. However, contact lens wear decreases the TBUT, so the test is not accurate just after lens removal.
2. Biomicroscopic evaluation of the tear prism would indicate whether an aqueous tear deficiency is present. The presence of inferior corneal and conjunctival fluorescein staining also indicates a dry-eye condition.
3. A tear volume test can also be performed.
4. Lissamine green is preferred over rose bengal when evaluating a dry-eye suspect for conjunctival staining because of the increased comfort with that dye.

■ FINAL CONSULTATION

Evaluation of Motivation

Motivation may be the most important factor in determining success versus failure of a contact lens wearer. A highly motivated patient can often tolerate discomfort and other problems that would be difficult for the patient who has only a superficial motivation.[39] Motivation can be tested by explaining that contact lenses are a healthcare device and must be cared for constantly and without error. The patient's motivation to wear them is twofold: the desire to see well and the desire to improve his or her appearance. The greater a patient's need for contact lenses, either visual or psychological, the more likely that motivation will be high.[40] Other factors to consider include the following:

1. Satisfaction with spectacles: is the patient exhibiting only a casual interest in contact lenses ("shopping")?

2. With a younger child, is it the child who really desires the contact lenses or is a vanity-conscious parent the only one who desires them? If the latter is true, the child is not ready for lens wear.
3. Limited wearing time (e.g., because of borderline dry eye) may decrease the patient's motivation to wear contact lenses.
4. If the patient has excessive concerns (e.g., high fees, discomfort, or possible complications), success is unlikely.
5. If the patient exhibits hypochondriac-like concerns about minor ailments, he or she may not be willing to tolerate the initial discomfort and adaptation associated with contact lens wear. Likewise, if the patient is quite timid, successful contact lens wear is much less probable than for patients who are independent and confident.[41]
6. If the patient does not agree with the practitioner's recommendations (e.g., GPs not soft, hydrogen peroxide not chemical disinfection, daily wear only not extended wear), lenses should not be ordered and careful documentation in the patient's record is required.

Benefits of Contact Lenses versus Spectacles

The benefits of contact lenses versus spectacles can also be explained to a new prospective contact lens candidate. Several studies have demonstrated that contact lens wearers are more outgoing, optimistic, athletic, and less self-conscious than their spectacle-wearing counterparts.[41] The following benefits can also be mentioned:

1. Contact lenses increase magnification of the retinal image for moderate to high myopes.
2. The contact lens wearer is free from obstruction by the spectacle frame.
3. A slight increase in light transmission is present. (This is also why some new contact lens wearers complain that they experience more photophobia in daylight conditions.)
4. Fewer optical aberrations are present because the patient views through the optical center of the lens at all times.

Comparison of Gas-Permeable and Soft Lenses

A discussion of which lens material is best for a given patient is important. The factors that can be considered when discussing this decision with a patient are presented in Tables 1.1 and 1.2.

TABLE 1.1 ADVANTAGES OF GAS-PERMEABLE AND SOFT LENSES

GP ADVANTAGES	SOFT LENS ADVANTAGES
Vision	Initial comfort
Ocular health	Oxygen transmission (silicone hydrogels)
High oxygen transmission	Variable wear
Wettability	Disposability = convenience
High astigmatic correction	No foreign body sensation
Ease of care/easier compliance	Athletes (see Table 1.2)
Long-term comfort	Ability to change eye color
Stability/durability	Residual cylinder with GPs
Benefit irregular cornea patient	Reduced initial chair time
Eye protection	

TABLE 1.2 PREFERRED CONTACT LENS CORRECTION IN SPORTS

	CONTACT LENS TYPE	
SPORT	SOFT	SOFT OR GP
Baseball		•
Contact sports	•	
Basketball		
Boxing		
Football		
Hockey		
Soccer		
Wrestling		
Golf	•	
Hunting		•
Jogging	•	
Mounting climbing		•
Racquet sports/handball		•
Handball		
Racquetball		
Squash		
Tennis		
Scuba diving	•	
Snow skiing		•
Swimming	•	

Comfort

Comfort is an important factor in the eventual decision. Discomfort is the number one reason for discontinuation of contact lens wear.[38,42] If the patient is very concerned about discomfort, soft lenses should be considered (assuming the patient is even motivated for contact lens wear in general). Always tell the patient what to expect before the diagnostic fitting process. The initial comfort can also be judged at this time. If the patient is a high reactor (e.g., if the patient is still tearing and has little desire to gaze straight ahead even after a 15- to 30-minute period), soft lenses should be considered. Likewise, if the patient demonstrates greater than average sensitivity during the examination (e.g., during drop instillation, lid eversion, tonometry), soft lenses are often preferable.

Myths

This is the perfect time to dispel any myths the patient may believe about contact lenses. Some of these include the following:

1. "The contact lens will get behind my eye."
2. "The contact lenses will break on my eye."
3. "I can't be fit because I have 'stigmatism.'"
4. "Contact lenses damage the eye."

5. "Shouldn't you be at least 16 years old to wear contact lenses?"
6. "Contact lenses HURT!"
7. "They don't make contacts for bifocal wearers."

Another myth to consider with employed patients is that contact lenses offer no protection to the eye. It is very likely that contact lenses can help protect the cornea from injury by various flying objects. One study reported on 125 cases that included sports, automobile, workshop, and chemical accidents in which eyes were protected by contact lens wear.[43] However, because of the trauma that can occur from a hard object in addition to substances that can result in toxicity reactions, contact lenses should never be substituted for the appropriate safety eyewear. Likewise, protective goggles should be worn in some sports, especially racquetball and squash.

■ OTHER CONSIDERATIONS

What about the −0.50 D Myope?

It is not uncommon for low ametropic patients to be told they are not good contact lens candidates. Often this results from the practitioner's preconception that the patient really does not need to wear any lenses and/or lacks motivation because of the low refractive error. In most cases, these patients are good contact lens candidates. If they appear to be motivated and/or have an occupational need for contact lenses, they should be fit with lenses. As a result of the low ametropia, soft lenses are often recommended, especially if occasional wear is desired.

How to Approach the Borderline Dry-Eye Patient

Dry eye is the most common problem associated with contact lens wear, and is one of the most common reasons that patients discontinue contact lens wear. As many as 50% of contact lens wearers report dry-eye symptoms, often worse later in the day.[44,45] Some borderline dry-eye patients present at the initial fitting visit with occasional dry-eye symptoms, whereas others are asymptomatic. In either case, contact lens wear usually aggravates dry-eye symptoms. It is often difficult to decide how to fit the borderline dry-eye patient (e.g., a patient with a low TBUT, reduced tear prism, or antihistamine use). There are several considerations that can help maximize the borderline dry-eye patient's likelihood for comfortable contact lens wear.[46]

Gas Permeable versus Soft

Hydrogel and silicone hydrogel lenses have the advantages of initial comfort and ability to rehydrate with application of rewetting drops. GP lenses often present a healthier alternative, in terms of oxygen availability to the corneal epithelium. The final decision may be determined by the case history and the prefitting evaluation. Would the patient benefit visually from GP lenses? Is the patient only interested in occasional wear? Is there a history of corneal infection or GPC? If the patient appears to be a patient for either GP or soft lenses, he or she may achieve a longer wearing time with soft lenses because of the ability to rehydrate the lenses, either by applying rewetting drops frequently or performing a 10-minute saline soak in the middle of the wearing period.

Soft Lens Selection

Among traditional hydrogel lenses, water content, lens thickness, and surface deposit resistance are the hydrogel material properties that help minimize dryness. Most agree that low-water-content lenses dehydrate less because there is less water to lose and that thicker lenses maintain a greater "reservoir" of water that dehydrates less than thinner lenses.[47] In one study, more borderline dry-eye patients preferred a low-water-content thick hydrogel lens (8) than low-water thin (5), GP (5), high-water thick (4), and high-water thin (4) lenses.[28] Lens surface treatments can also increase the on-eye wettability of soft lenses. Silicone hydrogel materials typically use surface treatments or internal wetting agents to improve wettability, thus providing another option for fitting the dry-eye patient. Several studies have shown that fitting dry-eye patients with silicone hydrogels improved dryness symptoms.[48,49]

Gas-Permeable Lens Selection

GP lenses have the advantage of not dehydrating and obtaining water from the postlens tear film. However, they may induce peripheral corneal desiccation in patients with dry eye. If a GP lens is desired, a highly wettable material, such as a medium-oxygen-permeability (Dk) fluoro-silicone acrylate, is recommended.

Care

Many care systems are available to patients, primarily preserved chemical disinfection systems. A patient who has been successfully using a particular care system should be kept with the same system. However, the care system of any patient who has shown a possible allergic reaction to a preservative or who has dry eye should be evaluated. It is important to be aware of the preservative in each care system to avoid giving that patient a similar system with the same preservative. Preservative-free care systems are an option for patients with possible allergies or dry eye. Daily cleaning with a good surfactant cleaner is recommended for dry eye because those patients tend to show more lens deposits. Cleaners with abrasive components may benefit patients who rapidly develop protein deposits. Patients who experience rapid protein deposition despite diligent cleaning may require a refit to weekly or daily disposable lenses.

Wearing Schedule

A reduced wearing schedule may be necessary for dry-eye patients. In addition, daily wear is mandatory. These recommendations should be made the first visit after tear film testing has been completed. Proactive education will prepare the patient for limited but successful lens wear.

Adjunct Therapy

The use of rewetting drops during lens wear is essential in maintaining good comfort and ocular surface health for dry-eye patients. Midday lens cleaning and saline soaks will allow the patient to prolong lens wear in the latter half of the day when dry-eye symptoms typically increase. If rewetting drops and saline soaks are not sufficient, punctal occlusion may be a good option. Initial diagnostic evaluation with dissolvable collagen plugs, followed by permanent occlusion with nondissolvable silicone plugs or cautery, can significantly increase tear retention and decrease dry-eye symptoms.

■ FINAL ANALYSIS

The goal of the preliminary evaluation is to be able to answer the question, "Is the patient a suitable candidate for contact lens wear?" In this final assessment, you must consider the patient's goals, history, refractive status, and ocular health. In addition to answering this question, you must determine the most appropriate contact lens option that will meet the patient's needs without creating clinical problems. Table 1.3 provides an overview of good, borderline, and poor candidates for contact lens wear.

■ SUMMARY

Careful patient selection is paramount to successful contact lens wear. If a comprehensive history, refractive and ocular evaluation, and assessment of suitability are performed, it is likely

TABLE 1.3 GOOD, BORDERLINE, AND POOR CONTACT LENS CANDIDATES

GOOD	BORDERLINE	POOR
1. Motivated	1. Borderline dry eye	1. Unmotivated
2. High ametropia	2. Allergies/occasional	2. Dusty, dirty
3. Children/adolescents	antihistamine use	environment
(if motivated/mature)	3. Excessive fear about	3. Poor hygiene
4. Aphakia	foreign body on eye	4. Diabetes
5. Refractive anisometropia	4. Lab workers/hairdressers	5. Pathologic dry eye
6. Irregular cornea	5. Mild (1–1.5 mm) limbal vessel	6. Active corneal infection
7. Good ocular/systemic	encroachment	(e.g., neovascularization,
health	6. Pinguecula	infiltrates, coalesced staining)
8. Normal binocular vision	7. Pre-existing corneal scars	7. Pterygium
9. Good manual dexterity	8. Entropion, ectropion,	8. Chronic blepharitis
	trichiasis	9. Endothelial dystrophy
	9. Patient under psychiatric care	10. Immunosuppressed patients
	10. Hypochondriasis	11. Lateral prism in correction
		12. Poor manual dexterity
		13. Chronic alcoholism

that the patient will be a successful contact lens wearer. Whether or not the patient is ultimately fit with contact lenses, providing an honest appraisal of the probability of successful contact lens wear will eventually benefit both doctor and patient.

■ CLINICAL CASES

CASE 1

A 38-year-old automobile mechanic visits the office for a complete eye examination. During the course of your examination he casually asks if you think he could wear contact lenses. His motivation results from having to clean his spectacles frequently because of oil, grease, and dirt coming in contact with them from a car and/or his hands. Otherwise he is quite pleased with the vision and wearing of spectacles. You observe that his hands appear to be quite dirty.

Should this patient be fitted with contact lenses?

SOLUTION: If this patient's dissatisfaction with his spectacles was greater and his hygiene was better, he may have been a good contact lens candidate. But his dirty hands and work environment would increase the risk of serious eye infection from lens contamination as compared to the general population. Therefore, it would be preferable to advise this patient that he is not a good contact lens candidate.

CASE 2

A 16-year-old woman visits the office for a complete eye examination and contact lens fitting. She has never worn contact lenses before but strongly dislikes wearing spectacles, which she needs to wear constantly because of her nearsightedness. During the case history she indicates to you that she has seasonal allergy problems necessitating occasional antihistamine use. You also observe that her palpebral conjunctiva has a grade 1 papillary hypertrophy. All other ocular health findings are normal. Her refraction is as follows:

$$OD -3.25 - 1.00 \times 170$$
$$OS -2.75 - 1.25 \times 005$$

Should this patient be fitted with contact lenses?

SOLUTION: Because this patient is very motivated and only uses antihistamines on an occasional basis, she is a good contact lens candidate. However, her allergies that have resulted in papillary hypertrophy may lead to dryness symptoms and lens deposits, especially during allergy season. For this reason, a daily-wear schedule is highly advisable. In addition, the patient should be warned that reduction in wearing time and possible temporary discontinuation of lens wear may be required during allergy season. Some patients can also be fitted with a daily disposable during allergy season, or all year, to avoid the excessive lens deposits often associated with allergies. For the same reason, a GP lens material which can be easily cleaned, may also be recommended.

CASE 3

A 21-year-old woman visits the office with a desire to be fitted with contact lenses. She wore GP lenses intermittently for 2 years but never could wear them for long periods of time because of dryness. When she visited her last doctor 1 year ago, he mentioned to her that she is not a good candidate for contact lenses because she has dry eyes. Nevertheless, she is very motivated for contact lens wear and is receptive to any recommendations on lens material and wearing time. She finds her spectacles to be unacceptable cosmetically while also being inconvenient during the many athletic activities in which she participates during her spare time. Her refraction is the following:

$$OD -4.00 - 1.25 \times 010$$
$$OS -3.50 - 1.00 \times 180$$

Slit-lamp evaluation shows an absence of staining and papillary hypertrophy. However, the tear breakup time is only 6 seconds.

Should this patient be fitted with contact lenses?

SOLUTION: Yes, this patient should become a satisfied contact lens wearer. Based on her motivation and past contact lens-wearing history, she should be fitted into either a disposable hydrogel or silicone hydrogel soft toric lens to minimize deposit-induced problems. She should also be warned not to expect all-day wear and to be careful about not overwearing the lenses. It may be desirable to add a cleaner to her care system to help keep the lenses clean, even on a 2-week disposable basis. Rewetting drops may also help with dryness symptoms later in the day. For some patients, removing the lenses and cleaning or soaking them briefly in saline may also help. In addition, a nonpreserved lens care system helps relieve dryness symptoms for some patients.

CASE 4

A 24-year-old patient enters the office inquiring about contact lenses. He is a professional musician who has never worn contact lenses before and wears spectacles only for reading music and night driving. He feels the spectacles are a hindrance while performing in the orchestra because he frequently has to shift fixation and they tend to obstruct his view. However, as excellent vision is critical for viewing both his music and the conductor, he feels a vision correction is necessary. The refraction results in the following:

$$OD -0.50 - 0.25 \times 180$$
$$OS -0.50 \ DS$$

Should this patient be fitted with contact lenses?

SOLUTION: Because of the critical vision demand required in his occupation, in combination with his dissatisfaction with spectacles, this patient would make a good contact lens candidate. However, as a result of his low refractive error, soft lenses would be recommended to accommodate a probable occasional lens-wearing schedule. Daily disposable lenses would be the best choice if he does wear them occasionally.

CASE 5

A 33-year-old woman inquires about contact lenses during her routine eye examination. She states that she has to wear her glasses constantly and would like to be able to see without having to wear them. She reports that she has never tried contact lenses before because she was afraid that they would damage her eyes. She asks many questions about the potential hazards of contact lens wear and seems overly concerned about discomfort during the adaptation process. She also appears very timid and nervous during your testing, particularly during tonometry and ophthalmoscopy. Her keratometry and refraction are as follows:

OD   41.00 @ 090; 41.75 @ 180   −0.50 − 0.75 × 090
OS   41.50 @ 090; 42.00 @ 180   −0.75 − 0.50 × 095

Should this patient be fitted with contact lenses?

SOLUTION: Although this patient seems motivated to wear contact lenses, her exaggerated concerns about potential risks reduce the likelihood that she will be a satisfied wearer. In addition, her apprehension during ocular testing may indicate that she will have difficulty learning application of contact lenses, which may further discourage her. Because of her concerns about initial comfort, a soft lens would be advisable; however, her refraction suggests that a spherical lens may not provide her with sharp acuity. A soft toric may provide better acuity but could be less comfortable initially. This patient is not a good candidate. However, if after a comprehensive discussion on the risks and benefits of contact lens wear she still desires to be fitted, proceed with caution.

CASE 6

A 54-year-old patient presents for his routine eye examination. During the examination, he expresses a desire to be fitted with contact lenses for his outdoor activities, which include golf, jogging, and working in his garden. His main complaint is that his glasses get dirty and fog up during these activities. He has never worn contact lenses before. His ocular history includes primary open-angle glaucoma, for which he takes timolol 0.5% b.i.d. in both eyes. His refraction is the following:

OD   −3.00 − 0.25 × 180
OS   −2.50 − 0.50 × 170
Add +1.75

Slit-lamp evaluation reveals normal ocular structures with no corneal staining or papillary hypertrophy. His TBUT is 10 seconds.

Should this patient be fitted with contact lenses?

SOLUTION: This patient is a good part-time contact lens candidate. Aside from his glaucoma, his ocular and systemic health are good, and he is motivated to eliminate spectacle wear during sports and other outdoor activities. The main concern is his use of topical medications. First, the contact lenses may alter the delivery of the medication to the eye, which may cause undue fluctuations in his intraocular pressure. Second, preservatives in the drops may discolor or damage the contact lenses. To address these concerns, a disposable soft lens (daily disposable being an excellent option) should be prescribed. This will allow the patient to replace his lenses frequently so that the drops do not adversely affect them. In addition, the patient should be instructed to wait 15 to 20 minutes after drop instillation before applying his lenses in the morning, and to wait until after removal to instill his drops in the evening. A soft lens also allows him to wear contact lenses on a part-time basis. Finally, the issue of single-vision versus multifocal options should be discussed (see Chapter 15).

CASE 7

A 14-year-old man presents for his annual eye examination. During the examination he reports that, although he wears sports goggles, they become dirty and limit his field of view during his junior high school football games. He has been told in the past that he can't wear contact lenses because of his astigmatism but inquires if he can wear them during practice and in games. Your keratometry and refraction reveal the following:

OD   43.25 @ 175; 45.50 @ 85 $-0.50 - 2.50 \times 175$
OS   43.75 @ 010; 45.50 @ 100 $-1.00 - 1.75 \times 010$

Slit-lamp examination reveals no corneal staining or tarsal abnormalities. His tear meniscus appears normal, and his TBUT is 15 seconds.

Should this patient be fitted with contact lenses?

SOLUTION: Yes, this patient is a great contact lens candidate. Most teenagers are mature enough to handle the responsibilities of contact lens wear and care, but it is important to individually assess each patient's maturity level. This patient has significant astigmatism and was told that he could not wear contact lenses. However, soft and GP lens designs are available that will be able to correct his vision quite well (see Chapter 14). Because of the physical nature of football, soft lenses should be fitted to avoid lens loss during games. In addition, a disposable or frequent replacement lens should be considered so that he can dispose of his lenses when they become soiled. This may occur as often as every game, so a disposable toric lens may be a good choice. He may even discover that his vision with contact lenses is good enough to consider full-time wear.

CASE 8

A 24-year-old architect presents for a contact lens fitting. He is currently earning his recreational pilot's license and is concerned that if he were to lose his glasses during turbulence, he would be unable to land his plane. Otherwise, he has no other complaints with his glasses. He reports that he had tried soft contact lenses in the past but did not continue with them because his work demands the sharpest vision possible. His keratometry and refraction are as follows:

OD   43.50 @ 175; 44.25 @ 085 $-1.50 - 0.75 - 175$
OS   43.75 @ 180; 44.25 @ 090 $-2.00 - 0.50 \times 180$

Should this patient be fitted with contact lenses?

SOLUTION: This patient is a good candidate for part-time soft lens wear. A spherical design should provide enough clarity for most visual tasks, including flying. If sharper vision is desired, a soft toric can be fitted in the right eye. A GP contact lens would provide sharper acuity, but they are not as suitable for part-time wear. In addition, the patient may experience dry eyes while flying, which can be minimized with proper soft lens selection.

CASE 9

A 38-year-old woman presents for a contact lens fitting. She reports that she would like the cosmetic benefit of not having to wear her glasses, which she wears full time. She reports that she has prism in her glasses, and without them she sees double. Lensometry reveals 2 prism diopters (pd) of base-out prism for both eyes. Your refraction is as follows:

OD -3.50 DS   20/20
OS $-1.75 - 1.50 \times 170$ 20/20

Binocular testing reveals an intermittent alternating esotropia of 10 pd. With 2 pd of base-out prism over each eye, she is able to fuse. Slit-lamp evaluation reveals good ocular health.

Should this patient be fitted with contact lenses?

SOLUTION: Because this patient requires lateral prism to prevent diplopia, contact lenses are not a good option. Even if her vision is correctable to 20/20 in each eye with contact lenses, she would require plano spectacles with the lateral prism to wear over her contact lenses. If the patient is mainly concerned about the poor cosmesis with thick myopic lenses with base-out prism, contact lens wear can significantly reduce the edge thickness of the glasses. A smaller frame size will further decrease edge thickness. However, the patient may decide over time that she is not appreciating much benefit from the contact lenses and discontinue wear. If the patient desires contact lens wear without spectacles, she should be advised that she is a poor candidate.

CASE 10

A 28-year-old man presents for a comprehensive eye examination and contact lens fitting. He is a salesman who feels that his glasses prevent him from making eye contact with his clients. He has never worn contact lenses in the past. He has no ocular complaints other than periodic redness and irritation. His general health is good. His refraction reveals the following:

OD -5.50 DS
OS $-5.75 - 0.25 \times 180$

Slit-lamp examination reveals flakes and crusts on his eyelashes, clogged meibomian gland orifices, mild conjunctival injection, and grade 1 inferior corneal staining. TBUT is 3 seconds.

Should this patient be fitted with contact lenses?

SOLUTION: This patient has a classic case of chronic blepharitis and meibomitis with mild conjunctival and corneal involvement. He should not be fitted with contact lenses at this time, although he may eventually become a good candidate once this condition is resolved. However, chronic blepharitis is very difficult to eradicate completely and will likely require continued maintenance treatment. The patient should be advised at this visit to begin a course of hot compresses and lid scrubs twice per day. The patient should then be re-evaluated in 2 weeks. If the condition has cleared sufficiently such that no injection or corneal staining is present, the patient can then be fitted. Either disposable soft or GP lenses can be fitted, and diligent cleaning and disinfection are crucial. This patient may suffer from dry-eye symptoms in contact lenses, even with treatment, so silicone hydrogels or daily disposables may be a good choice. Continued lid hygiene is also important in preventing future complications.

CLINICAL PROFICIENCY CHECKLIST

- Primary reasons for patient interest in contact lenses include cosmesis, inconvenience of spectacles, better vision, sports, and occupational considerations.
- Among the contraindications to contact lens wear are chronic allergies necessitating antihistamine use, dryness, juvenile diabetes, cardiovascular disorders, and pregnancy.
- If the patient is a current contact lens wearer, it is important to obtain a comprehensive contact lens history, including his or her satisfaction with current lenses and lens parameter verification.
- It is important to perform keratometry or videokeratography on all potential contact lens wearers. The use of videokeratography is especially beneficial for all high astigmatic and irregular cornea patients.
- A careful binocular refraction should be performed to predict the final lens power and determine residual astigmatism.
- The patient's binocular vision status should be evaluated; if lateral prism is necessary, the patient may not be a good contact lens candidate.
- Anatomic measurements such as corneal diameter, pupil diameter, and palpebral aperture height, in addition to determination of lid tension and blink rate, will help determine both the material to be used and the specific lens parameters.
- A comprehensive slit-lamp examination to evaluate eyelashes, tarsal and bulbar conjunctiva, and corneal integrity is important; a 360-degree evaluation of the limbus and fluorescein evaluation of the cornea are also important.

(continued)

(Continued)

- Preocular tear film quality and volume should be evaluated by a combination of tests such as tear breakup time, tear prism evaluation, corneal and conjunctival staining, and phenol red thread test.

- During the final consultation, the patient's motivation should be evaluated. In addition, it may be necessary to discuss the benefits of spectacles versus contact lenses and GP versus soft lens materials.

- The very low ametrope is a good contact lens candidate. Part-time daily wear is usually recommended for these patients.

- The borderline dry-eye patient may be an acceptable contact lens candidate; careful contact lens selection and patient education are keys to creating a successful contact lens wearer.

■ APPENDIX A

Dry-Eye Questionnaire

1. Age _____
2. Gender   Male   Female
3. Currently wearing (circle one) no contact lenses, rigid contact lenses, soft contact lenses.
4. If you wear contact lenses, do you have a modified wearing schedule because of dryness?
5. Are your eyes usually sensitive to cigarette smoke, smog, air conditioning, or central heating?
   Yes (2)   No (0)   Sometimes (1)
6. Do you take (please underline) antihistamine tablets (1); antihistamine eyedrops (1); diuretics (1); sleeping tablets (1); tranquilizers (1); oral contraceptives (1); medication for duodenal ulcer (1) or digestive problems (1), high blood pressure (1), hormone replacement pills (1), or other (write)?
7. Do you have arthritis?   Yes (2)   No (0)   Uncertain (1)
8. Do you have a connective tissues disorder?   Yes (2)   No (0)
9. Do you have a thyroid abnormality? Yes (2)   No (0)   Uncertain (1)
10. Do you experience dryness of the nose, mouth, throat, chest, or vagina?
    Never (0)   Sometimes (1)   Often (2)   Constantly (3)
11. Are you known to sleep with your eyes open?
    Yes (2)   No (0)   Sometimes (1)
12. Do you have eye irritation upon waking from sleep?
    Yes (2)   No (0)   Sometimes (1)
13. Have you ever had drops prescribed or other treatment for dry eyes?
    Yes (2)   No (0)

(Numbers in parentheses represent score for that answer.)

REFERENCES

1. Jaanus SD, Bartlett JD, Hiett JA. Ocular effects of systemic drugs. In: Bartlett JD, Jaanus SD, eds. Clinical Ocular Pharmacology, 3rd ed. Boston: Butterworth Heinemann, 1995:970–972.
2. Bartlett JD. Medications and contact lens wear. In: Silbert JA, ed. Anterior Segment Complications of Contact Lens Wear. New York: Churchill Livingstone Inc., 1994:474–482.
3. Carney LG, Mainstone JC, Carkeet A, et al. Rigid lens dynamics: lid effects. CLAO J 1997;23(1):69–77.
4. Josephson JE. Examination of the anterior ocular surface and tear film. In: Stein H, Slatt B, Stein R, eds. Fitting Guide for Rigid and Soft Contact Lenses, 3rd ed. St. Louis: CV Mosby, 1990:39–50.
5. Mandell RB. The enigma of the corneal contour. CLAO J 1992;18(4):267–273.
6. Rowsey JJ, Reynolds AE, Brown R. Corneal topography: corneascope. Arch Ophthalmol 1981;99:1093–1100.
7. Belin M, Litoff D, Strods S, et al. The PAR technology corneal topography system. Refract Corneal Surg 1992;8:88–96.

8. Snook RK. Pachymetry and true topography using the ORBSCAN System. In: Gills JP, Sanders DR, Thornton SP, et al., eds. Corneal Topography: The State of the Art. Thorofare, NJ: SLACK Inc., 1995:89–103.

9. Euclid Systems Corporation. Fourier profilometry [Web page]. http://www.euclidsys.com/efourier.html. Accessed January 12, 1999.

10. Chan JS, Mandell RB, Johnson L, et al. Contact lens base curve prediction from videokeratography. Optom Vis Sci 1998;75(6):445–449.

11. Jeandervin M. Computer-aided contact lens fitting with the corneal topographer. Contact Lens Spectrum 1998;13(3):21–24.

12. Szczotka L. Contact lenses for the irregular cornea. Contact Lens Spectrum 1998;13(6):21–27.

13. Allansmith MR, Korb DR, Greiner JV, et al. Giant papillary conjunctivitis in contact lens wearers. Am J Ophthalmol 1977;83(5):697–708.

14. Korb DR, Herman JP. Corneal staining subsequent to sequential fluorescein instillations. J Am Optom Assoc 1979;50(3):361–367.

15. Snyder C. Infiltrative keratitis with contact lens wear - a review. J Am Optom Assoc 1995;66(3):160–177.

16. Andres S, Henriques A, Garcia ML, et al. Factors of the precorneal fluid break time (BUT) and tolerance of contact lenses. Int Contact Lens Clin 1987;14(3):81–120.

17. Tomlinson A. Contact lens-induced dry eye. In Tomlinson A, ed. Complications of Contact Lens Wear. London: Mosby Year Book, 1992:195–218.

18. Mengher LS, Bron AJ, Tongue SR, et al. Noninvasive assessment of tear film stability. In Holly FJ, ed. Precocular Tear Film in Health, Disease, and Contact Lens Wear. Lubbock, TX: Dry Eye Institute, 1986:64.

19. Patel S, Murray D, McKenzie A, et al. Effects of fluorescein on tear breakup time and on tear thinning time. Am J Optom Physiol Opt 1985;62:188–190.

20. Guillon JP, Guillon M. Tear film examination of the contact lens patient. Optician 1993;206(5421):21–29.

21. Doane MG, Lee ME. Tear film interferometry as a diagnostic tool for evaluating normal and dry-eye tear film. Advances Exper Med Biol 1998;438:297–303.

22. Cho P, Yap M. Schirmer test. I. A review. Optom Vis Sci 1993;70(2):152–156.

23. Bennett ES, Gordon JM. The borderline dry-eye patient and contact lens wear. Contact Lens Forum 1989; 14(7):52–74.

24. Nichols, KK, Mitchell GL, Zadnik K. The repeatability of clinical measurements of dry eye. Cornea 2004;23(3): 272–285.

25. Methodologies to diagnose and monitor dry eye disease: report of the Diagnostic Methodology Subcommittee of the International Dry Eye Workshop (2007). Ocul Surf 2007;5(2):108–152.

26. Hamano T, Mitsunaga S, Kotani S, et al. Tear volume in relation to contact lens wear and age. CLAO J 1990;16(1):57–61.

27. Sakamoto R, Bennett ES, Henry VA, et al. The phenol red thread tear test: A cross-cultural study. Inv Ophthalmol Vis Sci 1993;34(13):3510–3514.

28. Elliott L, Henderson B, Bennett ES, et al. Comparison of overall performance of hydrogel and rigid gas permeable lens materials in the contact lens management of the borderline dry eye patient. Presented at the Annual Meeting of the American Academy of Optometry, Orlando, FL, December 1996.

29. Lupelli L. A review of lacrimal function tests in relation to contact lens practice: I. Contact Lens J 1988;16(7):4–17.

30. Feenstra RP, Tseng SC. What is actually stained by rose bengal? Arch Ophthalmol 1992;110(7):984–993.

31. Tseng SC, Zhang SH. Interaction between rose bengal and different protein components. Cornea 1995;14(4): 427–435.

32. Danjo Y, Watanabe H, Tisdale AS, et al. Alteration of mucin in human conjunctival epithelia in dry eye. Invest Ophthalmol Vis Sci 1998;39(13):2602–2609.

33. Argueso P, Tisdale A, Spurr-Michaud S, et al. Mucin characteristics of human corneal-limbal epithelial cells that exclude the rose bengal anionic dye. Invest Ophthalmol Vis Sci 2006;47(1):113–119.

34. Zuccaro VS. Rose bengal: a vital stain. Contact Lens Forum 1981;6:39–43.

35. Chodosh J, Dix RD, Howell RC, et al. Staining characteristics and antiviral activity of sulforhodamine B and lissamine green B. Invest Ophthalmol Vis Sci 1994;35(3):1046–1058.

36. Manning FJ, Wehrly SR, Foulks G, et al. Patient tolerance and ocular surface staining characteristics of lissamine green versus rose bengal. Ophthalmol 1995;102(12):1953–1957.

37. McMonnies CA, Ho A. Patient history in screening for dry eye patients. J Am Optom Assoc 1987;58(4):296–301.

38. Begley CG, Caffery B, Nichols KK, et al. Responses of contact lens wearers to a dry eye survey. Optom Vis Sci 2000;77(1):40–46.

39. Harris MG, Gilman EL. Consultation, examination and prognosis. In: Mandell RB, ed. Contact Lens Practice, 4th ed. Springfield, IL: 1988:136–172.

40. White PF, Gilman EL. Preliminary evaluation. In: Bennett ES, Weissman BA, eds. Clinical Contact Lens Practice. Philadelphia: Lippincott, 1992.

41. Terry R. The effect of glasses on personality perception. Contact Lens Spectrum 1989;4(7):58.

42. Hewett TT. A survey of contact lens wearers. II. Behaviors, experiences, attitudes, and expectations. Am J Optom Physiol Opt 1984;61(2):73–79.

43. Rengstorff RH, Black CJ. Eye protection from contact lenses. J Am Optom Assoc 1974;45(3):270–275.
44. Doughty MJ, Fonn D, Richter D, et al. A patient questionnaire approach to estimating the prevalence of dry eye symptoms in patients presenting to optometric practices across Canada. Optom Vis Sci 1997;74(8):624–631.
45. Begley CG, Chalmers RL, Mitchell L, et al. Characterization of ocular surface symptoms from optometric practices in North America. Cornea 2001;20(6):610–618.
46. Snyder C. Alleviating dryness in contact lens wear. Contact Lens Spectrum 1998;13(8):35–40.
47. Sorbara L, Talsky C. Contact lens wear in the dry eye patient: predicting success and achieving it. Can J Optom 1988;50(4):234–241.
48. Dillehay SM, Miller MB. Performance of lotrafilcon B silicone hydrogel contact lenses in experienced low-Dk/t daily lens wearers. Eye Contact Lens 2007;33(6 Pt 1):272–277.
49. Schafer J, Mitchell GL, Chalmers RL, et al. The stability of dryness symptoms after refitting with silicone hydrogel contact lenses over 3 years. Eye Contact Lens 2007;33(5):247–252.

CHAPTER 2

Companion for Contact Lens Optics

William J. Benjamin

Contact lenses are prescribed for their optical effects on vision, which have been extensively discussed in Chapters 26, 27, and 28 of *Borish's Clinical Refraction*.[1–3] In this chapter a practitioner's guide to the most essential optical formulae, key words, and clinical optics guidelines, with a worksheet for use in computing refractive powers of rigid contact lenses, especially those that are bitoric are presented. A set of 58 optical problems, accompanied by their answers, is also listed so that the busy practitioner or student of contact lens optics can relatively quickly prove his or her knowledge in this detailed and critical area. The four segments of this chapter, Formulae, Key Words, Clinical Guidelines, and Optics Problems, are intended to be practical companions of the more complete chapters already in print.

■ FORMULAE FOR CONTACT LENS OPTICS

Reflection for rays at near-normal incidence:

$$R = [(n' - n)/(n' + n)]^2$$

Back vertex power:

$$BVP = \frac{F_1}{1 - (t/n')F_1} + F_2$$

Front vertex power:

$$FVP = F_1 + \frac{F_2}{1 - (t/n')F_2}$$

where
  R = reflectance from 0 to 1.0
  n = refractive index of medium surrounding surface
  n' = refractive index of medium within lens
  t = center thickness of contact lens (m)

  BVP = back vertex power (D)
  FVP = front vertex power (D)
  F_1 = front surface power (D)
  F_2 = back surface power (D)

Surface power:*

$$F = \frac{n' - n}{r}$$

Law of Gladstone and Dale:

$$n_{hydrated} = n_p V_p + n_s V_s$$

Water content:

$$WC = \frac{n_{dehydrated} - n_{hydrated}}{n_{dehydrated} - n_{saline}} \times 100$$

where
      r = radius of curvature of contact lens surface (m)
      F = refractive power of surface
  V_p, V_s = fraction of material volume devoted to polymer, saline
  n_p, n_s = refractive indices for the polymer, saline in a hydrogel
    WC = water content, in %

---

*In *keratometric* diopters, n' = 1.3375 and n = 1.0000.

Astigmatic addition:

$$CPA = CA + IA$$

Fitting formulae:*

$$CPR = CLP + OR + LLP$$
and
$$FCLP = CPR - LLP$$

Diagnostic lens formula:

$$FCLP = DCLP + OR - \Delta LLP$$

Lacrimal lens power:

$$LLP = BC - K$$

where

CPA = astigmatism at corneal plane (DC)
CA = corneal astigmatism (DC)
IA = internal astigmatism (DC)
BC = base curve (D)
K = keratometry reading (D)
LLP = lacrimal lens power (D)

ΔLLP = change in LLP (D)
CPR = corneal plane refraction (D)
CLP = contact lens power (D)
$FCLP$ = final CLP (D)
$DCLP$ = diagnostic CLP (D)
OR = overrefraction (D)

Empirical effect of flexure on soft contact lens power:

$$\Delta F = -300(t)[(1/r_k{}^2) - (1/r_2{}^2)]$$

Prentice's rule:**

$$P = h(BVP)$$

Prism thickness formula:

$$P = \frac{100(n' - 1)(BT - AT)}{BAL}$$

Meniscus lens thickness formula:

$$CT + s_2 = ET + s_1$$

where

t, CT = center thickness of lens
r_k = radius of curvature of cornea
r_2 = base curve radius of lens
ΔF = change of refractive power (D)
ET = uncut edge thickness of lens
s_1, s_2 = front, back surface sagittal depths

Sagittal depth equations:

$$s = r - \sqrt{r^2 - h^2}$$

$$s_p = \left(\frac{r_{a-p}}{1-e^2}\right) - \sqrt{\left(\frac{r_{a-p}}{1-e^2}\right)^2 - \left(\frac{h^2}{1-e^2}\right)}$$

$$s_o = r_{a-o}\left(1-e^2\right) - \sqrt{\left[r_{a-o}\left(1-e^2\right)\right]^2 - h^2\left(1-e^2\right)}$$

$$s_p = \frac{h^2}{2r_{a-p}}$$

$$s_p = \left(\frac{r_{a-p}}{1-e^2}\right) + \sqrt{\left(\frac{r_{a-p}}{1-e^2}\right)^2 - \left(\frac{h^2}{1-e^2}\right)}$$

where

e = eccentricity
r_a = apical radius of curvature

P = prismatic power in prism diopters (Δ)
h = half of the chord diameter, 2h

*When an OR of zero is intended for the final lens order, these two equations are equivalent.
**Note that here, h is in *cm*.

r_{a-p} = prolate apical radius of curvature   BVP = back vertex power (D)
r_{a-o} = oblate apical radius of curvature   BT = thickness of prism base
s_p, s_o = prolate, oblate sagittal depths   AT = thickness of prism apex
                                                       BAL = length of the base–apex line

Relative Spectacle Magnification

Spectacle magnification:

$$SM = \frac{1}{1 - d(BVP)} \times \frac{1}{1 - (t/n')F_1}$$

(power factor)   (shape factor)

Axial anisometropia:

$$RSM = \frac{1}{1 + g(BVP)}$$

Refractive anisometropia:*

$$RSM = \frac{1}{1 - d(BVP)}$$

Comparison of contact lens to spectacle lens power factors:**

$$\frac{\text{Contact Lens Power Factor}}{\text{Spectacle Lens Power Factor}} = 1 - d(BVP)$$

where
   BVP = back vertex power (D)
       d = stop distance, from back vertex of correcting lens to entrance pupil of eye (m)***
       t = center thickness of correcting lens (m)
   SM = spectacle magnification relative to 1.0
   RSM = relative SM relative to 1.0
       g = distance from anterior focal point of eye to back vertex of correcting lens (m)

Magnification of spectacle–contact lens telescope:****

$$M_t = \frac{-Fe}{Fo} \times \frac{F_{add}}{4}$$

where
   M_t = magnification of telescope relative to 1.0
   F_o = power of objective, spectacle lens (D)
   F_e = power of eyepiece, contact lens (D)
   F_{add} = power of add in spectacle lens (D)

■ KEY WORDS OF CONTACT LENS OPTICS

Corneal reflex   Endothelial mosaic
Fresnel's formula of reflection   Guttata
Gullstrand exact schematic eye   Refractive index
Purkinje-Sanson images I–IV   Law of Gladstone and Dale
Specular reflection   Maurice's lattice theory
Tear fluid meniscus   Epithelial edema
Black line   Stromal edema
Sclerotic scatter   Central corneal clouding (CCC)

---

*Note similarity to power factor of spectacle magnification.
**BVP here is that of the spectacle lens.
***Stop distance = vertex distance + 3 mm.
****When no add is in the spectacle lens, the second factor (F_{add}/4) is omitted from this equation.

Sattler's veil
Fick's phenomenon
Birefringence
Optical anisotropy
Isochromes
Isoclinics or isogyres
"Against" motion
"With" motion
"Scissors" motion
Epithelial microcysts
Epithelial vacuoles
Epithelial bullae
Epithelial "microdeposits"
Keratometry limitations
Refractive index of keratometer
Corneal topography
Corneal apex
Visual axis
Central corneal cap
Elliptical surface
Regular and irregular toricity
"Semi-meridians"
Entrance pupil
Flare and glare
UVR: UV-A, UV-B, UV-C
Cobalt filter
Ultraviolet lamp
"Phantom fluorescein effect"
"Myopic creep"
Back vertex power
Front vertex power
"Sagittal depth effect"
Water content, equation
Blotting technique
Wet cell
Correction factor
Vertex distance
Effective power
"Lacrimal lens"
Lacrimal lens theory
K readings
"Steeper than K"
"Flatter than K"
"On K"
Masking of corneal shape
Overrefraction
Overkeratometry
With-the-rule
Against-the-rule
Residual astigmatism
Spherical rigid contact lens

Front toric rigid contact lens
Back toric rigid contact lens
Bitoric rigid contact lens
    Spherical power effect
    Cylindrical power effect
Rule of thumb for BCR changes
Flexure of soft lenses
"Equal change hypothesis"
Wrap factor
"Constant volume and thickness"
Flexure of rigid lenses
Warpage, regular and irregular
Back-surface bifocals
Crossed-cylinder effect
Sagittal depths
    Sphere
    Ellipse, prolate and oblate
    Parabola
    Hyperbola
Eccentricity
Shape factor $(1 - e^2)$
Accommodative demand
    At spectacle plane
    At corneal plane
    At lenticular plane
Prism diopter
Prentice's rule
Vergence demand
Pre-presbyopic myopes
Spectacle magnification
    Power factor
    Shape factor
    Stop distance
Relative spectacle magnification
    Axial ametropia
    Refractive ametropia
    Knapp's law
Field of view
Field of fixation
"Ring scotoma"
"Ring diplopia"
Off-axis aberrations
On-axis aberrations
Spherical aberration
Coma
Radial astigmatism
Curvature of field
Distortion
Chromatic aberration
Prismatic dispersion
Spectacle–contact lens telescope

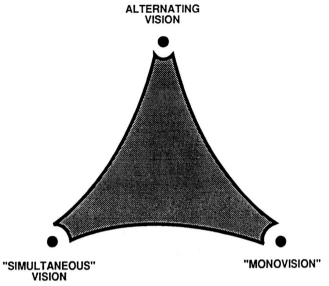

■ FIGURE 2.1 Achievement of presbyopic correction.

Alternating vision
Simultaneous vision
Monovision
Modified monovision
Diffractive bifocal contact lens
"Holographic" bifocal contact lens
Fresnel lens principle
Fresnel half-wavelength zones
"Full aperture" bifocal lenses

"Reduced aperture" lenses
Pupil dependence and independence
    Pupil size dependence
    Pupil location dependence
Coroneo effect
Rizzuti's sign
Liquid crystal
Polarization

■ CLINICAL GUIDELINES FROM CONTACT LENS OPTICS

Differences between Front and Back Vertex Powers for Rigid Lenses

BACK VERTEX POWER (D)	FRONT VERTEX POWER (D)	CENTER THICKNESS (mm)	POWER DISPARITY (D)
−10	−9.92	0.10	−0.08
−5	−4.95	0.12	−0.05
0	0.0	0.15	0.00
+5	+4.90	0.23	+0.10
+10	+9.71	0.32	+0.29
+15	+14.44	0.41	+0.56
+20	+19.06	0.50	+0.94

Effect of Vertex Distance at 15 mm

HYPEROPIC (+) CORRECTION AT SPECTACLE PLANE	AMOUNT OF EFFECTIVE CHANGE* WHEN REFERRED TO CORNEA (D)	MYOPIC (−) CORRECTION AT SPECTACLE PLANE
+4.00	±0.25	−4.25
+5.50	±0.50	−6.00
+6.75	±0.75	−7.50
+7.75	±1.00	−8.75
+9.25	±1.50	−10.75
+10.50	±2.00	−12.50
+12.75	±3.00	−15.75
+14.50	±4.00	−18.50
+16.00	±5.00	−21.00

*Referral of (+) refractive power to the cornea requires a net increase of power, whereas referral of (−) refractive power to the cornea requires a net decrease of power.

Changes of Radii for 0.25-D (0.05-mm) and 1.00-D (0.20-mm) Alteration in Keratometric* Diopters

BASE CURVE DIOPTERS (N = 1.3375)	mm	BASE-CURVE ALTERATION TO PRODUCE A 0.25-D CHANGE IN THE LACRIMAL LENS (mm)	BASE-CURVE ALTERATION TO PRODUCE A 1.00-D CHANGE IN THE LACRIMAL LENS (mm)
53.00	6.37	0.03	0.12
51.00	6.62	0.0325	0.13
49.00	6.89	0.035	0.14
47.00	7.18	0.04	0.16
45.00	7.50	0.04	0.16
43.00	7.85	0.045	0.18
41.00	8.23	0.05	0.20
39.00	8.65	0.055	0.22
37.00	9.12	0.06	0.24

Values have been computed for a range of base curves from 6.37 mm (53.00 D) to 9.12 mm (37.00 D). The rule of thumb specifying that 0.05 mm = 0.25 D is correct only for a limited range of base curves.

---

* $n' = 1.3375$.

Contact Lens Correction of Astigmatism*

CONDITION	CONTACT LENS OPTIONS
REFRACTIVE CYLINDER ≤0.75 DC	
Corneal toricity = Refractive cylinder	*Spherical rigid lens Spherical or aspheric soft lens
Corneal toricity ≠ Refractive cylinder	*Spherical or aspheric soft lens Spherical rigid lens
REFRACTIVE CYLINDER = CORNEAL TORICITY (WITHIN ±0.50 DC)	
Low astigmatism (0.75–2.00 DC)	*Spherical rigid lens Toric soft lens
High astigmatism (>2.00 DC)	*Bitoric "SPE" rigid lens Spherical rigid lens Custom toric soft lens
REFRACTIVE CYLINDER ≠ CORNEAL TORICITY (DIFFERENCE >0.50 DC)	
Low corneal toricity (≤2.00 DC)	*Toric soft lens Front toric rigid lens
High corneal toricity (>2.00 DC)	*Bitoric "CPE" rigid lens Custom toric soft lens

*Optimal option, on average, considering optical quality of correction, comfort, and fit of contact lenses.

Accommodative Demand at the Corneal Plane, Relative to Emmetropia for Near Object

DIFFERENCE IN CORNEAL PLANE ACCOMMODATIVE DEMAND COMPARED WITH EMMETROPIA (D)	BACK VERTEX POWER OF HYPEROPIC SPECTACLE LENS (D)	BACK VERTEX POWER OF MYOPIC SPECTACLE LENS (D)
±0.25	+3.25	−3.87
±0.50	+6.00	−8.37
±0.75	+8.62	−13.75
±1.00	+10.87	−20.87

Measurements of Gullstrand's simplified schematic eye have been assumed, as well as a near object distance 40 cm in front of a spectacle plane with a 15-mm vertex distance.

---

* Note the LARS Principle.
SPE, spherical power effect; CPE, cylindrical power effect.

Accommodative Demand at the Corneal Plane for Add Powers from 0 to Full Near Addition

SPECTACLE ADD	EMMETROPIC EYE	+6 D RIGHT EYE	−6 D LEFT EYE	CORNEAL PLANE ACCOMMODATIVE DEMAND IMBALANCE
No add	2.42	2.81	2.12	0.69 D
+1.00 D	1.47	1.71	1.29	0.42 D
+1.50 D	0.99	1.15	0.86	0.29 D
+2.00 D	0.50	0.58	0.43	0.15 D
+2.50 D	0	0	0	0

The spectacle refractions of the three eyes were plane (emmetropia), +6 D, and −6 D, respectively, at a vertex distance of 12 mm. The right column of the table shows corneal plane accommodative imbalances of an antimetrope with distance spectacle refraction R +6 D and L −6 D. Note that the accommodative demand imbalance decreases to zero as the bifocal add is increased to full correction for the 40-cm target distance.

Relative Spectacle Magnifications Compared with the Emmetropic Schematic Eye

	CORRECTION PLACEMENT		
	SPECTACLE PLANE	CORNEAL PLANE	LENTICULAR PLANE
Axial myopia	=E	>>E	>>E
Axial hyperopia	=E	<<E	<<E
Refractive myopia	<<E	<E	=E
Refractive hyperopia	>>E	>E	=E

E_o Emmetropia vertex distance = 15.7 mm.

Optical Aberrations of Correcting Lenses and Visual Deficits Produced During Lens Wear

ABERRATION	OBJECT POSITION	VISUAL DEFICIT	
		SPECTACLES	CONTACT LENSES
Spherical aberration	On axis	Central	Central
Coma	Off axis	Central and peripheral	Peripheral
Radial astigmatism	Off axis	Central and peripheral	Peripheral
Curvature of field	Off axis	Central and peripheral	Peripheral
Distortion	Off axis	Central and peripheral	Peripheral
Chromatic aberration	On and off axis	Central and peripheral	Central and peripheral
Prismatic dispersion	Off axis	Central and peripheral	Peripheral

Typical Tricurve Design: Rules of Thumb Concerning Peripheral Curves

LENS DIAMETERS (OAD/OZD, IN mm)	SECONDARY CURVE RADIUS (SCR)	PERIPHERAL CURVE RADIUS/WIDTH (PCR/PCW)
9.5/8.1	1.0 mm flatter than BC	2.0 mm flatter than BC/0.2 mm
9.0/7.8	1.5 mm flatter than BC	2.5 mm flatter than BC/0.2 mm
8.5/7.5	2.0 mm flatter than BC	3.0 mm flatter than BC/0.2 mm

BC, base curve; OAD, overall diameter; OZD, optical zone diameter.

■ CONTACT LENS OPTICS PROBLEMS AND ANSWERS

General Optical Concepts

1. A patient has a spectacle Rx of −11.00 DS at a vertex distance of 11 mm. What is the refractive error referred to the cornea?

   Answer: −9.81 DS

2. If the spectacle correction is +15.00 − 5.00 × 180 at a vertex distance of 12 mm, what correction is required at the cornea?

   Answer: +18.29 − 6.93 × 180

3. The following spectacle prescriptions for two ametropic eyes were obtained at a vertex distance of 12 mm: (A) −5.25 − 3.50 × 010; (B) +15.50 − 2.25 × 165. What are the powers referred to the cornea and rounded to the nearest eighth of a diopter?

   Answer: (A) −5.00 − 3.00 × 010   (B) +19.00 − 3.25 × 165

4. A contact lens has a back surface radius of 7.80 mm. (A) What is the refractive power of the surface in air if its refractive index is 1.49? (B) What would be the refractive power of the front surface of the tear film in air if it had the same radius of curvature as did the back surface of the contact lens (7.80 mm)? (C) How do these two values compare to the power of the posterior lens/tear film interface formed at the back surface of this lens?

   Answer: (A) −62.82 D   (B) +43.08 D

   (C) −19.74 D. Their sum is same as actual power calculated for the interface.

5. A polymethylmethacrylate (PMMA) contact lens has a back vertex power of −3.00 DS, a back surface radius of 8.00 mm, and a center thickness of 0.15 mm. What is the front surface radius of this lens?

   Answer: 8.46 mm

6. A contact lens has a back surface radius of 7.50 mm, a center thickness of 0.18 mm, a front optic radius of 7.95 mm, and a refractive index of 1.47. What are the vertex powers of this lens?

   Answer: BVP = −3.12 D   FVP = −3.07 D

7. You have measured a back surface bifocal contact lens in a wet cell, and know that for this particular lens material the refractive power in air is four times that in water. The lensometer measured −0.37 D when the distance image was in focus and measured +1.12 D when the near image was in focus. (A) What is the distance power in air? (B) What is the near "add" in air? (C) What is the true add that this lens will correct?

   Answer: (A) −1.50 DS   (B) +6.00 DS   (C) +1.50 DS

8. A back surface concentric bifocal contact lens is to have a +2.25 DS peripheral addition. What posterior peripheral radius is required if the base curve is 7.60 mm, center thickness is 0.21 mm, refractive index is 1.49, and central power is −1.00 DS?

   Answer: 8.55 mm

9. If a front surface concentric bifocal contact lens is to have a +2.25 D peripheral add, what anterior peripheral radius is required if the base curve is 7.60 mm, center thickness is 0.21 mm, refractive index is 1.49, and central power is −1.00 DS?

   Answer: 7.55 mm if "add" is generated by front vertex power, 7.59 mm if "add" is generated by back vertex power

10. A patient has a −9.00 DS spectacle correction at a vertex distance of 13 mm. (A) When fitted with contact lenses, will the patient require more or less accommodation for a 40-cm viewing distance than with spectacles? What dioptric amount of accommodation would this patient require with spectacles (B) and with contact lenses (C) when viewing a target 40 cm in front of the spectacle plane?

    Answer: (A) More accommodation required with contact lens
    (B) Corneal plane accommodation = +1.95 D
    (C) Corneal plane accommodation = +2.42 D

11. A spectacle–contact lens telescope was designed by adding −27.00 DS to a contact lens Rx to serve as an eyepiece. This now requires a +19.25 DS spectacle lens to serve as the objective lens for distance viewing. Calculate (A) the magnification of the telescope and (B) the vertex distance required by the spectacle lenses.

    Answer: (A) 1.4×   (B) 14.9 mm

12. A patient being fitted with a gel contact lens has the following Rx: −6.00 − 0.62 × 165 at a vertex distance of 15 mm. What is (A) the corneal plane refraction and (B) the expected equivalent sphere power required for the contact lens?

    Answer: (A) −5.50 − 0.50 × 165   (B) −5.75 DS

13. In the problem above, the spectacle Rx was made of resin (n = 1.50), +3.75 base curve, and 2.0-mm center thickness. The contact lens has a 0.08-mm center thickness, n = 1.45, and the base curve is 8.60 mm on the eye. Using equivalent spherical correction, calculate the spectacle magnification (A) when wearing spectacles and (B) when wearing contact lenses. (C) What is the net change in magnification when this eye switches from spectacles to contact lenses? (D) What is the net change in magnification attributable only to the power factors when switching from spectacles to contact lenses?

    Answer: (A) 0.902, or −9.8% (minification)   (B) 0.986, or −1.4% (minification)
    Note: Use power factor only.
    (C) +8.4% (magnification)   (D) 1.1035, or +10.35% (magnification)

14. Gullstrand's exact schematic eye has been fitted with a contact lens made of a material having a refractive index of 1.53. What is the increase of relative intensity, as a percentage, for the "corneal reflex" visible when the contact lens is worn in comparison to when it is not?

    Answer: 43% increase (3.0% vs. 2.1%)
    Hint: Use Fresnel's formula for reflection.

15. In its rigid form, unhydrated, a hydrophilic material has a refractive index of 1.49. The contact lens to be made of the material requires a water content of 37.5%. What will be the refractive index of the hydrated contact lens material?

    Answer: n' = 1.43

16. A patient's cornea has become swollen to the point that visual acuity has decreased. A biopsy of the stroma and resultant analysis shows the ground substance to have a refractive index of 1.348. Assuming that all other refractive indices and proportional contribu-

tions of stromal components remain the same as in a transparent cornea, what is the refractive index of the swollen stroma?

Answer: n′ = 1.368

> Hint: Use law of Gladstone and Dale.

17. K readings for an eye are 41.50/46.75 @ 180. (A) What is the actual refractive astigmatism at the cornea that is a result of the difference between primary meridians? (B) What is the estimated refractive astigmatism encountered at the *posterior* corneal surface?

Answer: (A) −5.85 DC × 090   (B) +0.60 DC × 090

> Hint: n = 1.3375 was used for the keratometer instead of n = 1.376 to account for the power of the posterior cornea.

18. A rigid gas-permeable contact lens has a base curve of 7.90 mm, center thickness of 0.15 mm, back vertex power of −4.00 D, and refractive index of 1.47. (A) What are the vertex focal lengths of this lens? (B) What would the front surface radius have to be for the lens to be of zero back vertex power?

Answer: (A) f_{BVP} = −250 mm; f_{FVP} = +253 mm   (B) 7.95 mm

19. The refractive index of a dry button of gel material is 1.49. It is to be made into a finished hydrophilic contact lens, which, when hydrated, will have a center thickness of 0.07 mm, back vertex power of −8.50 D, and base curve of 8.80 mm. (A) If the water content of hydrated material is 38.6%, what is the refractive index of the hydrated lens? (B) What is the radius of curvature of the front surface (hydrated)? (C) What is the front vertex power of the hydrated lens? (D) What would be the back vertex power of the lens (as if in air) when placed on a cornea having a K reading of 43.00 D? Assume that the front surface flexes an amount equal to that of the back surface and that the lens completely conforms to the cornea. (E) What would be the back vertex power of the lens (as if in air) when placed on the same cornea, but assuming flexure maintains equal center thickness and lens volume?

Answer: (A) n = 1.43   (B) 10.67 mm   (C) −8.45 D

> (D) −10.44 D. This is not representative of the real power of the lens on the eye.

> (E) −8.57 D. This is a small change, into the minus, which is more representative of the change that actually occurs.

20. A patient has a spectacle prescription of R +7.50 − 4.00 × 180 and L −5.00 DS at a vertex distance of 13 mm and views an object 40 cm in front of the spectacle plane. (A) What is the monocular accommodative imbalance at the corneal plane between primary meridians of the right eye? (B) What are the binocular accommodative imbalances at the corneal plane between eyes for the horizontal and vertical meridians? (C) If rigid contact lenses were fitted that excellently corrected the patient's ametropias, what accommodative imbalances would remain at the corneal plane between meridians and between eyes?

Answer: (A) 0.30 D (horizontal meridian greater)

> (B) 0.82 D and 0.52 D, respectively (R eye greater)

> (C) None would exist. However, slight accommodative imbalances would remain at the lenticular plane.

21. The same patient as in question 20 has presented to your office. Keratometry readings are R 44.50/49.12 @ 090 and L 44.50 DS. (A) What are the differences of relative spectacle magnification between the two eyes in the horizontal and vertical meridians when corrected with spectacles? (B) Spectacle base curves are R +13.00 DS and L +4.00 DS, and center thicknesses are R 5.5 mm and L 2.0 mm. The refractive index of these lenses is 1.49. What are the differences of spectacle magnification between eyes in the horizontal and vertical meridians? (C) If contact lenses are fitted that optimally correct the patient's ametropia, what are the differences of relative spectacle magnification between the two eyes in the horizontal and vertical meridians? (D) Considering only the power factor, what will be the differences of spectacle magnification between the two eyes in the horizontal and vertical meridians when corrected with contact lenses?

Answer: (A) 3.35% (R eye smaller), 13.3% (R eye larger), respectively, for horizontal and vertical

Hint: K readings indicate anisometropia to be of axial origin in horizontal meridian, but refractive in the vertical meridian. Note that vertex distance is not 15.7 mm; thus, slight aniseikonia exists even for axial anisometropia corrected with spectacles.

(B) 26.3% (R larger) and 18.2% (R larger), respectively

Hint: Use shape and power factors. Note that the origin of anisometropia does not enter into calculations.

(C) 19.5% (R eye smaller) horizontally and 2.5% (R eye larger) vertically

Hint: Refer power to the cornea. Note that contact lenses reduce aniseikonia for refractive anisometropes but do the opposite for axial problems.

(D) 3.9% (R larger) horizontally and 2.5% (R larger) vertically

Hint: Refer to cornea, and remember that d = 0.003 m.

22. A conventional monocurve rigid contact lens has a front surface sagitta of 1.80 mm and a diameter of 9.5 mm. Two prism diopters ($^\Delta$) are to be added to the Rx (base down). The thickness of the lens edge at the prism apex is to be 0.10 mm, refractive index is 1.49, and base curve is 7.80 mm. (A) What are the center thickness, thickness of the lens at the base of prism, and front surface radius? (B) What is the back vertex power at the apex, center, and base of the lens? (C) What is the prismatic power at the apex and base of the lens compared to the center?

Answer: (A) 0.49 mm, 0.49 mm, and 7.17 mm, respectively

Hint: Thicknesses are the result of contributions from prism and sagittas.

(B) +5.83 D, +7.09 D, and +7.09 D, respectively

Note: BVP alters vertically across lens because of thickness.

(C) 4.8$^\Delta$ BD, 2.0$^\Delta$ BD, and 1.4$^\Delta$ BU, respectively

Hint: Total prism is 2.0$^\Delta$ BD plus that added by Prentice's rule at each point.

Note: Prismatic power varies vertically across lens.

23. An emmetropic low-vision patient requires the use of a spectacle−contact lens telescope. You feel that 1.5× is an excellent magnification to obtain for this patient and have the availability of prescribing up to a −40 D contact lens. (A) The patient's spectacle frame allows only a 15-mm vertex distance. What is the maximum magnification that you can obtain, and with what power of spectacle lens? (B) If you fit the patient with a frame that has adjustable pads, in which a vertex distance of 20 mm is attainable, what is the lowest power of spectacle lens that you can use and still obtain 1.5× magnification?

Answer: (A) 1.×, with +25.00 D spectacle lens and −40.00 D contact lens

(B) +16.67 D, with contact lens of −25.00 D

Lacrimal Lens Problems

24. A patient who wears a rigid lens on one eye has come in for a checkup after 7 years without otherwise visiting your office. The lens was fitted over a central corneal graft, which originally had an average keratometry reading of 47.00 DS and now has a K reading of 43.00 DS, yet the patient still wears the same lens. For smaller amounts of corneal shape alteration, the lacrimal lens should "mask" nearly all refractive changes as long as the rigid lens is worn. But for very large K changes, the lacrimal lens theory may not completely predict changes in the overrefraction and the optimum rigid lens Rx. In this case, what overrefraction could have resulted from the K change noted?

Answer: +0.47 DS

25. If a patient has keratometer readings of 43.00 @ 180, 43.00 @ 090; has a spectacle Rx of −3.00 DS; and is fitted with a lens with a base curve of 7.60 mm, what power is needed in the contact lens?

Answer: −4.37 DS

26. If a patient has keratometer readings of 44.00 @ 180, 44.00 @ 090; has a spectacle Rx of −4.00 DS; and is fitted with a lens with a base curve of 7.60 mm, what power is needed in the contact lens?

Answer: −4.37 DS

27. A patient has on his eye a diagnostic lens with a 7.50-mm base curve and power of −1.50 DS. A refraction over the lens indicates the need for an additional −1.25 DS and the practitioner's analysis of the fit indicates that a base curve of 7.40 mm would be better. (A) What refractive power is required if the 7.40-mm base curve is ordered? (B) If the patient required a lens with a base curve of 7.55 mm, what refractive power would be needed?

    Answer: (A) −3.36 DS   (B) −2.47 DS

28. If a patient has keratometer readings of 45.00 @ 180, 47.00 @ 090; has a spectacle Rx of −1.00 − 2.00 × 180; and is fitted with a lens with a base curve of 7.50 mm, (A) what power is needed in the contact lens? (B) Did corneal toricity match refractive cylinder in this case?

    Answer: (A) −1.00 DS   (B) Yes

29. If a patient has keratometer readings of 46.00 @ 180, 47.50 @ 090; has a spectacle Rx of −2.00 − 1.50 × 180; and is fitted with a lens with a base curve of 7.18 mm, what power is needed in the contact lens?

    Answer: −3.00 DS

30. If a patient has keratometer readings of 44.00 @ 180, 45.50 @ 090; has a spectacle Rx of +2.00 − 2.00 × 180; and is fitted with a base curve of 7.50 mm, (A) what spherical power is needed in the contact lens and (B) what is the amount of residual astigmatism? (C) Did corneal toricity match refractive cylinder in this case?

    Answer: (A) +0.75 DS, equivalent sphere   (B) −0.50 DC × 180   (C) No

31. A patient has a K reading of 45.00 DS and a spectacle prescription of −2.00 DS, and is to be fitted with a rigid lens (n = 1.49) with a base curve of 7.40 mm. What power would be required in the contact lens?

    Answer: −2.61 DS

32. A patient has a spectacle prescription of −2.25 − 0.50 × 180 and keratometer readings of 45.00 @ 180, 45.50 @ 090. If a 7.40-mm base curve contact lens is fitted to this eye, (A) what power should be ordered and (B) how much residual astigmatism is expected? (C) Did corneal toricity match refractive cylinder?

    Answer: (A) −2.86 DS   (B) None   (C) Yes

33. The spectacle prescription of a patient is +12.00 DS measured at a vertex distance of 14 mm, and his keratometer reading is 42.00 DS. He is to be fitted with a contact lens with a base curve of 7.89 mm. What power should be ordered in the contact lens?

    Answer: +13.65 DS

34. If a patient is wearing a 7.85-mm base curve and −4.00 DS corneal lens, and the overrefraction is −1.25 DS, what power should be ordered in a new lens that has a 7.71-mm base curve?

    Answer: −6.03 DS

35. If a patient is wearing a 7.42-mm base curve and −2.50 DS lens, and the refraction over the lens is −0.75 DS, what power should be ordered in the new lens with a 7.50-mm base curve?

    Answer: −2.76 DS

36. A patient's K readings are 42.00 @ 180, 44.00 @ 090 and the spectacle Rx is −2.00 − 1.00 × 180. What is the predicted residual astigmatism with a spherical (A) rigid contact lens and with a spherical (B) soft contact lens?

    Answer: (A) −1.00 DC × 090   (B) −1.00 DC × 180

37. Find the predicted overrefraction when a diagnostic rigid contact lens having a base curve of 42.00 D and power of −2.00 D is used on a patient with a spectacle Rx of −3.00 − 0.50 × 175 and K readings of 41.75 @ 180, 43.00 @ 090.

    Answer: −0.50 − 0.75 × 095 or 090

38. A patient's eye has keratometer readings of 43.00 @ 180, 45.00 @ 090; has a spectacle Rx of −1.00 − 2.00 × 180, and is being fitted with a lens with a base curve of 7.76 mm. Your over-

keratometry readings are 42.50 @ 180, 43.50 @ 090. (A) What is your expected refraction over a −1.50 DS diagnostic lens? (B) Did corneal toricity match refractive cylinder in this case?

Answer: (A) pl − 1.00 × 180   (B) Yes

39. An eye has been fitted with a rigid contact lens having a base curve of 7.94 mm and of −3.00 DS power. The K readings are 42.50 @ 180, 44.00 @ 090 and the spectacle Rx is −2.00 − 0.75 × 180. (A) Assuming that this lens is inflexible, what is the expected over-refraction for the lens? (B) What would be your recommended refractive power if you were to correct the ametropia with (B) a front toric rigid lens or (C) a toric soft lens, ignoring rotational and orientational effects on the eye?

Answer: (A) +1.75 − 0.75 × 090   (B) −1.25 − 0.75 × 090   (C) −2.00 − 0.75 × 180

40. Surprise! You ordered a spherical rigid lens for the patient above with a power of −1.62 DS according to the spherical equivalent of your overrefraction at the fitting session, and your overkeratometry readings now show at dispensing that the lens is flexing on the eye with-the-rule by 0.75 D! (A) What is your expected overrefraction? (B) Given that you could order a lens of similar parameters that would flex in an identical manner, what spherical refractive power would you now order?

Answer: (A) −0.37 DS   (B) −2.00 DS

41. A patient has a spectacle prescription of −3.50 − 1.00 × 180. While wearing a rigid contact lens with a base curve of 7.70 mm and of −2.00 DS, the obtained overrefraction was −2.00 DS. What are this person's K readings?

Answer: 43.33 @ 180, 44.33 @ 090

42. A soft contact lens is fitted to a patient with K readings of 43.00 @ 180, 44.25 @ 090 and a spectacle Rx of −3.00 − 0.75 × 180. What residual astigmatism would be expected with the soft lens on the eye?

Answer: −0.75 DC × 180

43. A 1.00 DS myope with K readings of 45.00 DS is fit with a plano powered rigid contact lens. What base curve must be used to optimally correct this person's ametropia?

Answer: 7.67 mm

44. A patient was initially fit with a rigid contact lens having a base curve of 44.00 D and a power of −3.50 D. It was later necessary to change the base curve to 43.00 D. What power must now be ordered?

Answer: −2.50 DS

45. Calculate the corneal curvatures using the following:

Spec Rx: −2.50 − 0.75 × 180
Diagnostic rigid lens: 43.00 BC, −3.00 power
Overrefraction: +0.50 − 1.75 × 090

Answer: 41.25 @ 180, 43.75 @ 090

46. Find the predicted overrefraction when a rigid contact lens with a 42.25 BC and −3.00 D power is fitted on an eye having the following parameters:

Spec Rx: −4.50 − 1.00 × 172
Vertex distance: 13 mm
K readings: 44.50 @ 180, 46.25 @ 090

Answer: +1.87 − 0.87 × 090

47. Suppose that on the previous eye, the overrefraction was −1.25 − 1.50 × 180. What are the calculated K readings?

Answer: 42.25 @ 180, 41.63 @ 090

48. You have placed an inflexible rigid lens on a 43.50/44.00 @ 090 cornea from your fitting set of −3.00 DS lenses. You meant to place a lens with a 7.90-mm base curve on the eye, but found out just after the lens was on the patient that your set of trial lenses had been mixed up. (A) If the spectacle Rx was −2.00 − 1.25 × 180 and the overrefraction was +1.75 × 0.75 × 180, what was the base curve of the lens that you placed on the eye? (B) Suppose that you thought that the lens looked too "flat," and upon subsequent testing you found that a lens with a 7.70-mm base curve fitted the best. What should be your expected over-refraction with your 7.70-mm base curve trial lens, rounded to the nearest eighth of a diopter? (C) You could prescribe the "equivalent sphere" Rx and forget about the cylinder in the overrefraction, but you have the ability to increase flexure of the lens by making it thinner. If you could place a lens of the appropriate thickness on the eye such that it would flex to correct for the residual cylinder found with your inflexible trial lens, what amount of cylinder in the over-K readings would be ideal? Is this realistically achievable?

Answer: (A) 7.90 mm

> Hint: Use lacrimal lens theory applied to both meridians.

> Note: Lucky! The correct lens was on the cornea.

> (B) +0.62 − 0.75 × 180

> (C) 0.75 DC, steeper in the horizontal meridian. No. This cannot be reasonably expected.

> Hint: Flexure is attributed to the meridian of steepest corneal curvature. Lens power doesn't alter. Flexure can only correct for refractive astigmatism that is not the result of corneal toricity. Had the overrefraction been +0.62 − 0.75 × 090 and corneal curvature remained the same, flexure could correct for the refractive cylinder.

49. A patient's eye is +8.50 − 4.50 × 010 at a vertex distance of 14 mm, and has K readings of 43.50/48.00 @ 100. (A) A +5.00 D diagnostic rigid lens with 7.50-mm base curve seems to fit in a reasonable manner, for a spherical lens. What amount of residual astigmatism should show through the overrefraction? (B) The lens flexes on the eye such that 0.50 D of flexure is revealed in the overkeratometry readings. What is the expected over-refraction? (C) To obtain a better fit, you wish to order a bitoric rigid lens. Not having a bitoric diagnostic lens available, you estimate that about 2.50 D of back surface toricity should be correct, and order a lens with back surface radii of 7.60 mm and 7.20 mm. What refractive power should you order, assuming that this lens will not flex?

Answer: (A) −0.90 DC × 010

> Hint: Refer power to cornea before using lacrimal lens theory.

> Note: Although it appears that corneal toricity and refractive astigmatism are equal, once referred to the cornea they are not; therefore, astigmatism is not completely masked.

> (B) +3.14 − 1.40 × 010

> Hint: Flexure increases power of lacrimal lens into the plus/less minus in the steeper corneal meridian. Flexure in this case, as in most cases, worsens residual astigmatism.

> (C) +8.75 − 3.37 × 010. Note that in most bitoric fits, increasing back toricity necessitates an increase of refractive astigmatic correction in the lens.

Back Toric Contact Lens Problems

50. A patient has a spectacle prescription of −0.50 − 3.50 × 180 and keratometer readings 42.00 @ 180, 45.00 @ 090. If fitted with a toric base curve of 7.94/7.58 mm, what power must be ordered in the contact lens?

Answer: −1.00 − 2.50 × 180, or −1.00 D @ 180/−3.50 D @ 090

51. A refraction over a 7.70-mm base curve rigid diagnostic lens of −3.00 DS power is −1.75 − 1.00 × 090. The lens ordered has a toric back surface with radii of 7.50/7.90 mm (on a with-the-rule cornea). What lens power should be specified for this lens to correct the patient's refractive error?

Answer: −4.64 − 1.27 × 180, or −4.64 D @ 180/−5.91 D @ 090

52. A patient has keratometer readings of 42.00 @ 180, 46.00 @ 090; has a spectacle Rx of −2.00 − 5.00 × 180 at a vertex distance of 12 mm; and is fitted with a contact lens with base curve radii of 7.95/7.50 mm. What power is needed in the contact lens?

    Answer: −2.45 − 3.00 × 180, or −2.45 D @ 180/−5.45 D @ 090

53. A diagnostic lens with a base curve of 7.50 mm and −3.00 DS is placed on a patient's eye and a refraction over the lens indicates a need for the following additional power: −0.50 − 0.75 × 090. The lens to be ordered for this patient is to have a base curve of 7.35/7.70 mm (toric). What power is needed in the contact lens, assuming with-the-rule corneal toricity?

    Answer: −3.08 − 1.34 × 180, or −3.08 D @ 180/−4.42 D @ 090

54. A patient has keratometer readings of 43.00 @ 180, 46.25 @ 090; has a spectacle Rx of −8.00 − 3.50 × 180 at a vertex distance of 12 mm; and is fitted with a lens with base curve radii of 7.45/7.85 mm. The lens has a diameter of 9.50 mm, optic zone of 7.50 mm, secondary curve radii of 8.45/8.85 mm, and center thickness of 0.12 mm. The refractive index of the rigid lens is 1.52. (A) What power should be ordered in the lens and (B) what front radii are needed?

    Answer: (A) −7.30 − 1.86 × 180, or −7.30 D @ 180/−9.16 D @ 090

    (B) 8.86 mm @ 180 and 8.62 mm @ 090

55. A patient has a spectacle prescription of −10.00 − 5.00 × 180 at a vertex distance of 12 mm, and K readings of 44.00 @ 180, 49.00 @ 090. If the patient is fitted with a spherical rigid lens with a radius of 7.30 mm, (A) what spherical power would be required in the contact lens? (B) What residual astigmatism would be expected? (C) Does corneal toricity match refractive cylinder in this case? (D) Would lens flexure help or hinder in this case?

    Answer: (A) −10.55 DS, equivalent sphere   (B) −1.22 DC × 090

    (C) Actually, it does not. Once the refractive cylinder is referred to the cornea, it amounts to −3.78 DC × 180, which is less than corneal toricity.

    (D) Up to 1.25 DC of flexure would help correct the refractive astigmatism.

56. If the above eye is fitted with a toric base curve lens with radii of 7.55/6.96 mm, (A) what power would be required in each meridian to correct the patient's refractive error? (B) This lens is representative of what optical fitting effect? (C) How much cylinder rotates with this lens on the eye?

    Answer: (A) −9.63 D @ 180, −12.20 D @ 090   (B) Cylindrical power effect (CPE)

    (C) Approximately 1.25 DC

57. A patient's corneal toricity matches that of the refractive cylinder, yet the toricity does not allow a rigid contact lens with a spherical base curve to fit correctly. K readings are 40.00 @ 180, 44.50 @ 090 and the spectacle refraction is +1.00 − 4.50 × 180. With your office fitting set, you estimate that a bitoric lens having base curves of 8.33/7.76 would provide the best fit. (A) What would be the refractive power of the ordered lens (n = 1.47) in air? (B) What would be the power of the lens on the eye, its posterior surface immersed in tear fluid? (C) This lens is an example of what type of optical fitting effect? (D) How much cylinder rotates with this lens on the eye?

    Answer: (A) +0.50 − 3.00 × 180, or +0.50 D @ 180/−2.50 D @ 090

    (B) +40.79 @ 180, +40.83 @ 090 (essentially spherical)

    (C) Spherical power effect (SPE)

    (D) Almost none; zero

RIGID LENS "FORM 1040"

PATIENT NAME: _____   **DATE:** _____

1. **EYE: R or L**   **CPR =** [ ] – [ ] **X** [ ]

   sphere   minus cylinder   axis

BASIC INFORMATION

	FLAT MERIDIAN			STEEP MERIDIAN		

2. **K's** [ ] = [ ] @ [ ]   [ ] = [ ] @ [ ]
   mm   D   mm   D

3. **DIAG. CL BASE CURVE** [ ] = [ ] Verified? Y or N [ ] = [ ]
   mm   D   mm   D

4. **FINAL CL BASE CURVE** [ ] = [ ]   [ ] = [ ]
   mm   D   mm   D

Rx POWER ESTIMATE #1:   FINAL CLP = DIAG. CLP + OR – ΔLLP

FLAT MERIDIAN   STEEP MERIDIAN

5. **DIAG. CLP** [+ or – D]   Verified? Y or N   [+ or – D]
6. **OR** + [+ or – D]   + [+ or – D]
7. **ΔLLP** – [+ or – D]   Line 4 – Line 3 – [+ or – D]
8. **FINAL CLP EST. #1** [+ or – D] Line 5 + Line 6 – Line 7 [+ or – D]

Rx POWER ESTIMATE #2:   FINAL CLP = CPR – LLP

FLAT MERIDIAN   STEEP MERIDIAN

9. **CPR** [+ or – D]   From Line 1   [+ or – D]
10. **LLP** – [+ or – D]   Line 4 – Line 2 – [+ or – D]
11. **FINAL CLP EST. #2** [+ or – D] Line 9 – Line 10 [+ or – D]

CL REFRACTIVE POWER ADJUSTMENT WEIGHING ESTIMATES #1 and #2

FLAT MERIDIAN   STEEP MERIDIAN

12. **FINAL CLP** [+ or – D] From Lines 8 & 11 [+ or – D]

■ FIGURE 2.2 Rigid lens form.

CARL F. SHEPARD MEMORIAL LIBRARY
ILLINOIS COLLEGE OF OPTOMETRY
3241 S. MICHIGAN AVE.
CHICAGO ILL. 60616

58. A bitoric rigid contact lens has base curve radii of 8.03 mm and 7.67 mm and has back vertex powers of −1.00 D and −4.00 D in those meridians, respectively. What amount of cylinder power rotates with this lens as it varies rotational orientation on the eye?

Answer: 1.00 DC

NOTES FOR USE OF RIGID LENS "FORM 1040":

- Generally fit approximately two-thirds or three-quarters of the corneal toricity.
- Judge credibility of estimate no. 1 versus credibility of estimate no. 2 before adjusting power to that which will be ordered (final CLP).
- Bias toward the "spherical power effect" when appropriate, where back surface toricity in keratometric diopters (line 4) is equal to CLP refractive cylinder (line 12).

DEFINITIONS USED IN RIGID LENS "FORM 1040":

CPR = corneal plane refraction
Diag. CL = diagnostic contact lens
Diag. CLP = diagnostic contact lens (refractive) power
Final CL = the contact lens that will be ordered
Final CLP = final contact lens (refractive) power
LLP = lacrimal lens (refractive) power
ΔLLP = change of LLP to that of the final contact lens base curve from that of the diagnostic contact lens base curve
OR = overrefraction at the corneal plane

REFERENCES

1. Benjamin WJ. Contact lenses: applied optics of contact lens correction. In: Benjamin WJ, ed. Borish's Clinical Refraction, 2nd ed. St. Louis, MO: Elsevier Medical Publications, 2006:1188−1245.
2. Benjamin WJ. Clinical optics of contact lens prescription. In: Benjamin WJ, ed. Borish's Clinical Refraction, 2nd ed. St. Louis, MO: Elsevier Medical Publications, 2006:1246−1273.
3. Benjamin WJ, Borish IM. Correction of presbyopia with contact lenses. In: Benjamin WJ, ed. Borish's Clinical Refraction, 2nd ed. St. Louis, MO: Elsevier Medical Publications, 2006:1274−1319.

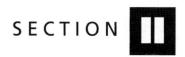
Gas-Permeable Lenses

CHAPTER 3

Corneal Topography

Eef van der Worp, John de Brabander, and Frans Jongsma

▓ INTRODUCTION

Contact lens practitioners have a high interest in the shape of the cornea. When this shape is known, a contact lens that will optimize the cornea–lens relationship can be selected, fitted, or designed. Generally, mimicking the shape of the cornea promotes comfort of lens wear and reduces mechanical effects of the lens on the cornea.

The standard procedure in contact lens practice is to measure the cornea with a keratometer. But what exactly does keratometry tell us? It typically measures the average curve of the central 3 mm of the cornea in two meridians. This includes, at minimum, three limitations. First, a keratometer measures curves and curves are not the equivalent of shape. Second, it estimates, rather than measures, the average central curves. This means it does not provide information about the exact central point (not to mention the top) of the cornea. Third, and most important: 3 mm is a very small area of a cornea. A typical cornea is 11 to 12 mm in diameter. Contact lenses, in general, cover a much larger part of the cornea than 3 mm (Fig. 3.1), and a keratometer does not provide information about the periphery of the cornea.

Corneal topography also has its limitations, all of which will be discussed in this chapter. However, when compared to the keratometer, it provides the practitioner with much more information about the geometry of the cornea and therefore can aid in optimizing the lens-to-cornea fitting relationship.

Interestingly, the principle of corneal topography is as old as that of keratometry, dating back to the late 19th century. Is it impossible to measure corneal shape with a keratometer? Theoretically, peripheral curve radii can be measured by performing keratometry over the lenses and having the subject view at an angle of 25 or 30 degrees nasally, temporally, superiorly, and inferiorly. If this information is related to the central curves of the cornea, some idea about the amount of flattening toward the periphery can be obtained. Apart from the fact that with a keratometer it is often challenging to obtain reliable peripheral curve data from the periphery of the cornea, computation of corneal shape from this data is difficult.

Overall, keratometry is not the best method to measure corneal shape, apart from being time consuming. Corneal topographers can provide information about thousands of data points on the cornea that will result in a better understanding about corneal shape. More and more, practitioners will have to rely on corneal shape data rather than corneal curves. This is crucial when managing refractive surgery, orthokeratology, and keratoconus patients, but also, for the design and manufacturing of any type of contact lens, information about the shape of the cornea is essential.

In this chapter history, principles, and recently developed devices to measure the shape of the eye front surface are discussed. The primary goal is to explain how corneal topographers work, and how these devices can be used optimally in the contact lens practice.

History

For centuries ophthalmologists, optometrists, and others involved in eye care have been using the reflection capacity of the first refractive surface of the eye to obtain a qualitative impression

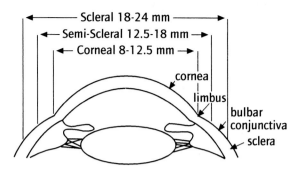

■ FIGURE 3.1 Contact lenses with various diameters in relationship to the eye dimensions.

of the integrity of the cornea. Historically it has been described to diagnose the integrity of the cornea by viewing the reflected image of a rectangle window (Fig. 3.2). This simple diagnostic tool is based on the fact that the boundary air–tear film acts as a mirror.

From this the basis for quantitative corneal topography was described by von Helmholtz, Placido, and Gullstrand in the late 19th century. Von Helmholtz[1] measured the local slope of the cornea by observing the reflection of a pair of objects positioned at a known place with respect to the subject's eye (Fig. 3.3). The virtual image obtained this way is called the *first Purkinje image*. On the basis that the cornea can be considered as an optical equivalent to a spherical mirror, Javal[2] designed an instrument in which the objects could be rotated around the optical axis. In this way it became possible to find the orientation of the flattest and steepest radius of curvature, so-called "principle meridians" of the cornea. With his device more precise measurements of the cornea were introduced. Although Javal called it *ophthalmometry*, this technique is known today as *keratometry* (from *keratos*, Greek for *cornea*).

Instead of pairs of objects, Placido[3] used a disk with concentric rings with a central hole through which he observed the image reflected by the subject's eye (Fig. 3.4).

This extended the observation to more meridians, and it evaluates an entire region rather than two or more points on the cornea. With this simple but ingenious invention (also called keratoscopy), the practitioner is able to make a qualitative diagnosis of corneal irregularities and, very importantly, to estimate the amount and direction of corneal astigmatism.

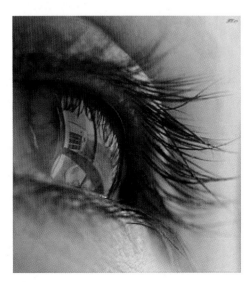

■ FIGURE 3.2 Image of a rectangle window as reflected by the cornea.

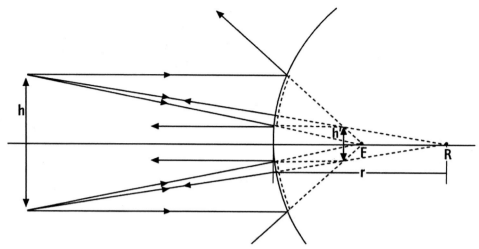

■ **FIGURE 3.3** The principle of keratometry is based on image formation as with a convex mirror. The radius of curvature of the cornea (*r*) determines the difference in distance between the object mires (*h*) and the same at the reflected image side (*h'*). Note that only two small and separated areas of the cornea actually contribute to the measurement. Note also that the longer the distance between the object mires (h) and the cornea is, the closer the h' is located to the focal plane of the cornea.

Gullstrand[4] took a major step in quantification of corneal topography by placing a photographic camera in the central hole of the Placido disk (Fig. 3.5). Measuring the size of the rings on the photographs enabled Gullstrand to estimate the corneal radius of curvature quantitatively. The technique, no longer in use today, was referred to as photokeratoscopy.

Placido disk photographs from an irregular cornea (Fig. 3.6A) and a cornea with a very steep apex, a flat superior area, and a steep inferior area, all associated with keratoconus (Fig. 3.6B), are shown. It can be observed that only a very small area of the cornea can be imaged and other areas cannot typically be interpreted or only with severe error.

A century after the invention of photography, the first television was developed, leading to the small and inexpensive charge coupled device (CCD) television systems that are common today. The modern personal computer has had a comparable history. Coupling these two devices has made it possible to collect and process a quarter of a million data points in a very brief time. After the development of algorithms for surface reconstruction, a translation of the acquired image into clinically relevant data in the 1980s, called computer-assisted video keratoscopy, was born.[5]

Today, these systems are simply called corneal topographers and many devices exist, but most of them are still based on the old Placido disk principle. The inherent limitations of imaging by specular reflection (see section Using a Corneal Topographer later in this chapter)

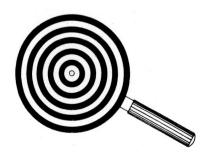

■ **FIGURE 3.4** Hand-held Placido disk.

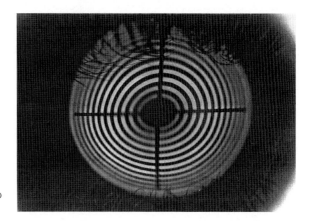

■ **FIGURE 3.5** Photographic image of a Placido disk reflected on an astigmatic cornea.

resulted in the development of alternatives. These topographic devices, based on different principles, opened new possibilities but also introduced other limitations. This has resulted in a somewhat confusing situation where it is not always possible for the practitioner to link modalities of a given device to what is desired and/or practical. This also accounts for the way image data are transformed into data of eye shape and even more how this is presented in numbers, indices, or color-coded maps.

Corneal topography has led to the publication of a vast number of papers and patents. In a study at the University of Maastricht by Jongsma et al.[6] information was found on 24 devices that were based on essentially different principles. Analyzing the principles of these devices

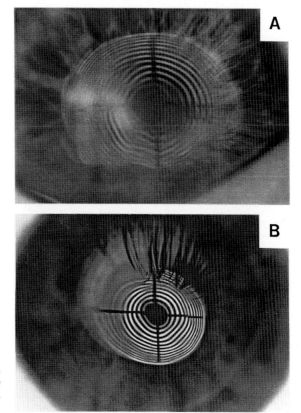

■ **FIGURE 3.6** Placido disk photograph from an irregular cornea **(A)** and a cornea with a very steep apex, a flat superior part, and a steep inferior part **(B,** keratoconus).

revealed that all devices would fit into a system that discriminates between the combinations of used light sources and the way they interact with the eye front surface (light–matter interaction). The literature descriptions yielded 12 modalities. The light source may be a light-emitting object (e.g., a Placido disk) or a projected image (e.g., a slit, lines, or a grid). The light used can be incoherent or coherent. The light matter interaction can be specular reflection, scattering, diffuse reflection, total reflection, or a combination. Not all combinations of these are technically feasible. Some are possible but rather expensive, or very difficult to use in clinical settings. Most widely used are devices based on reflection from a light-emitting object, such as the keratometer and the keratoscopes. Devices based on projection [e.g., a scanning slit or optical coherent tomography (OCT)] have entered the market recently. Generally, these devices are found to be most prevalent in ophthalmology clinics.

There are numerous new developments in the field of reflection corneal topographers, which will improve the accuracy and usefulness of the procedure. Collins et al.[7,8] in Brisbane, Australia, for example, researched dynamic corneal topography, via which multiple topography maps can be made within seconds, creating an almost live movie of the corneal topography showing its dynamic rather than static nature. Researchers in Amsterdam, the Netherlands, developed a modified Placido disk system using different colors.[9] They claim this system gives a more accurate representation about the periphery of the cornea.

In addition to this, corneal topographers are now integrated with wavefront aberrometers, which can be a major advantage in contact lens practice. Subtracting the anterior surface aberrations from the total aberrations will reveal the rest aberrations of the eye. Corneal topography then can be useful (see later section in this chapter) to aid in fitting contact lenses, and rest aberrations can be corrected on the front surface of the lens.[10]

Keratometry

In keratometry, the reflected image of small light-emitting targets, usually called *mires,* formed by the anterior surface of the cornea is used to determine the outer radius for one meridian (Fig. 3.3). By rotating the instrument about its optical axis, the principal meridians of the cornea (flattest and steepest) can be found. Actually, in keratometry it is not the size of an object that is compared with a formed image—the separation between the two mires at the object plane is compared with the measured separation in the image. To exactly measure the latter separation, keratometers have a built-in doubling system. As can be observed from Figure 3.3, only a very small area of the cornea is used to reflect the two mires. The angle between the incoming ray from the mires and the reflected ray from the cornea, called the *collimator angle,* is normally about 17 degrees. However, some autokeratometers work with different collimator angles to measure the asphericity along meridians. The keratometer actually presents an average measurement using two small areas that are separated from each other (depending on the device and the radius of curvature of the cornea, from 2.0 to 3.5 mm). So, the apex is not measured but estimated to be spherical between the measured areas. In irregular corneal surfaces and/or a decentered corneal apex (as in keratoconus), this may cause clinically relevant inaccuracies. Also, the range of corneal curvatures that ensure proper images for measurements is limited (usually from 6 to 9 mm). Furthermore, the periphery of the cornea is not measured using standard keratometric methods. A problem in keratometry is also that the measurement is observer dependent. Errors by the observer are misalignment, improper positioning of the mires, ambiguity by distorted mires, focusing, and, most important, accommodation by the observer. In most keratometers errors in focusing are restricted by using a Scheiner disk (double image if out of focus) or collimated mires and telecentric viewing systems (accommodation-independent systems).

Although strictly qualitative, the keratometer can still give the experienced user some information by judging the distortion of the imaged mires on corneal irregularities, tear film quality, and, indirectly, the fit and front surface quality of soft contact lenses. To decrease inaccuracies and also to reduce the inherent problem that the object is not placed in infinity and thus the image is not formed exactly at the focal plane of the cornea, Mandell[11] developed keratometers with a long working distance and small objects (small mire keratometry). With these devices he performed measurements of the peripheral corneal curvature by having the patient fixate on a movable off-axis light source. The need for extra information on the corneal periphery can be easily deducted from Figure 3.1, if one realizes that the smallest contact lens has a diameter of 8.0 mm and classic keratometry only provides information on an area of around 3.0 mm (around 8% of the corneal surface).

Using the principle of off-axis fixation devices, Wilms[12] developed a method that can be used with most ordinary keratometers and delivers an estimation of *e*-values at 30 or 25 degrees from the central axis (Fig. 3.7). Apart from the fact that it is often difficult to obtain reliable peripheral curve data from the periphery of the cornea, it also should be considered that two different methods are being postulated—tangential and sagittal curves—which are difficult to compare.[13]

In summary, the (auto-) keratometer is a relatively easy-to-use device that, in normal corneas, provides average information on corneal curvature, including amount and axis of astigmatism. In contact lens practice it is successfully used as an initial step to find parameters for a trial lens prior to evaluation by an experienced practitioner. More experienced users can also gain information on the quality of the central part of the corneal surface, the tear film, and the front surface of a soft contact lens.

Keratoscopy and Corneal Topography

Strictly, the name *keratoscopy* means viewing the cornea; therefore, the original Placido disk is a true keratoscope in the hands of the practitioner looking at the formed image. With photographing the image, the name of the device has historically been changed to *photokeratoscopy*. Examples of photokeratoscopic images are given in Figures 3.5 and 3.6.

When viewing these images, the qualitative information that can be gained is very evident for a trained clinician. Compared to the keratometer, the photokeratoscopic images give information on a relatively small area, but definitely a larger area than just two points.

With the replacement of the photo camera by a CCD camera, the name of the device was changed to a *videokeratoscope*. Over time, the name was changed to *videokeratograph* or, more

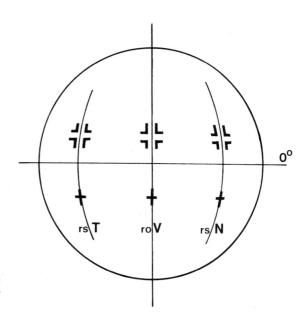

■ FIGURE 3.7 The areas measured using sagittal topography as proposed by Wilms. Note that the horizontal meridian is measured in the periphery with the keratometer mires in a vertical position.

common and most widely used, *corneal topographer* after the implementation of computer-assisted software algorithms to analyze the picture.

The name *corneal topography* implies that the topography of the cornea is exactly measured. Is this true? Is the picture that is displayed as a color-coded map the true shape (topography) of the entire cornea? The answer could be no or sometimes yes, but important for clinical applications, the correct answer is "we don't know." The reason for this lies in the inherent problem of using a reflected image of an unknown surface that, in itself, is the object of the measurement. Without discussing complicated optical mathematics, some understanding of these inherent problems is useful for practitioners to understand differences between the design of corneal topographers and the interpretation of corneal topographic maps as discussed later in this chapter. Recommended reading in this respect is the classic article by Mandell, "The Enigma of the Corneal Contour."[14]

Reflection Topography

Reflection follows the simple rules of Snell's law, where the incidence ray of light and the reflected ray of light form equal angles with the normal to the surface. In corneal topography, a picture is analyzed, from which it is known that the incident rays are coming from the Placido disk and the reflected rays are coming from the cornea. The advantage over keratometry is that with a flat Placido disk, a two-dimensional object is created so that more points can be evaluated. The problem is, however, that it is unknown where the image exactly was and where in space the reflection occurred. So finding the normal for multiple rays, which is essential for reconstruction of the corneal surface, becomes difficult. Furthermore, it is desired to measure as large an area of the cornea as possible. For this, the use of a large disk would be indicated. However, with large disks the peripheral rays will incident on a very skewed angle compared to the rays more centrally, and also most of these rays will be obscured by the eyelids. Even more complicated is that the image of a large disk is not flat but curved, so the image space becomes three-dimensional. For all of these reasons, modern corneal topographers use a curved or cone-shaped pattern of rings and try to diminish the working distance as much as possible. If the cornea happened to have a spherical shape, its shape would be easy to measure and actually keratometry would be satisfactory. The ironic fact is that the normal cornea is not spherical and that our specific aim is to actually measure the deviations from the sphere. To do so, the data must be fit to mathematically assumed shapes. The assumed shapes could be a sphere, an ellipse using *e*-values, various polynomials, or splines.

To measure the shape of the cornea with high resolution, one would think that as many as possible rings in the target would be beneficial. This is true, but as can been observed from Figure 3.6A,B compared to Figure 3.5, both the contrast and the order of the rings (lost rings or ring jam) in the image become problematic for software analysis. Some topographers analyze Placido ring borders by using different colors for the outer and the inner boundary of the ring. This way, confusion of rings may be reduced.

Another serious problem, as can be recognized from Figure 3.6A,B, is alignment of the ring target with the center of the cornea. Slight decentration would give an entirely different picture of the rings in the image. A normal cornea could, with decentered imaging, present as a keratoconus pattern. Also, shape algorithms do need a central reference point (with the exception of splines to some extent). In Placido ring imaging the real center is not imaged. This is not a problem for normal corneas, where it can be estimated, but in a keratoconic eye, where the top of the cone is usually not at the geometric center of the cornea, it can be problematic. Also, there is no such concept as a spherical apex area in keratoconus. Odd topographic maps may be seen as a result of this. More on this topic will be discussed later in this chapter under Indexes for Irregularity.

A problem in interpretation of topographic maps is that via viewing a map one could determine that the radius of curvature somewhere on the cornea is, for example, 7.5 mm (or if a dioptric map is used, 45.00 D). But what does this mean? Is the cornea steep, or is it a local steepness, or maybe a flatter area on a very steep cornea? Even more, what is the position of this steeper or flatter area on the slope of the cornea? It is like walking in an area with hills. You see the curve and you might feel the slope while walking, but are you on a mountain at 6,000 feet high, or on the hill next to your house at the beach? To have access to that knowledge, a height map is needed to really know where you are. The same is true with local corneal curvature data. Here the problem is that a Placido disk inherently estimates radii of curvature where ideally a height map would be desired. Therefore, most modern corneal topographers also present *height maps*. Although these maps are still derivatives from curvature, by using fast and smart algorithms combined with logical iterative/interpolation/extrapolation processes they can (given a reasonable starting point in the Placido disk image) be reasonably accurate. These data are ideal when designing and manufacturing custom contact lenses.

Reading of a height map is quite different from a curvature map. A height map representing the total, absolute sagittal height of the cornea actually would not give any detail at all. All it would show is that the central cornea is higher than the periphery, which is not really a surprise. It becomes useful only after matching the corneal surface with a so-called "best-fit sphere" (or sometimes "a best-fit oval"). Everything that is higher (meaning being closer to the observer) is color coded with warmer colors; everything that is positioned farther away from that shape is presented with cooler colors. Therefore, what the exact (and actual) shape of the cornea is can be immediately observed.

In summary, reflection corneal topographers, compared to keratometry, are ideal in obtaining more information on an extended area of the cornea, but still do not measure the complete corneal surface. They are not difficult to use, but care should be taken in obtaining both proper alignment and focusing. Looking at the image before processing is recommended, and proper interpretation of the different maps is a key consideration. This topic will be further discussed later in this chapter under How to Use a Corneal Topographer.

Projection Topography

Appreciating the disadvantages of reflection systems, alternatives to the Placido disk-based corneal topographers have been developed.[15–17] Most of these devices are more complicated in use, expensive, or more used in research settings than in routine clinical settings. To explain the principles of using a projecting light source, three different possibilities are described here. The first is projecting a set of lines on the cornea (Maastricht Shape Topographer, or MST); the second is the use of a scanning slit such as that used in Orbscan and Pentacam systems. The MST, based on Fourier profilometry, is able to present a height map of the total area composed to the instrument (Fig. 3.8A). The system projects from two directions a line pattern on the front surface of the eye in which fluorescein acts as diffusing medium. Because the line patterns are viewed by a central camera, they become, depending on the shape of the eye, curved in the image (Fig. 3.8B). Fourier analysis can transform this information to height data, and from there it is possible to create cross sections of the cornea and sclera including limbal topography (Fig. 3.8C). As with Placido disk devices, a good image is essential. Advantages of the MST include that it measures shape directly and—especially important in contact lens designing—presents height information on the entire eye front surface.

The principle of a scanning slit as in the Orbscan and Pentacam devices[15] can be easily appreciated from a cross section view of the cornea (Fig. 3.9A), routine for eye care practitioners. In the slit image the profile of the cornea front and back surface can be observed. Unfortunately, this is only one meridian and if the incidence angle of the slit were changed, a dramatic change would be observed. In the Orbscan device a scanning slit is used to obtain multiple images over many meridians. To overcome distortion by different incidence angles, a Scheimpflug correction system is built in (Fig. 3.9B). From the many imaged slits the corneal shape, both front and back surface, can be computed. So, actually indirect pachymetry

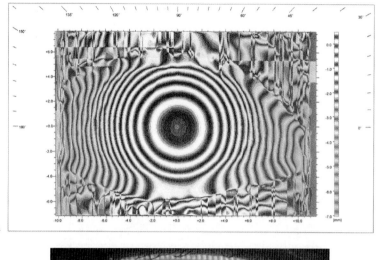

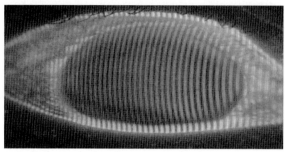

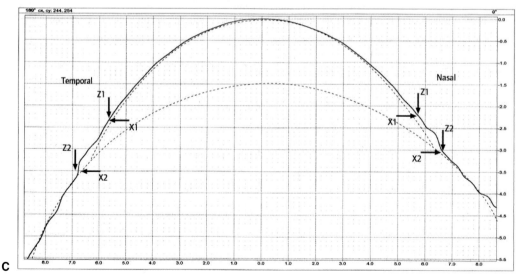

■ **FIGURE 3.8 (A)** Height contours obtained with the Maastricht Shape Topographer (MST). The contours represent lines of equal height that can be translated into x, y, and z coordinates to describe the complete eye surface as exposed to the device. **(B)** Projected lines at the eye surface with the MST device. **(C)** Cross section of a horizontal true height profile of a normal eye (OD) as obtained with the MST device. Topography of the entire eye surface including the limbal area and part of the sclera can be obtained.

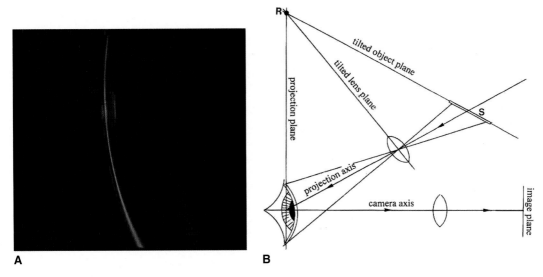

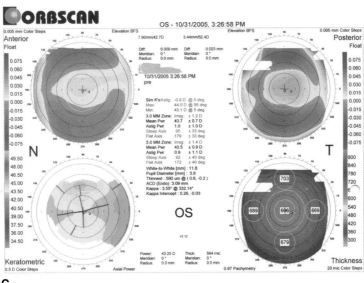

■ FIGURE 3.9 (A) Image cross section as obtained with the slit lamp, including the profile of the cornea front surface, gas-permeable contact lens back surface, and fluorescent tear layer. **(B)** Schematic view of a Scheimpflug correction. The tilted object plane (*S*) is conjugated with the projection plane when the tilted lens plane meets the object plane and projection plane at the same point (*R*). **(C)** Presentation of data with the Orbscan including corneal pachymetry.

is performed. The results are presented in color-coded maps, including corneal thickness data (Fig. 3.9C). Advantages of the Orbscan device are that it is able to present height data on both the front and back surface of the cornea.

Optical Coherent Tomography

Recently, devices have been developed that are able to image the front segment of the eye based on optical coherent tomography (OCT). The principle behind these devices is a Michelson interferometer, in which time differences using two imaging paths from the same target are used to compute distance data. One imaging path is calibrated for the device, and

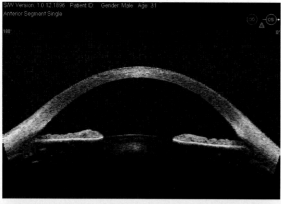

A

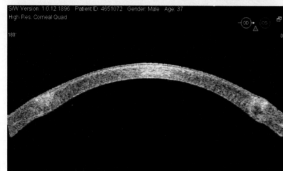

B

■ FIGURE 3.10 **(A)** Front segment optical coherent tomography (OCT). **(B)** Corneal high-resolution meridian topography with OCT.

the other path contains the object to measure (in this case the eye). Next to the front segment of the eye (Fig. 3.10A), the cornea can also be measured using so-called high-resolution imaging (Fig. 3.10B). From these images the real corneal height topography can be obtained. At present not much information on the accuracy and reproducibility of OCT for work in the contact lens field is available. It appears to be a promising device in the future, although it is still relatively expensive at the present time.

Clinical Potential of Devices

The question about which one of all the technologies mentioned is the best cannot be easily answered . It largely depends on the aim of the application. Corbett et al.[18] mentioned four considerations regarding this question: the kind of required measurement, the kind of eye surface, the kind of situation, and the kind of required presentation. If the corneal surface is considered to be an optical surface, a parametric measurement might be indicated with the advantage that considerable sensitivity is gained. Most devices based on specular reflection, including the Placido disk-based corneal topographers, measure parametrically. If the local corneal anatomy is important in the diagnosis, devices based on scattering can offer interesting modalities (e.g., pachymetry). Should it not be the optical performance but the shape that is the object of the diagnosis (e.g., pre- and postoperative evaluation or contact lens fitting), devices based on diffuse reflection offering direct height measurements can be more useful. Sometimes a diffusing membrane or simply a thin soft contact lens may be beneficial. Dry corneas, for example, exclude effective use of specular reflection, whereas during surgery no fluorescein can be used as this penetrates the stromal tissue.

For corneas with a regular surface, a mirrored image, which is easily acquired with a Placido disk-based corneal topographer, is adequate. For irregular corneas, of which the shape is to be determined, detailed height mapping might be more accurate when obtained with a nonparametric measurement using projection principles.

■ HOW TO USE A CORNEAL TOPOGRAPHER

A corneal topographer is a very powerful tool, and the primary limitation appears to be the amount of data that is provided, which might be too overwhelming to be of practical use. This part of the chapter on corneal topography will discuss the necessary insights in how to use the tools available in the giant toolbox that a topographer is, and how to optimize usage of the instrument.

Measuring Procedure

Most of the topographers, especially so in contact lens practices, are the reflection systems, and these will be further discussed in detail here. One of the primary disadvantages of a reflection system topographer is the limited area that typically can be measured. To measure the maximal surface area of the cornea, it is important to first minimize the upper eyelid interference, which can cause shadows on the cornea, leading to missing data points. This is typically accomplished by asking the subject to make "large eyes." If this is not sufficient, the eyelid can be held up by a cotton swab. However, it is important for there to be an absence of pressure on the eyeball, as pressure can easily cause corneal curvature changes. It is preferable to use the orbital rim as a resting point. The subject's nose also can cause shadows on the cornea, which may lead to missing data points. To avoid this, the patient can be asked to move his or her head slightly: if the right eye is being measured, ask the patient to rotate his or her head slightly to the left, while emphasizing the importance of fixation straight ahead. This way the nose will have a lesser impact on the topography picture that is taken.

In general, reflection system topographers have difficulty measuring the periphery of the cornea, and the area that is measured is limited. The more irregular a cornea is, the more data points are missing in the periphery.

Figure 3.11A shows a typical map of a keratoconus eye, with limited data points available. Figure 3.11B also shows a map of a keratoconus, but with the missing data points extrapolated. The topographer simply assumes that the cornea will continue farther out in the periphery in the same manner. As these are not actually measured data, but rather mathematically generated points, caution should be taken. In clinical practice extrapolation can still be of value as calculated data might be preferable to no data at all. Some topographers (see Fig. 3.11C) will show the extrapolated data (*dashed*) and the real measured data in the same picture, so that the practitioner knows exactly what the origin of all data points is.

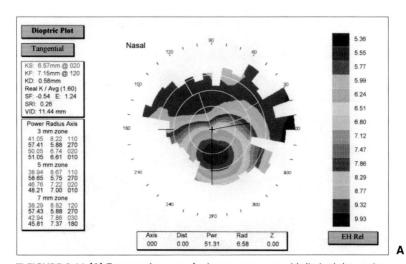

A

■ **FIGURE 3.11 (A)** Topography map of a keratoconus eye with limited data points available. **(B)** Topography map of a keratoconus eye with the missing data points extrapolated. **(C)** Some topographers will show the extrapolated data (*dashed*) and the real measured data in the same picture. *(continued)*

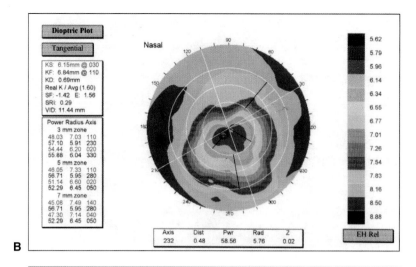

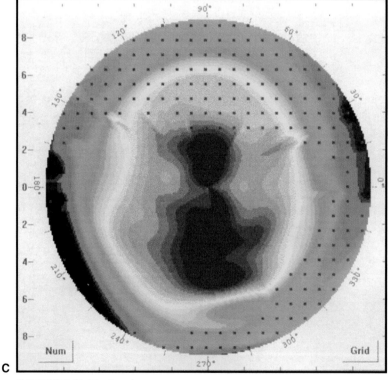

■ FIGURE 3.11 *(Continued)*

In addition to this it is crucial when using reflection systems to have a well-wetting ocular surface. Having the subject blink several times before measurement can help in achieving this. If this does not provide a well enough wetting ocular surface, tear supplements can be used to overcome the problem. It is suggested not to use viscous drops, as they can mimic corneal irregularities. Liquid eye drops or saline can alleviate the dryness issue. If the cornea is still not wetting properly, this could lead to an increase of missing data points in the dry areas. Conversely, excessive meibomian gland secretions can also alter corneal topography.[19] Figure 3.12 shows a topography map of a patient before and after treatment of the meibomian glands. It can be observed that the superior part of the cornea is less steep.

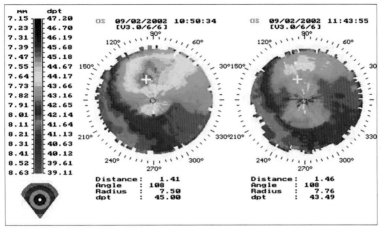

■ FIGURE 3.12 Topography map of a patient before and after treatment of the meibomian glands.

While the clinical implications are still a question mark, researchers in Brisbane, Australia, have found, using dynamic corneal topography, that the upper eyelid can also induce changes to the corneal topography.[20] While reading, the composition of the eyelids is different than when looking in primary eye gaze. The refractive power change to the cornea caused by the upper eyelid while reading was found to be significant: as a general rule it takes the cornea as long to recover to normal after reading as the length of time that was devoted to reading. Based on this, at least theoretically, it would be worth considering having patients not read in the reception room immediately before performing corneal topography.

Corneal staining and corneal scarring can also cause erroneous or missing topography data points. If corneal reflection rings overlap, corneal topographers can get confused and may assume that what started off as one ring will continue in a next ring, which is referred to as *ring jam*. It can occur with corneal staining and with dry spots, but also sometimes if the cornea is simply too irregular itself. That is why a higher ring density in a corneal topographer is not always better. As a result of these risks involved when performing corneal topography, it is advised to always take more than one picture and to compare the maps (which may include the original Placido image). In fact, taking three or four measurements is suggested, and maps that do not match the others should be excluded from further analysis. If the distortion of the rings is too severe and cannot be overcome, sometimes placing a thin, hydrogel contact lens over the cornea might help. Over this thin hydrogel lens corneal topography can be performed and, although the curvatures might not be very accurate, a good impression about the shape of the cornea can be achieved.[21]

Ring jam can also occur near the upper and lower eyelid margins. The tear prism present on these margins can cause such steep curves that the topographer is easily misled (Fig. 3.13). An increase in peripheral corneal astigmatism, which will be discussed in more detail later in this chapter, can sometimes be exaggerated this way. Some topographers will allow the practitioner to manually erase the areas of confusion to alleviate the problem. Again, trying to avoid interference of the eyelid (and its tear prism) by taking measurements with larger eyes is very important in performing topography.

Different Topography Maps

What Does a Map Tell Us?

On a typical curve map (Fig. 3.14), usually the following information is displayed: the simulated keratometry values, different colors representing the corneal curves, a representation of the pupil zone, and sometimes a millimeter grid overlapping the corneal map. The latter is

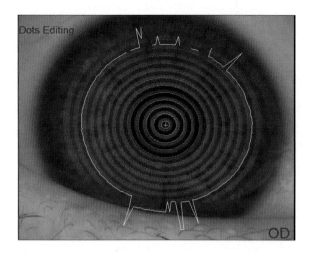

■ **FIGURE 3.13** Tear prism on the eyelid margins have steep curves that can mislead the corneal topographer.

useful to keep track of the size of the actual measured area of the cornea and the location of certain corneal distortions.

The pupil size is of limited value in most instruments, as certain light levels are required to perform the corneal topography (e.g., it is a reflection system, which requires light to be reflected off of the cornea). These lighting conditions will influence pupil diameter. Some instruments added infrared pupillometers that can measure the pupil diameter under various light conditions, which then can be assessed in relation to the topography data. Especially in orthokeratology and refractive surgery this can be a valuable tool, but also in normal rigid gas-permeable (GP) lens fitting and, for example, bifocal lens fitting this can be very beneficial in creating a successful fit.[22] With a normal topographer without an infrared pupillometer, the pupil diameter representation can give some idea about the pupil size relative to previously measured pupils if this is always measured under the exact same light conditions. This way it is rather a subjective tool than an objective instrument.

The simulated keratometry values are of questionable value. They might be of use to practitioners, who are accustomed to using a keratometer, and perhaps to compare these values to previously measured keratometry values, but they generally are not ideal since there is such a large amount of data points that are potentially available. They give no information about corneal shape and do not identify the top of the cornea. Notably in more irregular corneas it is misleading to use the simulated keratometry data.

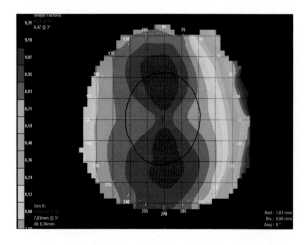

■ **FIGURE 3.14** A typical curve topographic map.

Instead of presenting all the individual curves of a cornea, colors are used to visualize the large amount of data. Cooler colors represent flatter curves, warmer colors steeper curves. Generally speaking, cooler colors are visible toward the periphery of the cornea, as the average cornea flattens in this region. Toward the center, warmer colors are present, but it is quite common that the warmest color is not necessarily the geometric center of the cornea. Another common finding is that the cornea nasally is flatter than peripherally.

The display of colors depends on the scale that is used. First of all, the steps representing different colors are typically set to 0.25 D. For irregular corneas it can be beneficial for the scale to be set to 0.50 D or 1.00 D steps to obtain a better general overview of the corneal shape.

Relative versus Absolute Scale

Whether an absolute or relative scale is used is critical to know for practitioners who are evaluating topography maps. Absolute scales are a representation of all curves available in normal corneas, and the available colors are evenly distributed over that range (in some topographers a customized absolute scale can be set by the practitioner). The relative scale represents curves that are available for that particular cornea and the colors available represent a much smaller range of curves. This means that much more detail is visible with this type of scale than with an absolute scale, which is usually preferred in contact lens practice. However, the relative scale will not allow practitioners to compare one cornea to another cornea, or even allow comparison of the same cornea over time, as the scale may vary. A "red" cornea on a relative scale does not mean this is a steep cornea. It only means that there is a relatively large steep (red) area within that particular cornea. Figure 3.15A and B are both postcorneal graft maps that, at first glance, look very similar. However, Figure 3.15A represents a 0.74-mm difference horizontally and vertically (or 3.7 D corneal astigmatism), whereas Figure 3.15B has a 3.46-mm difference or 17 D astigmatic cornea. This difference is not obvious by simply viewing the images as they are both relative scales. Typically, a normal cornea in a contact lens practice is best viewed on a relative scale as it provides the most details, as long as practitioners understand its limitations.

Tangential versus Sagittal Scale

Also of importance is the tangential versus sagittal representation of data. Sagittal curves make the assumption that the center of the radius of that curve is always on the central axis, hence the alternative name for this setting: an axial map. This will represent best the optical characteristics of a cornea. The tangential (or instantaneous) setting will typically show more detail than the sagittal setting of the same eye (Fig. 3.16A,B). Tangential maps are sometimes referred to as true curve data. Tangential curves do not make an assumption about where the center of the radius might be. They simply look at a certain part of the cornea and measure the radius of that point under 90 degrees (as a tangent), of which the center of the radius could be anywhere. This will give, especially in the periphery of the cornea, a much more detailed representation. In contact lens practice, where the periphery is of special interest, this is usually the preferred option. However, as with absolute versus relative scales, the sagittal map is more suitable for comparison between corneas as it has a standard reference point. In refractive surgery, axial maps are usually preferred over tangential maps for that reason.

Viewing both maps could be beneficial in some cases. In orthokeratology, for example, tangential maps are used to determine the overnight centration of the lens (as lens centration while sleeping cannot be evaluated behind a slit lamp), but to assess the optical state of a cornea and to follow the progression of the refractive change, axial maps are used.

Difference Maps

Difference maps are desired when evaluating the effect that lenses have on the cornea and are among the most useful of all maps in clinical practice. Difference maps take the original topographic data before contact lens fitting and subtract the topographic data of a certain

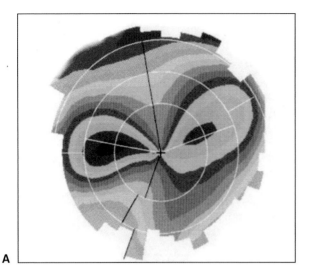

A

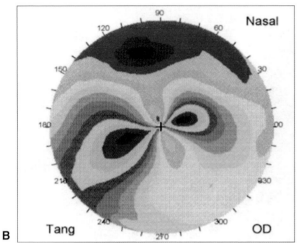

B

■ FIGURE 3.15 **(A)** Postcorneal graft cornea with 3.7 D astigmatism. **(B)** Postcorneal graft cornea with 17 D astigmatism.

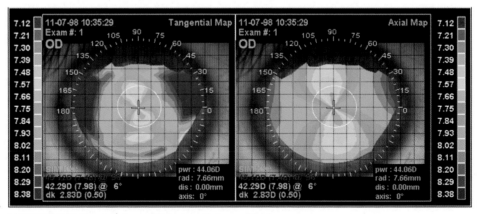

A

B

■ FIGURE 3.16 Tangential map **(A)** and sagittal map **(B)** of same eye.

time after lens fit. This could be 1 day (which is typically the case when fitting orthokeratology lenses), 1 week, or 1 month after lens fit (typically to evaluate the lens fit of normal GP or hydrogel lenses), or even years later (to evaluate the long-term effects of any lens and to evaluate the risk of developing corneal warpage and spectacle blur). Corneal topographers are beneficial in the initial fitting of the contact lenses—which can be somewhat confronting at times—and in showing how well the lens respects the shape of the cornea. Corneal changes in lens wear and the recovery of corneal changes will be discussed later in this chapter under Corneal Topography in Contact Lens Practice.

Indices for Corneal Irregularity

When evaluating topographic maps, practitioners should not focus too much on differences in colors, but primarily look for symmetry to determine whether or not a particular cornea is distorted. Figure 3.14 shows a standard topography map with warmer colors in the vertical meridian than in the horizontal meridian, representing corneal astigmatism. This is represented as a typical eight-shape pattern, which in this case shows symmetry. As the warmer colors represent steeper curves, this map represents with-the-rule corneal astigmatism. The differences between the horizontal and the vertical meridian are 0.36 mm or 2.13 D. In Figure 3.17, approximately the same difference between horizontal and vertical curves is seen (0.34 mm or 2.38 D), but within the vertical meridian alone there is also a 1.55 D difference. This topography map is not symmetric. This is an indication that this cornea is potentially irregular, whether existing or acquired. Corneas with a difference of 1.4 to 1.9 D within one meridian are moderately irregular but suspect for having keratoconus, while corneas with more than 1.9 D of asymmetry in one meridian are considered irregular and are highly suspect for having keratoconus.[23]

As it is not always obvious whether asymmetry of the corneal surface is clinically significant, corneal topographers provide indices that can help the practitioner in analyzing the corneal surface. The most commonly used index for the detection of irregularity and keratoconus is the I-S value (the inferior-superior value). It typically compares the cornea on five points in the superior half of the cornea with five points in the inferior half. Some topographers use the SAI value (surface asymmetry index), which evaluates the difference between opposite semi-meridians,

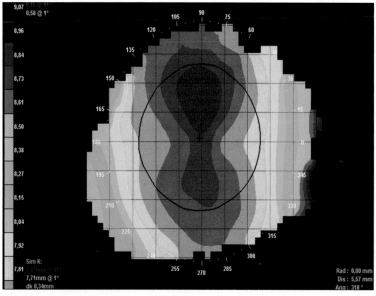

■ **FIGURE 3.17** Asymmetry in vertical meridian.

which is another way of comparing one part of the cornea with the opposite site. The modified Rabinowitz/McDonnell test that is used with some topographers does, in essence, the same (it uses the I-S value), but it adds the difference in corneal power between the right and the left eye. In keratoconus, one eye is usually more progressed than the other, and if there is more than 1 D of difference between the two corneas, this is also considered a risk for the condition.[24]

In addition to this, to detect irregular corneas it is also of interest to analyze the angle within one of the principal astigmatism axes. Astigmatism axes are usually fairly straight, although even in corneas that are considered normal, deviations from this can be observed. But if the angle within the astigmatism axis has a large deviation from straight, then the probability of an irregular cornea increases. The SRAX index considers a cornea to be irregular and keratoconus suspect if the astigmatism axis angle is more than 21 degrees diverged from straight, and combines this with the I-S value to give a prediction for the risk of keratoconus.[25]

KISA is another index, which is based on the just described astigmatism angle together with the I-S value, but this also takes the absolute keratometry values into account. Typically steeper curves are seen in patients with keratoconus than in normal corneas.[26]

Another way of detecting keratoconus is looking at *e*-values that corneal topographers provide (see more on this under Corneal Topography in Contact Lens Practice, Corneal Shape in this chapter). High *e*-values are common in keratoconus. Dao et al.[27] found that if the *e*-value of eyes was ≥0.8, the specificity (98%) and sensitivity (97%) were high for dealing with a keratoconus cornea. This abnormal *e*-value was observed in keratoconus eyes with a visual acuity of 1.0, whereas slit-lamp examination showed no abnormalities.

Pellucid marginal degeneration (PMD) is another corneal degeneration that can mimic many of the clinical signs and symptoms observed in keratoconus. The topography map of a PMD is different than that of keratoconus, in that the steeper curves are typically visible in the periphery of the cornea, sometimes shaped like a band of steepening parallel to the limbus. Centrally, this arc comes together toward the center of the cornea. This has been described as a pattern of two doves kissing. Typically, the distance from the center of the cornea (apex) to the steepest part of the cornea (the peak elevation index, PEI) is 1.95 mm in keratoconus, while it is, on average, 3.5 mm in eyes with PMD.[28] Differentiation between PMD and keratoconus is important as contact lens-fitting approaches are different in the two conditions.[29] In addition to topography, it is apparent that wavefront aberrometry, especially if combined with corneal topography, can be a valuable tool to predict early stages of keratoconus and/or PMD as well.[30]

When fitting contact lenses to keratoconus eyes, it is often difficult to obtain accurate curve data on the top of the cone. Typically, the top of the cone is not in the center of the cornea and central corneal curvatures (including simulated *k*-values) are not accurate. Moving the cursor to the top of the cone on the map and reading off the local *k*-values will provide a better idea. But this still has its limitations as corneal topographers assume that the top of the cornea is close to or on the geometric center of the cornea. As this is typically not the case in keratoconus, practitioners can ask the patient to look in the opposite direction of where the top of the cone is located to artificially create a situation where the top of the cone is centered in the map. Obviously this does not provide the real representation of the corneal geometry, but it will give the best possible curve values of the top of the cone.

When fitting bi- or multifocal contact lenses, it is also of importance to have information about the location of the exact top of the cornea. If this is not in line with the geometric center of the cornea, as in keratoconus, simultaneous lenses might be better avoided since the optical center of the lens needs to match the optical center of the cornea. If this is not the case, translating lenses might be preferred.

Other indices to evaluate corneal regularity are the SRI value (surface regularity index), which compares the power of each point within the central 4.5 mm (the pupil zone) to the points immediately surrounding it. This index correlates best with visual acuity. Normal corneas have low SRI values (<1.0). Other indices that attempt to do the same are the CIU (corneal uniformity index) and the PVA (potential visual acuity) index. The Holladay index fits a best-fit ellipse through the measured cornea, also to give a prediction of the potential visual acuity. These indices are widely used in refractive surgery management.

■ CORNEAL TOPOGRAPHY IN CONTACT LENS PRACTICE

Recently, the impact of contact lenses on the cornea has become clear within the framework of laser refractive surgery.[31,32] Contact lens wearers frequently need to cease lens wear for many weeks before surgery for the cornea to return to its baseline shape. One refractive surgery center in the Netherlands reported that 95% of all retreatments for refractive reasons were performed on previous contact lens wearers.[33]

Corneal Changes in Gas-Permeable Lens Wear

Alterations of corneal topography in GP contact lens wearers have been reported by many researchers.[34,35] With GP lenses it is more the mechanical pressure of the lens on the cornea rather than hypoxic stress that causes topographic changes. Hypoxic stress was a significant problem with polymethylmethacrylate (PMMA) lenses (causing up to 98% of corneas to have corneal edema),[36] which very often resulted in corneal distortion and corneal warpage. Still, patients who are wearing PMMA lenses are among the most difficult to be refitted with other lenses or to be treated with refractive surgery, but fortunately these cases are becoming rare today. First, refitting PMMA lens wearers with GP lenses before temporary cessation of lens wear seems advised in these cases. Currently, it is advised to stop GP lens wear for at least 8 weeks prior to laser surgery. After this, the cornea needs to be evaluated at 2-week intervals until a stable topography is reached, which is usually defined as 0.50 D change or less compared to the last visit. This also shows the importance of performing a baseline corneal topography before every single contact lens fit in your practice.

To avoid induced corneal changes, it is of importance to assess the fit of every GP lens wearer regularly, using fluorescein. Steep lens fits should be avoided at all times. It has been shown that GP lenses that are fitted 0.3 mm steeper than the flattest meridian induce corneal steepening after short-term lens wear.[37] In a recent orthokeratology study, patients showed significant central corneal flattening (-0.61 ± 0.35 D) within 10 minutes of open-eye lens wear, showing the vulnerable nature of the epithelium and the speed with which it can be altered.[38] Flat lenses can cause corneal changes as well and are, in addition, more prone to lead to decentration. A GP lens is designed and fitted on the central cornea. This means that decentration of the lens will cause a situation in which the lens and cornea are not in alignment with each other. Therefore, it is important to avoid decentration of lenses as much as possible as well. A map of a decentered GP lens can easily be confused for a keratoconus map. Typically, if a lens is decentered to a position lower on the cornea (a low rider), then in the inferior part of the cornea flatter curves will be observed while steeper curves will be present in the opposite direction of the cornea (superior).[35,39]

Another way the cornea might be altered by the GP lens is if a spherical lens geometry is used on a toric cornea. Mechanical pressure nasally and temporally in with-the-rule corneal astigmatism can cause significant corneal changes. The cornea always tries to mimic the shape of the back surface of the lens, which works as a mold. A corneal topography map that is taken immediately after GP lens removal is often quite inaccurate. Corneal astigmatism might be present, but suppressed by the GP lens. Typically, within a few days the original corneal astigmatism begins to reappear.

Some of the back aspheric bi- and multifocal contact lenses are an example of the GP lens fits that cause most corneal distortion. They are suggested to be fit 1 D, 2 D, or sometimes even 3 D steeper than K because of the nature of the high eccentricity of the back surface of the lens. While generally in GP lens wear fitting practitioners try to avoid steep fitting lens patterns, with these lenses it is interesting to note that apparently it is accepted to fit lenses steep. Corneal topography changes can be induced by this, and epithelial cells are typically suppressed in the midperiphery of the cornea and an increase in corneal thickness may even be observed centrally. Basically this is hyperopic orthokeratology, but with lenses that are not suitable for that purpose. Therefore, they can decenter and can cause severe corneal distortion. For corneas like this it can take several months to return to their baseline values.

Changes in Hydrogel Lens Wear

Less known than the GP changes during lens wear, and therefore more neglected, are the topographic changes underneath hydrogel lenses. If monitored closely, however, many changes can be detected. Schornack[40] estimated that 27% of all cases of corneal warpage are in patients wearing hydrogel lenses. These topographic changes are thought to be primarily the result of hypoxia, and indeed are observed more in patients wearing conventional lenses and especially in lenses that are thick and made of a low oxygen permeability (Dk) material. Topographic changes are, for example, regularly observed in prism ballasted toric hydrogels made out of conventional materials. At least 2 weeks of discontinuation of hydrogel contact lenses is advised, followed by 2-week-interval checkups to assess the corneal stability, before laser surgery can be considered. A change of <0.5 D is generally accepted as being within the margins of a stable cornea. The case at the end of this chapter is a good example of a patient exhibiting soft lens-induced corneal distortion, which dissipated after 2 weeks of non–lens wear. However, as a result of this ordeal, the patient decided not to return to contact lens wear.

The topographic changes under a hydrogel lens are often subtle and these patients also should be monitored on a routine basis. Distortion of keratometer mires can be the initial clinical sign, but these are limited to a small (usually 3 mm) central portion of the cornea and the changes cannot be classified.

Corneal topography covers a large, if not the total, area of the cornea and a difference map can identify subtle topographic changes promptly and accurately. Figure 3.18 shows a patient exhibiting an unusual case of severe peripheral corneal disruption underneath a conventional toric hydrogel lens, which is even visible without the use of a corneal topographer.

With the arrival of silicone hydrogel contact lens materials, the hypoxia-related corneal warpage cases have been reduced or essentially eliminated. However, the early versions of silicone hydrogel lenses brought on a different type of distortion because of the higher modality of the material compared to conventional hydrogels. Peripheral corneal changes, in particular, were not uncommon.

Interestingly, topographic changes to the cornea can also be used to the advantage of the lens wearer. Hydrogel lenses also have shown to be able to create orthokeratology-like patterns. Patients who accidentally wore silicone hydrogel lenses inside out reported changes in refraction, often leading to a decrease in myopia. This phenomenon was first described by Patrick

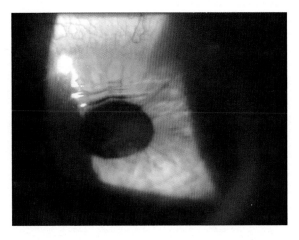

■ FIGURE 3.18 Unusual case of severe peripheral corneal disruption underneath a conventional toric hydrogel lens. (Courtesy of Hans Kloes, Kloes Eye Kliniek, the Netherlands.)

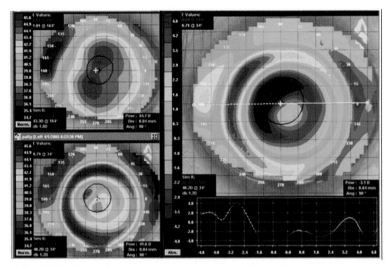

■ **FIGURE 3.19** A high minus silicone hydrogel contact lens that has been worn inside out purposely on a continuous-wear basis for 30 days, showing an orthokeratology-like difference map. (Courtesy of Patrick Caroline, Pacific University, Oregon.)

Caroline at the British Contact Lens Association Meeting in June 2003. Practitioners should be
aware of this effect, as apparently no decrease in lens-wearing comfort is noted when the
silicone hydrogel lenses are worn inside out. The effect is found to be more pronounced in
higher myopes wearing silicone hydrogel lenses, and the topographic effect is very difficult to
distinguish from a (successful) orthokeratology lens fit with GP lenses.

Figure 3.19 shows a CIBA Focus Night & Day lens (base curve 8.4, −10.00 D, diameter
13.8 mm) that has been worn inside out purposely on a continuous-wear basis for 30 days. The
difference map that is shown on the right of this figure shows a 3.12 D reduction in myopia in
the center of the topography. Research is under way to investigate whether these lenses can be
used to purposely change the shape of the cornea to temporarily reduce myopia.

Contact Lens Fitting Based on Corneal Topography

Careful lens selection while respecting the shape of the cornea with every lens fit is the basis
for every successful lens wearer. This is true for silicone hydrogel lenses and in conventional
lens wear, as shown in the previous section. With regard to fitting GP lenses, respecting the
shape of the cornea is of even more importance. Corneal topography can be a major help in
achieving this.

Respecting Corneal Shape

The primary goal in fitting GP lenses is to respect the shape of the cornea as much as possible
and to distribute pressure equally over the entire corneal epithelium. If the surface area of contact is maximized, the weight of the lens is distributed over the largest possible area of cornea.[41]
In this situation the force per unit of surface area applied to the cornea by the lens is minimized,
and the likelihood of corneal distortion is reduced.

The goal in normal GP lens wear is to avoid the induction of corneal change as much as possible. To do so, knowledge of the shape of the cornea is essential. By far the best instrument to
analyze this shape is the corneal topographer. Several attempts to modify manual keratometers
to carry out this analysis have proven to be of limited use. Although many of the Placido disk
systems are not able to measure curves in the far periphery of the cornea, they are usually able
to measure up to the point where the resting point of the lens will be positioned.

The shape of the average corneal surface is usually described as prolate ellipse, indicating a gradual flattening from center to periphery. This is one of first things that is obvious when looking at an average corneal topography map: relatively cooler colors in the periphery of the corneal map represent this flattening. The amount of flattening is traditionally designated as eccentricity, mostly noted as the *e*-value. The *e*-value of an ellipse can be calculated from the central curvature and the peripheral curvature plus the distance (angle) from the center where that peripheral curve was measured. The average cornea has been described as roughly 0.43, and typically is between 0.40 and 0.57.[42–44] But the *e*-value varies widely among individuals, and ideally it should be measured and evaluated on every single eye before fitting contact lenses. As an example, the Ohio State University looked at the corneal shape of 683 children's eyes (aged 8–15): the vast majority flattened toward the periphery, but two corneas actually steepened.[45] There seems to be a small correlation between ametropia and eccentricity (higher myopia showing reduced eccentricity).[42,46]

Not all meridians of the cornea have the same *e*-value. Most corneal topographers and automated keratometers will provide the average *e*-value of all meridians, although some will give *e*-values per meridian or quadrant. A major drawback with regard to *e*-value measurement is that manufacturers of topographers are very secretive about the way they calculate the *e*-value: it should be taken of the axial map, but neither the distance from the center nor the meridian used is usually revealed, which means that differences in *e*-values between topographers may occur. Unfortunately, there is no standard for defining corneal shape.

Besides this, another disadvantage of the *e*-value is that it can only describe prolate shapes. In corneas that are steeper in the periphery by default or in corneas that are reshaped that way by orthokeratology or laser surgery, an oblate shape is present. In these cases the *e*-value is useless, since mathematically it can only define shapes larger than zero (spherical). This problem can be overcome by using what has been called the *p*-value, which can be derived directly from the *e*-value: $p = 1 - e^2$. By using the *p*-value the exact same shape is described, but it should be borne in mind that a circle's value is now 1 instead of 0.[47] The *p*-value of all prolate shapes is <1, and in the case of peripheral steepening, the *p*-value is larger than 1, which is exactly the opposite of the *e*-value. Practitioners may be confronted with *p*-values as an alternative to *e*-values in the international literature, and should be aware of the opposite effect compared to the *e*-value.

Another approach to describe the asphericity of the cornea is to use the *Q*-value. This value can be derived as follows: $Q = p - 1$, or $Q = -e^2$. A negative *Q*-value describes prolate shapes and positive values an oblate shape, but the *Q*-value of a sphere remains 0, the same as the *e*-value.[46,47] Therefore, the *Q*-value has advantages over both the other shape descriptors and may be considered as a standard index for describing corneal shape,[48] especially in orthokeratology and refractive surgery practice.

In reality, however, the actual corneal shape is not as easily defined as a standard ellipse. Especially toward the periphery it becomes more complex and less predictable. The corneal shape is usually more spherical near the apex and it may flatten at a variable (usually progressive) rate toward the periphery. Zernike polynomials are often used to describe the corneal shape in more detail, but even these complex mathematical formulations have their limitations, and newer mathematical definitions of the corneal shape are being developed. However, the clinical usefulness of these complex formulations when manually fitting GP lenses seems limited. Therefore, to describe corneal eccentricity, shape parameters are still preferred and provide a good idea about the flattening of the cornea. The *e*-value is still the parameter most used in contact lens practice, and most topographers and automated keratometers currently use this.

As a rule of thumb, practitioners may square the *e*-value that was provided by the topographer or automated keratometer to have some idea of the amount of flattening in the periphery of average corneas. An *e*-value of 0.4 means that the flattening in the periphery at 30 degrees from the center is about 0.16 mm. An *e*-value of 0.6 describes a flattening of 0.36 mm, and a cornea with an *e*-value of 0.8 is 0.64 mm flatter in the periphery. From this it can be concluded that, as the *e*-value goes up, flattening increases progressively. This also means that small *e*-values are clinically of little importance, but the importance of *e*-values increases rapidly as the value gets higher.

To respect the shape of the cornea, the amount of flattening should be followed as much as possible. A spherical lens (tricurve, tetracurve, etc.) on an aspheric cornea could give friction in the midperiphery of the cornea. As most corneas flatten toward the periphery, theoretically most lenses should also be aspheric in nature.[41,49] In practice, this usually means choosing a lens with an *e*-value closest to the *e*-value of the cornea. If the exact *e*-value is not available, use a higher *e*-value lens (flatter lens fit appearance) rather than a smaller *e*-value lens. Usually aspheric GP lenses are manufactured with an *e*-value between 0.4 and 0.8 for normal corneas and higher *e*-values for keratoconus eyes. The common interval between *e*-values of available lenses is 0.15 or 0.2, but some manufacturers allow the practitioner to order the *e*-value in as little as 0.05 steps if desired.

By using aspheric lenses, the shape of the lens is followed accurately in an annular fashion. Also, in fitting bi- and multifocal contact lenses it is essential to know the *e*-value of the cornea. Back aspheric simultaneous lenses are designed for the average cornea (e.g., an *e*-value of 0.43). The lens is designed with a very high *e*-value (meaning more flattening toward the periphery). Because of this, the lens needs to be fitted steeper (as discussed before). However, if a cornea has an exceptional small or large *e*-value, then this can lead, respectively, to an exceptionally poor lens fit and/or to no near addition for the lens wearer.

Some lens design software programs allow the practitioner to choose different *e*-values for different zones. In this way the shape of the cornea can be followed even more closely (since the cornea is not usually a perfect ellipse). This can be very valuable when fitting keratoconus eyes, in which the differences in *e*-value in different meridians can be substantial.

In GP lens wear, 3 and 9 o'clock staining is one of the most often reported problems, and this complication is difficult to remedy. Several authors[50–52] have suggested that in theory an aspheric lens design could be beneficial in managing 3 and 9 o'clock staining. First, this is because aspheric back surface designs may follow the corneal shape closely, lessening areas of contact between the lens and (peripheral) cornea and thus enhancing tear fluid exchange and corneal wettability. Furthermore, aspheric lens designs are able to minimize lid–lens interaction, thereby decreasing discomfort and interference with blinking habits. Also, decreased edge lifts in aspheric lenses could lead to a reduction of the bridge effect (upper eyelid bridging the gap between lens edge and cornea) and tear meniscus formation around the edge of the lens[53]—all thought to be beneficial in 3 and 9 o'clock staining management.

To summarize, to avoid the induction of corneal topographic changes by GP lenses, the shape of the cornea should be followed as closely as possible. Matching the corneal shape with the lens shape by using aspheric lenses can be helpful in achieving this and also may aid in the management of 3 and 9 o'clock staining. Corneal topography is very useful for this purpose.

Corneal Astigmatism

The other major factor with regard to respecting the shape of the cornea is corneal toricity. Dealing with corneal toricity follows the same principle as dealing with corneal shape: the lens pressure should be evenly distributed over the corneal surface. Nontoric lenses on with-the-rule corneas will create pressure in the horizontal meridian.

Devising a general rule for the degree of corneal toricity that should be fitted with a toric back surface is not easy. Textbooks generally consider that toric designs are indicated when the corneal toricity is 2.5 to 3.0 D or more.[54] However, this could easily lead to topographic changes and spectacle blur. As stated above, 0.3-mm steep lenses (accounting roughly for a 1.5 D steep fit) can give significant corneal changes. In addition to this, corneal toricity may increase or decrease toward the periphery and thus influence fitting characteristics.[55] Szczotka et al.[55] found peripheral corneal toricity to be one of the major factors determining the success of toric hydrogel lens fitting. Since GP lenses rest mostly peripherally, this influence should not be

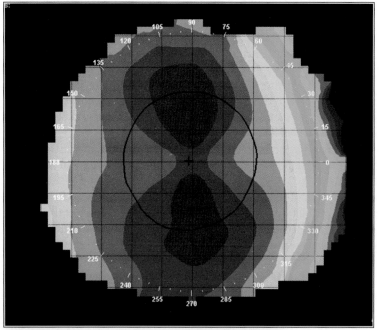

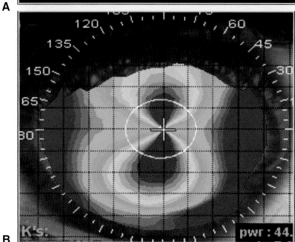

A

B

■ FIGURE 3.20 Central **(A)** versus peripheral **(B)** corneal astigmatism.

neglected in GP lenses either. Central corneal astigmatism is easier to deal with than limbal-to-limbal corneal astigmatism when fitting GP lenses (Fig. 3.20A,B). Corneal topographers can aid in assessing the degree of peripheral astigmatism. Researchers at the University of Brisbane Australia[56] looked at peripheral corneal astigmatism and found that 38% of cases showed a spherical central cornea with a spherical periphery. In 21% of cases a toric cornea was found with a stable astigmatism toward the periphery. However, 15% showed a spherical center with a toric periphery, 22% showed a toric center with a decrease of astigmatism toward the periphery, and in 4% the toricity increased toward the periphery. Although this was a small sample size, it clearly shows that different types of corneal astigmatism can be present. In addition to normal (GP and hydrogel) lens fitting, this is extremely important in orthokeratology practice and in bi- and multifocal lens fitting. In these cases it can predict the risk of lens decentration, and therefore it influences lens fit to a large degree. If a corneal topographer is not available, as an alternative a standard nontoric trial lens can be placed on the eye and the fluorescein pattern will tell the practitioner how much corneal toricity is present and whether or not this is acceptable.

When significant corneal toricity is noted, the first option is often to choose a full back toric lens design. The flattest meridian is usually fitted in alignment with the cornea or slightly flatter, taking radius of curvature and the *e*-value into account. The other meridian is generally fitted flatter than alignment to create a lens that moves well, but also to compensate for the difference in refractive index between tears and lens material and thus to prevent induced astigmatism. A popular rule of thumb is to take two-thirds of the corneal astigmatism and add this to the flattest meridian to calculate the steepest meridian. However, with the highly sophisticated lathing technology currently available, it is technically no problem to compensate the induced astigmatism on the front surface of the lens. Hence, practitioners should not worry about induced astigmatism when fitting the lens. Still, a slightly flatter back optic zone radius in the steepest meridian than alignment is desirable to promote movement, but should be limited to about 0.75 D.

Newly developed peripheral or edge toric back surface geometries with one spherical and one aspheric meridian can be used in lower degrees of corneal toricity, in particular when peripheral corneal toricity is present. Usually one meridian is fitted with a low or zero *e*-value, while the flattest meridian is fitted with an *e*-value between 0.6 and 0.8. Practical tips are to use fairly high *e*-values that provide more flattening and therefore more peripheral toricity. Also, use large diameters since the toric effect increases toward the periphery. It is important to be aware that, when evaluated with a radiuscope, these lenses are spherical centrally and only start to diverge toward the periphery. Some corneal topographers provide a lens holder, to be placed on the chin rest, to evaluate contact lens surfaces. However, most topographers use assumptions about the shape of the cornea and, since the back surface of a contact lens is hollow in contrast to the convex corneal shape, this could lead to erroneous values. The lenses are marked in the flattest meridian to make evaluation of the position of the lens on the eye possible; these lenses should show no or limited signs of rotation during lens wear.

Another reason for using back surface toric geometries on toric corneas is that this improves lens centration. Especially in with-the-rule toricity, there is a tendency for the lens to ride high or low.[54]

In summary, to reduce the influence of the contact lens on the corneal epithelium, corneal toricity should be respected. Textbooks generally advise practitioners to use back toric lens designs on corneas with an astigmatism of 2.5 or 3 D and higher, but this could easily lead to topographic corneal changes and spectacle blur. When fitting back toric lens designs, the amount of peripheral astigmatism should also be taken into account. Different types of back toric surface geometries are available to the practitioner to respect the shape of the cornea at all times.

Comfort, Corneal Topography, and Lens Fit

A study initiated by the University of Maastricht in the Netherlands[57] looked at the relation between GP lens fitting and comfort of wear. The first question this study sought to answer was what percentage of lens fits was acceptable when only central *k*-readings were used to fit the lenses. The second question in this study was related to corneal topography: can information derived from this technique be beneficial in finding the optimal lens fit? Finally, does accurate GP lens fitting improve comfort of wear?

Of all initial fits based on traditional computation, only 40% were acceptable (optimal or suboptimal). From the unacceptable fits, 15% needed an adaptation of the back optic zone ratios to be acceptable. In 28%, it was necessary to switch from a multicurve (MC) to an aspheric (AS) lens design to create an acceptable fit, and in 17% a toric back surface was necessary since the fluorescein pattern happened to be too toric. This was despite the fact that the maximum degree of central corneal astigmatism was only 1.83 D. The influence of peripheral astigmatism on lens fit was evident in these cases.

When the changes in lens fit that were made based on keratometry alone are compared with the topographic data, it can be concluded that in 88% of cases the reasons for changing the lens parameters originated from midperipheral differences between corneal shape, as established

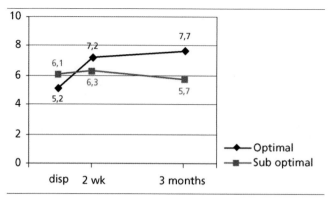

■ FIGURE 3.21 Comfort scores for optimal versus suboptimal fits.

with topography, and lens shape, as predicted from *k*-readings. In other words, in 88% of cases the lens fit could have been optimized before fitting by making use of corneal topography data.

The next question in the study was: does accurate lens fitting improve comfort? Figure 3.21 shows the comfort scores for optimal versus suboptimal fits. At the initial visit and at 2 weeks, there was no statistically significant difference between the two groups. In other words, initially (up to 2 weeks) the accuracy of the lens fit is not important for wearing comfort.

However, after 3 months of lens wear, the group of optimal fits scored 7.7 on the comfort scale, whereas comfort in the suboptimal group was 5.7. Also, the gain in comfort between the initial visit (5.2) and the visit 3 months later (7.7) was statistically significant in the group of optimal fits. In the group of suboptimal fits there was only a small temporary increase in comfort from dispensing (6.1) to the visit 2 weeks later (6.3), while after 3 months comfort had even slightly (but not statistically significantly) decreased to 5.7.

To analyze the aspect of comfort further, patients were subdivided into three groups on the basis of the lens geometry worn at 3 months (Fig. 3.22). No relationship between comfort and lens geometry was found at the initial visit. Within the aspheric lens geometry group (AS group), comfort increased significantly from dispensing (5.6) to the follow-up visit after 2 weeks of wear (7.5). Although there was also an increase in comfort over that same period in the multicurve lens geometry group (MC group) from 5.9 to 6.7, this increase was statistically not significant. Both groups did also show a significant increase in comfort between the initial visit and the follow-up visit 3 months later.

In contrast to the other two groups, comfort scarcely increased between dispensing (4.8) and a follow-up visit after 2 weeks (5.0) in the group with unacceptable toric fluorescein patterns with standard lens design. At this point the lens design was changed to a back toric lens. Because of the relatively low central difference in keratometry readings, a peripheral toric lens was chosen

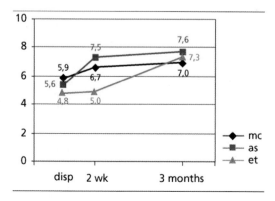

■ FIGURE 3.22 Comfort scores for a multicurve (MC), aspheric (AS), and edge toric (ET) lens design.

(two different *e*-values in two meridians). This resulted in an increase in comfort from the moment the lenses were introduced at the 2-week visit to the follow-up visit at 3 months. This increase (2.3 points) was statistically significant and resulted in a final comfort rate of 7.3, which is equal to the average comfort scores obtained with the other two lens designs.

In conclusion, there seems to be no difference in comfort within the first 2 weeks between optimally fitted lenses and suboptimally fitted lenses. However, after 3 months there is a 2-point difference on a 10-point scale between these two groups, which is a statistically and clinically significant difference. This implies that even small improvements in GP lens fits could influence comfort of wear.

Another interesting result of this study is that corneas with lesser degrees of central corneal astigmatism can show toric fluorescein patterns because of an increase in corneal astigmatism toward the periphery and would therefore benefit from modern back toric lens designs, leading to improved comfort compared to nontoric designs.

■ SUMMARY

The assessment of corneal topography is integral to successful contact lens design and wear. While keratometry provides some information—albeit quite limited—that can assist in determining the design to be used and in assessing corneal distortion, the use of a corneal topographer is invaluable in providing corneal shape information and allowing the examiner to observe subtle changes in topography over time. The continual improvements in corneal topography instrumentation have resulted in lens design software programs that can design contact lenses to fit even the most challenging corneas. The future in corneal topography assessment appears to be even more exciting.

■ CLINICAL CASE

A 49-year-old woman who wears hydrogel lenses came in for an eye examination, complaining of decreased visual acuity in her left eye. She was referred by an optician because her poor visual acuity could not be explained. She was wearing spherical monthly replacement lenses made of a conventional lens material. Figure 3.23 shows the topographic map of the left eye soon after lens removal. Her maximal visual acuity with lens was 20/50 and refraction without lenses did not improve her vision:

OS: $-4.75 - 1.75 \times 040$ 20/50

The cornea looked unremarkable behind the biomicroscope, but the irregularities in the center of the map easily explain her decrease in visual acuity.

Two weeks after lens removal, the cornea returned to baseline (Figure 3.24), showing a symmetric topographic map with limited central corneal astigmatism, and her visual acuity returned back to 20/20. Unfortunately, this patient discontinued contact lens wear because of this incident, which could have been prevented.

CLINICAL PROFICIENCY CHECKLIST

■ Many advances have occurred recently with corneal topographers. They are now integrated with wavefront aberrometers, which can be a major advantage in contact lens practice.

■ The keratometer can provide information that can be used for initial decisions for GP fitting as well as information—via assessment of distortion of imaged mires—on corneal irregularities, tear quality and, indirectly, the fit and front surface quality of soft contact lenses.

(continued)

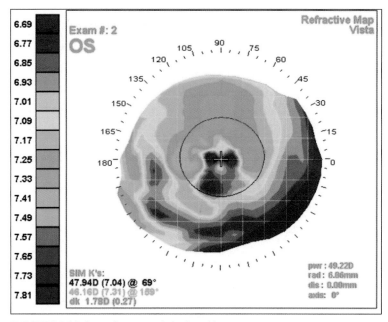

FIGURE 3.23 Corneal warpage in hydrogel lens wear.

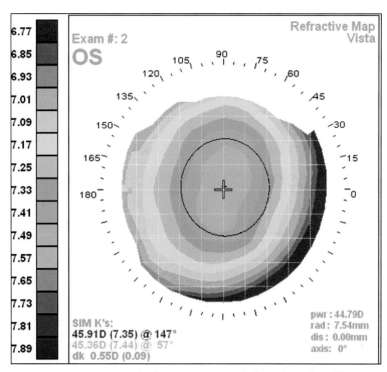

FIGURE 3.24 Same eye as in Figure 3.23 two weeks later. (Contributed by Marco van Beusekom [printed with permission].)

(Continued)

- Reflection corneal topographers, as compared to keratometry, result in much more information from an extended area of the cornea.

- When using a reflection corneal topographer, it is critical to have the patient blink several times immediately before the measurement to have a well-wetting ocular surface (i.e., no dry spots).

- Ring jam can occur near the upper and lower eyelid margins. The tear prism present on these margins can cause such steep curves that the resultant topography can be misleading.

- Sagittal maps are beneficial for comparison between corneas. Tangential maps represent true curve data and typically show more detail than a sagittal map. They have applications in orthokeratology to assess lens centration during sleep and in keratoconus.

- The topographic changes under a silicone hydrogel lens can often be observed peripherally.

- Corneal topography systems provide rate of flattening information (e-value or eccentricity). To avoid the induction of corneal topographic changes by GP lenses, the shape of the cornea should be followed as closely as possible. Matching the corneal shape with the lens shape by using aspheric lenses can be helpful in achieving this and also may aid in the management of 3 and 9 o'clock staining.

- It is important to assess peripheral corneal toricity before determining whether a back toric GP lens is indicated.

REFERENCES

1. Von Helmholtz H. Graefes Arch Clin Exp Ophthalmol 1854:3.
2. Javal E, Schiötz I. Un opthalmomètre practique. Ann Oculis 1881;84:5.
3. Placido A. Novo instrumento de exploracao da cornea. Periodico d'Ophthalmol Pract Lisbon 1880;5:27–30.
4. Gullstrand A. Photographisch-ophthalmometrische und klinische Untersuchungen ueber die Hornhautrefraction. Kongliga Svenska Vetenskap-Akademiens Handlinger 1896;28:7.
5. Klyce SD. Computer-assisted corneal topography. High-resolution graphic presentation and analysis of keratoscopy. Invest Ophthalmol Vis Sci 1984;25:1426–1435.
6. Jongsma F, de Brabander J, Hendrikse F. Review and classification of corneal topographers. Laser Med Sci 1999;14:2–19.
7. Iskander DR, Collins MJ. Applications of high-speed videokeratoscopy. Clin Exp Optom 2005;88:223–231.
8. Read SA, Collins MJ, Carney LG, et al. The topography of the central and peripheral cornea. Invest Ophthalmol Vis Sci 2006;47:1404–1415.
9. Sicam VA, van der Heijde RG. Topographer reconstruction of the nonrotation-symmetric anterior corneal surface features. Optom Vis Sci 2006;83:910–918.
10. de Brabander J, Chateau N, Marin G, et al. Simulated optical performance of custom wavefront soft contact lenses for keratoconus. Optom Vis Sci 2003;80:637–643.
11. Mandell R. Methods to measure the peripheral corneal curvature. J Am Optom Assoc 1962:889–892.
12. Wilms K, Rabbetts R. Practical concepts of corneal topometry. Optician 1977;Sept 16:7–11.
13. Meyer N. RGP-auswahl der ersten messlinse. Die Kontaktlinse 2001:27–33.
14. Mandell RB. Everett Kinsey Lecture. The enigma of the corneal contour. CLAO J 1992;18:267–273.
15. Swartz T, Marten L, Wang M. Measuring the cornea: the latest developments in corneal topography. Curr Opin Ophthalmol 2007;18:325–333.
16. Jongsma FH, de Brabander J, Hendrikse F, et al. Development of a wide field height eye topographer: validation on models of the anterior eye surface. Optom Vis Sci 1998;75:69–77.
17. Vos F, van der Heijde G, Spoelder H, et al. A new PRBA-based instrument to measure the shape of the cornea. IEEE Trans Instrum Meas 1997:794–797.
18. Corbett M, Marchall J, O'Brart D, et al. New and future technology in corneal topography. Eur J Implant Refr Surg 1995;7:372–386.
19. Markomanolakis MM, Kymionis GD, Aslanides IM, et al. Induced videokeratography alterations in patients with excessive meibomian secretions. Cornea 2005;24:16–19.
20. Buehren T, Collins MJ, Carney L. Corneal aberrations and reading. Optom Vis Sci 2003;80:159–166.

21. Kojima R. Validating corneal topography maps. Contact Lens Spectrum 2007;22(7):42–44.
22. Chateau N, De Brabander J, Bouchard F, et al. Infrared pupillometry in presbyopes fitted with soft contact lenses. Optom Vis Sci 1996;73:733–741.
23. Maeda N, Klyce SD, Smolek MK. Comparison of methods for detecting keratoconus using videokeratography. Arch Ophthalmol 1995;113:870–874.
24. Rabinowitz YS, McDonnell PJ. Computer-assisted corneal topography in keratoconus. Refract Corneal Surg 1989;5:400–408.
25. Li X, Rabinowitz YS, Rasheed K, et al. Longitudinal study of the normal eyes in unilateral keratoconus patients. Ophthalmol 2004;111:440–446.
26. Rabinowitz YS, Rasheed K. KISA% index: a quantitative videokeratography algorithm embodying minimal topographic criteria for diagnosing keratoconus. J Cat Refract Surg 1999;25:1327–1335.
27. Dao CL, Kok JH, Brinkman CJ, et al. Corneal eccentricity as a tool for the diagnosis of keratoconus. Cornea 1994; 13:339–344.
28. Anderson D KR. Topography: a clinical pearl. Optom Manage 2007;42(2):35–41.
29. Miller W. Treating PMD with contact lenses. Contact Lens Spectrum 2007;22:31.
30. Buhren J, Kuhne C, Kohnen T. Defining subclinical keratoconus using corneal first-surface higher-order aberrations. Am J Ophthalmol 2007;143:381–389.
31. Budak K, Hamed AM, Friedman NJ, et al. Preoperative screening of contact lens wearers before refractive surgery. J Cat Refract Surg 1999;25:1080–1086.
32. Wang X, McCulley JP, Bowman RW, et al. Time to resolution of contact lens-induced corneal warpage prior to refractive surgery. CLAO J 2002;28:169–171.
33. Lafeber R. Personal communication, 2004.
34. Ruiz-Montenegro J, Mafra CH, Wilson SE, et al. Corneal topographic alterations in normal contact lens wearers. Ophthalmol 1993;100:128–134.
35. Wilson SE, Lin DT, Klyce SD, et al. Topographic changes in contact lens-induced corneal warpage. Ophthalmol 1990;97:734–744.
36. Tomlinson A. Complications of Contact Lens Wear. St. Louis: Mosby Year Book, 1992.
37. Swarbrick HA, Hiew R, Kee AV, et al. Apical clearance rigid contact lenses induce corneal steepening. Optom Vis Sci 2004;81:427–435.
38. Sridharan R, Swarbrick H. Corneal response to short-term orthokeratology lens wear. Optom Vis Sci 2003;80: 200–206.
39. Wilson SE, Lin DT, Klyce SD, et al. Rigid contact lens decentration: a risk factor for corneal warpage. CLAO J 1990; 16:177–182.
40. Schornack M. Hydrogel contact lens-induced corneal warpage. Contact Lens Anterior Eye 2003;26:153–159.
41. Edwards K. Contact lens problem-solving: aspheric RGP lenses. Optician 2000;219:28–32.
42. Carney LG, Mainstone JC, Henderson BA. Corneal topography and myopia. A cross-sectional study. Invest Ophthalmol Vis Sci 1997;38:311–320.
43. Eghbali F, Hsui EH, Eghbali K, et al. Oxygen transmissibility at various locations in hydrogel toric prism-ballasted contact lenses. Optom Vis Sci 1996;73:164–168.
44. Guillon M, Lyndon D. Tear layer thickness characteristics of rigid gas permeable lenses. Am J Optom Physiol Opt 1986;63:527–535.
45. Walline JJ, Mutti DO, Jones LA, et al. The contact lens and myopia progression (CLAMP) study: design and baseline data. Optom Vis Sci 2001;78:223–233.
46. Horner DG, Soni PS, Vyas N, et al. Longitudinal changes in corneal asphericity in myopia. Optom Vis Sci 2000;77: 198–203.
47. Lindsay R, Smith G, Atchison D. Descriptors of corneal shape. Optom Vis Sci 1998;75:156–158.
48. Swarbrick HA. Mind your P's and Q's - Rodger Kame Award Lecture. In: Global Orthokeratology Symposium 2004, July 23–25 2004, Toronto, Ontario, Canada.
49. Kok J. New Developments in the Field of Contact Lenses. Amsterdam: University of Amsterdam, 1991.
50. Barr J. Aspheric update. Contact Lens Spectrum 1988:56–62.
51. Bennett E. DW investigation of aspheric posterior Boston IV lens design. Contact Lens Forum 1987;12(4):65–69.
52. Holden T, Bahr K, Koers D, et al. The effect of secondary curve lift-off on peripheral corneal desiccation. Poster presented at the Annual Meeting of the American Academy of Optometry, December 1987, Denver, CO.
53. van der Worp E, De Brabander J, Swarbrick H, et al. Corneal desiccation in rigid contact lens wear: 3- and 9-o'-clock staining. Optom Vis Sci 2003;80:280–290.
54. Grosvenor T. Fitting the astigmatic patient with rigid contact lenses. In: Ruben M, Guillon M, eds. Contact Lens Practice. London: Chapman & Hall, 1994:623–647.
55. Szczotka LB, Roberts C, Herderick EE, et al. Quantitative descriptors of corneal topography that influence soft toric contact lens fitting. Cornea 2002;21:249–255.
56. Franklin RJ, Morelande MR, Iskander DR, et al. Combining central and peripheral videokeratoscope maps to investigate total corneal topography. Eye Contact Lens 2006;32:27–32.
57. van der Worp E, de Brabander J, Lubberman B, et al. Optimising RGP lens fitting in normal eyes using 3D topographic data. Contact Lens Anterior Eye 2002;25:95–99.

CHAPTER 4

Gas-Permeable Material Selection

Edward S. Bennett

Before the fitting, evaluation, and patient education procedures, it is important to select the most appropriate lens material for a given patient. An understanding of gas-permeable (GP) advantages and applications as well as material properties and composition is important in assisting in this decision.

■ GAS-PERMEABLE LENS BENEFITS, APPLICATIONS, AND LIMITATIONS

Benefits

GP lenses have traditionally exhibited many benefits including quality of vision, ocular health, stability and durability, and patient retention and practice profitability.[1-3]

Quality of Vision

Studies comparing hydrogel and GP lenses have found significantly better visual performance with GP lenses. This includes both subjective patient preference[4,5] and contrast sensitivity function.[6,7] The superior optical quality provided by a stable refractive surface with little to no water content is the primary reason for this visual difference between contact lens types. In comparing both soft and GP lenses, it was found that whereas both soft and GP lenses induce more aberrations for the eyes that have low wavefront aberrations, soft lens wear tends to induce more higher-order aberrations and GP lens wear tends to reduce higher-order aberrations.[8-10] GP lenses also maintain surface wettability better than hydrogel lenses. This can lead to improved long-term comfort and less deposit formation, although the benefits of this is less with the popularity of disposable lenses, especially daily disposable lenses. GP lenses represent a very good option if the sphere-to-cylinder refractive error ratio is ≤2:1. When the corneal cylinder is 2.5 D or greater, a bitoric design often provides a stable and nonfluctuating vision correction.

Ocular Health

The benefits of a small overall diameter lens that does not compress the limbus, lens movement typically resulting in good tear exchange and debris with the blink, potentially (depending on the material) unparalleled oxygen permeability, and good surface wettability have resulted in numerous clinical studies that have found GP lenses to be a safer alternative to soft lenses. GP lenses have resulted in less corneal staining[4,11] and are less likely to result in peripheral corneal infiltrates, not uncommon with tight-fitting soft lenses.[12,13] The prevalence of microbial keratitis has been found to be less with GP lenses, with an incidence of 1 to 1.48 per 10,000 eyes as compared to 3.50 per 10,000 eyes with soft daily-wear lenses and 20 per 10,000 eyes with extended-wear soft lenses.[14,15] In several studies conducted in the United States in which the relative risk of wearing extended-wear lenses was evaluated, GP lenses resulted in the lowest rate of infectious keratitis.[16-18] There is also less binding of *Pseudomonas aeruginosa*[19,20] and acanthamoeba[21] to GP lenses than soft lenses. In addition, giant papillary conjunctivitis (GPC, also known as contact lens papillary conjunctivitis, CLPC) is less likely to occur with GP than with soft lenses.[22]

Stability/Durability

Unlike soft lenses, GP lenses do not tear or easily change shape or coloration; therefore, frequent lens replacement is not necessary.

Patient Retention/Profitability

One of the challenges facing contact lens practitioners today is patient retention and revenue from replacement contact lenses. The Fairness to Contact Lens Consumers Act (FCLCA) mandates that practitioners provide the contact lens prescription to their patients. With the increasing number of Internet sites offering replacement lenses, many patients think that they can bypass the professional care provided by eye care practitioners. However, as a custom device, GP lenses are much more difficult to obtain through these unconventional channels; in fact, it has been reported that only 1% of mail-order lenses were GP.[23] That percentage may not be any higher via the Internet for the same reason. The variety of parameters specified in a GP lens prescription (including base curve radius, overall and optical zone diameters, peripheral curve widths and radii) helps to demonstrate the specialty nature of the device to patients. Likewise, although the FCLCA requires that every contact lens patient is entitled to their prescription, they can only be provided this information once it has been determined, which may be as long as 1 to 3 months after dispensing for a GP patient.

It has been found that contact lens patients are approximately 50% more profitable to the eye care practice than non-contact lens wearers.[24] Further, it has been found that GP wearers generate greater revenue to the practice than soft lens wearers.[25] This was attributed to several factors, including the fact that GP lens patients return more frequently for eye examinations and purchase eyeglasses more often than soft lens patients.

Applications

Myopia Reduction

Several studies have found that GP lenses slow down the progression of myopia,[26–28] although this was not the conclusion of a recent study by Katz et al.[29] The most comprehensive and best controlled study was the Contact Lens and Myopia Progression (CLAMP) study.[28] In this study, children were adapted to GP lenses before being randomized to GP or soft lens groups. After 3 years, GP-wearing young patients increased by 1.56 D in myopia, whereas soft lens wearers increased by 2.19 D. However, most of the refractive error change occurred during the first year and no difference was found between soft and GP lens wearers in axial growth of the eyes. Therefore, it would be safe to conclude that GP lenses may slow down the progression in young people.

A more important benefit of GP lenses, particularly with—but not limited to—young people, pertains to overnight orthokeratology (OOK). Recent studies have found that OOK reduces myopia[30] and slows down axial growth.[31,32] In fact, both the Longitudinal Orthokeratology Research in Children (LORIC)[31] and the Corneal Reshaping and Yearly Observation of Nearsightedness (CRAYON) studies found that OOK subjects had 57% less axial growth than control subjects (i.e., consisting of spectacle wearers in LORIC and both soft lens and non-OOK GP wearers in CRAYON) over a 2-year period.

Postsurgical/Irregular Cornea

GP lenses are most often the material of choice when fitting postsurgical and irregular corneas. The optical quality and rigid nature of these lenses allow for a more regular refractive surface because of the ability of these lenses to exhibit some molding ability and sphericalization of an irregular cornea. It has been found in the Collaborative Longitudinal Evaluation of Keratoconus (CLEK) study, with over 1,100 keratoconus subjects, that 73% were GP lens wearers.[33] Patients who have undergone refractive surgery and still require an optical correction benefit from the increased oxygen delivery of GP lenses versus soft lenses. Numerous types of reverse geometry lens designs—incorporating a steep secondary curve radius—have been developed to allow a GP lens to align better and exhibit satisfactory centration on a postrefractive surgery patient who has a significantly flatter central than midperipheral cornea. Likewise, with the use of corneal topography instrumentation, it is possible for laboratories to fabricate a lens to closely match the corneal irregularity resulting from keratoconus, trauma, postpenetrating keratoplasty, postrefractive surgery, and other causes of irregular cornea. The availability of hyperpermeable GP lens materials also allows for optimum oxygen delivery to the cornea.

Presbyopia

Presbyopic patients benefit from any one of several GP presbyopic designs. Aspheric multifocal and segmented and annular translating designs have resulted in success rates of over 75%.[33–37] In addition, when compared to progressive addition lenses, monovision lenses, and soft bifocal lenses, aspheric GP multifocal lenses resulted in significantly better high- and low-contrast acuity and contrast sensitivity function as compared to the other contact lens options and exhibited visual parity to spectacle wear.[38] As a result of improvements in manufacturing technology, higher-add aspheric multifocal and segmented translating designs with an intermediate correction have been introduced.

Astigmatism

GP lenses have the natural ability to correct anterior corneal astigmatism by allowing the tear lens to compensate for the corneal astigmatism.

Soft Lens Refits

It has been reported that patients who failed with soft lens wear because of factors such as poor vision or giant papillary conjunctivitis (GPC) have been successfully refitted into GP lenses.[39,40] Likewise, individuals who have had a history of eye infections are also good candidates and often are motivated to be refitted into a potentially safer modality. Patients who are not satisfied with their vision from soft toric lenses are often successful with GPs. Practitioners who continue to fit a series of soft toric lenses on astigmatic patients—especially high astigmatic patients or individuals who have <2:1 sphere-to-cylinder ratio for their refraction—despite reduced vision because of lens rotation are doing a disservice to their patients. These patients often observe an immediate improvement in vision when refitted into GP lenses. As will be discussed in the next chapter, the use of a topical anesthetic before the initial lens application will be beneficial in minimizing initial awareness.

Limitations

The applications and benefits listed above would appear to position GP lenses as a primary modality; however, in 2007 they consisted of 8% of new fits worldwide and 7% of new fits in the United States.[41] There are several reasons for this low number, including the ease of fitting soft lenses as well as their disposability and availability of replacement lenses. Certainly, the increasing emphasis on consumerism and a desire to have immediate gratification has had an impact worldwide. However, the primary reason for the increasing use of soft lenses worldwide pertains to the difference in initial comfort between both modalities. This impacts the patients' interest in GP lenses and the confidence (or lack thereof) that a practitioner has in fitting patients into GP lenses.

Initial Comfort

The most commonly reported cause of discontinuation of GP lens wear is discomfort.[4,39,42] The initial sensation experienced by new GP wearers varies from mild awareness to much discomfort and tearing. Conversely, soft lenses are more comfortable initially, primarily a result of their larger overall diameter resulting in less movement with the blink. Andrasko and Billings[43] evaluated numerous factors in new GP lens wearers after 20 to 30 minutes of wear. If patients reported that they experienced either poor comfort or itching (or both) after this time period, they were deemed poor candidates for GP lenses. Whether discomfort is going to be problematic can sometimes be determined during the prefitting evaluation. If the patient exhibits apprehension during primary care examination procedures such as lid eversion, fluorescein application, or tonometry, soft lenses should be considered or the patient should be provided with a slow build-up schedule for adaptation. The authors have a three-step program to minimize initial awareness that consists of how GP lenses are presented to the patient, the use of a topical anesthetic before the initial application, and, if possible, allowing the patient to see optimally with the first lenses applied (i.e., via fitting empirically or from an inventory).[44] This will be explained in much more detail in the next chapter.

Lack of Disposability

GP wearers should always have a backup pair as lenses can be lost and, on occasion, warped or possibly broken. Soft lenses have the benefit of being available in, at minimum, six to a package in most cases.

Fitting Inventory

The simplicity of soft lens design lends itself very well to fitting from an inventory and being able to make small changes easily and determine if the lenses have successfully improved vision and/or fitting relationship. Patients can be sent home in trial lenses for which they experience good vision and can be assessed sometime afterward to determine the final lenses to be ordered. The custom nature of GP lenses often results in practitioners ordering lenses for the patient and, if changes are indicated, new lenses have to be ordered.

Occasional/Cosmetic Wear

Soft lenses have the benefit of allowing occasional or intermittent wear with relatively little effect on comfort. Soft lenses also can be used to change or enhance eye color, whereas the smaller overall diameter of GP lenses all but preclude iris color changes.

Environmental Limitations

Another limitation of GP lenses is increased susceptibility for dust and debris to become trapped underneath the lens. Patients who work exclusively outdoors in a dusty, windy environment may be better candidates for soft lenses. Likewise, individuals who participate in sports often benefit from soft lenses.[45] If GP lenses are indicated in these athletes, the use of a large overall diameter, low edge clearance design would be indicated.

Smaller Palpebral Size

It has been found that GP lenses can result in a smaller palpebral aperture size versus soft lens wearers and non-contact lens wearers.[46] In addition, one study reported 15 cases of long-term rigid lens wearers who presented with blepharoptosis.[47] It was hypothesized that this problem may be the result of chronic lens removal in which the pulling of the lids laterally over time may lead to levator aponeurosis dehiscence.

■ MATERIAL PROPERTIES

Oxygen Permeability/Transmission

Oxygen permeability (Dk) is a property of the lens material independent of the size, shape, or surface condition of a lens. Oxygen transmissibility (Dk/t) is a measure of the amount of oxygen transmitted through the lens. It is dependent on the Dk value of the material and thickness (typically center thickness for GP lenses) and is essentially equal to the Dk divided by the center thickness in millimeters × 10. For example, lenses manufactured in identical materials and Dk values with different thicknesses will result in a difference in oxygen transmission; the greater the lens thickness, the lower the oxygen transmission. For example, if the Dk value is 40 and the center thickness is 0.10 mm, the Dk/t is equal to 40; if the center thickness of this material is instead 0.20 mm, the Dk/t decreases in half to a value of 20 [the respective units are $(10^{-11} \text{ cm}^2 \times \text{mL O}_2)(\text{sec} \times \text{mL} \times \text{mm Hg})$ for Dk (which has also been termed "Fatt" units) and $10^{-9} \times$ same units for Dk/t]. Another method of evaluating oxygen transfer through a rigid lens is equivalent oxygen percentage (EOP). EOP is a measure of the amount of oxygen in the tears between the lens and the cornea and is determined in vivo; essentially, it is a predictor of how much oxygen will reach the anterior corneal surface with a particular lens material and design, the maximum value equaling 21%.[23]

Historically, there have been many methods to assess the oxygen permeability of a GP lens material. Early measures did not compensate for inaccuracies that could result from the so-called "boundary layer" and "edge effect."[48,49] As these effects often resulted in inflated Dk values, the marketing and promotion of contact lenses was often not consistent with the research behind these materials.[50,51] In addition, calibrations were often not performed via similar testing of reference lenses. These effects were resolved via the work of Benjamin and Cappelli[51] in 1998, which was funded by the Contact Lens Manufacturers Association (CLMA) and is often referred to as the *CLMA Method*.

Certainly there are advantages in potential oxygen transmission with GP versus hydrogel lenses. As a rule, GP lenses are able to deliver two to three times more oxygen to the cornea than hydrogel lenses of equal thickness.[52] This is a result of both the availability of higher-Dk materials and the fact that these lenses exchange up to 20% of the tear volume per blink.[53,54] Conversely, hydrogel lenses can exchange only approximately 1% of the tears per blink.[55] GP lenses having Dk values in the range of 18 to 25 have exhibited an amount of overnight corneal swelling (10%–12%) similar to that of many hydrogel extended-wear lenses.[56,57] However, upon awakening, the cornea deswells much faster with a rigid lens, and unlike hydrogel lenses, the cornea typically returns to the zero swelling level. The introduction of hyperpermeable silicone hydrogel lenses has closed the gap between the two modalities; however, recent research has found that a GP lens with a Dk/t of 90 is equivalent to a silicone hydrogel lens with a DK/t of 125.[58]

How much oxygen is necessary for corneal physiologic success? Research has shown that a Dk/t equal to 24 (10% EOP) should satisfy the daily-wear oxygen requirements of every patient.[59] Therefore, this value should be the goal of clinicians. A 30-Dk lens with a center thickness of 0.12 mm would meet this requirement, as would a 60-Dk material with a center thickness of 0.25 mm. For extended wear, however, this value is much higher. Originally established as a Dk/t of 87 (17.9% EOP),[59] it has more recently been increased to 125.[60–62] This makes it imperative to use hyperpermeable silicone hydrogel and GP materials for extended wear. It has been found that fitting plus power hydrogel lenses on a hyperopic extended-wear patient results in providing much less than half of the oxygen demand of the cornea.[63]

There have been several classifications of GP lens materials. Benjamin[64] has divided GP lenses into five categories based on Dk and using a standard thickness of 0.12 mm. The author simply divides the materials into three categories: low Dk (25–50), high Dk (51–99), and hyper-Dk (≥100).[65] These classifications are shown in Table 4.1.

TABLE 4.1 GAS-PERMEABLE OXYGEN PERMEABILITY/ TRANSMISSION CLASSIFICATIONS

BENJAMIN[a]	BENNETT
Low Dk: <15	Low Dk: 25–50
Medium Dk: 15–30	High Dk: 51–99
High Dk: 31–60	Hyper-Dk: ≥100
Super-Dk: 61–100	
Hyper-Dk: >100	

[a] Assuming a center thickness of 0.12 mm.
Dk, oxygen permeability.
From Benjamin and Cappelli (51) and Bennett (65).

The bottom line, however, is that oxygen transmission, although important to successful lens wear, should not be viewed apart from other lens performance factors, such as adequate movement, comfortable edge design, resistance to deposit buildup, flexural resistance, and dimensional stability.

Surface Wettability

Surface wettability is the ability of the blink to spread tear film mucin across the anterior contact lens surface. The mucin layer is essential for this purpose and its presence in the tear film raises the surface tension of the cornea to allow the spreading of tears. Good wetting properties are important for patient success as they enhance visual acuity, comfort, and corneal integrity.[66] This is of major importance to polymer chemists, manufacturers, and clinicians. In fact, a desire to have better wettable materials has been expressed as the number one request for desired rigid lens improvements in a nationwide survey of optometrists.[67] If the tear film over the lens surface evaporates rapidly after the blink, the mucin dries out and becomes more mucus-like, ultimately resulting in a mucoprotein film. Although the tear film wets the lens via three types of surface interactions—hydrogen bonding, hydrophobic interaction, and electrostatic interaction—the latter is the strongest of these forces.[68] The GP lens surface is negatively charged, making it a perfect complement for the positively charged tear protein, lysozyme.

Wetting agents within the lens enhance surface wettability and assist in overcoming the hydrophobic properties of silicone. The material polymer chemistry has to be carefully formulated as the excessive use of wetting agents can result in a material that is too soft and possibly too brittle. Wetting agents have included methacrylic acid, polyvinyl alcohol, hydroxyethylmethacrylate (HEMA), and N-vinyl pyrrolidone. Representative management of these wettability-related problems is discussed in Chapter 6.

A clinical predictor of how well a GP contact lens anterior surface spreads the tear film mucin has been via wetting angle measurements. In theory, the lower the wetting angle, the better the on-eye wetting performance will be. Methods that have been used to assess wetting angle have included Wilhelmy plate, sessile drop, and captive bubble. The difficulty has been the fact that different methods have been used and if low values result, these values are heavily promoted by the manufacturer. In reality, these tests have proven to not have a correlation with on-eye wetting and comfort.[69] The tear components, notably mucin, form a biofilm on the surface, which acts as a natural wetting agent to coat the lens within a few blinks. This reduces the lens wetting angle, contributing greatly to the surface wettability. Therefore, laboratory wetting angle measurements are typically not representative of on-eye performance.

Flexural Resistance

Flexural resistance pertains to the ability of a GP lens to resist the bending or flexing forces when a rigid lens is on a toric cornea. In other words, a lens with poor flexural resistance will tend to flex during the blinking process and therefore inadequately correct the patient's corneal astigmatism, resulting in reduced vision.[70] Factors that can influence flexure include amount of corneal toricity, lens material, optical zone diameter, center thickness, and lens-to-cornea fitting relationship. If the lens design increases in sagittal depth via a steeper base curve radius (BCR)[71–73] or larger optical zone diameter,[74] flexure is increased. Material flexibility via a high- or hyper-Dk material or from a thin center thickness in minus power lenses can contribute to lens flexure.[75,76] Modulus is another term that has been ascribed to the stiffness—or resistance to flexure—of a material. Higher-Dk GP lens materials have a much lower modulus rating than polymethylmethacrylate (PMMA).[69] Typically, flexure can be problematic for patients with corneal toricity ≥ 1.50 D.[77]

Specific Gravity

Specific gravity refers to the weight of a GP lens at a given temperature divided by the weight of an equal volume of water at the same temperature. It is often compared to water that has a specific gravity of 1.00. Specific gravity values for rigid lens materials can be divided into low (≤ 1.10), medium (1.11–1.20) or high (>1.20) values. These values can play an important role in the success of GP lenses as it is possible that the higher specific gravity (i.e., "heavier") lens materials may have more of a tendency to decenter inferiorly because of the forces of gravity.[78] In fact, if all other parameters are held constant, changing to a different lens material, with a different specific gravity, can produce as much as a 20% change in lens mass, therefore potentially impacting the lens-to-cornea fitting relationship.[79] This problem can be overcome by making higher specific gravity lenses thinner, thus resulting in an overall decreased lens weight. This should be particularly applicable in plus power and prism ballasted GP lenses.

Hardness

Other properties pertain to the so-called "softness" of a given material. Such factors as hardness value, scratch resistance, and optical quality have been described and compared. Hardness has been defined as resistance to penetration. If an indicator presses on the surface of the material being tested, the extent to which it compresses for a given pressure and time is an inverse measure of the hardness.[80] The Rockwell R hardness method is commonly used for testing the hardness of GP buttons; the Shore D hardness method is commonly used on finished lenses.

■ MATERIAL TYPES AND COMPOSITION

The materials in use today include (a) silicone/acrylate (S/A) and (b) fluoro-silicone/acrylate (F-S/A).

Silicone/Acrylate

The first successful GP lens materials were of silicone/acrylate (also termed siloxane-methacrylate) composition. Also referred to as "silicone" based, these copolymers actually contained the element silicon as siloxane bonds in side branches of the main carbon–carbon polymer chain. The silicon-containing side branches increase the free volume (space between the polymer chains), which allows the passage of oxygen.

The introduction of silicone-based copolymers in 1979 was a major breakthrough because silicone can greatly enhance the oxygen permeability characteristics of the material. Unlike PMMA lens materials, which are made up of a single component, S/A materials contain "silicone" methacrylate, wetting agents, and cross-linking agents. The latter two ingredients are important because their purpose is to neutralize both the hydrophobicity and the flexibility of the silicone component. Wetting agents, as previously indicated, achieve their effect by their strong affinity for water molecules. Most cross-linking agents strengthen the material, increasing its rigidity and making the material less sensitive to solvents.

However, the hydrophobicity of silicone resulted in a lens surface that was likely to attract both lipid and, notably, bound protein deposits.[69] This rapid drying of the tear film over the lens surface often resulted in patient complaints of redness, dryness, and fluctuating vision. The introduction of higher-Dk S/A lens materials often resulted in increased (or potential to increase) surface deposits,[69] warpage,[81–83] cracking,[84,85] and brittleness.[86]

Even with the aforementioned problems, there are several S/A materials in common use today. These include Boston II and Boston IV (Bausch & Lomb); Optacryl 60, Paraperm O2, and Paraperm EW (Paragon Vision Sciences); SA-18 and SA-32 (Lagado); and SGP and SGP II (LifeStyle).

Fluoro-Silicone/Acrylate

Fluoro-silicone/acrylate lens materials are similar to silicone/acrylates with the notable exception of the addition of fluorine. Fluorine, known for its nonstick properties in Teflon-coated cooking materials, increases the deposit resistance of the lens material, which is accomplished by fluorine promoting a tear film mucin interaction with the lens surface. In addition, low surface tension (energy) is present; in other words, there is a reduced affinity of polarized tear components to become adherent to the contact lens surface.[87] Therefore, the primary problem experienced with S/A lens materials, dryness, should be reduced with F-S/A materials. This has, in fact, been the case. Several comparison studies have concluded that F-S/A lenses are more wettable and are perceived as more comfortable by patients than S/A lenses.[82,88,89] In addition, it has been found that these materials are less prone to deposit buildup[90] and the rate of tear breakup is slower with the fluorinated material.[91]

The fluorinated component also assists in the transmission of oxygen through the lens material. This is accomplished by oxygen's preference to dissolve into fluorinated materials (i.e., oxygen transmission is achieved by solubility, not diffusion).[86,92] It is very apparent that although the ability of "silicone" to promote diffusion of oxygen through the lens material is very important, the additional permeability provided by fluorine will reduce the need for using excessive amounts of "silicone." Therefore, it has been found that the F-S/A materials are more dimensionally stable than S/A materials as well.[82,86]

As mentioned previously, F-S/A lenses can be divided into low-, high-, and hyper-Dk materials. All of the commonly available GP lens materials and their properties are provided in Table 4.2.[51,93–95] Low-Dk materials have become the lens of choice for most myopic daily-wear patients as a result of the benefits of surface wettability and dimensional stability.[96–99]

High-Dk F-S/A lens materials are typically the lens of choice for patients in need of higher oxygen transmission, although from an oxygen permeability level, they could be prescribed [if approved by the Food and Drug Administration (FDA) for overnight wear] for all but those individuals desiring continuous wear or hyperopes desiring extended wear. Hyper-Dk lens materials can be worn by all patients interested in GP wear but are definitely indicated for extended wear and represent the only option (i.e., Menicon Z, Menicon) for 30-day continuous wear. These applications are summarized in Table 4.3. It is not uncommon for practitioners to offer some form of annual replacement program for hyper-Dk lens materials as they often have a shorter life span than lower-Dk materials.

Improved material composition and manufacturing processes have resulted in the production of higher-Dk lenses that are durable, flexible, and maintain good wettability. Bausch & Lomb developed its Boston series of materials (ES, EO, XO) using the unique AERCOR technology, introduced in the mid-1990s. These materials contain an oxygen-permeable backbone and AER-

TABLE 4.2 COMMONLY AVAILABLE GP LENS MATERIALS AND THEIR PROPERTIES

NAME	MANUFACTURER	MATERIAL	DK	DK METHOD	REFRACTIVE INDEX	SPECIFIC GRAVITY
AccuCon	Innovision	F-S/A	25 (19.6)	Revised Fatt	1.458	1.16
Boston XO2	B & L	F-S/A	141	ISO/Fatt	1.424	1.19
Boston XO	B & L	F-S/A	100	ISO/Fatt	1.415	1.27
Boston Equalens II	B & L	F-S/A	85 (93–114.6)	ISO/Fatt	1.423	1.24
Boston EO	B & L	F-S/A	58	ISO/Fatt	1.429	1.23
Boston Equalens	B & L	F-S/A	47 (58)	ISO/Fatt	1.439	1.19
Boston RXD	B & L	F-S/A	24	ISO/Fatt	1.435	1.27
Boston IV	B & L	S/A	19 (20.8)	ISO/Fatt	1.469	1.10
Boston ES	B & L	F-S/A	18 (27.3)	ISO/Fatt	1.443	1.22
Boston II	B & L	S/A	12 (16.3)	ISO/Fatt	1.471	1.13
FLOSI	Lagado	F-S/A	26	ISO/Fatt	1.455	1.12
FluoroPerm 151	Paragon	F-S/A	151 (99.3)	Revised Fatt	1.422	1.1
FluoroPerm 92	Paragon	F-S/A	92 (64)	Revised Fatt	1.453	1.1
FluoroPerm 60	Paragon	F-S/A	60 (42.7)	Revised Fatt	1.453	1.15
Fluoroperm 30	Paragon	F-S/A	30 (30.3)	Revised Fatt	1.466	1.14
Hybrid FS	Contamac	F-S/A	31	Revised Fatt	1.4465	1.183
Hydro2	Innovision	F-S/A	50	Revised Fatt	1.463	1.145
Menicon Z	Menicon	F-S/A	163 (175.1)	ISO/DIS	1.436	1.20
ONSI-56	Lagado	F-S/A	56	ISO/ANSI	1.452	1.206
Optacryl 60	Paragon	S/A	18	Revised Fatt	1.467	1.13

(continued)

TABLE 4.2 (Continued)

NAME	MANUFACTURER	MATERIAL	DK	DK METHOD	REFRACTIVE INDEX	SPECIFIC GRAVITY
Optimum Extreme	Contamac E	Roflufocon	125	ISO/Fatt	1.4332	1.155
Optimum Extra	Contamac D	Roflufocon	100	ISO/Fatt	1.4333	1.166
Optimum Comfort	Contamac C	Roflufocon	65	ISO/Fatt	1.4406	1.178
Optimum Classic	Contamac A	Roflufocon	26	ISO/Fatt	1.4527	1.189
Paragon HDS 100	Paragon	F-S/A	100	ISO/ANSI	1.442	1.1
Paragon HDS	Paragon	F-S/A	58	Revised Fatt	1.449	1.16
Paraperm EW	Paragon	S/A	56	Revised Fatt	1.467	1.07
Paragon Thin	Paragon	F-S/A	29	Revised Fatt	1.463	1.14
Paraperm O_2	Paragon	F-S/A	16	Revised Fatt	1.473	1.12
SA-32	Lagado	S/A	32	Fatt	1.467	1.101
SA-18	Lagado	S/A	18	Fatt	1.469	1.126
SGP 3	LifeStyle	F-S/A	43.5 (33.5)	CLMA	N/A	1.13
SGP II	LifeStyle	S/A	43.5 (31.9) (13.8)	CLMA	N/A	1.13
SGP	LifeStyle	S/A	22(14.9)	CLMA	N/A	1.13
TYRO-97	Lagado	F-S/A	97	ISO/ANSI	1.440	1.187

B & L, Bausch & Lomb; Dk, oxygen permeability; F-S/A, fluoro-silicone/acrylate; S/A, silicone/acrylate.

From Rah (93), http://www.gpli.info (94), http://www.bausch.com (95), and Benjamin and Cappelli (51).

TABLE 4.3 GAS-PERMEABLE MATERIAL SELECTION (IN GENERAL)

LOW DK	HIGH DK	HYPER-DK
• Myopia	• Hyperopia	• Hyperopia
• Daily wear	• Flexible wear (hyperopia)	• Extended wear (myopia and hyperopia)
• Optimum wettability	• Extended wear (myopia)	
• Optimum stability	• Prism ballasted lens designs	

Dk, oxygen permeability.

From Bennett and Johnson (23).

COR O cross-linking agents, allowing more free volume within the lens and thus allowing more oxygen to reach the cornea. This allows the lens to be manufactured with a low level of silicone, thus potentially enhancing surface wettability. Soon thereafter Paragon Vision Sciences introduced its hyperpurification process that, in effect, sorts silicone molecules to select more oxygen-efficient silicone.[65,100] This resulted in the introduction of the Paragon Thin, Paragon HDS, and Paragon HDS 100. Not long after the new Paragon lenses were introduced, both Contamac and Lagado introduced F-S/A lenses with hydrophilic claims.[101] Contamac introduced the Optimum series of lens materials, which are polymerized via a proprietary new technology process that claims to not induce stress into the finished product. The "modified" F-S/A materials incorporate HEMA into the lens in an effort to optimize surface wettability and have been found to be successful in over 80% of GP wearers being refitted into the Optimum lenses.[102] Lagado introduced the Onsi-56 and Tyro-97 lens materials. These lens materials also contain HEMA and are modified F-S/A lens materials. They achieve their surface wettability via a combination of HEMA and a high proportion of fluoromonomer within the polymer formulation. Water is attracted to the lens surface but not absorbed into the interior of the lens.

Other Material Factors

Ultraviolet Blockers

Several GP lenses have ultraviolet (UV) blockers in the lens to reduce UV radiation exposure and the potential long-term complications such as cataracts, photokeratitis, and retinal degenerative changes.[69] UV-B (200–300 nm) are the rays that can be most problematic and UV absorbers in contact lenses do assist in providing some—but not total—protection to the eye. Sunglasses are still recommended for optimum protection. GP lenses with UV blockers also reduce fluorescence when evaluating the fluorescein pattern; therefore, an adjunct yellow filter over the observation system is recommended.

Plasma Treatment

The challenges involved in maintaining a clean surface as new—and higher-Dk—polymers are being introduced has resulted in the FDA approval of plasma treatment of almost all of the GP materials in common use today. This process is not a coating—like a wax—but is truly a treatment in which the front surface of the lens is sterilized via exposure to cold plasma gas in a reaction chamber.[103,104] Plasma is matter consisting of neutrons, positive ions, and electrons in a highly energized state. As the effect is localized to the surface, this form of plasma treatment does not adversely affect the material properties.

There are several benefits of plasma treatment. As it is not uncommon for polish residues to be attracted to the lens surface during the manufacturing process, plasma treatment results in removing all of these residues, resulting in an extremely clean and wettable surface. Although the clinical relevance of wetting angle measurements is debatable, it is evident that plasma treatment does greatly reduce the wetting angle of GP lenses. Paragon Vision Sciences, via their FDA approval process, has been able to claim that plasma treatment results in improved initial comfort.

The cost of this technology to the laboratory is quite high but, as a result of the aforementioned benefits, an increasing number of laboratories are providing plasma-treated lenses, often for a small additional fee. It is unknown at the current time how long the process lasts. However, the use of abrasive cleaners and in-office polishing are both not recommended with plasma-treated lenses.

■ MATERIAL SELECTION

The availability of all of these different rigid (or semirigid) lens materials presents myriad choices to the practitioner. What GP material is preferable to our patients? The answer depends on the particular patient to be fitted. In other words, it is recommended to use diagnostic sets of several different materials.

Figure 4.1 shows the authors' recommendations for material selection. It can be divided into five categories: (a) refractive error, (b) corneal topography, (c) refits, (d) occupation/hobbies, and (e) age.

Refractive Error

Because of the thin center thicknesses typically available in minus power lenses, most myopic patients would benefit from the dimensional stability provided by low-Dk F-S/A lenses while still meeting (or approximating) the cornea's daily-wear oxygen requirements. However, if edema is present with a low-Dk lens material, often the result of either a high corneal oxygen need (which varies between individual patients) or a tight-fitting lens, the patient should be refitted into a higher-Dk material. Hyperopic patients will benefit most from a high-Dk lens material because of the greater center thicknesses present in these lens powers. For the same reason, dimensional stability problems with high-Dk materials are less with plus (versus minus) powers.

Corneal Topography

Patients with moderate astigmatism (i.e., >1.50 D) benefit from the flexural resistance provided by low-Dk F-S/A lens materials. High astigmatic (i.e., ≥2.50 D) patients often benefit from bitoric designs, which benefit from the rigidity of low-Dk materials unless the patient is hyperopic. Likewise, for patients exhibiting high astigmatism associated with an irregular cornea, notably keratoconus, the greater rigidity of lower-DK lens materials can be beneficial. However, the decision-making process also has to take into consideration the amount of existing corneal compromise and fragility as well as patient compliance with wearing schedule (i.e., very compromised and fragile corneas as well as noncompliant patients would benefit from a higher-DK lens material).

Refits

Former PMMA and first-generation GP lens wearers should be refitted into low-Dk rigid lenses. Typically, these individuals have established care habits that could be damaging to the new softer lens materials. Surface scratches and warpage could occur (see Chapter 8), especially if these patients are not properly educated.

Previous soft wearers who have experienced deposit-related problems (redness, itching, decrease in wearing time) resulting in papillary hypertrophy would benefit from being refitted into essentially any GP material, preferably the most wettable available material. This may include a low-Dk F-S/A or any plasma-treated material. Patients with a history of eye infections

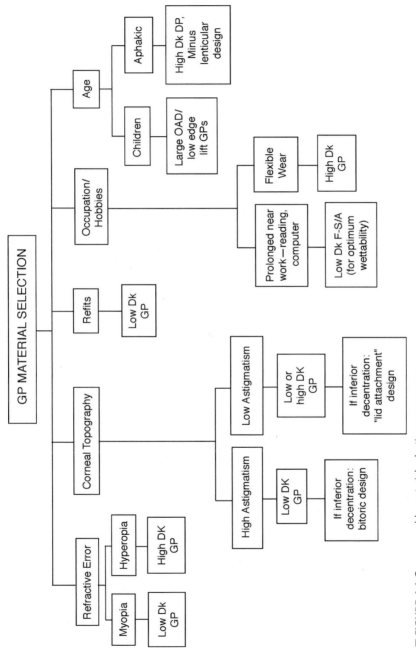

GP MATERIAL SELECTION

Refractive Error
- Myopia → Low Dk GP
- Hyperopia → High DK GP

Corneal Topography
- High Astigmatism → Low DK GP → If inferior decentration: bitoric design
- Low Astigmatism → Low or high DK GP → If inferior decentration: "lid attachment" design

Refits → Low Dk GP

Occupation/Hobbies
- Prolonged near work—reading, computer → Low Dk F-S/A (for optimum wettability)
- Flexible Wear → High Dk GP

Age
- Children → Large OAD/low edge lift GPs
- Aphakic → High Dk DP, Minus lenticular design

■ FIGURE 4.1 Gas-permeable material selection nomogram.

and peripheral soft lens-induced complications often benefit from the oxygen transmission and smaller diameter of GP lenses. These materials would also be recommended for all borderline dry-eye patients and mild allergy sufferers. In addition, spherical soft and soft toric lens wearers who are not satisfied with their vision are often good candidates for GP lenses.

Occupation

Individuals who perform much near work would benefit from the highest wettability materials available (similar to those for the aforementioned papillary hypertrophy patients) supplemented by frequent application of rewetting/reconditioning drops. Athletes benefit most from soft lenses; however, if this option is not satisfactory, a large hybrid material, such as SynergEyes (SynergEyes), which would less likely be displaced, would be recommended. Individuals who desire (or have a need) to wear their lenses on a flexible schedule or extended-wear basis (such as nurses, police, firefighters) would benefit from a high-Dk F-S/A material. Likewise, pilots and flight attendants, who are often exposed to less than optimum oxygen levels, would benefit from the higher-Dk materials.

Age

Pediatric aphakic children often benefit by being fitted with a silicone hydrogel lens. Phakic children would benefit from larger-diameter GP lenses, which should be less likely to dislodge. Initial comfort could be optimized by achieving an underneath-the-upper-lid fitting relationship and by the use of a rolled, tapered edge design. Aphakic patients would benefit from a high-Dk F-S/A material in a minus lenticular design and large (9.2–9.6 mm) overall diameter.

■ SUMMARY

GP lenses have numerous applications and benefits and, in fact, differentiate the novice practitioner from the practitioner who considers all options before making the decision about what type of contact lens to fit for any given patient. It is important to determine the patient's level of motivation, sensitivity to something approaching the eyes, and factors such as desired wearing time, occupation, and refractive error. Although no one GP material will be successful on every patient, the process for material selection does not have to be overly complicated. A close relationship with the independent GP fabricating laboratory consultant will be invaluable in deciding which material to use for any given patient.

■ CLINICAL CASES

CASE 1

A previously successful PMMA (12 years) and Polycon II (11 years) wearer is in your office complaining of blur through spectacles and a need to replace the contact lenses because they are "old and scratched." The patient has a tear breakup time (TBUT) equal to 7 seconds and a refraction equal to the following:

OD: $-5.00 - 1.75 \times 170$ 20/25
OS: $-5.50 - 1.50 \times 005$ 20/25

Keratometry was as follows:

OD: 42.75 @ 170; 44.25 @ 080
OS: 43.25 @ 005; 44.75 @ 095

SOLUTION: This patient is an ideal candidate for a low-Dk F-S/A material for several reasons: (a) Former PMMA wearers (and first-generation GP wearers) would benefit from the dimensional stability of a low-Dk material. If the corneal edema is not eliminated with the new material, a higher-Dk material can then be used. (b) Patients with borderline tear quality would benefit from the wettability provided by relatively low "silicone-containing" materials unless the material has a surface that has effectively neutralized the polarity and overcome the hydrophobicity of "silicone." (c) Myopic patients usually achieve sufficient oxygen transmission through the lens to meet the daily-wear requirements. (d) The presence of a moderate amount of corneal astigmatism would best be corrected by a low-Dk material to minimize the effects of flexure.

CASE 2

A first-time contact lens wearer desires good visual acuity since she is a nurse and has many critical demands on her vision. In addition, she works 18-hour shifts and would desire a lens that would be optimum for long periods of wear. Her refraction was:

$$OD: +4.25 - 1.00 \times 180$$
$$OS: +3.75 - 1.25 \times 175$$

SOLUTION: This patient would benefit from rigid lenses, in general, because of her critical vision demands. A high-Dk material (preferably F-S/A, although any other high-Dk lens materials with good surface wettability properties would be possible options) would be recommended for the following reasons: (a) she would benefit from the oxygen permeability and possible flexible-wear schedule allowed with these materials, and (b) as a result of the large center thicknesses required in her lenses, a high-Dk material would be necessary to provide sufficient oxygen through the center of the lens to meet the cornea's oxygen requirements.

CASE 3

A college baseball player comes to your office with complaints of foggy vision, itching, and redness from his hydrogel lenses, which have been bothering him for the past 6 months, gradually increasing in severity. He has decreased from a maximum of 14 hours to 8 hours of wearing time. He has been wearing his hydrogel lenses for a period of 12 months and has never been satisfied with his comfort or vision. The examination reveals the following:

VA (with CLs): OD: 20/20   OS: 20/25 + 1
SLE (OU): With lenses on
   Mucoprotein film
   <0.5-mm lens lag
  With lenses off
   6-second TBUT
   Grade 1 + conj. injection
   Grade 2 + papillary hypertrophy
Refraction: OD: −1.50 − 0.50 × 020
     OS: −1.25 − 0.50 × 172

SOLUTION: This patient would be a good candidate for a GP lens material, preferably a large-diameter wettable lens material that does not exhibit excessive lens lag after the blink. A large-diameter (9.6–10.2 mm) low-Dk F-S/A material would be recommended. Ordinarily, most athletes would be better hydrogel candidates; however, this patient would benefit from GPs because of (a) his dissatisfaction with hydrogels, (b) marginal tear quality, (c) surface deposits/papillary hypertrophy, (d) uncorrected refractive astigmatism, and (e) the limited amount of physical contact in baseball (typically much less than that of other major sports such as football and basketball). Initially, the patient will need to decrease or preferably discontinue wearing time to decrease the clinical signs of papillary hypertrophy and eliminate existing symptoms.

CASE 4

A 39-year-old woman who is a long-term GP wearer complains of dryness and redness with her GP lenses, especially late in the day. Her comfortable wearing time has decreased from

15 to 10 hours per day although the current lenses are only 12 months old. She is wearing a high-Dk F-S/A lens material. Her TBUT was 8 seconds OU and her refraction and keratometry values were as follows:

> OD: −3.25 − 1.25 × 180   20/20 + 2   43.25 @ 180; 44.25 @ 090
> OS: −3.00 − 1.00 × 173   20/20 + 1   43.00 @ 180; 43.75 @ 090

SLE (OU): Good centration and an alignment fluorescein pattern OU; mucoprotein film OU
VA (with CLs): OD: 20/25 + 1   OS: 20/20 − 2

SOLUTION: This patient could potentially benefit from being refitted into a plasma-treated low-Dk F-S/A lens material. The lens material may result in prolonging tear film interaction with the lens surface, and the plasma treatment should optimize short-term surface wettability. The patient was also provided with a combination (nonabrasive) cleaning/disinfection solution as well as a wetting solution. The wetting solution could also be used as a rewetting agent if needed.

CASE 5

An 8-year-old girl is interested in contact lenses. She has been a 2-year spectacle wearer and she does not enjoy wearing her spectacles for sports (she plays soccer and softball) and at school. Her refraction was as follows:

> OD: −2.00 − 0.75 × 175   20/20 + 2
> OS: −2.25 − 0.50 × 006   20/20

Her parents are highly myopic and they are concerned about the progression of her refractive error.

SOLUTION: It is important that the child has been a spectacle wearer first and that she—not just her parents—is motivated to wear contact lenses. There are two viable options for this young lady:

1. Daily-wear GP lenses. The GP modality may slow down the progression of her myopia. It would also be important to design the lenses such that they would have a large overall diameter (≥10mm) and low edge clearance to minimize the risk of displacement and loss during sports activities.
2. OOK. She would be an excellent candidate for OOK. This topic will be discussed in Chapter 20.

CASE 6

A 16-year-old high school student has been a soft toric lens wearer for 3 years. She indicates that she has never been satisfied with her vision. She has been refitted by three different practitioners, all of whom were determined for her to be successful with this modality. She indicated that she has probably worn six to seven different types of soft toric lenses but that they all resulted in fluctuating vision and her doctors all commented that the lenses tended to rotate on her eyes. Her mother had read about GP lenses on the Internet and mentioned this to her previous eye doctor; however, her doctor indicated that he does not fit GP lenses. Her refraction and keratometry readings were as follows:

> OD: −1.50 − 1.75 × 168   20/20   43.50 @ 165; 45.00 @ 075
> OS: −1.00 − 2.00 × 011   20/20 + 1   43.75 @ 180; 45.25 @ 090

SOLUTION: This patient is an excellent candidate for GP lenses. Although she will experience some initial awareness and will need to adapt to the lenses, the quality of vision she should experience with the GP lenses should result in a very satisfied patient.

CASE 7

A 25-year-old long-term highly myopic GP wearer expresses an interest in wearing his lenses extended wear. He's frustrated at how blurry his vision is when he awakens and his friends have discussed how satisfied they are with continuous wear of some of the new soft lenses. His refraction was as follows:

OD: $-6.75 - 1.25 \times 004$ 20/15
OS: $-7.00 - 1.00 \times 173$ 20/15 $-$ 2

His tear film and ocular health are normal.

SOLUTION: This patient would be a good candidate for continuous-wear GP lenses. A material that would be consistent with this desire would be Menicon Z.

CASE 8

A 23-year-old hyperopic patient enters your office and is greatly motivated to wear contact lenses. He is currently wearing spectacles, although he did have a history of wearing contact lenses. He indicated that he was fitted into spherical soft lenses when he was 12 but that he was never satisfied with his vision. He was fitted into soft toric lenses when he was 15 but he experienced an infection on two separate occasions, one of which was central and resulted in a slight loss of best corrected vision. Therefore, at age 19, he decided to return to spectacle wear. However, he is not pleased with the weight and the cosmetic appearance of spectacles. His refraction was as follows:

OD: $+4.50 - 1.50 \times 010$ 20/25 $+$ 1
OS: $+4.25 - 1.75 \times 173$ 20/20 $+$ 1

SOLUTION: A high-Dk F-S/A lens material would be a viable option for this patient. A low-Dk material would not meet the patient's corneal oxygen demands, but a high-Dk (or hyper-Dk) material would meet or exceed this requirement. The new generation of silicone hydrogel toric lenses would also represent a good option for this patient. However, because of the patient's history and expressed concern about soft lenses, the GP option would be recommended.

CLINICAL PROFICIENCY CHECKLIST

■ It is important to verify whether the lens material and design selected for a given patient meets the cornea's oxygen requirements. A minimum Dk/t (oxygen transmission or oxygen permeability/center thickness) of 24 is recommended for daily wear.

■ Recommended rigid lenses can be divided into low Dk (25–50), high Dk (51–99), and hyper Dk ($\geq$100)

■ Although good oxygen permeability is possible with these materials, silicone/acrylate materials can be compromised by the hydrophobic properties and flexibility of "silicone." This can result in desiccation, deposits, warpage, flexure, and subjective symptoms of dryness and decreased vision.

■ The addition of fluorine to silicone/acrylate-based copolymer materials promotes tear film mucin interaction with the lens surface. These materials—especially the low-Dk group—have become the lenses of choice for most rigid lens-wearing patients.

■ The SynergEyes family of hybrid lenses is revolutionary in that it, via molecular bonding, combines an outer hydrogel skirt with a hyper-GP center. It has the benefits of good initial comfort, astigmatic correction, and centration. The latter is especially important with patients having irregular corneas. Its problems include cost, adherence, tearing, and handling.

■ Hyperopes, individuals desiring extended/flexible wear, and those exhibiting edema with low-Dk lenses would all benefit from being fitted into high-Dk lens materials, preferably F-S/A.

■ Former PMMA wearers, borderline dry-eye patients, and myopes would all benefit from the dimensional stability and wettability of low-Dk F-S/A lens materials.

■ Athletes unable to wear soft lenses would benefit from a large diameter, low edge clearance GP lens.

REFERENCES

1. Bennett ES. Patient selection, evaluation, and consultation. In: Bennett ES, Hom MM, eds. Manual of Gas Permeable Contact Lenses, 2nd ed. St. Louis: Elsevier Science, 2004:58–85.
2. McMahon TT. The case for rigid lenses. Eye Contact Lens 2003;29(1S):S119–S121.
3. Van der Worp E, de Brabender J. Contact lens fitting today. Optom Today 2005;July 15:27–32.
4. Johnson TJ, Schnider C. Clinical performance and patient preference for hydrogel versus RGP lenses. Int Contact Lens Clin 1991;18(7,8):130.
5. Fonn D, Gauthier CA, Pritchard N. Patient preferences and comparative ocular responses to rigid and soft contact lenses. Optom Vis Sci 1995;72(12):857.
6. Ziel CJ, Gussler JR, Van Meter WS, et al. Contrast sensitivity in extended wear of the Boston IV lens. CLAO J 1990;16:276.
7. Timberlake GT, Doane MG, Bertera JH. Short-term low contrast visual acuity reduction associated with in vivo contact lens drying. Optom Vis Sci 1992;69(10):755.
8. Hong X, Himebaugh N, Thibos LN. On-eye evaluation of optical performance of rigid and soft contact lenses. Optom Vis Sci 2001;78(12):872–880.
9. Joslin CE, Wu SM, McMahon TT, et al. Higher-order wavefront aberrations in corneal refractive therapy. Optom Vis Sci 2003;80(12):805–811.
10. Dorronsoro C, Barbero S, Llorente L, et al. On-eye measurement of optical performance of rigid gas permeable contact lenses based on ocular and corneal aberrometry. Optom Vis Sci 2003;80:115–125.
11. Goldberg EP, Bhatia S, Enns JB. Hydrogel contact lens-corneal interactions: a new mechanism for deposit formation and corneal injury. CLAO J 1997;23:243.
12. Sucheki JK, Ehlers WH, Donshik PC. Peripheral corneal infiltrates associated with contact lens wear. CLAO J 1996;22:41.
13. Dart JK. The epidemiology of contact lens-related diseases in the United Kingdom. CLAO J 1993;19:241.
14. Cheng KH, Leung SL, Hoekman HW, et al. Incidence of contact lens-associated microbial keratitis and its related morbidity. Lancet 1999;354:181–185.
15. Dart JK, Stapleton F, Minassian D. Contact lenses and other risk factors in microbial keratitis. Lancet 1991;338(8768):650–653.
16. Schein OD, Buehler PO, Stamler JF, et al. The impact of overnight wear on the risk of contact lens-associated ulcerative keratitis. Arch Ophthalmol 1994;112(2):186–190.
17. Poggio EC, Glynn RJ, Schein OD, et al. The incidence of ulcerative keratitis among users of daily-wear and extended-wear soft contact lenses. N Engl J Med 1989;321(12):779–783.
18. Schein OD, Poggio EC. Ulcerative keratitis in contact lens wearers: incidence and risk factors. Cornea 1990;9:S55–S58; discussion S62–S63.
19. Ren D, Yamamoto K, Ladage P, et al. Adaptive effects of 30-night wear of hyper-O2 transmissible contact lenses on bacterial binding and corneal epithelium: a 1-year clinical trial. Ophthalmol 2002;109:27–40.
20. Ren DH, Petroll WM, Jester JV, et al. The relationship between contact lens oxygen permeability and binding of Pseudomonas aeruginosa to human corneal epithelial cells and after overnight and extended wear. CLAO J 1999;25(2):80–100.
21. Seal DV, Bennett ES, McFayden AK, et al. Differential adherence of Acanthamoeba to contact lenses: effects of material characteristics. Optom Vis Sci 1995;72:23–28.
22. Donshik PC. Giant papillary conjunctivitis. Trans Am Ophthalmol Soc 1994;92:687–744.
23. Bennett ES, Johnson JD. Material selection. In: Bennett ES, Weissman BA, eds. Clinical Contact Lens Practice. Philadelphia: Lippincott Williams & Wilkins, 2005:243–253.
24. Ritson M. Which patients are more profitable? Contact Lens Spectrum 2006;21(3):38–42.
25. Ames K. Rethink your approach to RGP lenses. Contact Lens Spectrum 1993;8(12):24–27.
26. Perrigin J, Perrigin D, Quinteros S, et al. Silicone-acrylate contact lenses for myopia control: 3-year old results. Optom Vis Sci 1990;67(10):764–769.
27. Khoo CY, Chong J, Rajan U. A 3-year study on the effect of RGP contact lenses on myopic children. Singapore Med J 1999;40:230–237.
28. Walline JJ, Jones LA, Mutti DO, et al. A randomized trial of the effects of rigid contact lenses on myopia progression. Arch Ophthalmol 2004;122(12):1760–1766.
29. Katz J, Schein OD, Levy B, et al. A randomized trial of rigid gas permeable contact lenses to reduce progression of children's myopia. Am J Ophthalmol 2003;136:82–89.
30. Walline JJ, Rah M, Jones LA. The Children's Overnight Orthokeratology Investigation (COOKI) Pilot Study. Optom Vis Sci 2004;81(6):407–413.
31. Cho P, Cheung SW, Edwards M. The Longitudinal Orthokeratology Research in Children (LORIC) in Hong Kong: a pilot study on refractive changes in myopic control. Curr Eye Res 2005;30:71–80.
32. Walline JJ. Slowing myopia progression with lenses. Contact Lens Spectrum 2007;22(6):22–27.
33. Lieblein JS. Finding success with multifocal contact lenses. Contact Lens Spectrum 2000;14(3):50–51.
34. Byrnes SP, Cannella A. An in-office evaluation of a multifocal RGP lens design. Contact Lens Spectrum 1999;14(11):29–33.

35. Remba MJ. The Tangent Streak rigid gas-permeable bifocal contact lens. J Am Optom Assoc 1988;59:212.
36. Gussler JR, Lin ES, Litteral G, et al. Clinical evaluation of the anterior constant focus (ACF) annular bifocal contact lens. CLAO J 1993;19:222.
37. Smith VM, Koffler BH, Litteral G. Evaluation of the ZEBRA 2000 (Z10) Breger Vision bifocal contact lens. CLAO J 2000;26(4):214–220.
38. Rajagopalan AS, Bennett ES, Lakshminarayanan V. Visual performance of subjects wearing presbyopic contact lenses. Optom Vis Sci 2006;83(8):611–615.
39. Connelly S. Why do patients want to be refit? Contact Lens Spectrum 1992;7:39.
40. Andrasko G, Smiley T, Nichold L, et al. Clinical recommendations for the management of symptomatic soft contact lens wearers. Contact Lens Spectrum 1993;8:24.
41. Morgan PB, Woods CA, Knajian R, et al. International contact lens prescribing in 2007. Contact Lens Spectrum 2008;23(1):36–41.
42. Hewitt TT. A survey of contact lens wearers, part II: behaviors, experiences, attitudes and expectations. Am J Optom Physiol Opt 1984;61:73.
43. Andrasko GJ, Billings R. A simple nomogram for RGP fitting success. Contact Lens Spectrum 1993;8:28.
44. Bennett ES. Be flexible about rigid lenses. Rev Cornea Contact Lens 2007;May:38–40.
45. Schwartz CA. New strategies for screening RGPs. Rev Optom 1994;131:29.
46. Fonn D, Pritchard N, Garnett B, et al. Palpebral aperture sizes of rigid and soft contact lens wearers compared with nonwearers. Optom Vis Sci 1996;73(3):211–214.
47. Thean JH, McNab AA. Blepharoptosis in RGP and PMMA hard contact lens wearers. Clin Exp Optom 2004;87(1):11.
48. Fatt I, Chaston J. Measurement of oxygen transmissibility and permeability of hydrogel lenses and materials. Int Contact Lens Clin 1982;9:76–88.
49. Fatt I, Rasson JE, Melpolder JB. Measuring oxygen permeability of gas permeable hard and hydrogel lenses and flat samples in air. Int Contact Lens Clin 1987;14:389–401.
50. Benjamin WJ. "Wiggle room" and the traditional Dk statistic. Int Contact Lens Clin 1998;25(7&8):118–120.
51. Benjamin WJ, Cappelli QA. Oxygen permeability (Dk) of thirty-seven rigid contact lens materials. Optom Vis Sci 2002;79(2):103–111.
52. Mandell RB, Liberman GL, Fatt I. Corneal oxygen supply: RGP versus soft lenses. Contact Lens Spectrum 1987;2(10):37–39.
53. Bennett ES, Ghormley NR. Rigid extended wear: an overview. Int Contact Lens Clin 1987;14(8):319–332.
54. Machara JR, Kastl PR. Rigid gas-permeable extended wear. CLAO J 1994;20:139.
55. Polse KA. Tear flow under hydrogel contact lenses. Invest Ophthalmol Vis Sci 1979;18:409.
56. O'Neal MR, Polse KA, Sarver MD. Corneal response to rigid and hydrogel lenses during eye closure. Invest Ophthalmol Vis Sci 1984;27(7):837–842.
57. Tomlinson A, Armitage B. Closed-eye corneal response to a tertiary butyl styrene gas-permeable lens. Int Eyecare 1985;1(4):320–323.
58. Ichijima H, Cavanagh HD. How rigid gas-permeable lenses supply more oxygen to the cornea than silicone hydrogels: a new model. Eye Contact Lens 2007;33(5):216–223.
59. Holden BA, Mertz GW. Critical oxygen levels to avoid corneal edema for daily and extended wear contact lenses. Invest Ophthalmol Vis Sci 1984;25:1161–1167.
60. Sweeney DF, Keay L, Jalbert I, et al. Clinical performance of silicone hydrogel lenses. In: Sweeney DF, ed. Silicone Hydrogels: The Rebirth of Continuous Wear Contact Lenses. Oxford: Butterworth-Heinemann, 2000:90.
61. Harvitt DM, Bonanno JA. Re-evaluation of the oxygen diffusion model for predicting minimum contact lens Dk/t values needed to avoid corneal anoxia. Optom Vis Sci 1999;76:712–719.
62. Papas E. On the relationship between soft contact lens oxygen transmissibility and induced limbal hyperemia. Exp Eye Res 1998;67:125–131.
63. Gordon JM, Bennett ES. Dk revisited: the hypoxic corneal environment. Presented at the Annual Meeting of the American Academy of Ophthalmology, Chicago, November 1993.
64. Benjamin WJ. EOP and Dk/L: the quest for hypertransmissibility. J Am Optom Assoc 1993;64:196.
65. Bennett ES. Gas permeable materials. In: Bennett ES, Hom MM, eds. Manual of Gas Permeable Contact Lenses, 2nd ed. St. Louis: Elsevier Science, 2004:48–56.
66. Benjamin WJ. Wettability. In: Bennett ES, Grohe RM, eds. Rigid Gas-Permeable Contact Lenses. New York: Professional Press, 1986:118–136.
67. Maruna C, Yoder M, Andrasko GJ. Attitudes toward RGPs among optometrists. Contact Lens Spectrum 1987;12(11):57.
68. Hom MM, Bruce AS. Material properties. In: Bennett ES, Hom MM, eds. Manual of Gas Permeable Contact Lenses, 2nd ed. St. Louis: Elsevier Science, 2004:30–47.
69. Cannella A, Bonafini JA. Polymer chemistry. In: Bennett ES, Weissman BA, eds. Clinical Contact Lens Practice. Philadelphia: Lippincott Williams & Wilkins, 2005:233–242.
70. Sorbara L, Fonn D, MacNeil K. Effect of rigid gas permeable lens flexure on vision. Optom Vis Sci 1992;69:953–958.

71. Corzine JC, Klein SA. Factors affecting rigid contact lens flexure. Optom Vis Sci 1997;74(8):639–645.

72. Herman JP. Flexure. In: Bennett ES, Grohe RM, eds. Rigid Gas-Permeable Contact Lenses. New York: Professional Press, 1986:137–150.

73. Herman JP. Flexure of rigid contact lenses on toric corneas as a function of base curve fitting relationship. J Am Optom Assoc 1983;54(3):209–213.

74. Brown S, Baldwin M, Pole J. Effect of the optic zone diameter on lens flexure and residual astigmatism. Int Contact Lens Clin 1984;11(12):759–766.

75. Bennett ES, Egan DJ. Rigid gas-permeable lens problem-solving. J Am Optom Assoc 1986;57:504–512.

76. Egan DJ, Bennett ES. Trouble-shooting rigid contact lens flexure - a case report. Int Contact Lens Clin 1985; 12:147.

77. Bennett ES. Problem solving. In: Bennett ES, Hom MM, eds. Manual of Gas Permeable Contact Lenses, 2nd ed. St. Louis: Elsevier Science, 2004:190–211.

78. Levitt AO. Specific gravity and RGP lens performance. Contact Lens Spectrum 1996;11(10):43.

79. Ghormley NR. Specific gravity - does it contribute to RGP lens adherence? Int Contact Lens Clin 1991;18:125.

80. Tighe BJ. Contact lens materials. In: Phillips AJ, Speedwell L, eds. Contact Lenses, 5th ed. London: Elsevier Butterworth-Heinemann, 2007:59–78.

81. Ghormley NR. Rigid EW lenses: complications. Int Contact Lens Clin 1987;14:219.

82. Bennett ES, Tomlinson A, Mirowitz MC, et al. Comparison of corneal overnight swelling and lens performance in RGP extended wear. CLAO J 1988;14:94.

83. Henry VA, Bennett ES, Forrest JF. Clinical investigation of the Paraperm EW rigid gas-permeable contact lens. Am J Optom Physiol Opt 1987;64:313–320.

84. Grohe RM, Caroline PJ, Norman CW. RGP surface cracking. Part I: clinical syndrome. Contact Lens Spectrum 1987;2(5):37–45.

85. Grohe RM, Caroline PJ, Norman CW. RGP surface cracking. Part II: clinical syndrome. Contact Lens Spectrum 1987;2(9):40–46.

86. Weinschenk JI. A look at the components of fluoro-silicone/acrylates. Contact Lens Spectrum 1989;4(10):61.

87. Feldman G, Yamane SJ, Herskowitz R. Fluorinated materials and the Boston Equalens. Contact Lens Forum 1987; 12:57.

88. Gelnar PV, Behnken BH. Paraperm EW vs. Fluoroperm 90 gas-permeable contact lens study. Contact Lens J 1989; 17:15.

89. Andrasko GJ. Comfort comparison between silicon acrylates and the Boston Equalens. Contact Lens Spectrum 1988;3(6):61.

90. Bark M, Hanson D, Grant R. A guide to rigid gas-permeable contact lens materials. Optician 1994;207:17.

91. Doane M, Gleason W. Tear film interaction with RGP contact lenses. Presented at the First International Material Science Symposium, St. Louis, March 1988.

92. Caroline PJ, Ellis EJ. Review of the mechanisms of oxygen transport through rigid gas-permeable lenses. Int Eyecare 1986;2:210.

93. Rah MJ. A GP materials guide. Contact Lens Spectrum 2007;22(7):19.

94. http://www.gpli.info. Accessed January, 2008.

95. http://www.bausch.com. Accessed January, 2008.

96. Quinn TQ. Clinical experience with Fluoroperm 30 lenses. Contact Lens Spectrum 1989;4(2):63.

97. Quinn TQ. Base curve stability of a fluoro-silicone-acrylate material of moderate permeability. Contact Lens Spectrum 1989;4(3):52.

98. Bennett ES. Basic fitting. In: Bennett ES, Weissman BA, eds. Clinical Contact Lens Practice. Philadelphia: Lippincott Williams & Wilkins, 2005:255–275.

99. Jackson JM. Prescribing GP lenses in a material world. Contact Lens Spectrum 2006;21(4):19.

100. Schachet JL, Rigel LE, Reeder KM, et al. Rethinking the link between RGP lens performance. Contact Lens Spectrum 1998;13(9):43–47.

101. Bennett ES. Optimizing GP wettability and performance. Contact Lens Spectrum 2006;21(2):21.

102. Knutson E, Young R. Assessing a new GP lens family. Contact Len Spectrum 2005;20(5):50–52.

103. Bennett ES. To plasma treat or not to plasma treat? Rev Cornea Contact Lenses 2006;Nov:9.

104. Schafer J. Plasma treatment for GP contact lenses. Contact Lens Spectrum 2006;21(11):19.

CHAPTER 5

Lens Design, Fitting, and Evaluation

Edward S. Bennett and Luigina Sorbara

The ability to successfully fit rigid gas-permeable (GP) contact lenses is often what separates the good contact lens practitioner from the average one. Certainly there are numerous patients who benefit from the quality of vision and ocular health provided by GP lenses. This chapter will discuss the importance of fitting GP lenses and the lens design, fitting, evaluation, and ordering procedures.

■ HOW TO OPTIMIZE INITIAL COMFORT

The first time a patient experiences contact lens wear can be quite traumatic. This is especially true with GP lenses because of the smaller diameter and greater lens movement with the blink as compared to soft lenses. This experience, in itself, can affect the fitting habits of practitioners who may decide to fit soft lenses—even when they are not the best option for patients—in an effort to provide a more initially comfortable and less time-consuming experience.

It is important, if not imperative, for the initial patient experience to be positive for the patient to be successful. The common perception by patients is that the initial comfort with GP lenses is poor, and this represents the primary reason why patients discontinue GP lens wear.[1] It is evident that if the patient has a poor initial experience with GP lenses, he or she will influence others away from considering this option. If the clinician—via his or her educational background (or lack thereof) or employment environment—is not motivated to fit GP lenses, it is likely that, despite the many benefits of GP lenses, patients will not be fitted into the mode of correction that would be indicated because of quality of vision, eye health, or some other reason.

The authors have recommended a fourfold approach to optimizing initial comfort.[2] These factors include (a) presentation, (b) topical anesthetic, (c) initial vision, and (d) lens design.

Initial Presentation

Most contact lens patients rely on their practitioner to recommend an appropriate lens material and design. It is important for practitioners to recognize that when presenting patients with a choice, they may, without realizing it, bias that choice. The doctor's language creates and colors patient perceptions. Such terms as *discomfort, pain,* or *always seems to feel like there is something on the eye* set up strong negative expectations. Prescribing practitioners are powerful authority figures. What they say and how they say it can easily influence patients.

Simple words like *soft, hard,* or *rigid* can influence a patient's contact lens preferences. Even nonverbal cues such as facial expression and eye contact can communicate an attitude to the patient. It is always important to begin with the assumption that a new patient has somewhere been given the impression that rigid lenses are uncomfortable. GP lenses can then be described in the following way: "GP lenses typically provide excellent vision and eye health. They are also quite wettable and durable. However, they do not feel the same way a soft lens does at first. Because they are smaller, they move more on the eye. The lids sense this movement initially and gradually adapt, typically resulting in comfortable lens wear." The use of the term *gas permeable* as compared to the previous *rigid gas permeable* terminology was recently proposed by the Contact Lens Manufacturers Association (CLMA) to minimize the focus on "rigid" lenses.

The impact of presentation methods was confirmed by a study in which subjects who were not previous contact lens wearers were divided into three groups before initiating GP lens wear.[3] Group one subjects, as part of the diagnostic fitting process, observed a videotape of a doctor discussing GP lenses with a new wearer using terms such as *discomfort, possible pain, intolerance,* and *failure* when describing GP lenses. Group two subjects observed a videotape of a doctor discussing GP lenses using neutral terms such as *lens awareness* and *initial lid sensation.* However, this doctor did not appear to be particularly positive about the GP lens option. In group three the doctor discussing GP lenses used the same terminology as in the videotape observed by group two but exhibited a positive attitude toward GP lenses. Eight subjects in this 1-month study discontinued lens wear; six of these subjects were in group one, and the other two were in group two. No subject provided with a neutral content and enthusiastic presentation discontinued lens wear. Likewise, the group three subjects were significantly more compliant in returning daily questionnaires than the other two groups.

It is important for patients to know the benefits of GP lenses, that they will adapt over time, and that good comfort is a very realistic goal.[4] Certainly experienced GP fitters do not have a problem with the comfort issue, and as one acquires more experience in fitting GP lenses, greater confidence in presenting this option in a positive but realistic manner results.

Topical Anesthetic Use

A second important technique for obtaining initial GP patient comfort and satisfaction is the use of a topical anesthetic during contact lens fitting. This has been considered somewhat controversial because of concerns pertaining to its potential for softening the epithelium, resulting in a greater incidence of corneal staining.[5,6] In addition, there is always the potential for misleading the patients who will ultimately experience the typical lens awareness with GP lenses. Fortunately, although these are legitimate concerns, they have not been confirmed by clinical research with GP lenses.[7,8]

With these issues in mind, an 80-subject multicenter study was performed to evaluate the effect of topical anesthetic use on initial comfort and patient satisfaction among first-time GP lens wearers.[7] Forty subjects were administered a topical anesthetic at the fitting visits, while a second group of 40 received a placebo. One month later, 70 of the 80 subjects were still wearing lenses. Eight of the 10 who discontinued lens wear were in the placebo group. In addition, at the completion of the study, subjects who had been given anesthetic rated their experience during adaptation, their comfort, and their overall satisfaction significantly higher than those subjects who had received placebo.

The benefits of topical anesthetic are significant. All patients are, at minimum, mildly apprehensive about the initial application of contact lenses. If the first few minutes of lens wear are acceptable, it makes sense that patient satisfaction, and the potential for successful long-term wear, will be greatly enhanced. The topical anesthetic should be allowed to wear off, and the patient will gradually experience lens awareness. In addition, in busy clinical practice environments, where time is a precious resource, the ability to evaluate the fluorescein pattern soon after diagnostic lens application is invaluable.[8] This is also important because of the fact that soft lenses often require little chair time during the fitting process and GPs benefit from being competitive with soft lenses whenever possible.

Nonsteroidal anti-inflammatory drugs (NSAIDs) have also been used to reduce awareness during adaptation.[9,10] Because NSAIDs reduce production of prostaglandins, which are mediators of pain, reducing their production reduces pain. The most effective drug within this class at inhibiting prostaglandin synthesis appears to be Voltaren. A recommended NSAID dosage for GP lens adaptation is as follows[10]:

- Instill one drop of Voltaren in each eye 30 minutes and then 15 minutes before lens insertion.
- Instill a third drop just before lens insertion.
- A fourth drop can be instilled 1 hour after insertion.
- This regimen can be maintained for 3 to 5 days or until adaptation is completed.

Topical anesthetic use is certainly not a requirement for GP fitting. However, for apprehensive practitioners as well as patients—particularly young people, people with keratoconus, and soft lens refits—anesthetic use can mean the difference between success and failure.

Initial Vision

Providing patients with an important benefit from GP lenses, good quality of vision, can be very important for initial patient satisfaction. When a patient is fitted with GP lenses in their correct power—either via empirical fitting or from an inventory—the resulting "wow" factor may reduce apprehension about lens awareness.

Lens Design

This will be discussed in more detail later in this chapter; however, a well-designed, alignment fitting lens with an optimum edge design and shape will contribute to a more positive initial patient experience.

■ FITTING AND EVALUATION

There are numerous important components to fitting lenses successfully. These include such factors as diagnostic fitting, fluorescein application and evaluation, and an accurate and compatible lens design.[11]

Methods of Fitting

Empirical Fitting

Empirical fitting refers specifically to designing lenses empirically or without using diagnostic lenses. Practitioners who utilize empirical fitting methodologies claim that manufacturers' recommendations (supplying the laboratory with such minimal prefitting information as keratometry values and refraction) and fitting guides provide effective means to obtain maximum lens performance and fit. Empirical fitting also means that a new, unworn lens will be fitted to one patient only. Empirical fitting has the attraction of eliminating a fitting visit and, consequently, enabling a simplistic fitting approach.[12] As indicated previously, however, empirical fitting often provides a very important benefit, good initial vision. The newer automated manufacturing equipment makes the success of empirical designs more likely than 10 to 20 years ago because of higher-quality lenses, aspheric and pseudoaspheric peripheries, thinner center thicknesses, and more consistent edge designs. Likewise, topography software programs allow the practitioner to better match corneal shape with the recommended computer-assisted design.[13–16]

Diagnostic Fitting

Diagnostic fitting is still a popular method of fitting GP lenses. It allows the practitioner to feel confident in the final lenses to be ordered as multiple diagnostic lenses can be applied (if necessary) and those that result in the best lens-to-cornea fitting relationship will be ordered. Greater patient compliance with the follow-up schedule in addition to significantly fewer reordered lenses have been found with diagnostic versus empirical fitting.[17] Although a fitting visit and a sufficient number of diagnostic lenses are required, diagnostic fitting allows practitioners the opportunity to evaluate the lens-to-cornea fitting relationship and to make the changes necessary to obtain a good fit and provide acceptable vision to the patient. It is also apparent that the fitting visit provides patients with an opportunity to become familiar with their particular lenses. Finally, such factors as lens centration and residual astigmatism can be evaluated.[18] The primary limitations pertain to (likely) not leaving the office with lenses, as compared with most soft lens patients, and the fact that, in most cases, satisfactory vision will not be obtained with the first pair of GP lenses applied. The 6 D myopic patient who is fitted with 3 D power diagnostic GP lenses will not only experience initial awareness, but also blurred vision. Nevertheless, with most special design GP lenses, including bifocal, keratoconic, and postsurgical designs, it is important to use diagnostic fitting sets because of the greater challenges involved in the fitting process and the more custom nature of the designs. When diagnostic fitting sets are to be used, it is important that the lenses are in the same design and material as the lenses to be ordered. A comparison of the factors involved in deciding between empirical and diagnostic fitting is provided in Table 5.1.

Diagnostic Fitting Sets/Inventories

Specific Fitting Sets

Having available several different diagnostic fitting sets is important, if not essential. For example, 20 lens diagnostic fitting sets in a −3.00 D power would be beneficial in materials of both low (<50) and high (≥50) oxygen permeability (Dk). An example of such a fitting set is provided in Table 5.2. In addition, similar diagnostic sets in a +3.00 D power in a high-Dk material with a minus lenticular edge design and in a −8.00 D power in a low-Dk material and a plus lenticular edge design would be recommended. Keratoconic, bitoric, aphakic, and bifocal diagnostic sets are also recommended and are discussed in other chapters of this text (Chapters 14, 15, 17, and 18).

For the diagnostic fitting sets, a good average overall diameter is 9.4 mm with an 8.0-mm optical zone diameter. However, for steeper than 44.50 D, you may find a 9.0/7.6-mm design to provide an optimum fitting relationship. Base curve radii can range from 40.75 D (8.28 mm) to 45.50 D (7.42 mm) in 0.25 D steps. A relatively constant edge lift of 0.09 to 0.11 mm is recommended for the diagnostic lenses; therefore, the flatter base curve radii will have a greater flattening of the peripheral curve radii, and steeper base curve radii will have a greater steepening. Finally, the appropriate center thickness should be ordered. For example, a low-Dk material may have a center thickness of approximately 0.14 mm in a −3.00 D power, although this can vary from material to material. All of the diagnostic lenses of the same power should have equal and

---

TABLE 5.1   DIAGNOSTIC FITTING VERSUS EMPIRICAL FITTING

Diagnostic Fitting Advantages
Fewer reorders
Practitioner confidence in fitting relationship
Greater patient satisfaction
Better patient compliance
Empirical Fitting Advantages
Good initial vision experience
Easier method
Minimizes transfer of diagnostic lens contaminants
Less initial chair time
Allows topography software to assist in lens design

TABLE 5.2   RECOMMENDED PARAMETERS FOR A 20-LENS DIAGNOSTIC SET, LOW-AND HIGH-DK GAS-PERMEABLE MATERIALS

Overall diameter	9.2 mm		
Optical zone diameter	7.8 mm		
Center thickness	0.14 mm		
Power	−3.00 D		
LENS	BCR (mm)	SCR/W	ICR/W	PCR/W
1.	7.42	8.00/.3	8.80/.2	10.00/.2
2.	7.46	8.10/.3	8.90/.2	10.10/.2
3.	7.50	8.20/.3	9.00/.2	10.20/.2
4.	7.54	8.20/.3	9.00/.2	10.20/.2
5.	7.58	8.30/.3	9.10/.2	10.30/.2
6.	7.63	8.30/.3	9.20/.2	10.40/.2
7.	7.67	8.40/.3	9.30/.2	10.50/.2
8.	7.71	8.50/.3	9.40/.2	10.60/.2
9.	7.76	8.50/.3	9.50/.2	10.60/.2
10.	7.81	8.60/.3	9.60/.2	10.70/.2
11.	7.85	8.60/.3	9.60/.2	10.80/.2
12.	7.89	8.70/.3	9.70/.2	10.80/.2
13.	7.94	8.70/.3	9.70/.2	10.90/.2
14.	7.99	8.80/.3	9.80/.2	11.00/.2
15.	8.04	8.80/.3	9.90/.2	11.10/.2
16.	8.08	8.90/.3	10.00/.2	11.20/.2
17.	8.13	8.90/.3	10.10/.2	11.30/.2
18.	8.18	9.00/.3	10.20/.2	11.40/.2
19.	8.23	9.10/.3	10.30/.2	11.50/.2
20.	8.28	9.20/.3	10.40/.2	11.60/.2

BCR, base curve radius; ICR/W, intermediate curve radius/width; PCR/W, peripheral curve radius/width; SCR/W, secondary curve radius/width.

appropriate center thicknesses; these parameters—and especially edge shape—should be verified upon receiving them from the laboratory. With the increasing popularity of ultrathin designs, a diagnostic set of this design in a minus power (i.e., −3.00 D) would be recommended as well.

Inventories

The use of a large (100–200 lenses) inventory system, which has been very popular with hydrogel lenses, is also an alternative available to practitioners. The advantages of using a large inventory to fit rigid lenses are many and include the following: (a) some patients can be fitted out of stock; (b) lens replacements can be provided to patients without delay, so patient satisfaction is enhanced; and (c) lens parameter changes can be made in the office without delay. Unlike hydrogel lenses, because of the custom or multiparameter design—especially base curve radius (BCR)–inherent with successful fitting of GP lenses, a minimum of 200 lenses is necessary to directly fit the majority of patients without having to order the lenses from a laboratory. Such a 200-lens inventory is given in Table 5.3.

TABLE 5.3   PARAMETERS FOR GAS-PERMEABLE INVENTORY LENS SET

RX	BASE CURVE RADIUS (mm)														
	7.42	7.50	7.54	7.58	7.63	7.67	7.71	7.76	7.80	7.85	7.89	7.94	7.99	8.04	8.13
−1.25								94	110	123	136	149	162	175	188
−1.50							79	95	111	124	137	150	163	176	189
−1.75							80	96	112	125	138	151	164	177	190
−2.00	1	14	27	40	53	66	81	97	113	126	139	152	165	178	191
−2.25	2	15	28	41	54	67	82	98	114	127	140	153	166	179	192
−2.50	3	16	29	42	55	68	83	99	115	128	141	154	167	180	193
−2.75	4	17	30	43	56	69	84	100	116	129	142	155	168	181	194
−3.00	5	18	31	44	57	70	85	101	117	130	143	156	169	182	195
−3.25	6	19	32	45	58	71	86	102	118	131	144	157	170	183	196
−3.50	7	20	33	46	59	72	87	103	119	132	145	158	171	184	197
−3.75	8	21	34	47	60	73	88	104	120	133	146	159	172	185	198
−4.00	9	22	35	48	61	74	89	105	121	134	147	160	173	186	199
−4.25	10	23	36	49	62	75	90	106	122	135	148	161	174	187	200
−4.50	11	24	37	50	63	76	91	107							
−4.75	12	25	38	51	64	77	92	108							
−5.00	13	26	39	52	65	78	93	109							

Overall diameter = 9.4

Optical zone diameter = 8.2

Secondary curve radius (SCR) = base curve radius (BCR) + 1.0 mm/0.3 mm wide; peripheral curve radius (PCR) = BCR + 3.0 mm/0.3 mm wide

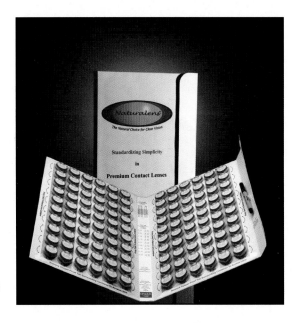

■ **FIGURE 5.1** The Naturalens inventory (Advanced Vision Technologies).

Some of the manufacturers, including those who manufacture the Boston Envision lens design (Bausch & Lomb) and the Naturalens (Advanced Vision Technologies, Fig. 5.1), can provide smaller inventories because of the philosophy that their respective designs can be successfully fitted to the great majority of patients with fewer base curve radii.[2]

Some GP lens manufacturers are unwilling to manufacture such large inventories because of the labor and expense necessary to do so. However, they are often available to practitioners who fit a high volume of GP lenses. As with soft lenses, the initial expense to the practitioner is minimal; however, the laboratory usually requires the practitioner to meet the following agreement provisions[19]: (a) maintain an inventory of lenses equal to the original consignment, (b) fit a certain number of lenses within a specified period, and (c) use manufacturer's lens design parameters. Nevertheless, it is a valuable alternative that can increase your success with GP lenses while also providing a valuable service to many GP patients.

Storage of Diagnostic Lenses

Storing diagnostic lenses in the hydrated state has the advantage of providing good initial wettability while maintaining the lenses in a somewhat sterile state. However, depending on the frequency with which the solution is changed, there are many advantages to keeping the lenses in the dry state.[20] It is both efficient and convenient to store the lenses dry because they can be kept in flat-pack cases that occupy very little space in the office. If the lenses are stored in the hydrated state, it is possible for the solution to either dry up in the case or leak out, both of these problems resulting in a lens that may adhere to the case or even change in base curve radius because of variation between the hydrated and unhydrated states. In addition, the dried solution may be difficult to remove from the lens surface. Whenever a diagnostic lens has been applied, however, it is recommended to carefully clean the lens and blot it dry with a soft tissue prior to disinfection and placement in the case and into the appropriate diagnostic lens set. The Centers for Disease Control and Prevention (CDC) recommends ophthalmic-grade hydrogen peroxide for GP lenses; therefore, AOSept or Clear Care (Ciba Vision) for a 5- to 10-minute soak has been recommended.[21] GP lenses that are going to be dispensed to a patient should be hydrated for a minimum of 24 hours prior to application to enhance surface wettability and maintain the base curve radius in the hydrated state (similar to the "on-eye" condition as the back surface rests against the tear film). Obviously, patients should likewise be advised to maintain the lenses in the appropriate soaking/disinfecting solution upon removal (see Chapter 6).

Fluorescein Application and Evaluation

Description

Sodium fluorescein is an organic compound that is inert and harmless to tissue.[22] The application of fluorescein enables the practitioner to evaluate the lens-to-cornea fitting relationship. In fact, it would be appropriate to indicate that fluorescein has an invaluable, if not essential, role in rigid lens fit assessment.

To perform the procedure, the fluorescein strip is wetted with an ophthalmic irrigating solution. The strip is then gently applied against the superior bulbar conjunctiva with the patient viewing inferiorly. It is important to reassure the patient that this procedure is painless. In addition, the thumb should carefully pin back the upper lid to prevent the possibility of the lid pushing the strip toward the superior cornea, which could result in superior corneal staining and accompanying subjective discomfort.

The use of an ophthalmic irrigating solution has numerous advantages for wetting the fluorescein strip, including the following:

• Sterility.
• Slightly alkaline in pH, which assists in fluorescence.
• Reduced risk of burning and stinging caused by pH.
• Less viscous than use of a wetting solution (which may result in an abnormally thick tear layer).

However, for optimum fluorescence, the use of liquid fluorescein has been recommended.[23]

Methods of Observation

The fluorescein pattern can be evaluated with both a Burton lamp and a biomicroscope.

Burton Lamp: The traditional method of evaluating the fluorescein pattern is by use of an ultraviolet fluorescent lamp that utilizes a +5.00 D magnification lens to assist in viewing (Fig. 5.2). This method has the following advantages:

• Inexpensive.
• Easy to use.
• Overall field of view and ability to directly compare fluorescein pattern of both eyes simultaneously.

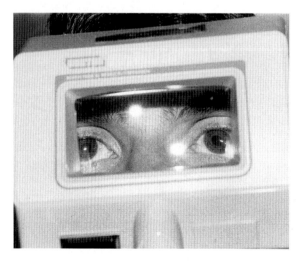

■ **FIGURE 5.2** The Burton lamp for fluorescein pattern evaluation.

However, the Burton lamp is very limited in its abilities. It does not allow for variable magnification or illumination. In addition, it is an ineffective method of observing the fluorescein pattern of rigid lens materials with ultraviolet-absorbing capabilities. Therefore, it would not be advantageous or appropriate to use this as the only method to evaluate a fluorescein pattern. However, it is a useful adjunct to the biomicroscope because of the overall field of view. This is especially beneficial in observing some of the more distinctive patterns, such as those pertaining to high corneal toricity and keratoconus.

Biomicroscope: The most popular method of evaluating the fluorescein pattern of a rigid lens is with the biomicroscope. The primary advantage of this over other observational methods is flexibility. It allows the practitioner the opportunity to vary the magnification, illumination, and slit-beam width while observing the fluorescein pattern. Proper use of a biomicroscope for GP fitting and evaluation is essential for patient success.

As biomicroscopes vary considerably from manufacturer to manufacturer, it is important for a good illumination source and variable magnification to be present to effectively evaluate the fluorescein pattern. In fact, it has been determined that with many biomicroscopes it is not possible to use >10× magnification and still retain an adequate field of view.[24]

Once fluorescein has been properly instilled, the patient should be instructed to blink several times for adequate distribution on the eye. The fluorescein pattern should be initially observed under low magnification with a wide (diffuse) slit-beam and high-intensity illumination. The central and peripheral fluorescein pattern should be relatively easy to determine after several seconds. An optic section with the angle of illumination equal to 45 to 60 degrees can also be used to observe the pooling of tears in relation to the contact lens. It will appear as a green layer representing the outer layer of tears on the lens; then a wider dark layer, which is the contact lens; next another green layer, which represents the tear layer between the lens and cornea; and finally a bright grayish layer, the cornea.[22] The lens-to-cornea fitting relationship can be evaluated by viewing the thickness of the tear layer along the optic section.

Typically, the fluorescein pattern is viewed with the assistance of a cobalt blue filter, which, in effect, transmits blue light that will activate the fluorescein dye. It is important to use a Wratten no. 12 yellow filter (or equivalent) that can be attached to the observation system to serve as a barrier filter, screening out all but the wavelengths of interest.[25] The importance of the yellow filter cannot be underestimated since it makes an easily observable improvement in fluorescein pattern evaluation. The use of a yellow filter, in combination with a good illumination source, is especially important in the evaluation of GP materials that contain ultraviolet inhibitors because, as the material absorbs wavelengths that correspond to the illumination source, there is an apparent reduction or even absence of fluorescence behind the lens unless the appropriate filters and illumination source are used. It is hoped that biomicroscopic manufacturers will begin to incorporate the yellow filter into their respective instruments.

Pattern Evaluation: The fluorescein pattern assumes a variety of forms. Areas of fluorescein pooling appear green; areas in which fluorescein is absent or where the tear layer is too thin to detect, having the contact lens in direct contact with the cornea, appear as dark or black. In between these extremes, the varying thickness of the tear layer is observed as varying shades of green.

An alignment fit is observed when the lens evenly contours the cornea with a light, even tear pooling (Fig. 5.3). Apical clearance exists when a steep central fit with excessive fluorescence or central tear pooling is present (Fig. 5.4). This can result in midperipheral bearing and seal-off with a reduced ability to remove cellular debris and mucus that may be an important precursor to rigid lens adherence to the cornea. Apical clearance has also been found to induce corneal steepening, even after short-term wear.[26] Apical bearing exists when there is direct contact of the lens against the central cornea or the amount of tear pooling is too shallow to detect

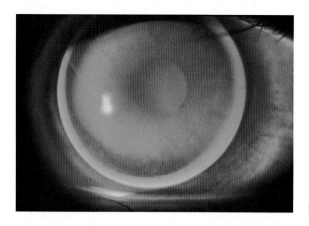

■ FIGURE 5.3 An alignment fluorescein pattern.

with the instillation of fluorescein (Fig. 5.5). Excessive apical bearing can potentially result in corneal molding with resultant distortion or warpage. In addition, the gradual formation of a central corneal abrasion is also possible.

With corneal astigmatism greater than one diopter, a dumbbell-shaped fluorescein pattern will be observed (Fig. 5.6). Typically, along the steeper meridian of the cornea, the tear layer thickness gradually increases toward the edge and the lens does not touch the cornea.

Along the flatter meridian, however, the tear layer thickness decreases toward the periphery and the lens comes in contact with the cornea at the edge of the optical zone. As corneal astigmatism increases, the difference in tear layer thickness between the two primary meridians becomes greater, the area of alignment becomes smaller, and the astigmatic, or dumbbell-shaped, fluorescein pattern becomes exaggerated.[27] If the cornea exhibits with-the-rule corneal astigmatism, the pooling is in the vertical meridian with alignment or bearing in the horizontal meridian. If the cornea exhibits against-the-rule astigmatism, the opposite is true: the pooling is in the horizontal meridian with alignment or bearing in the vertical meridian. In high corneal astigmatism—typically greater than two diopters—the use of a high-Dk material with a steeper than K base curve radius will result in excessive flexure and reduced visual acuity. In addition, the "rocking" of the lens during the blink process may result in discomfort, mechanical corneal staining, and possible lens adherence. The selection of a lower oxygen-permeable material, and perhaps a flatter base curve radius, is recommended. Another option would be a bitoric design, especially if the high amount of corneal toricity results in inferior decentration of the lens (see Chapter 14).

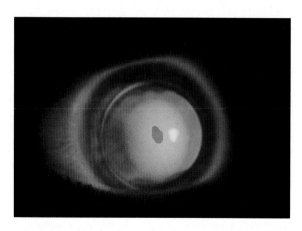

■ FIGURE 5.4 An apical clearance fluorescein pattern.

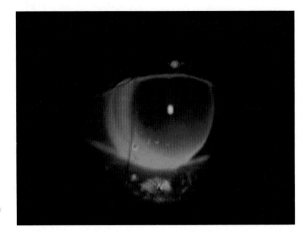

■ **FIGURE 5.5** An apical bearing fluorescein pattern.

It is important to evaluate the fluorescein pattern after the blink since the amount of pooling and bearing will vary during the blink process. If the lens is decentered, the position of the lens relative to the cornea must be considered prior to evaluating the fluorescein pattern. For example, an inferior decentering lens will typically exhibit excessive superior pooling since the flatter peripheral bevel is adjacent to the steeper central cornea.

The evaluation of the fluorescein pattern at the lens periphery is also beneficial. There should be sufficient clearance peripherally—typically greater than apically—to allow sufficient tear exchange and debris removal while avoiding mechanical irritation as the lens moves across the cornea. If fluorescein pooling is minimal or absent peripherally and seal-off exists, the peripheral curve(s) should be flattened.

Fluorescein pattern evaluation of the rigid lens-to-cornea fitting relationship should be performed both at the fitting visit and at all subsequent follow-up visits. A practitioner's ability to properly assess fluorescein patterns occurs with experience and frequent evaluation. There are several educational resources available from the GP Lens Institute (www.gpli.info) including an educational CD-ROM entitled "GP Fitting, Evaluation, and Problem-Solving," a GP Lens Management Guide, and a Fluorescein Pattern Identification laminated card. It would be erroneous to believe that fluorescein pattern evaluation is not as important with GP materials as with polymethylmethacrylate (PMMA) as a result of the reduction in edema-related complications. The lens material is only as good as the practitioner's ability to properly evaluate it; a poor lens-to-cornea fitting relationship can result in numerous problems, including desiccation, adhesion, and abrasion. In particular, the fluorescein pattern evaluation is invaluable in the difficult-to-fit cases such as high corneal toricity, irregular/distorted corneas, and keratoconus.[28]

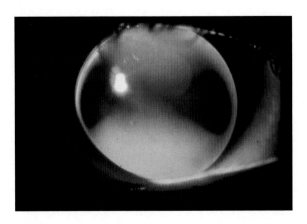

■ **FIGURE 5.6** The dumbbell-shaped fluorescein pattern present with a highly astigmatic patient.

False Fluorescein Patterns: Occasionally, the fluorescein pattern is contrary to the expected appearance. This phenomenon can occur as a result of a variety of causes:

1. Corneal topography. This varies between patients; for example, a patient with a small corneal cap (defined as the region within 0.50 D of the corneal apex) will exhibit a somewhat steeper fluorescein pattern than a patient with a larger-than-average cap.[29,30]
2. Selection of a steep BCR may result in poor tear exchange and a misleading small amount of fluorescein centrally.
3. If the peripheral curve is too steep, peripheral seal-off can occur and the fluorescein pattern can exhibit apical clearance.
4. In certain individuals—particularly dry-eye patients—the fluorescein will dissipate quickly and may create a "pseudoapical flat" relationship; therefore, the pattern should be evaluated immediately after fluorescein instillation.
5. A "pseudosteep" pattern has been reported in high minus fluoro-silicone/acrylate (F-S/A) lenses.[31] Apparently the edge thickness blocks the fluorescence, giving an appearance of central pooling. Likewise, one would expect that a high plus lens may demonstrate a flatter than actual base curve fitting relationship because the thick center would attenuate the light more.

Designs/Fitting Philosophies

There are numerous available methods for determining the rigid lens design parameters for diagnostic fitting. In this section of the chapter two fitting philosophies will be presented.

There are two primary fitting philosophies for designing and fitting GP lenses, both based on lens position on the eye. The first approach is to design a lens so that it positions consistently under the upper eyelid (i.e., a lid-attached fit) and the second is to design a lens that achieves an interpalpebral fit on the eye.

Studies have been done to compare these two lens designs with respect to comfort, vision, and physiologic response.[32–34] Results are mixed about which design performs the best because of individual variation in corneal topography, lid/cornea interaction, and lid tension.

Lid-Attachment Fitting and Design

Overall/Optical Zone Diameter: The overall diameter (OAD) of a rigid lens should be large enough to allow for a sufficient optical zone while providing good lag with the blink. The optical zone diameter (OZD) typically encompasses anywhere from 65% to 80% of the lens diameter.[35] The size of both OAD and OZD depends on the following factors:

Palpebral Aperture Size/Lid Position: The palpebral aperture size refers to the vertical separation of the lids in the normal state. An average amount of separation is 9.0 to 10.5 mm. If the difference is greater, a larger-diameter lens should be considered; if less, a smaller-diameter lens can be used.

The position of the lids, however, is more important. This varies between patients, and it has been demonstrated that if the upper edge of the lens rides underneath the upper lid when gazing straight ahead, it will be more comfortable than an interpalpebral fitting relationship.[36,37] The reason for this is that the initial rigid lens sensation is usually the result of the lid margin.[38,39] During the blink process the upper lid moves over the upper edge of the lens; if the position of the upper lid is above the edge of the lens, there will be contact between the two, creating an initial awareness or sensation. However, if the upper lid is positioned at or above the superior limbus, a position not easily obtainable, it may be preferable to select a smaller-diameter lens and a fit steeper than K, and to obtain a well-centered lens that positions, at minimum, 1 mm below the upper lid.

Pupil Size: The diameter of the pupil should be measured in both high and low illumination. Assuming a good lens-to-cornea fitting relationship, the optical zone diameter should be greater than the pupil size in dim illumination to minimize the risk of subjective symptoms of flare at night.

Refractive Power: It is often necessary to select a larger OAD/OZD with hyperopic lens powers to provide adequate pupil coverage with the thicker, higher-mass lens. This large OAD, however, should be in combination with a minus lenticular edge design. In addition, although not always the case, it is not uncommon for hyperopia to be accompanied by flatter keratometry values (and myopia by steeper K values); therefore, the same principle as indicated in the following section holds true.

Corneal Curvature: It is recommended to select a larger than average overall diameter with flatter corneal curvatures (e.g., flatter than 41 D) and a smaller than average overall diameter with steeper curvatures (e.g., steeper than 45 D) to maintain an optimum centering lens. A good rule of thumb has been proposed by Caroline and Norman[34]: Select an optical zone diameter equal to the base curve radius in millimeters. In other words, a 41.75 D (8.09 mm) base curve radius would be accompanied by an OZD equal to 8.1 mm, and a 45.50 D (7.42 mm) base curve radius would be accompanied by an optical zone equal to 7.4 mm.

Lid Tension: The amount of lid tension will play a prominent role in diameter selection. Lid tension can be determined by lid eversion. As this should be performed both at the prefitting evaluation and at all subsequent follow-up visits, one can obtain a good idea of which patients have loose lids (i.e., upper lid everts very easily) and which have tight lids (i.e., upper lid everts with much effort, if at all). Since a loose upper lid will provide little assistance in raising a lens during the blink process, a larger than average overall diameter is recommended in this case.

What are good overall diameter/optical zone diameters to use? Average values are typically in the 9.2- to 9.4-mm range for an overall diameter and 7.6- to 8.2-mm range for an optical zone diameter. A 9.4/8.0-mm design is a good starting point in many custom-designed lenses. When a larger OAD/OZD is indicated, a 9.8/8.4-mm design is recommended; when a smaller OAD/OZD is indicated, an 9.0/7.6-mm design is recommended.

Bottom Line: The current trend with new GP materials is for manufacturers to recommend larger overall diameters (i.e., typically in the 9.6- to 10.2-mm range) to optimize initial comfort. This often occurs because of less initial lens movement and good centration.[40] A word of caution is indicated here. A larger lens tends to exhibit more of an effect on the cornea, possibly resulting in molding and distortion. In addition, in a highly flexible material, the potential for limited lens lag and adherence exists; therefore, debris removal and additional oxygen flow are limited. Likewise, selecting a large optical zone diameter may result in limited lateral lens movement with the blink since the junction between the base curve radius and the secondary curve radius is located at a more peripheral region of the cornea. This may encourage peripheral corneal desiccation since the lens does not move over the peripheral cornea.[38] Some practitioners prefer to use a large overall diameter (e.g., 9.6 mm) with a small optical zone diameter (e.g., 7.4 mm) for the purpose of creating an optimum midperipheral corneal alignment. This design would be acceptable assuming that both sufficient lens lag and pupil coverage exist. In addition, when making a change in diameter, it is important that this change is a significant one, which has been found to be a minimum of 0.4 mm in overall diameter and 0.3 mm in optical zone diameter.[41]

Base Curve Radius: The primary purpose of the base curve radius is to optimize the fitting relationship of the lens to the central and midperipheral cornea. The base curve radius to be selected depends on several factors, including corneal curvature, the observed fluorescein pattern, and

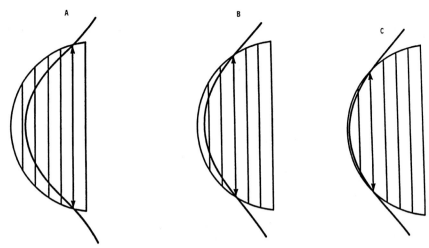

■ **FIGURE 5.7** The fitting relationship of various optical zone diameters. If optical zone diameter **A** or **B** is chosen, a steep fitting relationship will result. The smaller optical zone **C** will provide an alignment fitting relationship [From Caroline PJ, Norman CW. A blueprint for rigid lens design. I. Contact Lens Spectrum 1988;3(11).]

the desired lens-to-cornea fitting relationship. It can be specified in diopters or millimeters (see Appendix 1).

It is important to emphasize that the selection of a given base curve radius (e.g., "on K") on several patients will result in differences in the observed fluorescein patterns because of differences in corneal topography (apical area, rate of flattening, etc.) and lens design. Typically, a lens fit "on K" will provide an apical clearance fitting relationship since the optical zone is often much larger than the corneal cap or apex (Fig. 5.7).[38] Therefore, to maintain an alignment fitting relationship it is necessary in most cases to select a base curve radius flatter than K. In addition, a flatter base curve radius will minimize both lens-induced flexure and the potential for seal-off of tear exchange, which can potentially occur with an "on K" fit on a spherical cornea.[42]

What base curve radius should you select? A philosophy for diameter and base curve radius selection is provided in Table 5.4.[11]

It is important to mention that if the optical zone diameter is smaller than normal, a slightly steeper base curve radius is necessary. For example, with steeper than 45 D corneal curvatures, a smaller optical zone diameter is necessary to maintain alignment. Conversely, if the optical zone diameter is larger than normal, a slightly flatter base curve radius than recommended in Table 5.4

TABLE 5.4   GAS-PERMEABLE DIAMETER AND BASE CURVE SELECTION CRITERIA (LID ATTACHMENT)

CORNEAL CYLINDER (D) (KERATOMETRY)	OAD/OZD	
	9.4/8.0 mm (LID ATTACHMENT)	9.8/8.4 mm (LARGE PUPILS/ATHLETES)
0.0−0.75	0.50 D FTK	0.75 D FTK
1.00−1.25	0.25 D FTK	0.50 D FTK
1.50−1.75	"On K"	0.25 D FTK
2.00−2.25 D	0.25 D STK	"On K"
≥2.50	Bitoric design	Bitoric design

FTK, flatter than K; OAD, overall diameter; OZD, optical zone diameter; STK, steeper than K.

may be indicated. For example, with flatter than 41 D corneal curvature values, a larger optical zone diameter is necessary to maintain alignment; in addition, patients with large pupil diameters will need a larger optical zone diameter to minimize flare. A simple rule to remember is: flatten the base curve radius 0.25 D for each increase in optical zone diameter of 0.5 mm and steepen the base curve radius 0.25 D for each decrease in optical zone diameter equal to 0.5 mm.[34] Of course, the specific base curve radius to be selected will depend primarily on the fluorescein pattern, especially if an instrument to measure eccentricity or shape factor of the cornea (i.e., from central to, at minimum, midperipheral cornea) is not available.

A steeper base curve radius may be necessary with high rather than low astigmatic patients because of many factors, the most important of which is to increase the probability of obtaining an optimum lens-to-cornea fitting relationship. Typically, with high astigmatic patients (i.e., corneal astigmatism >2 D), the base curve radius has to be steepened, or a bitoric design can be used to obtain the best distribution of lens alignment over the largest area.[22] An "on K" base curve radius fitted on a highly astigmatic cornea will not only provide very little corneal alignment and subsequent decentration, but the resulting areas of bearing and excessive clearance may also result in lens "rocking" on the cornea with the blink, discomfort caused by an increase in edge contact with the upper lid, and corneal desiccation.

A steeper than K base curve radius is also often necessary with hyperopic patients since the center thickness is greater and the center of gravity is located more anteriorly; therefore, the lens would have a greater tendency to drop inferiorly after the blink. A steeper than K base curve radius would be more likely to provide a well-centered lens position.

The geometric center of the lens should coincide or be positioned slightly above the patient's line of sight. A slightly superiorly positioned (tucked underneath the lid) lens-to-cornea fitting relationship should maximize patient comfort by minimizing the interaction of the lens edge with the upper lid. This is the basis behind the "lid attachment" design philosophy developed by Korb and Korb.[36] In addition, this fitting relationship has been found to result in less corneal desiccation than interpalpebral and inferiorly positioned lenses.[43]

The amount of lens lag or downward movement after the blink should be, at minimum, 1 mm and, at maximum, 3 mm. A larger amount of lens lag may result in fluctuation in vision because of flare and possible lens awareness, while a smaller amount of lag could cause adherence with resultant trapped debris and edema. Good pupillary coverage by the optical zone diameter should be present throughout the blink process.

What is the bottom line? Although recommendations have been made, it is important to mention that no single base curve radius selection philosophy can accurately predict the resultant lens positioning on a given patient. Therefore, trial and error, supplemented by fluorescein pattern evaluation, is an important factor in deciding on the appropriate base curve radius.

Peripheral Curve Radii/Width: The peripheral curve radii, which typically encompass the outer 20% to 35% of the lens, surround the optical zone diameter of the lens. Designs in common use have either one (i.e., bicurve), two [i.e., tricurve with a secondary curve radius (SCR) and a peripheral curve radius (PCR)], or three [i.e., tetracurve with an SCR and intermediate curve radius (ICR) and a PCR] peripheral curves. In addition, some lens designs utilize an aspheric periphery with a continuous flattening of the peripheral region of the lens. Each curve must be progressively flatter than the adjacent, more centrally positioned curve to provide proper lens clearance from the cornea. The peripheral curve, in particular, serves the following three functions[44]:

- To prevent the edge of the lens from digging into the corneal surface during lens movement.
- To permit proper circulation of the tears beneath the lens to maintain the metabolism of the cornea.
- To support a meniscus at the edge of the lens to provide forces that cause the lens to center.

The peripheral curves serve no optical purpose. If the contact lens is decentered such that the peripheral curves are directly in front of the visual axis, flare will result.[45]

The application of peripheral curves creates a sharp ridge between the curves. This ridge can prevent adequate circulation of tears to the central cornea and can also impair the removal of metabolic debris from under the lens. Therefore, the application of a blend will result in a more even tear flow. Typically the blend, which is performed with a radius tool midway between the peripheral curve radii values (see Chapter 9), can either be light, medium, or heavy. At minimum, a medium blend should be performed to enhance debris removal. Blending the peripheral curve radii junction will increase lens lag caused by the smoother surface and may also increase initial comfort.[46]

The distance from the lens edge perpendicular to the peripheral cornea is termed *edge clearance*. A geometric and therefore quantifiable term, *edge lift,* has also been used to approximate edge clearance; this pertains to the distance between the lens edge and an extension of the base curve radius of the lens (therefore, it is a slightly larger value than clearance). If the peripheral curve radius is flattened and/or the peripheral curve width is increased, edge clearance will increase, all other lens parameters being held constant. Changing the peripheral curve radius and/or width has more of an effect on edge clearance than changing the secondary or intermediate curves.[47]

Lens positioning can be influenced by the amount of edge lift. Essentially, as the edge lift increases, the interaction with the upper lid will increase.[48] A high edge lift/clearance design will result in excessive interaction with the upper lid and a superiorly decentered lens. An excessively low edge lift/clearance design will result in very little, if any, interaction with the upper lid and potentially position inferiorly. To provide good tear circulation and debris removal, the use of a flat, wide peripheral curve has been customarily used in traditional PMMA lens designs because of enhanced oxygen flow to the cornea. These philosophies typically used either a bicurve design or a tricurve design with an SCR approximately 1.0 to 1.5 mm flatter than the BCR and a PCR equal to 12.00 to 12.25 mm. For example, a lens design equal to 7.8 mm BCR, 9.2/0.3 mm SCR/W, and 12.25/0.4 mm PCR/W was not uncommon. However, excessive edge clearance may result in lens decentration, lens awareness, and corneal desiccation.[38,49–51] The latter problem may result from a combination of a receding tear meniscus as it is pulled underneath the lens edge from the adjacent peripheral cornea and a possible alteration in the normal blink pattern caused by the upper lid contacting the anteriorly positioned edge.[44,52,53] The decentration may result from either inferior displacement caused by the increased contact between edge and lid or actual superior displacement caused by an alignment of the flatter part of the lens with the flatter corneal region.[38]

What peripheral curve system should we use? As gas-permeable lenses are not as dependent on the tear pump as PMMA and since many of these materials are silicone-based, presenting the possibility of a short over-the-lens tear breakup time[54] and evaporation of the peripheral tear pool,[52] a lower edge clearance design should be advantageous. Most aspheric designs (to be discussed later in this chapter) align well with the paracentral and midperipheral cornea and, therefore, have a relatively low edge clearance. If such an option is not feasible, the following peripheral curve system is recommended by the first author:

TETRACURVE

$$SCR/W = BCR + 0.8/0.3 \text{ mm}$$

$$ICR/W = SCR + 1.0/0.2 \text{ mm}$$

$$PCR/W = ICR + 1.4/0.2 \text{ mm}$$

For example, if the BCR = 7.8 mm:

$$SCR/W = 7.8 + 0.8 = 8.6/0.3 \text{ mm}$$

$$ICR/W = 8.6 + 1.0 = 9.6/0.2 \text{ mm}$$

$$PCR/W = 9.6 + 1.4 = 11.0/0.2 \text{ mm}$$

However, to maintain a fairly constant edge clearance, the peripheral curve system must be flattened at a greater rate with flat base curve radii and flattened at a lesser rate for steep base curve radii. Therefore, the aforementioned peripheral curve design philosophy can be used for the average base curve radii; however, slightly flatter than recommended values should be used with flatter BCRs and slightly steeper values with steeper BCRs.

Lenses having steeper than recommended peripheral curve radii (i.e., low edge clearance) are often more difficult to remove and may also trap debris.[55] In addition, increased risk of lens adherence[56,57] and vascularized limbal keratitis (VLK)[58] have been associated with the use of low edge lift designs.

What is the bottom line? It is important to avoid excessively flat/wide peripheral curves and especially a limited curve design (i.e., bicurve), which can provide poor midperipheral alignment with the cornea. Likewise, it is important to verify the number and width of the peripheral curves (radius is extremely difficult to verify) and the quality and accuracy of the blends.

Center Thickness: Center thickness is dependent on many other lens parameters, but primarily lens power and overall diameter. The center thickness is greater and the center of gravity more anterior for plus lenses, while the edge thickness is greater and the center of gravity more posterior for minus lenses.[35]

There is a fine line between a lens that is too thin and a lens that is too thick. A lens that is too thin will likely be too unstable and could flex significantly on the eye as well as be prone to warpage. Therefore, standard-thickness designs are recommended in moderate-to-high corneal astigmatism (i.e., >1.50 D). A lens that is too thick, however, may result in inferior decentration, with accompanying variable vision, corneal desiccation, and injection.[59]

The introduction of ultrathin lenses in many of the new lower-Dk lens materials has resulted in reducing the incidence of decentration and increasing patient satisfaction,[60–62] although initial comfort may not be better.[63] These lenses are as much as 50% thinner than standard designs. For example, a −3.00 D lens may be made as thin as 0.10 mm in a −3.00 D power as compared to a standard thickness of approximately 0.14 mm.

What center thickness should be ordered? Recommended center thickness values for standard (not ultrathin) designs are given in Table 5.5. The recommended center thickness values vary from material to material and from manufacturer to manufacturer.

What is the bottom line? It is extremely important to verify center thickness because an inaccurate value may affect lens performance. Often, it is easier for the laboratory to manufacture

TABLE 5.5   CUSTOM DESIGN GAS-PERMEABLE CENTER THICKNESS VALUES (MILLIMETERS)[a]

	DK VALUE	
POWER (D)	20–49	50+
−1.00	0.18	0.19
−2.00	0.16	0.18
−3.00	0.14	0.16
−4.00	0.14	0.15
−5.00	0.13	0.14
≥ −6.00	0.13	0.14

[a] Standard thickness.

Dk, oxygen permeability.

a thicker than necessary lens to reduce the probability of breakage during the procedure. In fact, in a study in which center and edge thickness values were the only parameters not provided to the laboratory (lenses of four different powers were ordered from eight laboratories selected at random), the differences in center thickness, overall thickness, and lens mass were significant for a given power.[64] A decision on center thickness should not be made on the basis of oxygen permeability alone but on factors such as vision, lens stability, and positioning. For example, increasing center thickness by 0.04 mm will increase mass by 24% but will only decrease equivalent oxygen percentage by <1%.[65]

The sign of a good laboratory is the ability to consistently manufacture thin lens designs. Likewise, although Table 5.5 is a recommended guide, it is a good idea to obtain the recommended center thickness table from the manufacturer for every GP material to be used in your practice.

Edge Thickness/Design: The edge design is an extremely important and often underestimated parameter that can be the primary variable affecting comfort and lens positioning. A thin, tapered, rolled-edge design is desirable. The edge can be divided into three zones.[66] The anterior zone interacts with the upper lid during blinking. The posterior zone is often a narrow reverse curve that is placed onto the posterior lens surface to flare the edge away from the cornea. This assists in allowing free movement of the lens across the cornea. The junction between the anterior and posterior zones is the lens apex, which must be well rounded to minimize lens awareness during the blink.

The shape of the lens edge is important as well. As indicated previously, Korb and Korb[36] recommend an edge design that has its apex anteriorly to assist the upper lid in lifting and attaching to the upper lens edge. Likewise, it has been found that lenses with well-rounded anterior edge profiles were significantly more comfortable than lenses with square anterior edges; there was no significant difference between a rounded and square posterior edge profile.[67] Therefore, it was concluded that the interaction of the edge with the eyelid is more important in determining comfort than edge effects on the cornea.

Several studies have demonstrated the inconsistency of edge design with GP materials.[67–69] One study found that not only was there much inconsistency between materials, but also there were large differences within lenses of the same material from the same manufacturer with identical parameters.[68] Typically, as a material increases in oxygen permeability, it also increases in softness and potential for chipping and breakage. If, in fact, an unverified lens is defective from an edge that is either too sharp, too blunt, or chipped, but is nevertheless dispensed to the patient, the result may be a dissatisfied patient who may never again desire to wear GP lenses. However, because of the advanced manufacturing and polishing methods in common use today, inconsistent and defective edges are much less common. Nevertheless, edge verification, as recommended in Chapter 7, is important. One device that is commercially available only to evaluate the edge is the Contact Lens Edge Profile Analyzer (CLEPA, from Valley Contax, Springfield, OR) (Fig. 5.8).

What about the interaction of center thickness and edge thickness? Both center thickness and edge thickness change with changes in overall diameter and with different lens powers.[70] Edge thickness is greater in medium-to-high minus powers and center thickness is greater in low minus and all plus powers. Edge and center thicknesses are not equal at plano but at approximately –2.00 D power.[38,70]

What are lenticular designs? As a result of the variance in edge thickness with lens power and overall diameter, the use of a lenticular design is sometimes indicated. In a lenticulated lens, the front surface consists of a central optical portion surrounded by a peripheral carrier portion that is thinner and flatter.[45] The thickness of the lens at the junction of the optic cap and carrier portion should equal 0.12 to 0.14 mm.[37,71] If it is thicker, lens mass is unnecessarily added to the lens; if thinner, the lens can break at this junction.

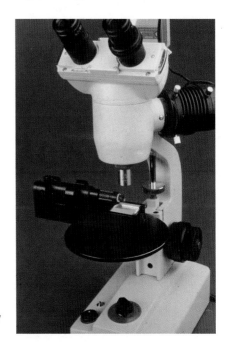

■ FIGURE 5.8 The Contact Lens Edge Profile Analyzer (Valley Contax, Springfield, OR).

In high minus powers, either an anterior CN bevel (Fig. 5.9) or plus lenticular design (Fig. 5.10) can be used to reduce edge thickness, with the latter option most often used. Plus lenticular designs are often used because they minimize problems associated with thick edges such as lens awareness, inferior positioning caused by lid–lens interaction, and corneal desiccation resulting from compromise in the normal blinking process. In addition, plus lenticular designs reduce center thickness and overall lens mass. Typically, minus lens powers of ≥ 5 diopters are lenticulated because the edge thickness is ≥ 0.20 mm without this modification.[38]

A minus lenticular design to increase edge thickness is also very important to enhance lid interaction with the edge and minimize inferior decentration. A minus lenticular design is recommended with minus powers ≤ -1.50 D and all plus power lenses. A summary of minus versus plus lens design parameters is given in Table 5.6.

What is the bottom line? The importance of verifying every lens edge cannot be emphasized enough. This is the number one means of reducing the initial discomfort while also ensuring that your laboratory has good quality control. The hallmark of any given laboratory is its ability to

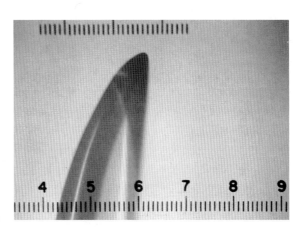

■ FIGURE 5.9 Anterior CN bevel.

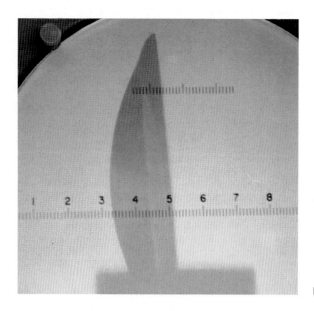

■ **FIGURE 5.10** Plus lenticular design.

fabricate a good edge. The use of a lenticular edge design, when appropriate, is a win-win situation as it typically improves lens centration while increasing oxygen transmission.

What Is the Bottom Line on Lens Design? A summary of important factors in GP lens design and fitting is given in Figure 5.11.

One factor that is especially important to adhere to is as follows: whenever you make a change in lens design, make sure it is a significant one. In other words, merely increasing the diameter 0.1 to 0.2 mm, decreasing the center thickness by 0.01 mm, or changing the base curve by 0.25 D will rarely have the desired effect on the lens-to-cornea fitting relationship. The parameter changes necessary to have a significant effect on the fitting relationship are given in Table 5.7.[41]

Interpalpebral Fitting

There are many similarities to lid-attachment fitting in selecting the proper lens design. The following is an outline of the particular differences.

Overall Lens Diameter: The overall lens diameter is determined by the average corneal diameter [horizontal visible iris diameter (HVID)] of the patient, the interpalpebral aperture height, and the contact lens power. These factors affect the contact lens center of gravity and thus lens

TABLE 5.6 MINUS VERSUS PLUS LENS DESIGN PARAMETERS

PARAMETER	MINUS POWER	PLUS POWER
BCR	Flatter than K	Steeper than K
OAD	Smaller (8.8–9.6 mm)	Larger (9.2–9.8 mm)
CT	Lesser (<0.20 mm)	Greater (>0.20 mm)
Edge design	Thicker—plus lenticular for all high (> −5 D) powers; minus lenticular for all powers with low (<1.50 D) powers	Thinner—minus lenticular necessary

BCR, base curve radius; CT, center thickness; OAD, overall diameter.

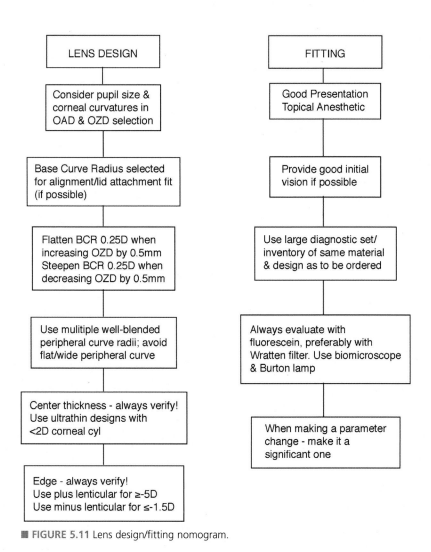

FIGURE 5.11 Lens design/fitting nomogram.

TABLE 5.7 CLINICALLY SIGNIFICANT PARAMETER CHANGES

PARAMETER	CHANGE FOR CLINICAL SIGNIFICANCE
Base curve radius	0.50 D (approximately 0.1 mm)
Overall/optical zone diameter	0.4/0.3 mm
Peripheral curve radius	0.5 mm
Center thickness (high Dk)	0.02 mm

Dk, oxygen permeability.
From Szczotka (41).

TABLE 5.8 GAS-PERMEABLE LENS DIAMETER SELECTION (INTERPALPEBRAL)

FACTOR	MEASUREMENT	PREDICTED DIAMETER
PA	<8.0 mm	9.0–9.3 mm
	8.5–11.0 mm	9.4–9.6 mm
	>11.5 mm	9.7–9.9 mm
HVID	10.0–11.0 mm	9.2–9.4 mm
	11.5–12.5 mm	9.5–9.7 mm
	>12.5 mm	9.8–10.0 mm
PS	PS + (3.5–4.0 mm) = BOZD	BOZD + (1.2–1.4 mm)

BOZD, back optic zone diameter; HVID, horizontal visible iris diameter; PA, palpebral aperture; PS, pupil size.

position, lens stability, the option to have larger back and front optic zone diameters (BOZDs and FOZDs), lens comfort, and the physiologic response to the lens (i.e., 3 and 9 o'clock staining and palpebral conjunctival response).

The center of gravity of contact lenses and thus the lens position can be moved anteriorly (lower position) with smaller-diameter lenses and posteriorly (higher-riding lens position) with larger-diameter lenses. Selection of overall lens diameter is based on Table 5.8, taking into account interpalpebral aperture height, HVID, and pupil size. Normally, the selection for an interpalpebral fit is based on the HVID, unless the interpalpebral aperture height is unusually small or if the pupil size is unusually large (Table 5.8).

Adjustments to the lens diameter can be made based on the contact lens power. The power has an effect on lens position because of the location of the center of gravity (CG). Generally, plus lenses whose CG is forward because of thick center thickness result in a low lens position. Plus lenses should be designed with larger overall diameters (with lenticulated minus carriers and thinner center thickness designs) to move the CG back and toward a more centered interpalpebral position. Conversely, high minus lenses tend to be high riding because of the CG being too far backward and so should be designed with a smaller diameter (with lenticulated plus carriers and slightly thicker CT designs) to move the CG forward to achieve an interpalpebral lens fitting relationship.

What is the bottom line? A lens that is too small may result in decentration and exposure of the pupil (especially in the dark), causing flare, a visual disturbance resulting in visual discomfort. A lens that is too large may initially feel more comfortable but may result in conjunctival (CT) staining if the lens overlaps the limbus in any position with movement on the blink.

Base Curve Radius Selection: In interpalpebral fitting lens design, an aligned lens-to-cornea relationship needs to be achieved. Corneal topography, to check for regularity of the corneal astigmatism, whether the astigmatism is centrally located or extends out to the limbus, the eccentricity values (e-value), and the simulated K readings, are essential to determine the base curve [or back optic zone radius (BOZR)] that will result in an aligned fluorescein pattern according to the amount of corneal astigmatism and lens diameter. Figure 5.12A,B shows corneal topographies demonstrating regular astigmatism that is only located centrally versus regular astigmatism extending from limbus-to-limbus.

It is important to note that the shape of the cornea resembles a prolate ellipse. The e-value is a measure of the rate of flattening from the center of the cornea to the periphery.

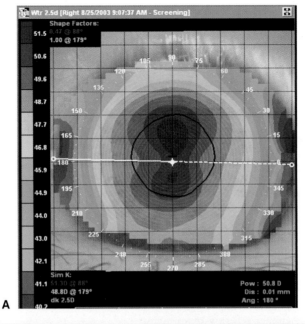

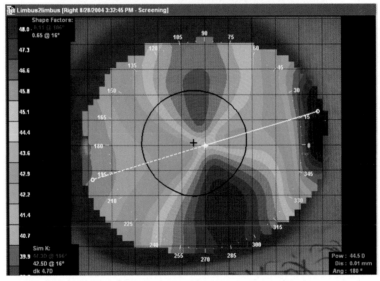

■ FIGURE 5.12 Corneal topographies demonstrating regular astigmatism that is only located centrally **(A)** versus regular astigmatism extending from limbus to limbus **(B)**. (Photographs courtesy of Randy Kojima, Precision Technology, BE Enterprises.)

TABLE 5.9 BASE CURVE RADIUS SELECTION FOR A 9.2- TO 9.4-MM OVERALL DIAMETER LENS

CORNEAL CYLINDER	BASE CURVE RADIUS
0.00 to −1.00 D	On K
−1.12 to −2.00 D	1/4 delta K + flat K
−2.12 to −2.87 D	1/3 delta K + flat K
> −3.00 D	Back surface/bitoric lens

The selection of the BCR varies with the lens diameter that was initially chosen and depends on the amount of corneal astigmatism. Table 5.9 shows the relationship between the amount of corneal astigmatism and the BCR to choose for an interpalpebral, aligned fitting relationship for lens diameters of 9.2 to 9.4 mm.

If the lens diameter that was chosen was <9.2 mm (i.e., 8.8–9.1 mm), then the rules of thumb based on the ΔK from Table 5.9 can be used and the BCR that was calculated can be steepened by an additional 0.25 D. If the selected OAD is >9.6 mm (i.e., 9.7–9.9 mm), then the calculated BCR from the table can be flattened by 0.25 D. These adjustments for smaller and larger lens diameters will ensure that an aligned fitting relationship is still maintained to result in an interpalpebral positioned lens by maintaining the same sag. One will know that the proper lens-to-cornea fitting relationship has been achieved by instilling fluorescein and interpreting the fluorescein pattern. An aligned fitting relationship in the central pattern must be achieved. Lenses that are either fitting too flat or too steep cannot be accepted and adjustments must be made.

What is the bottom line? Proper selection of the BCR according to the amount of corneal astigmatism that is present and with an average lens diameter will ensure that the lens-to-cornea fitting relationship will result in an interpalpebral fitting lens as the BCR steepens with increasing astigmatism. In addition, proper assessment and interpretation of the fluorescein pattern in ensuring that the lens-to-cornea relationship is neither too steep nor too flat will result in an ideal interpalpebral fitting relationship.

Peripheral Curve Radii/Width and Optical Zone Diameter: The selection of the widths and radii of the peripheral curves and resultant back optic zone diameters will strongly determine the amount of peripheral edge clearance that determines the lens position (and final comfort) and the central lens-to-cornea fitting relationship (from OZD), respectively.

To achieve an interpalpebral lens positioning, one must design the periphery (and BOZD or BOZR) to maintain an axial edge lift (AEL) and resultant axial edge clearance (AEC) of 0.10 to 0.12 mm and >0.08 to 0.10 mm, respectively.[72] These values assume that the average cornea has an e-value between 0.45 and 0.55.

As defined earlier, AEL is the vertical distance from the lens edge to an extension of the back optic zone radius of the lens. Radial edge lift is the extension of the lens edge perpendicular to the extension of the BCR. AEC is the vertical distance from the lens edge to the peripheral cornea and is usually less than the AEL (Fig. 5.13).

Regardless of the diameter of the lens and the BCR, a constant amount of AEL/AEC is desired and is to be maintained when fitting the average patient. On average (i.e., for an average e-value), this amount is 0.10 to 0.12 mm for AEC (usually reported in micrometers). This amount of AEC should result in a 0.50-mm-wide band around the lens periphery as seen with fluorescein instilled in the eye.

Constant Axial Edge Lift: If the same radius value is added to the BCR for the SCR and PCR, the resulting AEL will not be a constant but will be higher for steep lenses (6.5–7.3 mm) and lower for flat lenses (7.9–8.3 mm). Thus, a computer program aids the practitioner and the laboratories in manufacturing lenses with constant AELs regardless of the BCR. Most diagnostic lens sets have made the adjustments in SCR and PCR to maintain a constant AEL.

Once the lens is inserted, the subject's individual corneal topography in the periphery will determine the appearance of the fluorescein pattern in the periphery (i.e., the AEC). Adaptations in AEL can then be made to either increase or decrease the AEL to achieve the ideal AEC after central alignment is achieved. Also, when changes in overall diameter, OZD, and BCR are made, care must be taken to first maintain the AEL/AEC. Once these new parameters are ordered and with this new trial lens an alignment fit is achieved, then adjustments to the periphery can be made.

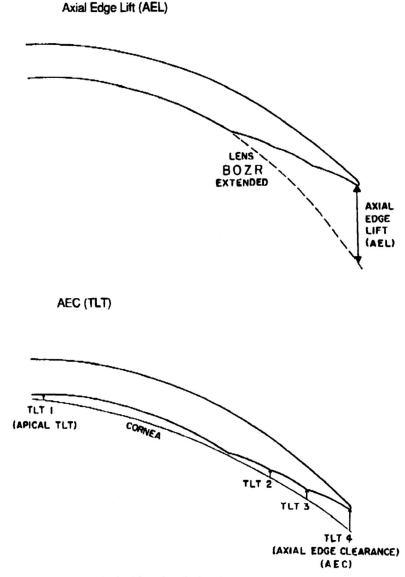

Axial Edge Lift (AEL)

AEC (TLT)

■ FIGURE 5.13 Axial edge lift and axial edge clearance.

Changes in AEL/AEC are made only after the central fluorescein pattern demonstrates an alignment fitting relationship.

Table 5.10 provides an average selection amount for the secondary and peripheral curve widths and BCR. Table 5.11 outlines the average amount that the BCR needs to be flattened to result in the radii of the secondary and peripheral curves to maintain an approximate AEL of 0.12 mm.

What is the bottom line? Only adjust the axial edge clearance as seen with the fluorescein pattern by adjusting either the SCR or PCR or SCW or PCW after an aligned central fluorescein pattern is achieved. These average values of AEL (plus AEC) are based on an average corneal eccentricity (as measured via a corneal topographer). Corneal *e*-values that are well outside that average will result in an aligned central fluorescein pattern but may demonstrate

TABLE 5.10 SCW, PCW, AND BCR SELECTION TO MAINTAIN AN APPROXIMATE AEL OF 0.12 MM

LENS DESIGN	WIDTHS
Tricurve	SCW = 0.25–0.35 mm
(lens diameter: 9.0–9.6 mm)	PCW = 0.30–0.40 mm
Tetracurve	SCW − 1 = 0.20 mm
(lens diameter: 9.7–10.2 mm)	PCW − 2 = 0.30 mm
OZD	= OAD − 1.1–1.6 mm

AEL, axial edge lift; BCR, base curve radius; OAD, overall diameter; OZD, optical zone diameter; PCW, peripheral curve width; SCW, secondary curve width.

either an insufficient (if *e*-value is much higher, 0.65–1.0) or excessive (if *e*-value is much lower, 0.25–0.40) axial edge clearance.

Center Thickness: As a general rule of thumb for lenses of high-Dk values, Table 5.12 offers some further suggestions to select center thickness (CT).

What is the bottom line? In choosing the most appropriate CT of a lens, consideration of the material Dk and thus resultant transmission of oxygen must be considered along with the factors that control lens flexure, including the amount of corneal astigmatism, lens-to-cornea fitting relationship, and material rigidity.

Edge Thickness Design: To maintain comfort with an interpalpebral lens design, the edge contour must be as thin and as smooth as possible. All plus lenses and high (>-4.00D) minus lenses are lenticulated with minus or plus carriers, respectively, to achieve the proper lens positioning to counter the forces of the center of gravity. This will allow plus lenses to sit up and more centrally and minus lenses to sit lower and more centrally from their usual positions on the eye. Excessively flat minus carriers (combined with excessive edge clearance) will result in superior lens positioning.

What is the bottom line? Look at the comfort of the patient and lens position to determine if an interpalpebral fitting has been achieved. If not, the FOZD that controls the size of the lenticular carrier and the edge thickness to improve both comfort and centration can be adjusted. The smaller the FOZD for a plus lens, the larger and more effect that the minus carrier will have in lifting the lens position. Conversely, the larger the FOZD for a minus lens, the

TABLE 5.11 SCR AND PCR TO MAINTAIN AN APPROXIMATE AEL OF 0.12 MM

LENS DESIGN	SCR/PCR
Tricurve	SCR = BCR + 0.8–1.0 mm (flatter)
(lens diameter = 9.0–9.6 mm)	PCR = BCR + 1.5–2.5 mm (flatter)
Tetracurve	SCR − 1 = BCR + 0.8–1 mm (flatter)
(lens diameter = 9.7–10.2 mm)	SCR − 2 = BCR + 1.5–2.5 mm (flatter)
	PCR = BCR + 2.5–3.5 mm (flatter)

AEL, axial edge lift; BCR, base curve radius; PCR, peripheral curve radius; SCR, secondary curve radius.

TABLE 5.12 CENTER THICKNESS (DK >50)

POWER	CT
Plano	0.02 mm
Minus	Subtract 0.02 mm per diopter of power from initial 0.20 mm up to a limit of CT = 0.10 mm
Plus	Add 0.20 mm per diopter of power from initial 0.20 mm up to a limit of CT = 0.30 mm, then lenticulate to keep CT low

CT, center thickness; Dk, oxygen permeability.

larger the effect of the plus carrier in lowering the lens position. Parameters of a typical inter-palpebral fitting set are provided in Table 5.13.

Power Determination and Lens Order

Once the proper lens design and an optimum lens-to-cornea fitting relationship have been achieved, determination of the final lens power can occur. This is obtained by a comprehensive overrefraction and an understanding of both tear layer optics and vertex distance.

TABLE 5.13 PARAMETERS OF A REPRESENTATIVE INTERPALPEBRAL FITTING SET

BCR	SCR/W	PCR/W	OAD/OZD	RX	AEL	REL	CT
8.55	9.44/.3	12.00/.4	9.8/8.4	−3.00	0.115	.094	.14
8.44	9.24/.3	11.75/.4	9.8/8.4	−3.00	0.114	.093	.14
8.33	9.10/.3	11.50/.4	9.8/8.4	−3.00	0.115	.093	.14
8.23	9.00/.3	11.50/.4	9.6/8.2	−3.00	0.115	.094	.14
8.13	8.90/.3	11.15/.4	9.6/8.2	−3.00	0.114	.093	.14
8.08	8.85/.3	11.00/.4	9.6/8.2	−3.00	0.114	.092	.11
8.04	8.80/.3	10.89/.4	9.6/8.2	−3.00	0.115	.092	.14
7.99	8.78/.3	10.70/.4	9.6/8.2	−3.00	0.114	.092	.11
7.94	8.75/.3	10.60/.4	9.6/8.2	−3.00	0.115	.092	.14
7.90	8.65/.3	10.50/.4	9.6/8.2	−3.00	0.114	.091	.11
7.85	8.55/.3	10.45/.4	9.6/8.2	−3.00	0.114	.091	.14
7.80	8.45/.3	10.40/.4	9.6/8.2	−3.00	0.115	.091	.11
7.76	8.50/.3	10.35/.4	9.4/8.0	−3.00	0.114	.091	.11
7.67	8.37/.3	10.15/.4	9.4/8.0	−3.00	0.114	.090	.11
7.58	8.20/.3	10.00/.4	9.4/8.0	−3.00	0.114	.090	.10
7.50	8.00/.3	9.95/.4	9.4/8.0	−3.00	0.114	.087	.11
7.42	8.32/.3	10.30/.3	9.2/8.0	−3.00	0.111	.087	.10
7.34	8.15/.3	10.45/.3	9.2/8.0	−3.00	0.116	.091	.11
7.18	7.87/.3	10.20/.3	9.2/8.0	−5.00	0.122	.094	.12
7.03	7.85/.3	9.95/.3	9.2/8.0	−5.00	0.128	.097	.12

AEL = 0.11 mm. Rx is in diopters; all other parameters are in millimeters.

AEL, axial edge lift; BCR, base curve radius; CT, center thickness; OAD, overall diameter; OZD, optical zone diameter; PCR/W, peripheral curve radius/width; REL, radial edge lift; SCR/W, secondary curve radius/width.

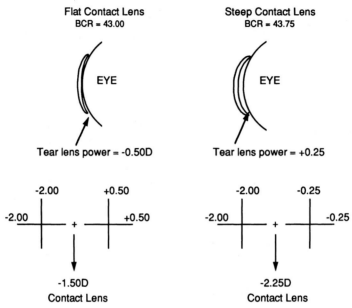

Refraction: -2.00 - 1.00 x 180

Keratometry Readings: 43.50 @ 180, 44.50 @ 90

■ FIGURE 5.14 Tear lens calculations in determining the final lens power.

Tear Layer Power: Tear layer power effects are important when a rigid contact lens is fitted either flatter or steeper than flat K. If a rigid lens is fitted flatter than flat K, a minus tear lens power is created; therefore, a correcting plus power is necessary. If a lens is fitted steeper than flat K, a plus tear lens power is created; therefore, a correcting minus power is indicated. For example, if a lens is fitted 0.50 D flatter than flat K on a cornea with a flat keratometry reading of 43.50 D, the tear layer power is equal to −0.50 D; therefore, +0.50 D is necessary to correct for the tear layer. If the spherical refractive value is equal to −2.00 D, the final predicted lens power is equal to −2.00 + (+0.50) = −1.50 D (Fig. 5.14).

If a lens is fitted 0.25 D steeper than the flat keratometry reading on a patient, a +0.25 D tear layer power is created; therefore, −0.25 D is necessary to correct it. If the spherical refractive value is equal to −2.00 D, the final predicted lens power will equal −2.00 + (−0.25) = −2.25 D. If a rigid lens is fitted on flat K or equal to the flat keratometry reading, the tear lens power is equal to zero. The predicted lens power is then equal to the spherical refractive value if the latter is < ±4 diopters. It is *incorrect* to assume that the final predicted lens power will be equal to the spherical equivalent (as is often true with soft lenses), unless the lens is being fitted one-half of the difference steeper than flat K.

Vertex Distance: Determination of the effective power at the corneal plane is another important factor to consider when fitting patients exhibiting either high myopia or hyperopia; specifically, the effective power difference becomes significant at ≥4 diopters of ametropia. The effective power at the corneal plane in all cases is always increased in plus relative to the spectacle plane. The first step in any contact lens-fitting process is to vertex the powers of both the flat and steep meridians to the corneal plane, assuming either a standard vertex distance or measuring it precisely.

Appendix 2 presents the difference in effective power from the spectacle to the corneal plane, assuming a 12-mm vertex distance. The formula for determining the effective power is as follows:

$$Fc = \frac{Fs}{1 - d(Fs)}$$

where

Fc = contact lens power
Fs = spectacle lens power
 d = distance between the spectacle lens and the contact lens in meters

If, for example, a 12-mm vertex distance is present and the patient's refractive error is equal to $-6.50 - 1.00 \times 180$, at the corneal plane this will equal the following:

$$\frac{-6.50}{1 - (0.012) \times -6.50} = -6.03 \text{ D}$$

$$\frac{-7.50}{1 - (0.012) \times -7.50} = -6.88 \text{ D}$$

Therefore, the spectacle prescription at the corneal plane is equal to $-6.03 - 0.85 \times 180$ or $-6.00 - 0.75 \times 180$. Especially for aphakic patients, this effective power difference becomes quite significant. For example:

$$\frac{+14.50}{1 - (0.012) \times +14.50} = +17.55 \text{ D}$$

$$\frac{+11.50}{1 - (0.012) \times +11.50} = +13.34 \text{ D}$$

It is important to measure vertex distance because it can vary between patients; this factor increases in importance as the ametropia increases.

Ordering: Before fitting GP diagnostic lenses, it is desirable to indicate the predicted vertexed lens powers on the fitting form. In addition, information pertaining to the diagnostic lens parameters, lens-to-cornea fitting relationship, and overrefraction should also be provided. Table 5.14 shows an example of the fitting information and resultant order for a high myopic patient.

The predicted lens power can be obtained from simply adding the best sphere overrefraction value to the contact lens power. For example:

Keratometry:	42.50 @ 180; 42.75 @ 090
Spectacle refraction:	$-6.50 - 0.25 \times 180$
Effective power:	$-6.00 - 0.25 \times 180$
Base curve radius:	42.00 D or 0.50 D flatter than K (using aforementioned lid attachment philosophy)
Predicted lens power:	Spherical refractive value at the corneal plane – tear lens power
	$= -6.00 - (-0.50)$
	$= -5.50$ D

TABLE 5.14 FITTING FORM AND FINAL LENS ORDER

Patient data (OD only):	
Keratometry readings: 42.50 @ 180/42.75 @ 090	
Spectacle refraction: −6.50 − 0.25 × 180 20/20	
Vertexed to corneal plane: −6.00 − 0.25 × 180	
Predicted Lenses (OD only): BCR 8.04, OAD 9.4, Power −5.50	
Diagnostic lens	FP 30
BCR/OAD/Rx/CT	8.04/9.4/−4.00/.14
Fluorescein pattern	Mild apical touch/alignment pattern
Position and lag	Superior central with 2-mm lag
Retinoscopy/VA	−1.50 20/20
Best sphere/VA	−1.50 20/20
Final Design and Order (OD only)	
BCR	8.04 mm
SCR/W	8.9/.03 mm
ICR/W	9.9/0.2 mm
PCR/W	11.3/0.2 mm
OZD	8.0 mm
OAD	9.4 mm
Power	−5.50 D
CT	0.14 mm
Blend	Medium
Lenticular	Plus
Tint	Blue
Material	FP 30

BCR, base curve radius; CT, center thickness; ICR/W, intermediate curve radius/width; OAD, overall diameter; OZD, optical zone diameter; PCR/W, peripheral curve radius/width; SCR/W, secondary curve radius/width; VA, visual acuity.

In the previous example, the overrefraction values equaled the predicted. In many cases this does not occur because of several factors, including the following:

1. Inaccurate refraction.
2. Inaccurate keratometry values.
3. Base curve radius not equal to desired.
4. Lens power not as ordered.
5. Flexure.
6. Lens decentration.

If this discrepancy is only 0.25 D, it is probably not significant; if it is a higher amount, the other factors should be ruled out prior to ordering the lenses. This is one of many important reasons for using diagnostic lenses as opposed to fitting empirically since the final power derived from adding the overrefraction with the diagnostic lens power will usually be more successful than selecting the lens power based on the predicted values. In addition, in some cases a large amount of residual astigmatism is predicted; therefore, spherical rigid lenses may not be desirable. However, on performing an overrefraction, if very little or no cylinder is present and the patient is satisfied with the vision obtained with a spherical overrefraction, success should be achieved.

Other Important Design/Fitting Considerations

Standard Versus Custom Lens Design

Many practitioners order lenses using a standard design. Typically, the base curve radius, over-all diameter, and power are ordered with the manufacturer using its own design to determine such parameters as thicknesses, peripheral curves, and optical zone. This method has the advantage of being less time consuming, and if difficulty is experienced by the practitioner in determining what other parameter specifications to provide, an experienced laboratory should be able to assist in developing an effective design for a given GP material. The disadvantages of this option versus custom lens design are that it takes some control away from the practitioner and no one parameter such as overall diameter, optical zone diameter, center thickness, or peripheral curve system will be successful on every patient. Nevertheless, with the ability to manufacture thin designs in aspheric and pseudoaspheric designs, the current generation of standard designs has been quite successful and practically every laboratory has, at minimum, one standard design available to practitioners.

Aspheric Design

Although knowledge of the role and design of specific base curve radii, peripheral curve radii, and optical zone diameter is important, the use of aspheric designs is increasing in popularity. This section will discuss the benefits, applications, and fitting considerations of the various types of aspheric lens designs.

Definitions: The term *aspheric* can simply be described as "not spherical" as it pertains to the cornea. In other words, the cornea is not a sphere but gradually flattens from center to periphery. Therefore, an aspheric lens design typically consists of a design that gradually flattens, often at a similar—if not greater—rate than the cornea.

The term *eccentricity*, which has been loosely defined as the rate of corneal flattening, is actually the deviation from a circular path. A circle has an eccentricity value equal to zero. A value between zero and one is termed an *ellipse*. With this definition, the cornea would be an ellipse as it has an average eccentricity value of about 0.4.[73] Some corneas exhibit a greater rate of paracentral flattening, therefore having a higher eccentricity (or *e*) value. An eccentricity value >1.0 is termed a *hyperbola*. Some presbyopic lens designs, as a result of the greater plus power generated with higher than 1.0 eccentricity, use hyperbolic aspheric designs. In addition, some single-vision aspheric designs have a hyperbolic periphery to allow for good tear exchange.

Benefits/Disadvantages: The benefits of aspheric designs include the following:

- An alignment lens-to-cornea fitting relationship resulting from the posterior lens design shape approximating the corneal shape.[74,75]
- Better initial comfort resulting from the elimination of both localized bearing areas on the cornea and peripheral curve junctions.[75,76]
- Better centration on against-the-rule and irregular astigmatic corneas.[77]
- Easier to fit and design because of the reduced number of parameters and the reduced importance of the base curve radius in most aspheric designs.[78]

Some of the perceived/experienced problems with aspheric designs include the following[76]:

- Reduced vision because of poor-quality optics.
- Variable vision if lens decentration is present.
- Difficult to verify because of variable optical quality.

Applications: There are numerous applications for aspheric designs, including the following[77,78]:

- Patients experiencing decentration with other spherical lens designs.
- Patients with irregular corneas or against-the-rule astigmatism.

- Pre-presbyopic and incipient presbyopic patients.
- Computer users.
- Myopic patients with a poor accommodation convergence/accommodation (AC/A) relationship.

Lens Designs: There are many types of aspheric and "pseudoaspheric" lens designs.[78] It is important for practitioners to understand the differences between these designs, which can be placed into the following four categories:

Pseudoaspheric: These designs typically consist of a series of well-blended peripheral curves. If well manufactured, these designs have benefits over other more conventional spherical lens designs. These designs tend to vary in their effectiveness, and a recent study found no difference in performance between a conventional design and a pseudoaspheric design.[79] It is important for practitioners to use good judgment when considering use of these designs, which are often advertised as being "aspheric-like."

Spherical Optical Zone/Aspheric Periphery: These are typically designs in which the aspheric periphery is tangential to the spherical optical zone diameter (in other words, the transition from the optical zone to the periphery is a continuous curve). The optical zone is rarely larger than 6 mm in these lenses, and the clinical performance is typically superior to blended bicurve and tricurve lens designs. An aspheric periphery, while similar to a well-blended spherical periphery, provides a more uniform edge lift and can be maintained with greater consistency and accuracy on replacement lenses.

Aspheric Optical Zone/Aspheric Periphery: These lenses have a totally aspheric posterior surface; however, the optical zone and the periphery are two different curves. This design should, in theory, provide more uniform alignment by means of a more uniform tear layer both centrally and midperipherally.

The EnVision (Bausch & Lomb) has an elliptical optical zone equal to approximately 0.4 and a hyperbolic periphery that is tangential to the optical zone. The term *bi-aspheric* has been used to describe this design configuration. The clinical results with the EnVision and its early-generation predecessors have been favorable. It is apparent that the selection of base curve radii in 0.1-mm steps is sufficient. It has provided better initial comfort than spherical lens designs,[75] and it is claimed to have excellent centration characteristics.[74] In addition, as a result of the limited parameters necessary with this design, the ability to inventory this lens is easily obtained.

Single Aspheric Curve Posterior Surface: These conicoid lenses are typically elliptical in design. More information about these designs will be forthcoming in the future.

Fitting Considerations: Several lens design and fitting considerations are important:

- The importance of using a diagnostic set is essential as a result of the design characteristics of every type of aspheric lens.
- Dependence on central keratometry readings is not recommended with these designs as the fitting relationship of a lens of any given base curve radius is determined by the shape of the paracentral, not the central, cornea.
- Because of the proximity of posterior lens design to cornea and the corresponding uniform tear layer thickness, small incremental changes in base curve radius are usually unnecessary.
- As a result of all of the differing types of aspheric designs with variations in posterior surface geometry, eccentricity, and manufacturing methods, one should not make generalizations about aspheric designs without referring to a specific aspheric design.[75]

Topography-Assisted Lens Design

Corneal topography, to check for regularity of the corneal astigmatism, whether the astigmatism is centrally located or extends out to the limbus, the eccentricity values (*e*-values), and the simulated K readings, is essential to determine the base curve (or BOZR) that will result in an aligned fluorescein pattern according to the amount of corneal astigmatism and lens diameter. The shape of the cornea resembles a prolate ellipse. The *e*-value is a measure of the rate of flattening from the center of the cornea to the periphery. For an average eye, this value is between 0.40 and 0.57.[80–82]

The use of corneal topography instrumentation can be a valuable asset for any practitioner desiring to increase contact lens patient satisfaction and success. This is especially important as it has been found that only 40% of lenses fitted empirically, using keratometry and refraction only, resulted in first fit success.[83,84] However, it was also found that in 88% of the cases in which lenses were changed, the change in lens parameters originated from midperipheral differences between corneal shape as originated with corneal topography and lens shape as predicted from keratometry readings. In other words, the great majority of lens-to-cornea fitting relationships could have been optimized before fitting if corneal topography data would have been used.

Corneal topography instrumentation can provide the practitioner with much more information about the cornea (apex location, rate of flattening, irregularity) while simplifying the fitting process via obtaining recommended lens design information based on corneal topography. The lens design parameters can be changed and their effect on a simulated fluorescein pattern viewed. These software programs typically have a recommended design philosophy, which should result in an alignment or near-alignment simulated fluorescein pattern. The practitioner often has the option of custom designing the lenses as well. One of the most important benefits of all such programs is the ability to view a simulated fluorescein pattern before diagnostic lens application. The proximity of the posterior lens surface to the anterior surface of the cornea and the thickness of the layer of tear fluid in between can be viewed in various shades of green. This allows lens fitting with a pre-evaluation of the actual lens base curve-to-cornea fitting relationship via the tear lens thickness, rather than a numeric estimate provided by keratometry. Often it is possible to make lens design changes and then, by recalculating, the revised simulated fluorescein pattern can be observed. Therefore, changes in peripheral curve radii and widths (i.e., edge clearance), diameter, and base curve radius can be made and the revised fluorescein pattern determined before lens application. There have been reports of ≥90% patients having a similar fluorescein pattern with their actual lens as that simulated with topography-based contact lens software.[85–87] When differences do exist, they may be attributed to software limitations such as an absence of simulated lens movement, flexure, lid position and tension, and corneal periphery topographic data inaccuracy.[88,89] However, the programs continue to improve and some programs provide the ability to simulate such factors as lens decentration and tilt. Several software programs have the capability of sending information, including contact lens orders, topography information, etc., to contact lens laboratories or other practitioners. In addition, several manufacturers are interfacing their CNC computer-driven lathes with topography software programs so that the practitioner can send topography information and lens parameters directly to the manufacturer.

The Laboratory Consultant

One of the greatest underutilized resources is the GP laboratory consultant. These individuals can assist in such factors as advising on which material(s) to recommend, providing diagnostic fitting sets and inventories, and offering lens design advice on specific cases. An experienced consultant will often provide an opinion based on the experience of designing thousands of lenses for similar patients. The specialty lens designs and custom fits are typically the consultant's specialty. Likewise, with increasing use of corneal topography to assist in GP specialty fits, many laboratories are set up to assist practitioners in interpreting the maps and making recommendations. Many consultants are familiar with the software and pertinent data from multiple topographers, and those data are influential in choosing a specific design.

■ SUMMARY

The importance of diagnostic fitting, comprehensive fluorescein evaluation, and selection of the appropriate lens design parameters for a given material are paramount to successful fitting of gas-permeable lenses. As shown in Figure 5.10, there are several important factors to consider when determining the final lens parameters for a given patient. If careful attention is devoted to proper design and evaluation, a high success rate with GP lenses should be expected.

■ CLINICAL CASES

CASE 1

A 12-year-old progressive myopic patient had complaints of peripheral corneal ulcers as well as blurred vision from her (nonsilicone hydrogel) soft toric lenses. She had been fitted into soft torics 2 years previously because that was the recommendation of her practitioner. In addition, she plays soccer throughout the year. Her manifest refraction was the following:

$$OD: -3.25 - 2.25 \times 007$$
$$OS: -2.75 - 2.00 \times 177$$

Slit-lamp evaluation: Both lenses tended to rotate approximately 10 to 15 degrees with the blink and were slow to return to a set position.

SOLUTION: GP lenses were mentioned as a viable option. The patient commented that she has heard that "hard lenses hurt." She was reassured that there is some initial lid awareness because of the smaller size and the greater movement present with the blink, but that she will adapt and should achieve total comfort with the lenses. In addition, she was advised that this is both a healthier alternative and one that should provide improved, and more consistent, vision. A topical anesthetic was applied immediately before fitting her from the Naturalens inventory. This type of design is very good for young athletes because of the large overall diameter and low edge lift, both combining to minimize decentration and loss. Fitting from an inventory also allowed the patient to experience good vision after the initial application of GP lenses. If an inventory is not available, empirical fitting would be recommended to provide the same benefit, good initial vision.

CASE 2

The practitioner uses PMMA lenses of the following design for diagnostic fitting purposes, and a good lens-to-cornea fitting relationship is obtained OU:

BCR: 7.81 mm
OAD/OZD: 8.8 mm/7.4 mm
PCR/W: 12.25 mm/0.7 mm
CT: 0.12 mm

The lenses are ordered with only BCR, power, and diameter indicated to the laboratory. When the lenses arrive, they decenter inferiorly on the patient.

The laboratory has provided lenses in a 60-Dk material in the following parameters:

BCR: 7.81 mm
OAD/OZD: 8.8 mm/7.8 mm
SCR/W: 9.0 mm/0.3 mm; PCR/W: 11.00 mm/0.2 mm
CT: 0.17 mm

SOLUTION: This is an example in which the use of a different material and design for diagnostic fitting from what was ordered occurred, resulting in a less than desirable fitting relationship.

The lenses received from the laboratory were much thicker, which contributed to a change in the fit. In addition, the optical zone diameter was larger and the edge clearance was less. Diagnostic fitting of GP lenses should be with the same (or similar) material and design as that to be ordered. In this particular case, another diagnostic fitting with the same material is indicated.

CASE 3

An alignment lens-to-cornea fitting relationship and good centration has been achieved with the following lens design:

BCR: 7.89 mm
OAD/OZD: 8.8 mm/7.2 mm

However, good pupillary coverage is not present because of the patient's large pupil size. A larger diagnostic lens in this material is not available. An approximate 0.5-mm larger optical zone should be necessary to avoid subjective complaints of flare.

What base curve radius should be ordered?

SOLUTION: To maintain an alignment lens-to-cornea fitting relationship, for every 0.5-mm increase in optical zone, a 0.25 D flatter base curve radius should be selected. Therefore, the following design should be ordered:

BCR: 7.94 mm
OAD/OZD: 9.3 mm/7.7 mm

CASE 4

What material, diagnostic lens, and predicted overrefraction would you expect with the following daily-wear patient?

OD Keratometry: 42.00 @ 180; 42.50 @ 090
Refraction: $-2.50 - 0.50 \times 180$

SOLUTION: A low-Dk (25–50) lens material is recommended. According to the authors' recommended design philosophy, a base curve radius 0.50 D flatter than K or equal to 41.50 (8.13 mm) should be used. If this diagnostic lens has a power equal to −3.00 D, the predicted overrefraction is equal to the following:

$$[-2.50 \text{ D (sphere value)} - (-)0.50 \text{ D (tear lens)}]$$
$$- (-)3.00 \text{ D (diagnostic lens)} = +1.00 \text{ D}$$

CASE 5

What material, diagnostic lens, and predicted overrefraction would you expect with the following daily-wear patient?

OS Keratometry: 41.00 @ 180; 42.25 @ 090
Refraction: $+3.00 - 1.25 \times 180$

If the overrefraction equals the predicted values and an optimum fitting relationship is obtained, using the authors' recommended design philosophy, what final lens design parameters would you recommend?

SOLUTION: Since hyperopic patients benefit from a higher-Dk material for optimum oxygen transmission, selecting a >50-Dk GP lens material is recommended. A slightly steep base curve radius equal to 0.25 D steeper than K or 41.25 (8.18 mm) is recommended for diagnostic purposes. If this lens has a power equal to +3.00 D, the predicted overrefraction is equal to the following:

$$[+3.00 \text{ D (sphere value)} - (+)0.25 \text{ D (tear lens)}]$$
$$- (+)3.00 \text{ D (diagnostic lens)} = -0.25 \text{ D}$$

The lens power would equal the diagnostic lens + overrefraction = +3.00 D + (−)0.25 D = +2.75 D. The final order would be the following:

Material	BCR	OAD/OZD	Power	SCR/W	ICR/W	PCR/W	CT	Edge
Fluoroperm 60	8.18 mm	9.4/8.0 mm	+2.75 D	9.00/0.3	10.00/0.2	11.40/0.2	Min.	−Lent.

CASE 6

What diagnostic lens and predicted overrefraction would you expect with this patient?

OD Keratometry: 43.50 @ 180; 44.50 @ 090
Refraction: −6.75 − 1.25 × 180

If the overrefraction equals the expected values and an optimum fitting relationship is obtained, using the authors' recommended design philosophy, what are the recommended final lens design parameters?

SOLUTION: The first step is to vertex the refraction to the corneal plane:

Vertexed refraction: −6.25 − 1.00 × 180

Next, select a base curve radius 0.25 D flatter than K or equal to 43.25 (7.81 mm). The predicted overrefraction for a −6.00 D diagnostic lens power would equal the following:

[−6.25 D (sphere value) − (−)0.25 D (tear lens)]
− (−)6.00 D (diagnostic lens) = plano

The final lens parameters would equal the following:

BCR	OAD/OZD	Power	SCR/W	ICR/W	PCR/W	CT	Edge
7.81 mm	9.2/7.8 mm	−6.00 D	8.60/0.3	9.60/0.2	11.00/0.2	0.13	+Lent.

CASE 7

A 45-year-old female came in for a progress check on her GP lenses. She has been a GP lens wearer for many years, and her current pair of Boston ES is 2 years old. She wears her lenses 14 hours a day, 7 days a week. Her vision has always been better in her left eye than right eye when wearing contact lenses.

Lenses off:

Keratometry: OD 41.50 @ 180; 42.00 @ 090 −0.50 × 180
OS 42.50 @ 180; 42.12 @ 090 −0.62 × 180
Subjective refraction: OD −2.75 − 0.75 × 090
OS: −3.00 DS

Present GP parameters:

Material	BCR	SCR/W	PCR/W	OZD	OAD	Power	CT	AEL	Blend
OD Boston ES	8.15	9.10/0.3	11.60/0.4	8.2	9.6	−3.00	0.16	0.12	med
OS Boston ES	8.15	9.10/0.3	11.60/.04	8.2	9.6	−2.50	0.16	0.12	med

Biomicroscopy:

Current lens appearance (OD and OS)
Lag = 1.5 mm
Well centered; held in place with upper lid
Some scratches and film observed on lens surface
Fluorescein pattern: center thin, even layer of fluorescein; midperiphery has slight bearing; edge clearance of approximately 0.5 mm
Visual acuity (VA): OD 6/7.5 − 1 OS 6/6

OVERKERATOMETRY (GP):

OD: 39.50 @ 180/39.00 @ 090
OS: 39.87 @ 180/39.50 @ 090 Ret (sph/cyl):

OD: pl − 1.25 × 090 VA 6/4.5
OS: +0.25 − 0.50 × 090 VA 6/4.5

Problems include the following:

1. Reduced visual acuity OD because of uncorrected residual astigmatism

$$\text{OD: CRA} = \text{spectacle cyl} - \text{delta K}$$
$$= -0.75 \times 090 + (-0.50 \times 180) = -1.25 \times 090$$

$$\text{OS: CRA} = \text{spectacle cyl} - \text{delta K}$$
$$= 0.00 + (-0.62 \times 180) = -0.62 \times 090$$

2. Scratched and deposited lenses OU

SOLUTION:

1. Correct for the residual astigmatism by ordering new lenses with decreased center thickness to increase flexure.
2. Order new lenses.

Final lens parameters

Material	BCR	SCR/W	PCR/W	OZD	OAD	Power	CT	AEL	Blend
OD Optimum Extreme	8.15	9.10/0.3	11.60/0.4	8.2	9.6	−3.00	0.13	0.12	med
OS Optimum Extreme	8.15	9.10/0.3	11.60/0.4	8.2	9.6	−2.50	0.14	0.12	med

CLINICAL PROFICIENCY CHECKLIST

- It is important to discuss GPs with all new patients in a neutral, nonthreatening manner.

- Topical anesthetic use can be very beneficial in assisting the patient over the initial psychological hurdle of wearing GPs while accelerating the fitting process.

- The use of GP diagnostic lenses will reduce lens replacement and increase both patient compliance and patient confidence in the practitioner. However, many patients, especially those apprehensive about GP lenses, would benefit from experiencing the clear vision obtained from lenses received via empirical fitting or from an inventory.

- Standard GP diagnostic fits should include −3.00 D power lenses in both low-Dk (<50) and high-Dk (>50) materials, +3.00 D power lenses with a minus lenticular edge in a high-Dk material, and −8.00 D power lenses with a plus lenticular edge in a low-Dk material. A good average OAD/OZD is 9.2 mm/7.8 mm; a BCR range from 40.75 to 45.50 D in 0.25 D steps is also recommended.

- The use of fluorescein is essential for rigid lens assessment. Educational resources are available from the GP Lens Institute, the educational division of the CLMA.

- The use of a larger OAD with flatter BCR (i.e., <41 D) and a smaller OAD with steeper BCR (i.e., >45 D) is recommended. In addition, the BCR should be flattened by 0.25 D for each 0.5-mm increase in OZD; likewise, the BCR should be steepened by 0.25 D for each 0.5-mm decrease in OZD.

- The use of several peripheral curve radii (i.e., tetracurve or aspheric design) is recommended to better align the lens periphery with the cornea. Prevent possible corneal desiccation and edge awareness by the use of a wide, flat peripheral curve with the traditional PMMA bicurve design.

- It is important to verify center thickness; often the contact lenses may be thicker than requested, which results in increased lens mass and possibly inferior decentration.

- Edge verification is essential as a rolled, tapered edge will optimize patient comfort.

- The use of a minus lenticular edge design is recommended for <−1.50 D and all plus powers; a plus lenticular edge design is recommended for all lenses with −5.00 D and higher lens powers.

(continued)

(Continued)

■ The tear lens power and vertex distance must be considered when determining contact lens power.

■ Modern low eccentricity single-vision aspheric designs have the potential benefits of enhancing centration, better initial comfort, and ease of fit.

■ Topography-assisted designs have several benefits including making the design process simpler, simulating lens fitting characteristics on the eye, and on-line transmission of order and topography information to the laboratory.

■ The laboratory consultant can be invaluable in assisting with GP lens design, material, and fitting.

REFERENCES

1. Polse KA, Graham AD, Fusaro RE, et al. Predicting RGP daily wear success. CLAO J 1999;25:152–158.
2. Bennett ES. Be flexible about rigid lenses. Rev Cornea Contact Lenses 2007;May:38–40.
3. Bennett ES, Stulc S, Bassi CJ, et al. Effect of patient personality profile and verbal presentation on successful rigid contact lens adaptation, satisfaction and compliance. Optom Vis Sci 1998;75(7):500–505.
4. Quinn TG. Presenting the GP lens option. Contact Lens Spectrum 2004;19(10):41.
5. Jervey JW. Topical anesthetic for the eye: a comparative study. South J Med 1989;48:770–774.
6. Lyle WM, Page C. Possible adverse effects from local anesthetics and the treatment of these reactions. Am J Optom Physiol Opt 1975;52:736–744.
7. Bennett ES, Smythe J, Henry VA, et al. The effect of topical anesthetic use on initial patient satisfaction and overall success with rigid gas permeable contact lenses. Optom Vis Sci 1998;75:800–805.
8. Schnider CM. Anesthetics and RGPs: crossing the controversial line. Rev Optom 1996;133:41–43.
9. Gordon A, Bartlett JD, Lin M. The effect of diclofenac sodium on the initial comfort of RGP contact lenses: a pilot study. J Am Optom Assoc 1999;70:509–512.
10. Caroline PJ, Andre MP. NSAIDs in RGP adaptation. Contact Lens Spectrum 2001;16(5):56.
11. Bennett ES. Basic fitting. In: Bennett ES, Weissman BA, eds. Clinical Contact Lens Practice, 2nd ed. Philadelphia: Lippincott Williams & Wilkins, 2005:255–275.
12. Ames K. Rethink your approach to RGP lenses. Contact Lens Spectrum 1993;8:24–27.
13. Lebow KA. Fitting accuracy of an arc step-based contact lens module. Contact Lens Spectrum 1997;12(11):25–30.
14. Soper B, Shovlin J, Bennett ES. Evaluating a topography software based program for fitting RGPs. Contact Lens Spectrum 1996;11(10):37–40.
15. Szczotka LB. Clinical evaluation of a topographically based contact lens fitting software. Optom Vis Sci 1997;74: 14–19.
16. Evardson WT, Douthwaite WA. Contact lens back surface specification from the EyeSys videokeratoscope. Contact Lens Ant Eye 1999;22:76–82.
17. Bennett ES, Henry VA, Davis LJ, et al. Comparing empirical and diagnostic fitting of daily wear fluoro-silicone/acrylate contact lenses. Contact Lens Forum 1989;14:38–44.
18. Davis R, Keech P, Dubow B, et al. Making RGP fitting efficient and successful. Contact Lens Spectrum 2000; 15(10):40–47.
19. Keech P. The top 10 reasons to inventory RGPs. Contact Lens Spectrum 1996;11(10):32–36.
20. Snyder C, Daum KM, Campbell JB. Rigid contact lens base curve constancy between wet and dry lens storage conditions. J Am Optom Assoc 1990;61(3):184–187.
21. Szczotka LB. In-office RGP lens disinfection. Contact Lens Spectrum 2001;16(11):17.
22. Mandell RB. Trial lens method. In: Mandell RB, ed. Contact Lens Practice, 4th ed. Springfield, IL: Charles C. Thomas, 1988:243–264.
23. Herman JP. Managing the delayed allergic response in CL patients. Presented at the annual American Optometric Association Contact Lens Section Symposium, Williamsburg, VA, October 1990.
24. Korb DR. Recent developments in the observation of the cornea-lens relationship. In: Encyclopedia of Contact Lens Practice, vol. 3. South Bend, IN: International Optics, 1959–1963:98–101.
25. Courtney RC, Lee JM. Predicting ocular intolerance of a contact lens solution by use of a filter system enhancing fluorescein staining detection. Int Contact Lens Clin 1982;9(5):302–310.
26. Swarbrick HA, Hiew R, Kee AV, et al. Apical clearance rigid contact lenses induce corneal steepening. Optom Vis Sci 2004;81(6):427–435.
27. Young G. Fluorescein in rigid lens fit evaluation. Int Contact Lens Clin 1988;15(3):95–100.

28. Bennett ES, Barr JT, Johnson J. Unmasking the RGP fit with fluorescein. Contact Lens Spectrum 1998;13(10): 31–38.
29. Edmund C. Location of the corneal apex and its influence on the stability of the central corneal curvature. A photokeratoscopy study. Am J Optom Physiol Opt 1987;64(11):846–852.
30. Rowsey JJ, Reynolds AE, Brown R. Corneal topography. Corneascope. Arch Ophthalmol 1981;99:1093–1100.
31. Davis LJ, Bennett ES. Fluorescein patterns in UV-absorbing rigid contact lenses. Contact Lens Spectrum 1989; 4(8):49.
32. Sorbara L, Fonn D, Holden BA, et al. Centrally fitted versus upper lid-attached rigid gas permeable lenses. Part I. Design parameters affecting vertical decentration. Int Contact Lens Clin 1996;23(5&6):99–104.
33. Sorbara L, Fonn D, Holden BA, et al. Centrally fitted versus upper lid-attached rigid gas permeable lenses. Part II: a comparison of the clinical performance. Int Contact Lens Clin 1996;23(7&8):121–126.
34. Caroline PJ, Norman CW. A blueprint for RGP design. Part 1. Contact Lens Spectrum 1988;3(11):39–49.
35. Bennett ES. Lens design, fitting and troubleshooting. In: Bennett ES, Grohe RM, eds. Rigid Gas-Permeable Contact Lenses. Boston: Butterworths, 1986:189–224.
36. Korb DR, Korb JE. A new concept in contact lens design. I and II. J Am Optom Assoc 1970;41(2):1023–1032.
37. Bier N, Lowther GE. Lens design. In: Bier N, Lowther GE, eds. Contact Lens Correction. London: Butterworths, 1977:207–225.
38. Lowther GE. Review of rigid contact lens design and effects of design and lens fit. Int Contact Lens Clin 1988; 15(12):378–389.
39. Lowther GE, Hill RM. Sensitivity thresholds of the lower lid margin in the course of adaptation to contact lenses. Am J Optom 1968;45:587–594.
40. Hazlett R. Custom designing large-diameter rigid gas permeable contact lenses: a clinical approach intended to optimize lens comfort. Int Contact Lens Clin 1997;24(1):5–9.
41. Szczotka LB. RGP parameter changes: how much change is significant? Contact Lens Spectrum 2001;16(4):18.
42. Herman JP. Flexure of rigid contact lenses on toric lenses as a function of base curve fitting relationship. J Am Optom Assoc 1983;54(3):209–213.
43. Henry VA, Bennett ES, Forrest JF. A clinical investigation of the Paraperm EW rigid gas permeable contact lens. Am J Optom Physiol Opt 1987;14(8):313–320.
44. Bibby MM. Factors affecting peripheral curve design. Am J Optom Physiol Opt 1979;56(1):2–9.
45. Honan PR, Morgan JF, Dabezies OH. Nomenclature, lens design, and fitting parameters. In: Dabezies OH, ed. CLAO Guide to Contact Lenses. Orlando, FL: Grune & Stratton, 1984:22.1–22.17.
45a. Picciano S, Andrasko GJ. Which factors influence RGP lens comfort? Contact Lens Spectrum 1989;4(5):31–33.
45b. Young G. The effect of rigid lens design on fluorescein fit. Contact Lens Ant Eye 1998;21(2):41–46.
46. Atkinson TCO. The design of the back surface of gas permeable lenses. J Br Contact Lens Assoc 1982;5(1):16–30.
47. Bennett ES. Silicone/acrylate lens design. Int Contact Lens Clinic 1985;12(1):45–53.
48. Jackson JM. We have (edge) liftoff. Contact Lens Spectrum 2005;20(4):21.
49. van der Worp E, de Brabander J. Contact lens fitting today part one: modern RGP lens fitting. Optom Today 2005;July:27–32.
50. Edrington T, Barr JT. We have edge lift. Contact Lens Spectrum 2002;17(10):49.
51. Stone J. Designing hard lenses in the 1980s. J Br Contact Lens Assoc 1982;4(4):130–137.
52. Poster MG. Clinical evaluation of the Polycon 8.5 design. J Am Optom Assoc 1981;52(3):243–246.
53. Doane M, Gleason W. Tear film interaction with RGP contact lenses. Presented at the First International Material Science Symposium, St. Louis, March 1988.
54. Williams CE. New design concepts for permeable rigid contact lenses. J Am Optom Assoc 1979;50(3):331–336.
55. Swarbrick HA, Holden BA. Rigid gas permeable lens binding: significance and contributing factors. Am J Optom Physiol Opt 1987;64(11):815–823.
56. Zabkiewicz KR, Terry R, Holden BA, et al. The frequency of rigid lens binding in extended wear increases with time. Am J Optom Physiol Opt 1987;64:110P.
57. Grohe RM, Lebow KA. Vascularized limbal keratitis. Int Contact Lens Clin 1989;16(7,8):197–209.
58. Andrasko G. Center thickness: an important RGP parameter. Contact Lens Forum 1989;14(6):40–41.
59. Toscano F, Bridgewater B. A comparative study of RGP materials in thin lens designs. Contact Lens Spectrum 1997;12(10):25–28.
60. Croatt C, Wing F. An RGP lens with a soft lens fit. Contact Lens Spectrum 2000;15(6):49–52.
61. Norman C. Today's RGPs: better performance through innovative technology. Contact Lens Spectrum 1996;11(11).
62. Achiron LR. Custom-designed ultra-thin RGP lenses. Contact Lens Spectrum 2001;16(5):40–45.
63. Cornish R, Sulaiman S. Do thinner rigid gas permeable contact lenses provide superior initial comfort? Optom Vis Sci 1996;73(3):139–143.
64. Nelson JM, Huff J, Bennett ES, et al. Evaluation of variation in oxygen transmission in rigid contact lens extended wear. CLAO J 1989;15:125–133.
65. Hill RM, Brezinski SD. The center thickness factor. Contact Lens Spectrum 1987;2(10):52–54.
66. Campbell R, Caroline P. Don't take RGP lens edge design for granted. Contact Lens Spectrum 1997;12(7):56.

67. Andrasko GJ. Keeping your eye on edge quality. Contact Lens Spectrum 1991;6(9):37–39.
68. Morris DS, Lowther GE. A comparison of different rigid contact lenses: edge thickness and contours. J Am Optom Assoc 1981;52(3):247–249.
69. LaHood D. The edge shape and comfort of rigid lenses. Am J Optom Physiol Opt 1988;65(8):613.
70. Andrasko GJ, Stahl B. Hard choices made easy. Rev Optom 1986;123(4):85–86.
71. Snyder C. Designing minus carrier RGP lenses. Contact Lens Spectrum 1998;13(12):20.
72. Atkinson TCO. A computer assisted and clinical assessment of current trends in gas-permeable lens design. Optician 1985;Jan:16–22.
73. Editorial staff. Hard gas permeable elliptical lenses. Optician 1986;5075(192):19–20.
74. Bennett ES, Henry VA, Seibel DB, et al. Clinical evaluation of the Boston Equacurve. Contact Lens Forum 1987;12(4):65.
75. Andrasko GJ. A comfort comparison. Contact Lens Spectrum 1989;4(4):49–52.
76. Ames KS, Erickson P. Optimizing aspheric and spheric rigid lens performance. CLAO J 1987;13(3):165–170.
77. Goldberg JB. Aspheric corneal lenses for nonpresbyopic and presbyopic patients. Contact Lens Spectrum 1990;5(4):71–74.
78. Feldman GE, Bennett ES. Aspheric lens designs. In: Bennett ES, Weissman BA, eds. Clinical Contact Lens Practice. Philadelphia: JB Lippincott, 1991:1–10.
79. Snyder C, Poling T. Does the Starlens clinically differ from a conventional tricurve design? Contact Lens Spectrum 1990;5(4):33–38.
80. Carney LG, Mainstone JC, Henderson BA. Corneal topography and myopia: a cross-sectional study. Invest Ophthalmol Vis Sci 1997;38:311–320.
81. Eghbali F, Yeung KK, Maloney RK. Topographic determination of corneal asphericity and its lack of effect on the refractive outcome of radial keratotomy. Am J Ophthalmol 1995;119:275–280.
82. Guillon M, Lydon DP, Wilson C. Corneal topography: a clinical model. Ophthalmol Physiol Opt 1986;6:47–56.
83. van der Worp E. Respecting the shape of the cornea in RGP fitting. Optom Pract 2004;5:153–162.
84. van der worp E, de Brabander J, Lubberman B, et al. Optimising RGP fitting in normal eyes using 3D topography data. Contact Lens Ant Eye 2002;11:1–5.
85. Dubow B. Corneal topography and RGP fitting in a managed care world. Eyecare Technol 1996;6(1):61–63.
86. Soper B, Shovlin J, Bennett ES. Evaluating a topography software based program for fitting RGPs. Contact Lens Spectrum 1996;11(10):37–40.
87. Szczotka LB. Clinical evaluation of a topographically based contact lens fitting software. Optom Vis Sci 1997;74(1):14–19.
88. Roberts C. Characteristics of the inherent error in a spherically-biased corneal topography system in mapping a radially aspheric surface. J Refract Corneal Surg 1994;10:103–116.
89. Szczotka LB, Reinhart W. Computerized videokeratoscopy contact lens software for RGP fitting in a bilateral postkeratoplasty patient: a clinical case report. CLAO J 1995;21(1):52–56.

CHAPTER 6

Lens Care and Patient Education

Edward S. Bennett and Heidi Wagner

The ability to care for and handle rigid gas-permeable (GP) contact lenses properly depends on several factors. First, the patient must be provided with several methods of insertion and removal, and proficiency in these methods must be demonstrated before leaving the office. Second, the patient must be aware of the function of each solution in the recommended care regimen, the importance of performing each function properly and regularly, and the basis for which other solutions are not compatible with the particular material. Third, several methods should be provided to both educate the patient and reinforce the education. The patient must know the "do's and don'ts" of the newest GP lenses; in other words, the patient must recognize the limitations of the lenses and the problems that can occur through noncompliance. The purpose of this chapter is to provide an overview of the ways in which these important factors can be satisfied, thereby enhancing the probability of patient success.

■ CARE REGIMEN

Wetting and Soaking

The majority of solutions used for wetting and soaking GP lenses combine several functions into one solution. These solutions have four major functions[1]:

1. To temporarily enhance the lens surface wettability.
2. To maintain the lens in a hydrated state similar to that achieved on the eye.
3. To disinfect the lens.
4. To act as a mechanical buffer between the lens and cornea.

The specific formulation of the ingredients in these solutions, especially the preservatives and wetting agents, is very important.

Preservatives

Preservatives are capable of either killing microorganisms (bactericidal agents) or inhibiting their growth (bacteriostatic agents).[2] They are the active ingredients in these solutions (and all other GP care solutions) that should perform the following functions[3]:

- Provide the necessary degree of disinfection.
- Preclude toxic reactions.
- Avoid adverse effects on lens surface wettability and parameters.
- Enhance compatibility with the tear film.

There are numerous preservatives currently in common use, all differing in their mode of action and effectiveness. The most common preservatives include benzalkonium chloride (BAK), chlorhexidine, thimerosal, ethylenediamine tetraacetate (EDTA), polyaminopropyl biguanide (PAPB), polyquarternium-1 (polyquad), and benzyl alcohol (Tables 6.1 and 6.2).

139

TABLE 6.1 STORAGE AND DISINFECTION SOLUTIONS

MANUFACTURER	NAME	PRESERVATIVE(S)
Bausch & Lomb	Boston Advance® Comfort Formula Conditioning Solution	Chlorhexidine gluconate, polyaminopropyl biguanide
Bausch & Lomb	Original Formula Boston® Conditioning Solution	Chlorhexidine

Benzalkonium Chloride: Benzalkonium chloride is a quaternary ammonium compound that is effective against a wide spectrum of bacteria and fungi and normally is used at a concentration of 0.004%. It was first introduced as a preservative in the late 1940s and is currently used in the majority of ophthalmic preparations. The effectiveness of BAK is enhanced when it is used in combination with EDTA, allowing a lower concentration than otherwise necessary.[4] It is not used as a preservative with soft lens solutions because the soft polymer will bind the preservative and actually concentrate it, thereby allowing it potentially to reach toxic levels and cause ocular injury.[5]

Chlorhexidine: Chlorhexidine is bactericidal in action and traditionally has been used in a concentration of 0.0005% in soft lens chemical disinfection solutions. However, unlike soft lenses, the binding capacity of chlorhexidine to GP lenses appears to be limited because of the wettability of GP lenses and chlorhexidine's large molecular structure.[6] Although chlorhexidine has been reported to have an excellent spectrum of antimicrobial activity, it has limited effectiveness against yeast and fungi; therefore, it often has been combined with EDTA for greater effectiveness. In addition, chlorhexidine has been found to be relatively ineffective against *Serratia marcescens*.[7]

Thimerosal: Thimerosal is a bactericidal organic mercurial compound that at one time was a commonly used soft lens solution preservative. However, some patients are sensitive to organic mercurial compounds and experience a burning sensation and associated clinical signs of redness and superficial punctate keratitis.[8,9] In addition, it is slow-acting in nature and, in low concentrations, may be ineffective against *Pseudomonas*.[2,10] Although thimerosal has been found to be compatible with GP lenses, exhibiting only rare sensitivity reactions, for optimal antimicrobial effectiveness it should be used in combination with another preservative such as chlorhexidine.[11] It has largely been eliminated from contact lens care systems.

Ethylenediamine Tetraacetate: EDTA is a chelating agent and not a true preservative. However, it is commonly used in combination with BAK and other preservatives in GP contact lens solutions because of its synergistic ability to enhance the bacterial action of pure preservatives against *Pseudomonas*.[12]

TABLE 6.2 COMBINATION SOLUTIONS

MANUFACTURER	NAME	PRESERVATIVE
Alcon	Unique pH Multipurpose Solution	Polyquaternium-1
Lobob	Optimum by Lobob	Benzyl alcohol
Bausch & Lomb	Boston Simplus Multi-Action Solution	Chlorhexidine gluconate, polyaminopropyl biguanide

Polyaminopropyl Biguanide: PAPB has been used as a preservative in soft disinfection regimens because of its low sensitivity rate. It has supplemented chlorhexidine as a preservative in one of the GP care systems because it exhibits greater antimicrobial effectiveness, notably against *Serratia marcescens*.[7] However, in the concentration used in GP lens solutions, which is 30 to 50 times the concentration used in soft lens solutions, the potential for toxicity reactions has been documented.[13,14] However, when reduced in concentration by one-third, it has demonstrated excellent antimicrobial activity in comparison with other systems.[15] It has also demonstrated effectiveness against *Acanthamoeba*.[16]

Polyquaternium-1: Polyquaternium-1 is a large cationic (+) polymer that also is similar in molecular structure to chlorhexidine. The quaternary ammonium group has a lower cationic (+) charge than polyhexamethylene biguanide and, as a result, is used at higher concentrations.[17] It is less likely to produce toxic or allergic reactions than previously developed preservatives such as benzalkonium chloride and thimerosal.[17]

Benzyl Alcohol: Benzyl alcohol originally was considered for use as a solvent for contact lens materials; however, it was also found to have good disinfection capabilities. Pure benzyl alcohol possesses certain physicochemical characteristics that are regarded as ideal for an ophthalmic preservative, including low molecular weight, bipolarity, and water solubility.[19] Benzyl alcohol exhibits negligible binding to the surface of GP lenses, especially fluoro-silicone/acrylate (F-S/A) lens materials.[18] In addition to its properties as a disinfectant, benzyl alcohol is effective in lipid removal.[19]

All commonly used preservatives in GP lens solutions appear to be safe and exhibit far fewer sensitivity reactions than soft lens disinfecting solutions. Certainly, it is possible for an occasional patient to exhibit a sensitivity reaction to any one of the aforementioned preservatives. This sensitivity is manifested, as with any allergic reaction, in the form of itching, burning, and redness. If this reaction occurs, it is often eliminated by switching to a care regimen using a different preservative.

Wetting Agents

Wetting/soaking solutions typically contain either polyvinyl alcohol or a methylcellulose derivative as a wetting agent.

Polyvinyl alcohol has several properties that make it a beneficial additive to GP lens solutions.[2] It is water soluble and is relatively nonviscous and nontoxic to ocular tissues. It has good viscosity-building properties and exhibits good spreading and wettability on the eye and lens surfaces.[20,21] Also, unlike methylcellulose, polyvinyl alcohol does not retard regeneration of corneal epithelium.[22] Methylcellulose derivatives have been used successfully as wetting agents in more viscous GP solutions.

Cleaning

Several types of cleaners are available for use by GP lens wearers, including nonabrasive surfactants, abrasive surfactants, and surfactant soaking solutions, enzymes, and laboratory cleaners.

Nonabrasive Surfactants

GP cleaners and traditional hard lens cleaners may contain nonabrasive surfactant (detergent) cleaning agents to remove contaminants (e.g., mucoproteins, lipids, and debris) from the lens surface. The use of digital pressure or friction during the cleaning process is important in removing deposits from rigid lenses. Optimum Extra Strength Cleaner (Lobob Laboratories, Inc.) is an example of a nonabrasive surfactant lens cleaner.

Abrasive Surfactants

Abrasive particulate matter has been used in cleaners as an effective adjunct in removing adherent mucoproteinaceous deposits from the lens that may be resistant to use of the surfactant alone. The daily use of abrasive cleaning regimens has been demonstrated to be more effective than the use of nonabrasive cleaners.[23] However, two problems have been described with abrasive cleaners. First, small surface scratches have been observed under high magnification.[24] Second, inducing minus lens power while reducing center thickness can result.[25–27] These problems have been minimized by the introduction of small-particle abrasive cleaners; however, abrasive lens cleaners may be contraindicated for lens materials with hyper-oxygen permeability (Dk) as well as for lens materials that have been plasma treated (discussed below). Examples include Boston Cleaner and Boston Advance Cleaner (Bausch & Lomb) and Opti-Free Daily Cleaner (Alcon Laboratories, Inc.).

Surfactant Soaking Solutions

GP lens care systems have traditionally embraced two-bottle regimens composed of separate cleaning and soaking solutions. One-bottle GP systems, combining these procedures, are a more recent innovation. These solutions use surfactant soaking, intended to dissolve deposits during the overnight soaking cycle; therefore, little digital pressure is necessary and warpage is less likely.[28] Optimum Soaking Solution (Lobob Laboratories, Inc.) contains nonabrasive surfactants; it is used for both cleaning and disinfection. It should be rinsed before insertion to remove the benzyl alcohol and facilitate the mechanical removal of lens debris. Boston Simplus (Bausch & Lomb) and Unique pH (Alcon Laboratories, Inc.) are examples of multipurpose lens care products that do not require rinsing before insertion.

The lens care system should be prescribed for the needs of the patient. For example, Boston Original was formulated specifically for silicone/acrylate lens materials that are predisposed to protein deposition. Boston Advance Comfort Care was designed for fluoro-silicone/acrylate lens materials that are more likely to attract lipids. Multipurpose lens care systems may be most appropriate for patients who do not tend to deposit lenses or who are not compliant with two-bottle lens care regimens. Patients who exhibit sensitivity to one formulation may be better served by a system using a different preservative.

Enzymes

The use of a weekly enzymatic cleaning regimen for GP lens wearers has been proven to be a beneficial adjunct to surfactant cleaning in protein removal from the lens surface.[29] In addition, enzyme use has not been reported to cause any adverse effects for GP lens wearers.[30]

More recently developed protein removal products are in liquid, rather than tablet, form and may be used with the manufacturers' accompanying storage solution. Boston One-Step Liquid Enzymatic Cleaner (Bausch & Lomb) is added to the storage solution weekly, whereas SupraClens (Alcon Laboratories, Inc.) is added to the storage solution daily. Both products should be rinsed before insertion. Boston One-Step is composed of subtilisin; SupraClens is a pancreatin derivative. Both products are designed to promote patient compliance and meet the patient's desire for convenience.[31,32]

Laboratory Cleaners and Solvents

The use of laboratory-approved, extra-strength cleaners such as the Boston Lens Laboratory Cleaner (Polymer Technology Corporation) or Fluoro-Solve (Paragon Vision Sciences) can be beneficial. The Boston Lens Laboratory Cleaner, a solution consisting of several surfactants, can be beneficial for in-office cleaning of lenses that either exhibit poor initial wettability or have acquired a heavy film over time. However, surface debris that is more tenacious and difficult to remove, such as pitch or wax, can be removed only with Fluoro-Solve, which is a mild solvent.

TABLE 6.3 DAILY CLEANERS

MANUFACTURER	NAME
Alcon	Opti-Free DailyCleaner
Bausch & Lomb	Original Boston® Formula Cleaner
Bausch & Lomb	Boston Advance® Cleaner

MiraFlow (Ciba Vision), not approved for routine GP use, can be an excellent restorer of lens surface wetting. Since prolonged and repeated exposure to MiraFlow may result in permanent damage because of parameter changes,[33] brittleness, and cracking caused by isopropyl alcohol,[34] it should be used for no more than 30 seconds and then thoroughly rinsed off. Menicon PROGENT Intensive Protein remover is a further example of lens care products intended for professional in-office use. Available GP lens cleaners are listed in Table 6.3.

Plasma Treatment

Plasma treatment for GP lenses removes residue from the manufacturing process and imparts an ultra-clean lens surface. This can enhance lens wettability and patient comfort and vision, particularly upon initial dispensing and early lens wear. Certain lens materials (Menicon Z) are routinely manufactured with plasma treatment, whereas other materials (Boston and Paragon) utilize plasma treatment at the discretion of the laboratory or practitioner.[35]

Rewetting and Relubricating

A solution that is used to rewet a GP lens surface while it is still on the eye should perform the following functions[36]:

1. Rewet the lens surface.
2. Stabilize the tear film.
3. Rinse away trapped debris.
4. Break up loosely attached deposits.

Ideally, this solution should clean the lenses of any debris while rewetting them for an extended period. Because the key to rewetting a GP lens is contact time, polyvinyl alcohol (PVA) often is added to increase the length of contact time. Some solutions contain hydroxyethylcellulose, methylcellulose, or other cellulose derivatives to aid surface wetting by increasing viscosity. Several rewetting solutions also contain a mild, nonionic detergent to loosen and solubilize mucus and debris and keep it from adhering tenaciously to the lens surface.[36] Available rewetting/relubricating drops formulated specifically for GP lenses are listed in Table 6.4.

TABLE 6.4 WETTING AND LUBRICATION SOLUTIONS

MANUFACTURER	NAME
Bausch & Lomb	Boston® Rewetting Drops
Lobob	Optimum by Lobob Wetting and Rewetting Drops

▩ DISPENSING VISIT

Procedures

Knowledge about the available care regimens and their respective functions, applications, and benefits becomes especially important at the dispensing visit. Before dispensing new lenses to a patient, it may be beneficial to apply fluorescein dye to the tear film to rule out any baseline staining with the biomicroscope. Once GP lenses have been inserted, an adaptation period is necessary before performing any test procedures. When the patient's awareness has decreased and he or she is able to gaze in the straight-ahead position with minimal difficulty (a variable period, typically 10 to 45 minutes), visual acuity and lens evaluation can be performed. The use of a topical anesthetic immediately before initial lens application may result in the ability to assess both vision and the lens-to-cornea fitting relationship much more readily.

Visual Acuity

The patient's vision should be assessed. Biomicroscopy should then be performed to evaluate lens position and surface wettability. If both good lens centration and surface wettability are present, an overrefraction can be performed to determine the necessary additional correction.

Overrefraction

If the visual acuity is equal to the expected value, typically a spherical over-refraction only is indicated. If a reduction of one line or greater is present, a spherocylindrical over-refraction should be performed. Just as the diagnostic fitting is imperative, both for obtaining a proper fit and for enhancing patient motivation (by the knowledge that contact lenses can be tolerated), so too is the dispensing visit important in continuing this momentum toward eventual patient success by the ability to see, handle, and care for the new GP lenses.

If an uncorrected cylinder that is not residual in nature is causing reduced visual acuity, overkeratometry should be performed to determine if the lens is flexing. If the keratometry readings are not spherical, flexure is present. This induced flexure can be minimized by selecting a flatter base curve radius (e.g., 0.50 D minimum) or increasing center thickness by a minimum of 0.02 mm.[37]

Slit-Lamp Biomicroscopy

The use of a biomicroscope is essential for evaluating lens centration, lag, fluorescein pattern, and surface wettability (although a Burton lamp would be a valuable adjunct for assessing fluorescein pattern). The lens-to-cornea fitting relationship initially should be evaluated using a wide beam with low-intensity white light and low magnification to scan the lens surface. In addition, the lens can be evaluated for regions of poor wettability or hazing. If the patient experiences variable visual acuity in combination with poor initial wettability, this problem can be minimized by presoaking the lenses for at least 24 hours to precondition the surface before insertion.

If poor wettability is present after presoaking the lenses, an in-office cleaner can be used or approved laboratory solvents should eliminate the problem. Polishing the front surface of the lens also may be beneficial; however, this should be performed after the lens is initially cleaned with an in-office cleaner and only if the lens has not been plasma treated.

Comprehensive evaluation of the fluorescein pattern is also important. Is the pattern similar to that observed at the diagnostic fitting visit? The use of high illumination, low magnification, and a moderate-to-wide beam width with cobalt filter should be beneficial when observation is by biomicroscope. If there is difficulty in observing the pattern, a Wratten no. 12 or similar filter can be used, especially if the lens material contains an ultraviolet inhibitor. In addition, if lower magnification is necessary to evaluate the pattern accurately, or to view both eyes simultaneously, a Burton lamp can be used.

Patient Education

Handling

The key to teaching patients to handle GP lenses successfully is *reassurance*. No matter how frustrating it is to the person performing the instruction, that feeling of frustration must not be conveyed to the patient. The instructions must be provided slowly and one at a time. Performing group instruction is distracting and denies the patient the necessary one-on-one personal instruction. The patient should not have the perception that the eye care provider or assistants have lost confidence in the patient's ability to learn how to handle the lenses properly; otherwise, feelings of failure and surrender may result, possibly leading to the attitude that contact lenses will never be worn again. Conversely, if the patient feels confident about handling the lenses, a perception of satisfaction and success is often present. A minimum of three successful insertions and removals is recommended, although the number depends on how confident the patient feels. If it takes two or three visits (closely spaced to maximize memory of techniques and to minimize further anxiety) for the patient to master lens handling, it is often worth the effort. This is more often a problem with presbyopic patients, who not only are experiencing blurred vision at near, but also may have lived 40 or more years without having a foreign body placed on their eye, thereby increasing anxiety.

Patients should be instructed to insert and remove the lenses over a cloth or paper towel spread on a table (not over a sink drain). In addition, patients should be asked and reminded to avoid oily substances such as hand creams, lotions, or cosmetics, and their hands should be washed and rinsed thoroughly prior to handling the lenses. It is important for both practitioner and staff members to set a good example by washing hands before handling lenses in the office and requiring patients to do likewise.

Insertion by the Patient: Insertion of lenses by the patient is a three-step procedure.

Positioning. The patient should be encouraged to use an adjustable mirror when inserting the lenses. This will help to ensure that the lens is positioned properly on the finger and to view the position of the lens; the latter is especially important because patients may consistently bring the lens in contact with the upper or lower lid.

Lid Retraction: For the right eye, the lens should be placed on the right index finger. The middle finger of the left hand should be placed *over* the upper lashes to lift up the upper lid. The middle finger of the right hand should be placed directly *over* the lower lashes to depress the lower lid (Fig. 6.1). The ability to retract the lashes successfully is essential.

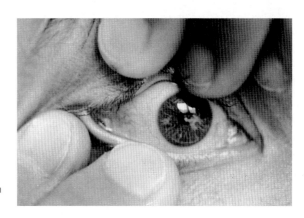

■ **FIGURE 6.1** Proper lid retraction for insertion of a gas-permeable lens.

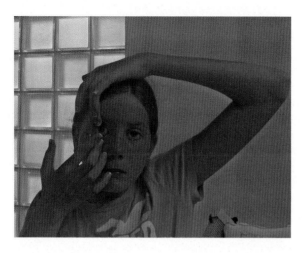

■ **FIGURE 6.2** Proper insertion of a gas-permeable lens by the patient.

Placement: The patient should be looking straight ahead (Fig. 6.2), typically at a mirror on a table or counter. Often, the new rigid lens patient will experience difficulty maintaining proper fixation as the lens approaches the eye; therefore, it is important to assure the patient that the lens will not damage the eye. Finally, once the lens has made contact with the eye, the patient should be instructed first to release the finger holding the lens, then the lower lid, and finally the upper lid. This procedure then can be performed in reverse for the other eye (i.e., use the index finger of the left hand for holding the lens, the middle finger of the right hand for holding the upper lid, and the middle finger of the left hand for holding the lower lid).

Insertion by the Practitioner or Assistant: The procedure is similar if performed by an office member. If the lens is to be placed on the right eye, the lens will be placed on the index finger of the right hand, with the left middle finger holding the upper lid and the right middle finger holding the lower lid (Fig. 6.3). Because the patient may become especially apprehensive with someone else inserting the lens, it is very important to apply pressure underneath the lashes to ensure that they will not move during this process. In this case, the patient can be instructed to view a distant target, for example, a letter on the acuity chart.

Removal by the Patient: There are at least three methods of removing a GP lens. Which method is used depends on such factors as lid tension, lens design, and personal preference.

The easiest method is to use the index finger of the same hand as the eye from which the lens is to be removed to eject the lens. The finger is placed at the junction of the lateral edge of

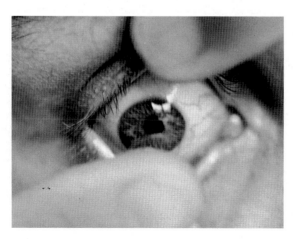

■ **FIGURE 6.3** Proper insertion of a gas-permeable lens by the practitioner.

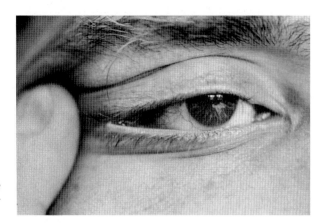

■ **FIGURE 6.4** Removal of a gas-permeable lens by having the patient place the index finger at the lateral edge of the lids.

the lids (Fig. 6.4). With the eye opened wide, the lids are pulled laterally; at the same time, the patient blinks and the lens should be ejected. This procedure can be performed with both the middle and index fingers of the same hand to enhance the possibility of lens ejection. The other hand can be positioned underneath the eye to catch the lens if it fails to adhere to the lower eyelashes. For patients who experience difficulty with the first method because of such factors as loose lid tension, low edge lift, and large overall lens diameter, a more forceful method to remove the lens is to use both hands. The middle and index fingers of the same hand are positioned over the lower lid; the middle and index fingers of the opposite hand hold up the upper lid. As with the first method, the lids are pulled laterally and, while the patient blinks, the lens is ejected (Fig. 6.5A–C). As with all methods of removal, the most important factor is allowing

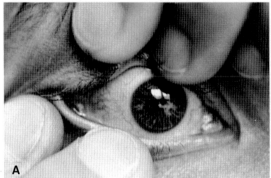

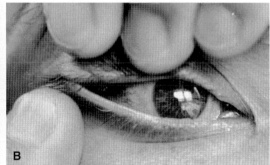

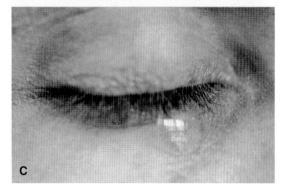

■ **FIGURE 6.5 (A)** With proper position of fingers over lid margins, **(B)** as the lids are pulled laterally, **(C)** the lens is ejected.

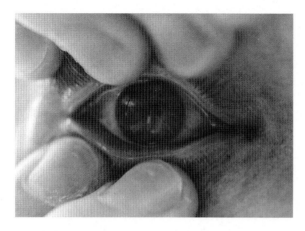

■ **FIGURE 6.6** Improper lid retraction can result in lid eversion and inability to remove the lens.

the lid margins to eject the lens. Figure 6.6 shows that if the lids are not retracted properly (i.e., if the finger is not placed *over* the lashes), the lid can evert and, therefore, apply very little pressure toward ejecting the lens.

Another forceful method of removing the lens is to eject the lens with a vertical (not lateral) motion. The fingers are positioned as in the second method (i.e., fingers of the opposite hand holding the upper lid, fingers of the same hand positioned on the lower lid). The lower lid is pushed superiorly and the lens is then ejected.

Removal by the Practitioner: The same methods for removal by the patient can be used by the practitioner. In the first method, the lids are pulled laterally (Fig. 6.7). In the second method (i.e., fingers of one hand holding the upper lid, fingers of the other hand positioned on the lower lid), the lens is ejected with a vertical motion (Fig. 6.8).

The fear of being unable to remove a GP lens is perhaps the greatest cause of anxiety with a new wearer. Every patient should be able to remove his or her lenses easily before leaving the office. Although the temptation exists to allow the patient to practice at home, this may eventually result in a frustrated and dissatisfied patient. Both practitioners and assistants should be skilled at all of these removal methods.

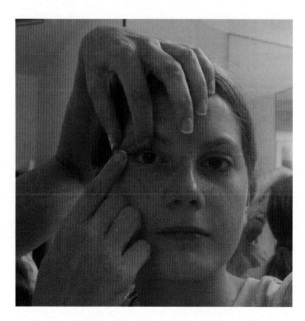

■ **FIGURE 6.7** Practitioner or office staff member removal by pulling laterally with the index finger and having the patient blink.

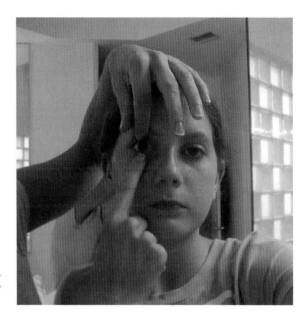

■ **FIGURE 6.8** Another effective method of gas-permeable lens removal is for the practitioner or assistant to push the lids in a vertical motion.

A suction cup should not be used as a crutch for patients unless the practitioner deems it essential. However, in an emergency situation in which a suction cup is unavailable, the patient's head can be placed in sink filled with water and his or her eyes opened, allowing the lenses to dislodge from the eye.

Recentration: It is extremely important to demonstrate to new GP lens wearers how to recognize when a lens has decentered off the cornea and how to reposition it. This often occurs during adaptation, when lenses tend to drop further on the cornea after the blink.

If the patient notices a unilateral blurring of vision, the eye should be evaluated for the possibility of a decentered lens. Location can be determined by the use of a mirror, or if this is not possible, a finger can be placed gently over different regions of the lids to feel any region that may be overlying the lens. Once the lens has been located, it can be manipulated through the lids. The patient should look away from the lens and, after placing a finger on the opposite side of the lens, should look toward the direction of the lens, repositioning it on the cornea (Fig. 6.9A,B). Often, the patient will develop the confidence to reposition the lens gently without the

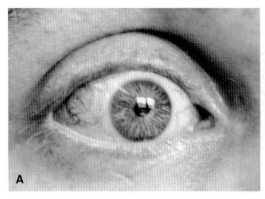
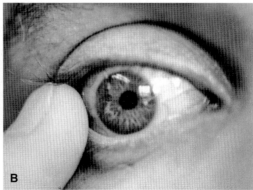

■ **FIGURE 6.9 (A)** To properly recenter a gas-permeable lens, the patient must first look in the opposite direction of the lens. **(B)** Next, the lens is gently nudged onto the cornea as the patient shifts his or her gaze toward the lens.

benefit of the lids. If the lens is difficult for the patient to locate, it most likely is superior. If the lens is decentered during the dispensing/educational session, fluorescein can be applied to determine the specific location.

Cleaning

Patients should be told what specific brand of cleaning solution(s) should be used, when to use it, and how to clean the lens properly. Cleaning with a surfactant cleaner should be performed *immediately* upon removal at the end of the day, not before insertion the next morning. This is important in maintaining good surface wettability, because the lens is inserted directly from the wetting/soaking solution and debris is removed more easily after the lens has been in recent contact with the tear film. It is very difficult for any patient to exhibit compliance if the lenses are not cleaned upon removal and are placed in an empty case. Any mucoproteinaceous and other deposits may adhere to the lens surface if the lenses are stored dry; therefore, deposit removal will become more difficult to perform.

Cleaning should be performed carefully in the palm of the hand (not between the fingers). Excessive digital pressure can result in lens warpage or lens fracture, especially with the more flexible hyper-Dk lens materials.[25] This has been shown to be a much greater problem in former polymethylmethacrylate (PMMA) wearers.[38] These patients may be accustomed to lens care habits (i.e., cleaning between the fingers, storing in a dry state, carelessness in handling). An exception to the rule may, in fact, be the Menicon Z lens, which has been found not to exhibit greater warpage when cleaned digitally versus in the palm of the hand.[39] Patients should also be advised to rub their lenses, with the recommended cleaner or multipurpose solution, for a minimum of 20 seconds after removal.[40] In general, patients should be warned about what can occur with noncompliance, and the proper cleaning techniques should be reviewed at the follow-up visits.

It is also important to note that patients should be told what *not* to use in cleaning the lenses and why. Former PMMA wearers may have used such products as baking soda, toothpaste, baby shampoo, or dishwashing liquid to clean their lenses. It should be emphasized that these products are not approved with GP lenses and may be both irritating and harmful to surface wettability.

Patients should also be warned of the so-called "left lens syndrome." This pertains to the problem of patients who clean the right lens first and more thoroughly than the left. Eventually, the left lens becomes more deposit bound and problematic to the patient. Simply bringing this potential problem to the patient's attention should be sufficient to prevent its eventual occurrence.

In addition to a surfactant cleaner, the use of an enzymatic cleaner for one 2-hour cycle every week should be recommended with some patients. Both extended-wear and borderline dry-eye patients should be started with an enzyme cleaner. Other patients also may benefit from enzymatic cleaning, which can be provided once it has been established that surface deposits have become problematic.

Care Regimen

Every patient should know what solutions they can and cannot use with their lenses and why. For example, it must be emphasized that although other solutions may cost less and appear to have similar functions, changing to such a solution may cause redness, burning, and reduced surface wettability. The specific recommended solutions and any acceptable alternative solutions should be provided as part of the patient instruction materials (Fig. 6.10). In addition, the progress evaluation forms should have a space for solutions such that patients can be asked to provide the brand names of their care regimens at each visit.

Every product in the care kit provided to a new GP lens patient should be explained to the patient as they pertain to everyday use (i.e., inserting, removing, cleaning and disinfection, etc.). The patient should then repeat the care instructions to ensure understanding and aid

NEW PATIENT INFORMATION

We appreciate your choice of the Eye Institute for your contact lens needs. Contact lens wear can improve the quality of your life. However, you must take proper care of your lenses and know what to do in the event of a problem. This information sheet provides important instructions and information. Please read it completely and refer to it if you have any questions.

EMERGENCY INFORMATION

- **In an emergency we can be reached at (954) 262 -4200 for 24 hours a day.**
- **Remove your lenses and call our office for assistance if you experience any of the following:**
  - ☎ **EYE PAIN**
  - ☎ **SENSITIVITY TO LIGHT**
  - ☎ **REDNESS OF YOUR EYES**
  - ☎ **EXCESSIVE TEARING OR DISCHARGE**
  - ☎ **CLOUDY, FOGGY OR REDUCED VISION**

GENERAL INFORMATION

- Contact lenses are medical devices that are regulated by the U.S. Food and Drug Administration. The recommended wearing, replacement and follow-up schedules are indicated below.
- Different types of lenses have varied risk. For example: lenses worn overnight have a higher risk of complications than do lenses removed on a nightly basis. This risk is greater after swimming with lenses.
- For all types it is best to remove contact lenses before swimming in fresh, salt or pool water. If lenses are mistakenly worn during this period, they should be removed and disinfected as soon as possible.
- It is best not to wear lenses during periods of illness or in situations where you will not be able to properly care for your lenses.
- Contact lenses must never be shared. Glasses and sunglasses should be maintained for wear as needed.
- As with prescription medications, contact lenses can only be dispensed pursuant to a prescription of an eye care practitioner, with a limit on the supply of lenses to be purchased before an expiration date.

LENS WEAR SCHEDULES AND REPLACEMENT INFORMATION

- Maintaining healthy eyes and proper vision includes regular evaluations by your doctor every:
  - ❏ 3 mos ❏ 6 mos ❏ 12 mos ❏ other _____ ❏ Please wear your lenses into your next visit
- Your lenses are designed to be worn on the following schedule:
  - ❏ Daily wear, up to ___ hours with removal before sleeping ❏ Continuous wear, up to ____ nights
- Your lenses are designed to be replaced on the following basis:
  - ❏ daily ❏ weekly ❏ biweekly ❏ monthly ❏ every 3 mos ❏ every 6 mos ❏ every 12 mos ❏ other _____

IMPORTANT: Wearing your lenses beyond this schedule may expose you to additional risk. Should you purchase your contact lenses elsewhere, your lens wear schedule, care regimen, lens replacement cycle, and periodic examinations will remain unchanged.

LENS CARE INFORMATION

To a large extent, lens wear success will depend on carefully following the care instructions we reviewed, and following common-sense instructions concerning hand-washing prior to lens handling, and lens case cleaning or frequent replacement.
To best meet your needs we have recommended the following lens care products:

- ❏ Care System: _____ ❏ Contact Lens Cleaner: _____
- ❏ Rewetting Drop _____ ❏ Other _____

IMPORTANT: Please do not change care products unless you are specifically instructed to do so by our office, as products are not all the same. Some may be incompatible with your lenses/eyes, thus substitution without approval from your doctor is discouraged.

ACKNOWLEDGEMENT

I have read this document carefully, and fully understand the importance of the doctor's recommendations. I have been trained in the care and handling of my contact lenses. I understand the policies of this office and understand that I am free to purchase lenses from a dispenser of my choosing. I understand the importance of following all directions, caring for my lenses as instructed and returning for all recommended, periodic examinations. I have been given the opportunity to have all of my questions answered and concerns addressed.

_____	_____
Patient Name (Print)	Doctor/Assistant Signature
_____ _____	_____ _____
Patient Signature Date	Parent/Guardian Signature Date

■ FIGURE 6.10 A form from Nova Southeastern used for providing important information to new contact lens patients.

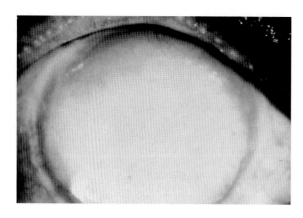

■ FIGURE 6.11 A *Pseudomonas* ulcer in which "topping off" of solution was implicated as the probable cause. (Courtesy of Larry J. Davis, OD.)

compliance. What the assistant and practitioner believe is common sense may be confusing to the patient. It cannot be assumed that every patient will carefully read and understand product labels and care instructions. If each product is explained and the patient still appears to be confused, the specific care instructions for each care product can be provided in written form. In addition, the function(s) of each bottle can be applied on a large label taped to the solution. The latter is especially beneficial for presbyopic patients who may experience difficulty with small print.

Rewetting or relubricating drops do provide some important functions with GP lenses. Specifically, these solutions can be used on an as-needed basis to rewet the lens surface while also rinsing loosely adherent debris off the lens surfaces.

Patients should be advised *always* to soak the lenses in the recommended disinfecting solution, not in the dry state. Soaking the lenses overnight has numerous benefits, including the following:

1. Disinfection.
2. Enhanced surface wettability because these solutions contain wetting agents.
3. Maintenance of hydrated state—the lenses are in this state during wear because they are in contact with the tear film.
4. Minimization of "case" scratches—a dry, dirty case can result in damage to a GP lens surface.

Patients should not allow their disinfecting solution to remain in the case for longer than 30 days without replacement.[41] It has been found that not only is contamination an issue, but also solutions lose their effectiveness over time.[42] In addition, the patient should be advised against "topping off" their disinfecting solution. Instead of replacing the solution every night, the patient simply adds a small amount to top off what is already in the case. The resulting contaminated solution may cause potential sight-threatening ocular complications (Fig. 6.11).

Lens Case

The lens case should have several important features to be effective for GP lens storage. It should easily differentiate left from right lenses. Many cases have an "L" and an "R" in the lens well or on the cap (Fig. 6.12). A hard plastic, ribbed, and deep-welled case is recommended, both to allow sufficient solution in the wells and to minimize leakage. The more flexible, hyper-Dk lens materials can adhere to a smooth-welled case if placed improperly in the case (e.g., convex side up), possibly resulting in warpage caused by the force required to remove the lens from the case. In addition, lenses that adhere to the bottom of a smooth-surface case may experience edge chipping from the excessive digital pressure needed to dislodge the lens. Both of these problems can be eliminated by using a case that has ridges or holes in the wells. As the lens

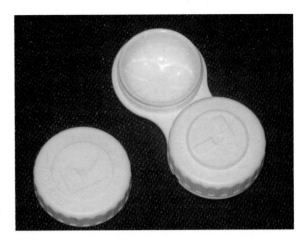

■ **FIGURE 6.12** Easy differentiation of "L" versus "R" results from having these initials on the lens caps and within the wells of the case.

case is an excellent source of microorganisms (Fig. 6.13), it should be washed every morning and allowed to air dry, using a clean toothbrush in combination with soap or surfactant cleaner and water[43,44] (Fig. 6.14). The soap can be rinsed off with fresh saline and the case allowed to air dry. Weekly cleaning, to include rinsing out the case with boiling hot water and allowing the case to air dry without replacing the tops, is also recommended.[45] Patients should be encouraged to replace their case on a regular basis (i.e., every 1–3 months). To reinforce the importance of a clean case, a new one can be provided at every progress evaluation.

Scratches

Every patient should be warned about the softness of these materials, especially the hyper-Dk lens materials. Lenses should be handled over a towel or soft tissue. If the lens is exposed to a hard surface, a drop of wetting solution can be placed on a finger and the lens can be gently lifted off the surface.

Foreign-Body Particles

GP lens patients should be informed about the possibility of dust or debris becoming trapped underneath the lens and irritating the cornea. Using rewetting drops in this situation is very ben-

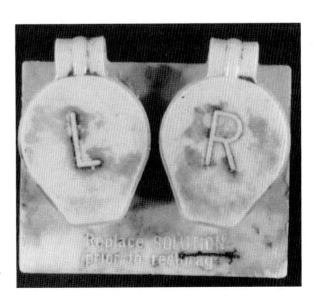

■ **FIGURE 6.13** A contaminated gas-permeable lens case.

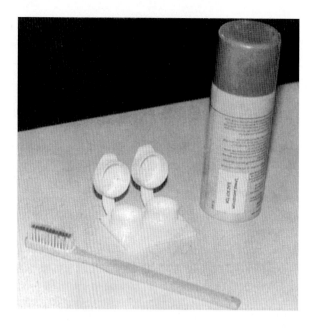

■ **FIGURE 6.14** The use of a toothbrush in combination with soap and water in addition to spray saline is important in the daily cleaning of a gas-permeable lens case. Rinsing with hot tap water and air drying is also an option.

eficial. If it results in greater than momentary discomfort, the patient should be told to remove the lens and clean it. If discomfort persists, the patient should call the practitioner's office.

Cosmetics

Every contact lens patient should be thoroughly educated about proper use of cosmetics. Cosmetics can be the cause of lens discoloration, damage, and surface deposition. Because many popular cosmetics contain ingredients such as preservatives, pigments, oils, and solvents, subjective discomfort and eye infection can result from their use.[46]

Cosmetics should be applied after lenses have been inserted. Mascara can flake off into the tear film, resulting in corneal abrasion. This is especially problematic with rigid extended-wear patients in whom these flakes are trapped underneath an adherent lens during sleep.[47]

Bacterial infection is also a problem.[48] A patient may transfer infectious organisms from the lashes to the mascara wand and then to the mascara tube, where they colonize. In addition, eyeliner should not be applied to the inner lid margin because it may clog the meibomian glands, possibly resulting in blepharitis, hordeolum, or chalazion.

Numerous cosmetic products on the market are recommended for contact lens wearers. They are water soluble and contain little, if any, fragrances or fillers. It is important to note again that cosmetics should be applied after lenses have been inserted.

Any cream or oil that is used on the face or hands can be transferred to the contact lenses, resulting in discomfort and blurred vision; therefore, these substances should be applied after the lenses have been inserted. Any contaminant or residual oils on the hands can be transferred to the lens and possibly be absorbed into the lens matrix. Hand soaps contain additives such as oils, perfumes, dyes, deodorants, and abrasives that can complicate the problem.[49] The addition to the care regimen of an optical-compatible hand cleaner developed specifically for contact lens wearers will minimize discoloration and deposit build-up on contact lenses.

Swimming

GP lens patients should be advised not to swim with their contact lenses unless they wear goggles. If a patient swims with the GP lenses but without goggles, he or she should know about the likelihood of lens ejection. Swimming in contact lenses may also place the patient at risk for infection. Likewise, with the recent concerns about *Acanthamoeba* keratitis, patients should be advised to insert their contact lenses after showering.

TABLE 6.5 NORMAL AND ABNORMAL GAS-PERMEABLE LENS ADAPTATION SYMPTOMS

Normal Adaptation Symptoms (Diminish Gradually)
1. Tearing
2. Minor irritation
3. Intermittent blurry vision
4. Light sensitivity as well as extra sensitivity to wind, smoke, and dust
5. Mild redness
Abnormal Symptoms (Occur Suddenly)
1. Sudden pain or burning (greater than minor irritation)
2. Severe or persistent haloes seen around lights
3. Severe redness or irritation
4. Blurry vision through spectacles for over 1 hr
5. Increasing eye discharge or mattering

Adaptation

Patients should be told that adaptation varies from person to person with an average of 10 to 14 days before the achievement of no lens awareness. This period can be estimated by how much tearing and discomfort is experienced at the dispensing visit. However, the patient should also know that it could last as long as 4 weeks in some patients. The patient should be reassured that comfort typically will improve on a daily basis. Avoiding the use of sensitizing words like pain and discomfort is helpful in reassuring the patient. Normal and abnormal adaptation symptoms are described for the patient in Table 6.5.

In addition, the patient should be told that, if lens wear must temporarily be discontinued (e.g., because of irritation or a lost lens), wearing time will need to be rebuilt gradually. A typical wearing schedule is below:

Day 1   4 hours
Day 2   4 hours
Day 3   6 hours
Day 4   6 hours
Day 5   8 hours
Day 6   8 hours
Day 7   10 hours
Day 8   10 hours

Current all-day rigid lens wearers should be able to go immediately into a full 12-hour wearing schedule after receiving their new GP lenses. Some practitioners prefer to have daily-wear patients wear their lenses a minimum of 4 hours prior to their scheduled progress evaluation; therefore, it is important to schedule these visits in the afternoon or evening. Exceptions to this are GP extended-wear patients, who should be seen in the morning. Typically, orthokeratology patients are evaluated in the morning after the first night of wear and then later in the day for subsequent visits to monitor residual refractive error at the end of the day.

Progress visits for a new daily-wear patient should be scheduled as follows:

Visit one   1 week after dispensing
Visit two   1 month after visit one

Visit three   3 months after visit two
Visit four   6 months after visit three

After the 6-month visit, patients should be scheduled at regular 6-month intervals.
   For continuous-wear patients, visits should be scheduled as follows:

Visit one   1 week after dispensing (daily wear)
Visit two   24 hours after initiating extended wear
Visit three   1 week after initiating extended wear
Visit four   1 month after visit four
Visit five   3 months after visit five

After the initial five visits, progress evaluations should be scheduled every 3 months for the extended-wear patient.

Educational Methods

The educational process should be a four-step process: (a) written, (b) verbal, (c) audio-visual, and (d) reinforcement.

Written: A patient instructional manual is beneficial in the educational process. It should be comprehensive and should contain the information provided in Table 6.6. In addition, it should be written in layperson's language with a print quality that makes it easy for a patient to read, understand, and comply with the information presented. The manual also can have a patient agreement form that has important information such as the after-hours contact information and care regimen (see Fig. 6.10). This should be signed in duplicate; for example, the second form can be attached by perforation and easily removed for the patient's permanent record. This manual can include customized inserts on such information as a fee or compliance agreement, cosmetic use, and continuous wear. The assistant can discuss the most important information with the patient and encourage the patient to ask questions. It also should be noted that from

---

TABLE 6.6 CHECKLIST FOR GAS-PERMEABLE (GP) PATIENT INSTRUCTION MANUAL

1. Composition, benefits, and applications of a GP lens
2. Insertion, removal, and decentration
3. Cleaning techniques
4. Normal and abnormal adaptation symptoms
5. Importance of adhering to prescribed wearing schedule
6. Causes of reduced wear (e.g., colds, hay fever, medications)
7. Importance of using the recommended care regimen (not saliva or other brands); alternative acceptable solutions
8. How to minimize loss and surface damage
9. Benefits of a spare pair of lenses or spectacles
10. Swimming and showering
11. Cosmetic use
12. Caring for the lens case
13. Possible contact lens-induced complications (i.e., redness, reduced vision, pain, etc.) and what to do
14. Visit schedule
15. Fee and refund policy
16. Service agreement, if applicable

a medical-legal point of view, an informed consent document listing wearing schedule and solution brands should be signed and dated by the patient.[50]

Verbal: The verbal educational process is much more important than the written because patients cannot be expected to understand all the information provided and, on occasion, the manual may not be read at all. In addition to handling information, a well-trained assistant can review important care information provided in the manual.

Audio-Visual: A more innovative and effective method of patient education is the use of audio-visual materials. For example, an instructional DVD produced by the Contact Lens Manufacturers Association (CLMA) and the GP Lens Institute (GPLI) is available from the CLMA (1-800-344-9060). Video segments demonstrating lens handling as well as a care and handling patient brochure are also available on the GPLI website (http://www.gpli.info). If any reservations exist pertaining to a patient's ability to handle or care for contact lenses, audio-visual materials reviewed together in the office or for frequent viewing at home would be an excellent supplement to the instruction manual.

Reinforcement: Important care instructions should be reviewed with the patient at *every* progress evaluation visit. They can include such information as the following:

1. What solutions are being used? Are the solutions the same as originally dispensed?
2. How often is the patient cleaning the lenses?
3. What method is being used for cleaning?
4. What is the current wearing schedule?
5. What is the current condition of the lens case?
6. Does the patient have any questions?

   In one large clinical study, asymptomatic contact lens wearers who did not have their lens care instructions reinforced at progress visits over a 3-month period ended up with over 50% contamination of their solution samples.[51] A second group, who had their care instructions reviewed with them at every follow-up visit, ended up with only 6% contamination of their solution samples.

■ IMPORTANT ISSUES

Compliance

Several recent studies have found a low patient compliance rate with contact lenses in general.[52,53] In fact, when over 1,400 lens wearers were asked to complete a 14-question compliance questionnaire, only 0.3% admitted compliance with all steps.[53] Ocular complications associated with noncompliance are more common with soft lens wearers.[54–56] However, GP lens wearers who do not comply with the recommended care guidelines may experience problems as well. Some of the more frequent causes of noncompliance problems with GP lens wearers include the following:

1. Patient does not clean the lenses as often or as comprehensively as desired (if at all).
2. Patient does not adhere to the prescribed wearing schedule.
3. Patient does not use disinfection solution or, if used, does not replace it regularly.
4. Patient does not wash hands before handling the lenses.
5. An inappropriate wetting solution such as saliva or tap water is used.
6. Expired solutions are used.
7. Case is not cleaned regularly.
8. Patient substitutes originally recommended solution with another brand.

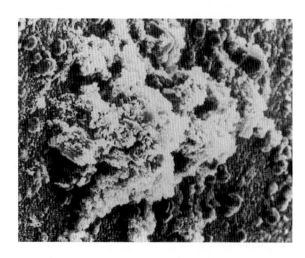

■ **FIGURE 6.15** Bacteria biofilm formation. (Courtesy of Patrick J. Caroline.)

One study found that approximately 50% of rigid lens care solutions were contaminated.[55] In addition, a much higher percentage of patients who admitted noncompliance were found to have contaminated care regimens than compliant patients. It is important to note that all solutions that were <21 days old were uncontaminated.

Certainly, by optimizing patient compliance, the probability of ocular complications and liability problems will be minimized. A three-step approach has been recommended[57]:

1. Inspect the lens care products that you use in your office or sell—look for contamination, tampering, and expired bottles.
2. Assume patients know nothing; document your instructions and warnings in patient files.
3. Inspect patients' solutions at follow-up visits, and question patients about any solution substitutions while reinforcing proper care procedures.

One important problem resulting from poor compliance is the development of a *microbial biofilm* within the case, attached to the lenses and/or the solutions.[58–60] Bacteria in a nutrient-deprived environment, such as the contact lens case, initiate a survival strategy to make them more resistant to disinfectants. The principal strategy is the development of a bacteria biofilm, which is a collection of bacterial cells in an exopolysaccharide glycocalyx slime secreted by the bacterial cell (Fig. 6.15).

This glycocalyx slime can serve as protection for the bacteria against certain preservatives. A notable example is the resistance of *Serratia marcescens* against chlorhexidine. It has been found that PAPB's performance is superior to that of chlorhexidine- and benzalkonium-preserved solutions with respect to preservative efficacy and prevention of biofilm formation in contact lens cases.[61] In addition, the combination of benzyl alcohol and a surfactant mixture should provide good effectiveness against biofilm formation. To minimize biofilm formation, cases should be designed with minimal hard-to-clean areas and replaced on an every 1- to 3-month basis as noted before. Disposing of cases on a regular basis may be as—or more—important than disposing of lenses as recommended. Microbial keratitis associated with a contaminated case is certainly possible (Fig. 6.16).

Appropriate cleaning and disinfection practices should also be executed on a daily basis. A summary nomogram on management of patient noncompliance is provided in Figure 6.17.

Tap Water

The use of tap water with GP lenses remains a contentious issue because of the association of contact lens wear with *Acanthamoeba* keratitis.[62–64] Although the condition is rare, the

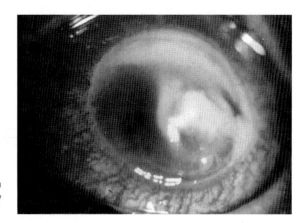

■ **FIGURE 6.16** A corneal ulcer resulting from a contaminated lens case. (Courtesy of Randy McLaughlin.)

prognosis for visual rehabilitation is poor, and the treatment regimen expensive and prolonged.[65,66] *Acanthamoeba* is a ubiquitous, free-living protozoan organism that is present in water, soil, sewage systems, and air.[67] The scientific literature first documents case reports of *Acanthamoeba* keratitis in 1974.[68] Disease incidence increased slightly over the following decade, with an outbreak in the mid-1980s associated with homemade saline and inconsistent hydrogel contact lens disinfection practices.[62,69] In the most recent outbreak, the Centers for Disease Control and Prevention determined that the risk for *Acanthamoeba* keratitis was seven times greater for consumers who used Complete MoisturePlus Solution (Advanced Medical Optics) as compared to individuals who did not use it.[70] Although Advanced Medical Optics has since issued a voluntary recall,[71] recent research implicates other environmental factors such as contaminated water.[72] Hence, contact lens wear appears to be a primary risk factor with inappropriate contact lens cleaning and/or disinfection practices, swimming or showering with contact lens wear, improper lens case care, and pre-existing corneal compromise predisposing factors. Furthermore, several recent cases are in conjunction with GP lenses prescribed for overnight orthokeratology.[73–75] Therefore, it is beneficial to avoid the potential for contamination through good lens care practices, with the use of tap water contraindicated in GP, as well as soft lens regimens.[76] The mechanical effect of digital rubbing, accompanied by rinsing, has been found to dislodge *Acanthamoeba* from the lens surface.[77,78] Important steps in optimizing compliance and minimizing the incidence of *Acanthamoeba* keratitis are provided in Table 6.7.[79]

Solution Confusion

The large number of currently available GP and soft lens care products also makes patient compliance more challenging. Frequently, patients cannot recall the name of the product(s) and may inadvertently select a similar-appearing but incorrect (and possibly ill-advised) solution. This may be further confused by competitive contact lens solution marketing, which may result in companies' adopting similar-appearing label colors, print styles, and bottle sizes and shapes.[80] Finally, solution substitution may simply be a result of pricing—the patient may buy the solution simply because it is less expensive.

Solution confusion can be minimized by the following steps:

1. Thoroughly educate patients about what solutions they can use, including alternatives.
2. Emphasize *why* you are recommending specific solutions to discourage price shopping.
3. Inquire about what solutions are being used at progress evaluation visits to ensure that solution switching has not occurred. To obtain an honest response, it is important for the

GP Patient Compliance Nomogram

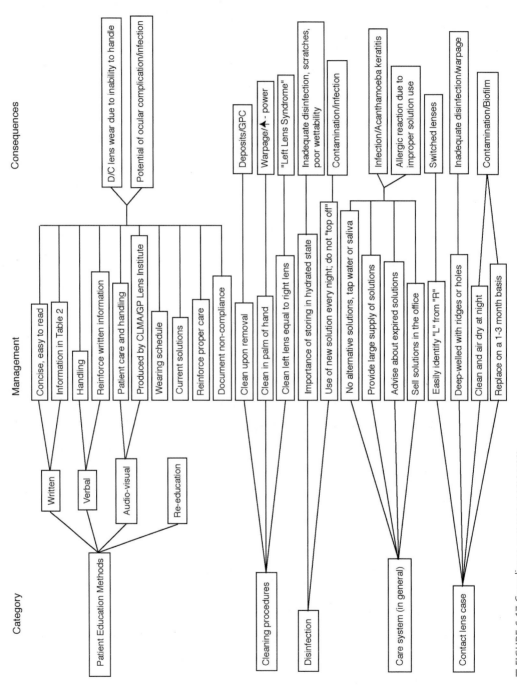

■ FIGURE 6.17 Compliance summary nomogram.

TABLE 6.7 GUIDELINES TO MINIMIZE RISK OF ACANTHAMOEBA KERATITIS

1. Solution Use

• Use fresh disinfecting solution every day. Do not reuse or top off solution.

• Use only products recommended by your eye care practitioner. The use of saline solution (not intended for disinfection) and rewetting drops should be used for soaking the lenses.

• Tap water should not be used in the wetting, rewetting, or soaking of contact lenses.

2. Care and Compliance

• Always wash your hands before handling contact lenses.

• Unless daily disposable lenses are being worn, always clean the lenses or—at minimum—utilize a rub-and-rinse action upon removal.

3. The Lens Case

• Replace the lens case, at minimum, every 3 mo, although preferably every month.

• Rinse the case every day with sterile disinfecting solution, and allow to air dry (exception: Proguard lens case with Aquify solution has antimicrobial properties with lens caps on).

• The lens case should be sterilized on a regular basis (weekly recommended), either via boiling the case in hot water or microwaving the case (in dry form) for 3 min.

4. The Environment

• Do not swim while wearing your contact lenses. If so, dispose of the lenses immediately after swimming (use rewetting drops to loosen lenses first). It would be preferable to wear airtight goggles over the lenses if they are to be worn during swimming.

• Do not wear contact lenses while showering, while in a hot tub, or during exposure to well water.

practitioner or assistant to use neutral questioning, such as "What is the name of the solution you are using?" Otherwise, if patients are asked if they are still using the recommended solution, they may sheepishly answer "yes."

4. Provide a large (3-month) supply of solutions initially to minimize solution substitution.

5. Sell solutions in the office or provide them at no extra cost—put the cost into the office fees, for example.

■ SUMMARY

GP lenses provide less risk of surface contamination and preservative sensitivity than soft lenses. Nevertheless, comprehensive and effective patient education is extremely important for the eventual success of the patient.

■ CLINICAL CASES

CASE 1

A GP patient enters your office for her 1-week progress evaluation with her 45-Dk GP lenses. She has complaints of mild itching, burning, and redness that occur for a few minutes after insertion of her lenses. She is using a PAPB-preserved care system. The slit-lamp examination reveals mild diffuse punctate staining and grade 1+ conjunctival injection in both eyes.

SOLUTION: Most likely, this is the result of an allergic reaction to the preservative in this system. This patient can be switched to another preserved system such as BAK, chlorhexidine, or benzyl alcohol.

CASE 2

Your patient returns for a 1-month evaluation of his 60-Dk F-S/A lenses. He complains of "foggy vision," which began in the past week. Your slit-lamp evaluation shows a mucoprotein film on the lens surface. In addition, he has grade 1 conjunctival injection and mild (grade 1+) papillary hypertrophy. He is currently using a nonabrasive surfactant cleaner, although he admits that the lenses are not being cleaned every night.

SOLUTION: Review proper lens care procedures with the patient and indicate why these procedures are important. Emphasize proper cleaning upon removal every night followed by storage of the lens in the recommended soaking solution. In addition, an abrasive cleaner supplemented by liquid enzymatic cleaning (as often as every night) should be recommended (unless the lens is plasma treated).

CASE 3

Your patient is motivated for GP lenses and you are able to achieve a successful fit, although some difficulty is experienced with placing the lenses on the patient's eyes because she is apprehensive about anything touching her eyes; in addition, her eyes are somewhat deep set. The lenses have arrived from the laboratory, and the patient is in your office for the dispensing visit. Your assistant is experiencing difficulty with teaching the patient proper lens insertion. How do you handle this situation?

SOLUTION: In this case, emphasizing the importance of lid retraction accompanied by *much* reassurance is very important. It should be demonstrated to the patient how to pin back the lashes to minimize the lid closure effect not uncommon with new patients. Likewise, with removal, the lashes should be pinned back to eliminate the possibility of lid eversion. The use of an instructional video, which can be viewed repeatedly, if desired, would also be beneficial. If the patient is still experiencing difficulty, she can be asked to return for a second visit to continue learning how to handle the lenses; in the interim she can practice bringing her finger (with a warm drop of water, which will have a numbing effect) up to her eye. The patient can also be provided with an educational DVD to reinforce proper handling.

CASE 4

A patient enters your office for a 3-month GP lens evaluation. It is readily apparent that the patient's hygiene is less than ideal; in addition, upon removal of the lenses, it is observed that his case is contaminated.

SOLUTION: Comprehensive patient re-education and a regular case replacement program are important in this case. If his case is contaminated, it is very likely his solutions are as well (e.g., cap off the bottle, hands not washed before handling lenses, "topping off" solution). It is important to review proper care procedures and the possible ramifications if noncompliance continues. Reviewing daily and weekly case cleaning methods is important. The patient can be provided with several new cases to reinforce the importance of using clean cases. A photo album illustrating compliance-induced complications would be very beneficial in this case as well.

CASE 5

Your GP patient enters for his 6-month progress evaluation. His only complaint is intermittent blurred or foggy vision in his left eye. Slit-lamp evaluation shows a good lens-to-cornea fitting relationship in both eyes; however, the left lens shows a mucoprotein film. In addition, the left bulbar conjunctiva is slightly injected, whereas it is clear in the right eye. Upon lid eversion, the right upper tarsal conjunctiva exhibits a grade 1− papillary hypertrophy, whereas the left lid is grade 2.

SOLUTION: Very likely, this is "left lens syndrome." The patient will need to be educated to clean the left lens as well as the right. In addition, in-office cleaning with a compatible laboratory cleaner or solvent should assist in cleaning the left lens.

CASE 6

Your long-term PMMA and very-low-Dk silicone-acrylate lens wearer, who has been refit into high-Dk F-S/A GPs, is in your office for dispensing of his new lenses. During the patient education process, he admits to your assistant that he often uses tap water as a wetting solution for insertion of the lenses. In addition, when asked, he also admitted occasionally rewetting the lenses with saliva. What do you tell this individual?

SOLUTION: This patient is similar to many former PMMA patients who developed poor care habits with their hard lenses. Since the durability and wettability of hard lenses typically are superior to GP lenses, the patient needs to be told to adhere to the recommended care instructions to minimize the incidence of problems such as warpage, scratches, and deposits. In addition, the possibility of ocular infection (e.g., corneal ulcer, *Acanthamoeba* keratitis) should be mentioned as well, especially if an inappropriate wetting solution is used. The fact that the incidence of *Acanthamoeba* keratitis has increased recently, often resulting in vision loss and a corneal transplant, should be indicated as well.

CASE 7

A GP patient enters your office complaining of redness, itching, and burning, which began right after she purchased her new solutions. Upon questioning, she admitted that she bought a generic brand of solution, which was on sale at the pharmacy. In addition, she admitted some difficulty in remembering the specific solutions she is supposed to use. Upon performing slit-lamp evaluation, she exhibited the same signs of a preservative-induced solution reaction as experienced by the patient in Case 1.

SOLUTION: Patient re-education is important in this case. She can (once again) be provided with a form giving the specific recommended solutions. In addition, the possible problems resulting from the use of inappropriate (including "bargain") solutions should be discussed. If she is experiencing much difficulty in remembering the solution names, she can be provided with a generous supply of the solutions. If she also admits difficulty with using a solution appropriately (e.g., using wetting/soaking solution for cleaning the lens), large labels can be placed over the bottles, each indicating the specific function of that particular solution.

CLINICAL PROFICIENCY CHECKLIST

- PAPB and benzyl alcohol are examples of GP lens preservatives that have demonstrated an ability to minimize microbial biofilm formation.
- The use of a small particulate abrasive cleaner (unless a plasma-treated lens) or surfactant-soaking regimen, supplemented by liquid enzyme use, is effective for deposit-prone patients.
- In-office use of a laboratory cleaner, compatible solvent, or alcohol-based cleaner is recommended for both poor initial wettability and long-term acquired deposit build-up problems.
- Patients should clean their lenses immediately upon removal in the palm of the hand and then place them in the recommended disinfecting solution.
- At the dispensing visit, visual acuity, overrefraction, and a comprehensive slit-lamp examination (i.e., lens position and lag, fluorescein pattern, and surface wettability) should be performed.
- As GP lenses typically have a lower edge lift design, patients need to be educated about alternative methods of lens removal, with an emphasis on lid pressure against the lens edge.

(continued)

(Continued)

■ Comprehensive patient education is essential. A four-step approach is recommended: (a) verbal instruction, (b) written education manual, (c) audio-visual observation, and (d) reinforcement of care at follow-up visits. Patients should be advised to restate the important care instructions.

■ The lens case is an important component of the care regimen. Patients should be instructed to clean the case every night and dispose of it on a regular (every 1–3 months) basis.

■ Tap water should not be used with GP lenses, especially for wetting/rewetting purposes. *Acanthamoeba* keratitis has been implicated with tap water use when caring for GP lenses.

REFERENCES

1. Bennett ES, Grohe RM. Lens care and solutions. In: Bennett ES, Grohe RM, eds. Rigid Gas-Permeable Contact Lenses. New York: Professional Press, 1986:225–244.
2. Mandell RB. Lens care and storage. In: Mandell RB, ed. Contact Lens Practice. Springfield, IL: Charles C. Thomas, 1988:326–351.
3. Hopkins GA. The formulation of rigid lens care systems. Optician. 1986;191(5038):18–22.
4. Brown MRW, Richards RME. Effect of ethylenediaminetetracatate on the resistance of Pseudomonas aeruginosa to antibacterial agents. Nature 1965;207:1391.
5. MacKeen GD, Bulle K. Buffers and preservatives in contact lens solutions. Contacto 1977;21(6):33–36.
6. Lieblein JS. Overview of soft contact lens hygiene. Rev Optom 1978;115(4):29–32.
7. McLaughlin R, Barr JT, Rosenthal P, et al. The new generation of RGP solutions meet increasing demands. Contact Lens Spectrum 1990;5(1):45–50.
8. Witten EM, Molinari JF. Allergic keratoconjunctivitis from thimerosal in soft contact lens solutions. South J Optom 1981;23(7):12–20.
9. Binder PS, Rasmussen DM, Gordon M. Keratoconjunctivitis and soft contact lens solutions. Arch Ophthalmol 1981;99(1):87–90.
10. Erikson S, et al. Suitability of thimerosal as a preservative in soft lens soaking solutions. In: Bitonte JL, Keates RH, eds. Symposium on the Flexible Lens. St. Louis: Mosby, 1972.
11. Huth S, et al. Care products for silicone-copolymer lens materials. Optician 1981;181(4701):16–18.
12. Mac Gregor DR, Elliker PR. A comparison of some properties of strains of Pseudomonas aeruginosa sensitive and resistant to quaternary ammonium compounds. Can J Microbial 1968;4:449–503.
13. Begley CG, Weirich B, Benak J, et al. Effects of rigid gas permeable contact lens solutions on the human corneal epithelium. Optom Vis Sci 1992;69(5):347–353.
14. Begley CG, Waggoner PJ, Hafner GS, et al. Effect of rigid gas permeable contact lens wetting solutions on the rabbit corneal epithelium. Optom Vis Sci 1991;68(3):189–197.
15. Keeven J, Wrobel S, Portoles M, et al. Evaluating the preservative effectiveness of RGP lens care solutions. CLAO J 1995;21:238–241.
16. Hiti K, Walochnik J, Haller-Schober E, et al. Efficacy of contact lens storage solutions against different acanthamoeba strains. Cornea 2006;25(4):423–427.
17. Hom MM. Current multi-purpose solution concepts. Contact Lens Spectrum 2001;16(9):33–39.
18. Gasson A, Morris J. Care systems. In: Gasson A, Morris J, eds. The Contact Lens Manual. Oxford, England: Butterworth-Heinemann, 1992:234–244.
19. Feldman GL. Benzyl alcohol: new life as an ophthalmic preservative. Contact Lens Spectrum 1989;4(5):41–44.
20. Weisbarth RE. Hydrogel lens care regimens and patient education In: Bennett ES, Weissman BA, eds. Clinical Contact Lens Practice. Philadelphia: Lippincott, 1993:34-1–34-27.
21. Hill RM, Terry JE. Ophthalmic solutions: viscosity builders. Am J Optom Physiol Opt 1974;51:847–851.
22. Krishna N, Brow F. Polyvinyl alcohol as an ophthalmic vehicle. Am J Ophthalmol 1964;57:99–106.
23. Chou MH, Rosenthal P, Salamone JC. Which cleaning solution works best? Contact Lens Forum 1985;10(8):41–47.
24. Doell GB, Palombi DL, Egan DJ, et al. Contact lens surface changes after exposure to surfactant and abrasive cleaning procedures. Am J Optom Physiol Opt 1986;63(6):399–402.
25. Carrell B, Bennett ES, Henry VA, et al. The effect of abrasive cleaning on RGP lens performance. J Am Optom Assoc 1992;63(3):193–198.
26. Boltz KD. The overzealous contact lens cleaner. Contact Lens Spectrum 1989;4(12):53–56.

27. Bennett ES, Henry VA. RGP lens power change with abrasive cleaner use. Int Contact Lens Clin 1990; 17(3):152–154.
28. Feldman G. Manufacturer's report: a new system for RGP lens care. Contact Lens Forum 1989;14(6):48.
29. Lasswell LA, Tarantino N, Kono D. Enzymatic cleaning of extended-wear lenses: papain vs. pancreatin. Int Eyecare 1986;2(2):101–105.
30. Lowther GE. Caring for hard GP lenses. Int Contact Lens Clin 1984;11(2):75.
31. Morgan P. A new liquid enzyme cleaner for daily use. Optician 1998;215(5654):30–33.
32. Misel JP. Reviewing today's lens care systems. Optom Today 1998;6(6):32–34.
33. Lowther GE. Effect of some solutions on HGP contact lens parameters. J Am Optom Assoc 1987;58(3):188–192.
34. Rakow PL. Solution incompatibilities and confusion: observations and caveats. Contact Lens Forum 1989;14(9): 60–66.
35. Schafer J. Plasma treatment for GP contact lenses. Contact Lens Spectrum 2006;21(11):19.
36. Greco A. Lubricating drops for hard and soft contact lenses. Int Contact Lens Clin 1985;12(4):205–211.
37. Herman JP. Flexure of rigid contact lenses on toric corneas as a function of base curve fitting relationship. J Am Optom Assoc 1983;54(3):209–213.
38. Henry VA, Bennett ES, Forrest J. Clinical investigation of the Paraperm EW rigid gas-permeable contact lens. Am J Optom Physiol Opt 1987;64(5):313–320.
39. Cho P, Ng H, Chan I, et al. Effect of two different cleaning methods on the back optic zone radii and surface smoothness of menicon rigid gas permeable lenses. Optom Vis Sci 2004;81(6):461–467.
40. Walline JJ, Rah MJ. Emphasizing lens care. Contact Lens Spectrum 2008;23(1):51.
41. Ward MA. Maintaining and disinfecting GP diagnostic lenses. Contact Lens Spectrum 2006;21(9):24.
42. Boost M, Cho P, Lai S. Efficacy of multipurpose solutions for rigid gas permeable lenses. Ophthalm Physiol Opt 2006;26(5):468–475.
43. Smythe JL. The forgotten lens care step. Contact Lens Spectrum 2003;18(9):21.
44. Caroline PJ, Andre MP. Combating the dreaded contact lens case. Contact lens case reports. Contact Lens Spectrum 2000;15(4):57.
45. Ward MA. Keeping clean cases. Contact Lens Spectrum 2004;19(1):27.
46. Baldwin JS. Cosmetics: too long concealed as culprit in eye problems. Contact Lens Forum 1986;11(6):38–41.
47. Bennett ES, Ghormley NR. Rigid extended wear: an overview. Int Contact Lens Clin 1987;14(8):319–331.
48. Ng A, Mostardi B, Mandell RB. Adherence of mascara to soft contact lenses. Int Contact Lens Clin 1988;15(2): 64–68.
49. Hoffman WC, Cook SA. Reducing lens spoilage via CL wearers' hand soap. Contact Lens Forum 1986; 11(5): 44–45.
50. Harris MG. Is your CL practice vulnerable to legal action? Contact Lens Forum 1990;5(1):51–52.
51. Wilson LA, Sawant AO, Simmons RB, et al. Microbial contamination of contact lens storage cases and solutions. Am J Ophthalmol 1990;109(2):193.
52. Donshik PC, Ehlers WH, Anderson LD, et al. Strategies to better engage, educate, and empower patient compliance and safe lens wear: compliance what we know, what we do not know, and what we need to know. Eye Contact Lens 2007;33(6):430–434.
53. Morgan P. Contact lens compliance and reducing the risk of keratitis. Optician 2007;June:20–25.
54. Ky W, Scherick K, Stenson S. Clinical survey of lens care in contact lens patients. CLAO J 1998;24(4):216–219.
55. Donzis PB, Mondino BJ, Weissman BA, et al. Microbial contamination of contact lens care systems. Am J Ophthalmol 1987;104(4):325–333.
56. Smith RE, MacRae SM. Contact lenses: convenience and complications. N Engl J Med 1989;321(12):824–826.
57. Harris MG. Save yourself from lens care lawsuits. Rev Optom 1990;127(4):69–71.
58. Caroline PJ, Campbell RC. Strategies of microbial cell survival in contact lens cases. Contact Lens Forum 1990;15(9):27–36.
59. Campbell RC, Caroline PJ. Inefficacy of soft contact lens disinfection techniques in the home environment. Contact Lens Forum 1990;15(9):17–25.
60. Caroline PJ, Andre MP. Searching for an antimicrobial contact lens case. Contact Lens Spectrum 2005;20(1):56.
61. Chou MH, DeCicco BT, Keeven JK, et al. The mechanism of survival of bacteria in contact lens cases. Presented at the Annual Meeting of the Contact Lens Association of Ophthalmologists, New Orleans, LA, January 1989.
62. Acanthamoeba keratitis associated with contact lenses. Morb Mortal Wkly Rep 1986;35:405–408.
63. Stehr-Green JK, Bailey TM, Visvesvara GS. The epidemiology of Acanthamoeaba keratitis in the United States. Am J Ophthalmol 1989;107:331–336.
64. Stehr-Green JK, Bailey TM, Brandt FH, et al. Acanthamoeba keratitis in soft contact lens wearers: a case-control study. JAMA 1987;258:57–60.
65. Kumar R, Lloyd D. Recent advances in the treatment of Acanthamoeba keratitis. Clin Infect Dis 2002;35:434–441.
66. Mathers W. Acanthamoeba: a difficult pathogen to evaluate and treat. Cornea 2004;23:325.
67. Kilvington S, Larkin DF. Acanthamoeba adherence to contact lenses and removal by cleaning agents. Eye 1990; 4:589–594.

68. Naginton J, Watson PG, Playfair TJ, et al. Amoebic infections of the eye. Lancet 1974;2:1537–1540.
69. Acanthamoeba keratitis in soft-contact-lens wearers. Morb Mortal Wkly Rep 1987;36:397–398.
70. Acanthamoeba keratitis — multiple states. Morb Mortal Wkly Rep 2007;56:1–3.
71. Advanced Medical Optics voluntarily recalls Complete MoisturePlus contact lens solution. FDA News May 26, 2007.
72. Joslin CE, Tu EY, Shoff ME, et al. The association of contact lens use and Acanthamoeba keratitis. Am J Ophthalmol 2007;144:169–180.
73. Xuguang S, Lin C, Yan Z, et al. Acanthamoeba keratitis as a complication of orthokeratology. Am J Ophthalmol 2003;136:1159–1161.
74. Yepes N, Lee SB, Hill V, et al. Infectious keratitis after overnight orthokeratology. Cornea 2005;24:857–860.
75. Wilhelmus KR. Acanthamoeba keratitis during orthokeratology. Cornea 2005;24:7.
76. Davis L. Lens hygiene and care system contamination of asymptomatic rigid gas permeable lens wearers. Int Contact Lens Clin 1995;22:217–221.
77. Snyder C. Lens care complications – where's the rub? Contact Lens Anterior Eye 2006;29:161–162.
78. Shih KL, Hu JC, Sibley MJ. The microbiological benefit of cleaning and rinsing contact lenses. Int Contact Lens Clin 1985;12(4):235–242.
79. Bennett ES. Contact lens care and compliance: Has it changed since the *fusarium* scare. Rev Optom 2007;144(5):34–42.
80. Berenblatt AJ. Lens care systems: a practitioner's wish list. Contact Lens Forum 1988;13(3):37–38.

CHAPTER 7

Verification of Gas-Permeable Lenses

Vinita Allee Henry

■ VERIFICATION OF RADIUS

Base Curve Radius

The base curve radius (BCR) is one of the most important lens parameters to verify because it affects the lens-to-cornea fitting relationship. The most commonly used method of determining the BCR is the radiuscope or radiusgauge. The BCR is determined by the distance between the real and aerial images observed in the radiuscope (Fig. 7.1).

Following are the steps for determination of the BCR.

1. Place a small amount of water in the depression of the lens mount.
2. The lens should be clean and dry when placed in this depression, concave side upward. Caution should be taken to avoid submerging the entire lens or allowing any fluid on the concave surface as this will result in an inaccurate reading or a poor-quality image (Fig. 7.2).
3. Center and position the lens mount so that a small green beam of light can be observed reflected in the lens. The aperture selector should be in the large aperture position at the back of the instrument.
4. Viewed in the oculars, the real and aerial images will be observed as a spoke or star pattern (Fig. 7.3). The real image will appear at the lower end of the scale at approximately zero and will be centered; however, the aerial image will be located approximately 6 to 9 mm on the scale and may not be centered. This aerial image should be centered, and the lens mount should not be moved again before setting the instrument at zero and a reading is taken. Note that between the two images, the light filament (Fig. 7.4) will be observed.
5. On obtaining a clear, sharp spoke pattern of the real image at the lower end of the scale, place the needle on zero. This can be accomplished by using the knob located at the left side of most radiuscopes and the back of most radiusgauges (Fig. 7.5). The manual provided with the instrument should provide this information.
6. The objective should be adjusted with the coarse adjustment knob to obtain a clear, sharp image of the aerial image. As the scale increases in value, the light filament will be observed before the aerial image is viewed. The BCR will be the reading taken from the zero point to the clear, sharp image of the aerial image.
7. The BCR is read off the millimeter scale to the nearest hundredth. The millimeter scale is located in the ocular of the radiuscope and on a clock dial at the back of the radiusgauge. For example, a typical BCR would be recorded as 8.20 mm.

If the needle of the instrument will not position at zero when the real image is in focus, the nearest whole number should be used. This whole number will be added or subtracted from the final reading. For example, if the real image is in focus at +1.0 and the final reading is 7.0 mm, the BCR is 8.0 mm.

Verification of the BCR of gas-permeable (GP) contact lenses is also possible with several automated keratometers. These devices have been found to accurately measure the base curve radius within tolerance.[1]

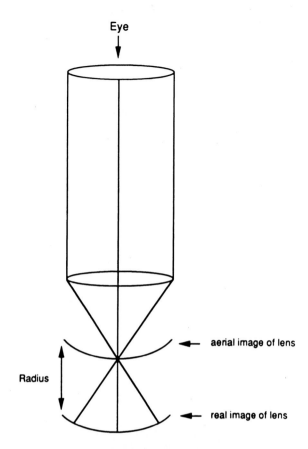

Eye

aerial image of lens

Radius

real image of lens

■ **FIGURE 7.1** Diagram demonstrating that base curve radius is the difference between real image and aerial image.

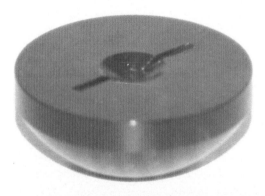

■ **FIGURE 7.2** Lens mount for determining base curve radius.

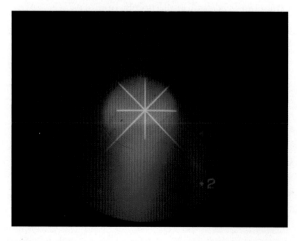

■ **FIGURE 7.3** Spoke pattern observed in the radiuscope.

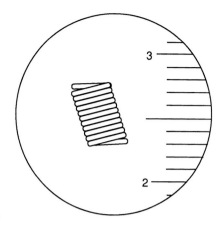

■ **FIGURE 7.4** Diagram of light filament observed in the radiuscope.

Verification of the BCR should be performed before dispensing and after 12 to 24 hours of soaking the lenses in an approved disinfecting solution. GP lenses may flatten on hydration, and verification is necessary to determine if the lens is still within tolerance.[2,3]

Front (Convex) Curve Radius

In addition to measuring the BCR, it may be necessary to measure the convex radius—for example, with front toric and bitoric lenses. A different lens mount is used to determine the convex radius (Fig. 7.6). The procedure is similar to determining the BCR with the exception that the real image is now the upper image and the aerial image is now the lower image. The needle should be set at the nearest whole number when the real image is in focus. When the aerial

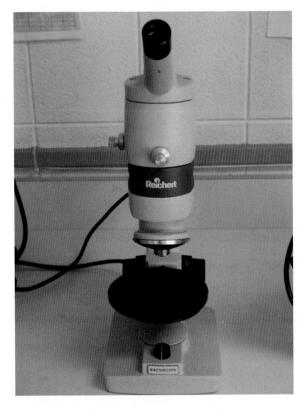

■ **FIGURE 7.5** Radiuscope.

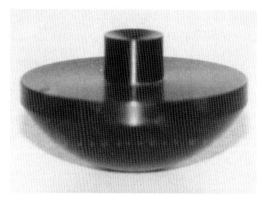

■ **FIGURE 7.6** Lens mount used to measure the convex surface.

image is in focus, the number is read from the scale and subtracted from the whole number. For example, if the real image is in focus at 8.00 mm and the aerial image is in focus at 1.00 mm, the resulting front curve radius would be 7.00 mm.

Toric or Warped Lenses

The steps for determining a toric or warped lens are similar to those for determining the BCR; however, the spokes of the image will not all be in focus at the same time. First, one set of spokes will come in sharp focus; this will represent the steeper curve. The spokes 90 degrees away from the first set of spokes will next come in focus, and this is the flatter curve. The symptoms of a patient wearing a warped lens will vary from no subjective symptoms but slightly reduced visual acuity to subjective symptoms of blur and decreased visual acuity, accompanied by a spherocylindrical over-refraction. These symptoms alone will not indicate a warped lens. Verification of the BCR is necessary as lens flexure may also produce these symptoms. A lens that is flexing may appear warped immediately on removal; however, typically it will return to the original spherical state soon after removal. Patients exhibiting lenses that are warped will require re-education in the proper care and handling of GP lenses because poor care habits, such as cleaning the lenses between the index finger and thumb instead of the palm of the hand, will greatly increase the likelihood of lens warpage.

Peripheral Curve Radius

The peripheral curve radius can be determined by the same method as BCR; however, if the peripheral curve is not ≥1 mm in width, it is unlikely that it can be obtained. Typically, this is not a parameter that the practitioner can verify.

■ VERIFICATION OF LENS POWER

Spherical Lenses

Back vertex power is typically the method by which power is determined for contact lenses. For low-power lenses, there is very little difference in back and front vertex power; however, there can be as much as 1 D difference in back and front vertex lenses in high prescriptions.[4] If there is doubt about which surface power to verify, it would be best to check with the laboratory that supplies the lenses.

Back vertex power of contact lenses is determined similarly to spectacles. The lensometer should be adjusted for the individual user before the lens power is verified as specified in the instrument manual. The lens is placed concave side against the lens stop of the lensometer, and the power drum is adjusted until a clear image is achieved. The lens should be clean and dry.

It will be necessary to tilt the lensometer upward into a vertical position to allow the lens to rest on the lens stop or for the lens to be gently held on the lens stop with the thumb and forefinger. Caution should be taken not to flex the lens. Most lensometers have a contact lens accessory device that can be placed on the lens stop to aid in more accurate measurements.

Prism

To measure prism on a contact lens, the lens must be centered with the concave side against the lens stop. The reticule inside the ocular consists of concentric black rings designating 1 to 5 prism diopters. For example, when the center of the target is on the first concentric ring of the reticule, it corresponds to one prism diopter (Fig. 7.7). Prism is primarily used in front toric lenses to reduce rotation.

Toric Lenses

Front toric lenses should be placed on the lensometer with the prism in the base-down direction. The resulting power will be recorded in a spherocylindrical notation. For example, if the lens is positioned so the prism indicates one prism diopter base down and the power drum indicates powers of −1.00 D and −3.00 D at 90, the power would be recorded as −1.00 − 2.00 × 90.

In toric lenses with no prism, such as bitorics and back torics, the power is not recorded in the spherocylindrical form, but as the values found in each meridian. An example of this is as follows:

BCR: 7.50/8.04 mm
Powers: Pl/−3.00 D

■ VERIFICATION OF CENTER/EDGE THICKNESS

A dial gauge is the most frequently used method of determining lens thickness. The lens is positioned on the gauge, and a plunger is lowered onto the lens with the thumb (Fig. 7.8). The center thickness (CT) or edge thickness can be measured by changing the portion of the lens beneath the plunger. The thickness is read directly off the gauge; for example, if the needle is on 23, then the thickness is recorded as 0.23 mm. Lens thickness can also be determined with the Marco radiusgauge because a thickness gauge is incorporated into the instrument itself. It is important to verify this parameter in cases pertaining to flexure, oxygen transmission, comfort, and lens position.[5]

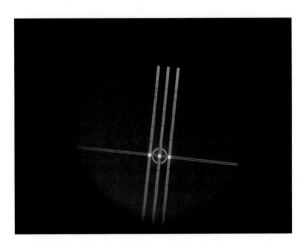

■ FIGURE 7.7 Prism as shown on a lensometer.

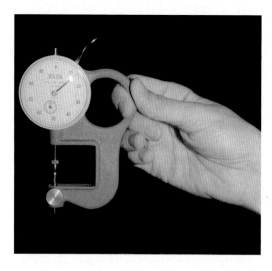

■ **FIGURE 7.8** Center thickness gauge.

■ INSPECTION OF THE LENS EDGE

The shape and condition of the lens edge can represent the most important factor in providing patient comfort. If the edge is not inspected before the lens is dispensed to the patient, symptoms of foreign-body sensation or scratchy, irritated eyes, for example, may result from edge defects. The use of the "palm test," in combination with one of the methods of projection magnification, makes this parameter relatively easy to inspect. To perform the palm test, the lens is placed concave side down in the palm of the hand and gently pushed across the palm (Fig. 7.9). A good edge will glide easily and feel smooth. A poor edge will feel scratchy, will show resistance to movement, and may make an audible scratchy sound. A projection magnifier provides a magnified image of the lens, allowing inspection of the edges. The lens is positioned so that it can be viewed from both the straight-ahead and the profile positions (Fig. 7.10).

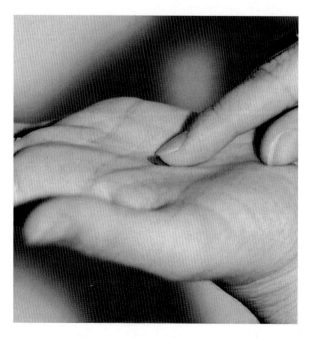

■ **FIGURE 7.9** Palm test used to determine the quality of the edge.

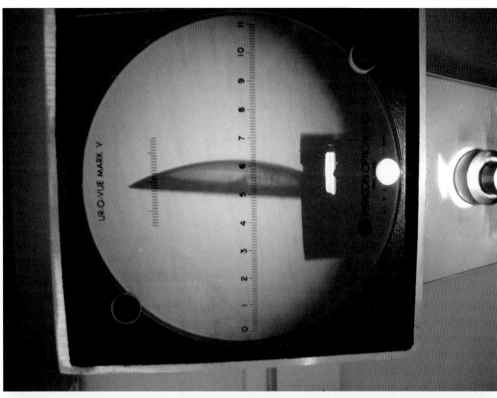

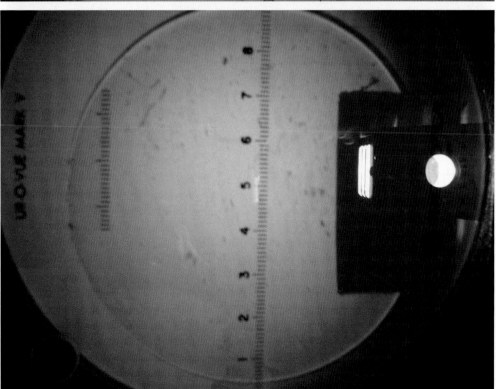

FIGURE 7.10 **(A)** Front view of edge with projection magnifier. **(B)** Side edge profile.

■ VERIFICATION OF LINEAR DIMENSIONS

Overall Diameter

The overall diameter (OAD) of a lens can be determined by several methods. The projection magnifier, a PD stick (used to measure interpupillary distance), a V-channel gauge, and a dial gauge can all be used to determine OAD (Fig. 7.11). The most common and practical method, as it can be used for measuring other parameters and for inspection, is the use of the measuring magnifier or reticule. On the back of the measuring magnifier there is a scale ranging from 0 to 20 mm. The lens is placed on the measuring magnifier and held up to a background light source (Fig. 7.12A). By positioning the lens on the scale, the diameter can be easily measured (Fig. 7.12B).

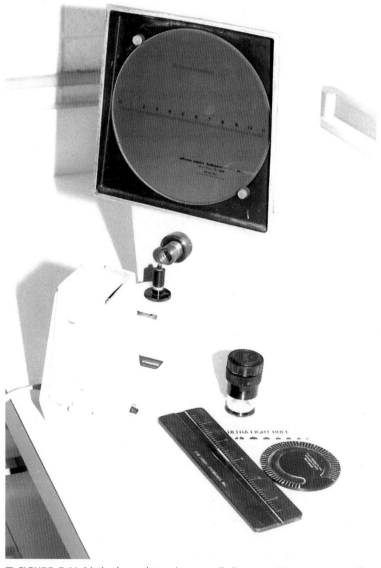

■ **FIGURE 7.11** Methods to determine overall diameter: Measuring magnifier, V-channel gauge, dial gauge, projection magnifier, and PD stick.

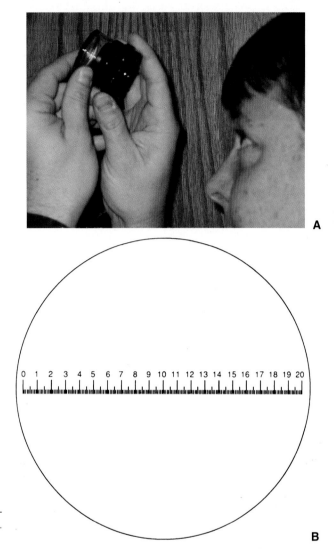

■ **FIGURE 7.12 (A)** Demonstration of viewing a lens through a measuring magnifier. **(B)** Diagram of measuring magnifier scale.

B

Optical Zone Diameter

The optical zone diameter (OZD) is the area between the innermost peripheral curve on each edge of the lens (Fig. 7.13). Like the OAD, the OZD can be determined by using the measuring magnifier. It can also be determined by the formula OZD = OAD − 2(PCW), where OZD is the optical zone diameter, OAD is the overall diameter, and PCW is the total width of the peripheral curves on one side of the lens. With some lens designs, the optical zone will be oval, making it necessary to rotate the lens and check the OZD 90 degrees away. Some examples of this are a spherical base curve with toric peripheral curves, a toric base curve with spherical peripheral curves, and a toric base curve and toric secondary curve in which the differences in curvature of the major meridians are not equal.[6]

Peripheral Curve Widths

Contact lenses are typically manufactured in a bicurve (base curve and peripheral curve), a tricurve (base curve, secondary curve, and peripheral curve), or tetracurve (base curve, secondary curve, intermediate curve, and peripheral curve) design. The measuring magnifier is the

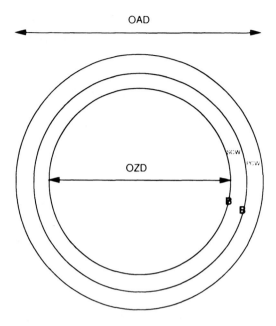

■ **FIGURE 7.13** Diagram showing overall diameter (OAD), overall zone diameter (OZD), and peripheral curve widths.

preferable method to measure the widths of these curves. The lens is placed on the measuring magnifier as specified for the OAD; however, the measuring magnifier may need to be moved back and forth slightly in the light source to determine where the curve exists. The junctions of the peripheral curves are typically blended. As the blend time is increased, determination of the specific peripheral curve width becomes more difficult (Fig. 7.14A–C).

■ SURFACE QUALITY

The surface quality of a lens is best determined by the projection magnifier or the biomicroscope. A measuring magnifier can be used; however, the magnification may not be high enough to reveal small surface defects. Examination of the lens surface may reveal surface scratches, cracking/crazing, residual pitch, deposits, or film (Fig. 7.15).

■ VERIFICATION OF SOFT LENSES

Because of the challenges of verifying soft lenses, this process is often overlooked. When soft lenses are ordered and arrive packaged in sterile vials or blister packs, the parameters should be verified from the package label. However, there are times when being able to verify a soft lens is beneficial to the practitioner. The parameters that are simplest to verify are power, OAD, surface and edge inspection, and any identification markings. Other parameters that can be verified but are more difficult and may require special equipment are BCR and CT.[7]

Lens Power

The power of a soft lens can be verified either in a dry or wet state. The simplest method is to blot the lens dry on a lint-free tissue and place the lens concave side against the lensometer stop, identical to the method used for GP lenses. The power is read from the lensometer. A wet cell can also be used in the same manner, except the lens is floating in saline to keep it hydrated (Fig. 7.16). With this method, a correction factor must be used to find the correct power because of the lens being immersed in saline, which has a similar index of refraction as the lens. For low-water-content lenses, the correction factor is 4.6.[8] The correction factor is higher for high-water-content lenses.

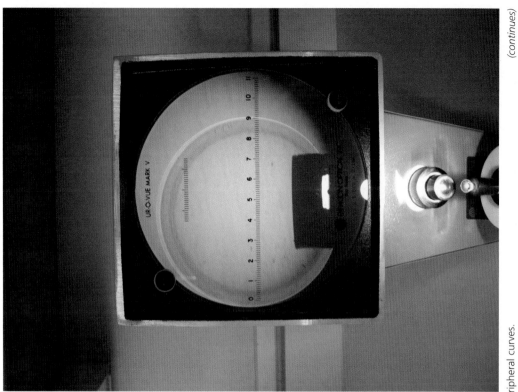

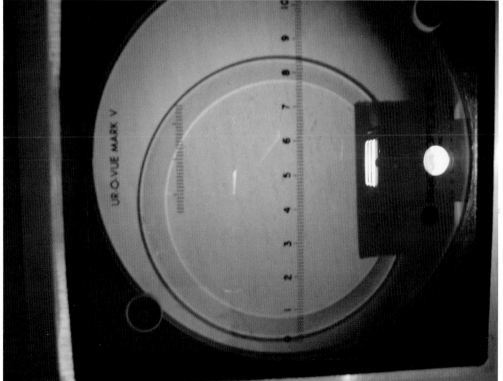

■ **FIGURE 7.14 (A)** Light blend of the peripheral curves. **(B)** Medium blend of the peripheral curves.

(continues)

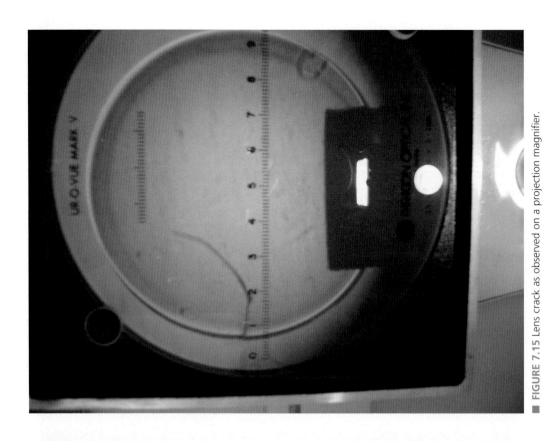

■ FIGURE 7.15 Lens crack as observed on a projection magnifier.

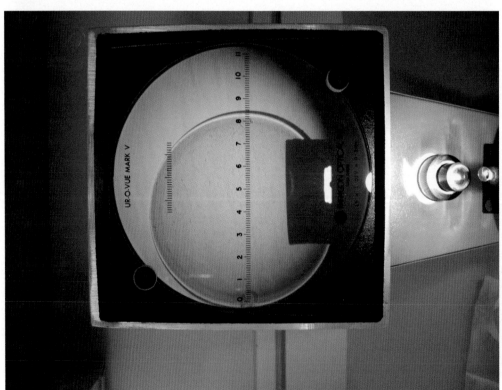

■ FIGURE 7.14 (*Continued*) (**C**) Heavy blend of the peripheral curves.

C

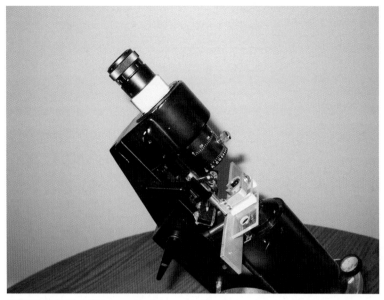

■ FIGURE 7.16 Soft lens wet cell power verification on lensometer.

Diameter

The diameter of a soft contact lens can be measured on a measuring magnifier or reticule. The lens should be blotted gently with a lint-free tissue and quickly measured on the reticule concave side down before dehydration occurs. Dehydration will cause the diameter to be smaller than the actual OAD.

Surface and Edge Inspection

Inspection of the surface and edge of a soft contact lens will be performed each time the lens is examined on the patient's eye with a slit-lamp biomicroscope. This is the easiest way to inspect the lens. The lens may also be held with soft lens tweezers behind the slit lamp while off the eye. Other methods of inspecting the lens surface are holding the lens up behind the light source of a projection magnifier or viewing the lens through a measuring magnifier. During the inspection of the lens surface, any identification markings on the lens can be viewed and recorded. The markings may identify the manufacturer, the type of lens, inversion indicators, or toric lens laser marks.

▓ SUMMARY

A summary of verification procedures is provided in Figure 7.17.

■ CLINICAL CASES

CASE 1

A previous GP wearer [oxygen permeability (Dk) = 18] is refit into a GP lens material with a higher Dk of 100. At the 6-month visit, the patient returns, complaining of slightly blurry vision. The examination reveals a visual acuity equal to 20/40 (OD) and 20/30 (OS), a spherocylindrical over-refraction (OU) that improves the visual acuity through the lenses, and normal ocular health. The patient admits to cleaning the lenses between the index finger and thumb.

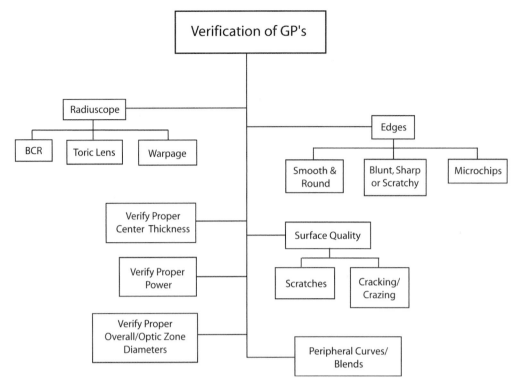

■ FIGURE 7.17 Summary nomogram of gas-permeable verification.

SOLUTION: Verification of the BCR of the lens reveals warpage for both eyes. The patient is re-educated on proper care procedures such as cleaning the lenses in the palm of the hand with the little finger and, if tap water is used, to rinse the lenses before disinfection, keeping the temperature lukewarm.

CASE 2

A patient is dispensed a GP extended-wear lens material with a Dk of 151. The lens parameters (OU) include an OAD of 9.2 mm, Rx of −3.50 D, CT of 0.15 mm, and BCR of 7.50 mm. The patient's keratometry readings are OU 44.50 @ 180/47.00 @ 90. At the 1-month visit, the patient's visual acuity is decreased to 20/25−3. The overrefraction is +0.50 − 1.00 × 180 OU, and over-keratometry is 44.00 @ 180, 45.00 @ 90. Verification of the BCR reveals no toricity.

SOLUTION: The reduced visual acuity is caused by flexure. Typically, a flatter base curve may be used to reduce flexure; however, in this case a flatter base curve would most likely compromise the fit. Lens materials with the higher Dk values used for extended wear are prone to flexure and need to be made slightly thicker than a low-Dk lens of the same power. This patient may have been fitted with a low-Dk diagnostic lens that did not exhibit flexure. In addition, this patient has 2.50 D of corneal astigmatism, which warrants a thicker lens than is required for a patient with little to no corneal astigmatism. The lens should be reordered with an increase in CT or at least 0.03 mm thicker, or a CT of 0.18 mm, which is recommended for this lens power with this amount of corneal astigmatism.[9]

CASE 3

A previously successful patient is refitted with a new pair of 30-Dk GP lenses and returns 2 weeks later complaining of discomfort. On biomicroscopic examination, the lenses are de-centering inferiorly, resting on the lower lid, with superficial staining above the lens on the superior cornea. Verification of the lenses results in parameters identical to those ordered with the exception of CT. The lenses were ordered "ultrathin," which is typically about 0.11 mm in this material and design (power = −5.50 D OU) and were verified as 0.15 mm.

SOLUTION: The lenses are too thick. The increased mass is most likely pulling the lenses to an inferior position, resulting in staining superiorly and discomfort when the lenses batter the lower lid after a blink. If the lenses had been verified before dispensing, this problem would have been prevented. The lenses should be returned and a CT of 0.11 mm ordered, as the patient has little to no corneal astigmatism.

CASE 4

A patient is dispensed a new pair of high-Dk GP lenses (BCR = 7.71 mm/43.75 D OU). The fit appears to be optimum and the visual acuity is good. At the 1-week visit the lenses appear to exhibit an apical bearing pattern with a lag of approximately 3 to 4 mm. The lenses were not soaked before dispensing.

SOLUTION: The lenses have flattened on hydration. The BCR was found to be within tolerance before dispensing; however, the lenses were not hydrated. Now the lenses are too flat (i.e., verified as 7.89 mm/42.75 D), and they exhibit an apical bearing pattern and excessive movement. The lenses need to be reordered in the correct BCR. Although this is most likely the result of excessive heat generated during the manufacturing process, CT should also be verified to rule out that the lenses are too thin.

CASE 5

A patient is dispensed GP lenses for the first time. The patient returns at the 1-week visit complaining of discomfort. The patient is told that an adaptation period is normal; generally, at minimum, 2 weeks is necessary. The patient returns at 2 weeks requesting a refund as the lenses are intolerable.

SOLUTION: Inspection reveals sharp, "scratchy" edges with small edge defects or microchips in both lenses. If the lenses had been verified before dispensing, the edges could have been polished or the lenses returned to the laboratory. At this time, the only option is to explain the problem to the patient and to indicate that it can be easily solved.

CASE 6

A patient comes for a follow-up examination on his Menicon Z lenses. Upon slit-lamp examination, the practitioner observes scratches on the lens surface. The patient had depleted his supply of the solutions dispensed and purchased Boston Original Formula (Conditioning and Cleaner from Bausch & Lomb).

SOLUTION: The Boston Cleaner is too abrasive for use on the Menicon lenses and it is not a recommended cleaner. The lens material is a hyper-Dk, soft material; therefore, the abrasive cleaner scratches the lenses. The recommended care regimen is a nonabrasive system—for example, Claris (Menicon/Allergan), Optimum (Lobob), or Boston Simplus (Bausch & Lomb/Boston). The patient should be re-educated on proper care and handling of his lenses.

CASE 7

A patient is fitted with a new pair of soft contact lenses. The powers and brand of his previous lenses are unknown. At the follow-up examination, he complains of poor vision. His vision is 20/20 OU. The new lenses are −1.50 D OU.

SOLUTION: The powers of his previous lenses are verified. The previous lenses verify as −2.00 D OU. The red-green test shows that he is overminused in the previous lenses. The patient is educated to try the new powers, and if he does not adapt, a compromise between the old and the new powers will be attempted.

CASE 8

A patient comes for an examination reporting discomfort in the left eye with her soft lens on. The discomfort has been present for about 1 week.

SOLUTION: Inspection of the soft lens on the eye reveals a central tear in the left lens, which has caused superficial corneal staining upon lens removal.

CASE 9

A new patient comes to your office to be fit with soft lenses. She does not remember what her previous soft lenses are, but she thinks they are some kind of Vistakon lens.

SOLUTION: When the lenses are viewed with the slit-lamp biomicroscope, the marking "AV" is found on the lenses. "AV" was an inversion indicator manufactured onto Acuvue lenses. The other Vistakon lenses have a "123" on the lens.

CLINICAL PROFICIENCY CHECKLIST

- It is imperative that GP lenses be verified before dispensing to ensure that, at minimum, the appropriate BCR, power, OAD and OZD, CT, and edge design have been received.

- It is necessary to soak GP lenses in an approved disinfecting solution for at least 12 hours before base curve verification and dispensing.

- Overkeratometry readings, BCR, and power verification are all necessary procedures to determine the difference between a lens that is flexing and one that is warped.

- It is important for the lens edge to be inspected in both the frontal and side (profile) views on a projection magnifier before dispensing or whenever the edge design or condition may be in question. In addition, the "palm test" may be used as an initial screening procedure before the aforementioned method of projection magnification is performed to determine the condition of the edge.

- With toric lens designs, it is possible to differentiate between spherical and toric designs and front, back, and bitoric designs by verifying the BCR, the front curve, and the power of the lens.

- If a patient complains of soft lens irritation, the soft lens should be inspected on or off the eye for tears, deposits, or other lens damage.

- The easiest parameters to verify on a soft lens are power, OAD, surface inspection, and identification markings.

REFERENCES

1. Jurkus JM, Kelly SA. Automated and manual base curve assessment of rigid gas permeable contact lenses. Int Contact Lens Clin 1996;23(7–8):138–141.
2. Henry VA, Bennett ES. Inspection and verification of gas-permeable contact lenses. In: Bennett ES, Weissman BA, eds. Clinical Contact Lens Practice. Philadelphia: Lippincott Williams & Wilkins, 2005:294–305.
3. Barr JT, Hettler DH. Boston II base curve changes with hydration. Contact Lens Forum 1984;9:65–67.
4. Sarver MD. Verification of contact lens power. J Am Optom Assoc 1963;34(16):1304–1306.
5. DeKinder JO, Henry VA. Verifying GP contact lenses. Contact Lens Spectrum 2005;20(4):51.
6. Lowther GE. Inspection and verification. In: Lowther GE, ed. Contact Lenses: Procedures and Techniques. Boston: Butterworths, 1982:153–192.
7. Jameson M. Verifying soft contact lens parameters. Contact Lens Spectrum 2003;18(8):47.
8. Janoff LE. Hydrogel lens verification. In: Bennett ES, Weissman BA, eds. Clinical Contact Lens Practice. Philadelphia: JB Lippincott Co, 1991:37-1–37-13.
9. Bennett ES. Hydrogel versus rigid gas permeable lenses for extended wear: criteria and difference. J Am Optom Assoc 1986;57(7):500–502.

CHAPTER 8

Gas-Permeable Lens Problem Solving

Edward S. Bennett and Terry Scheid

Although rigid gas-permeable (GP) lenses can induce subjective and physiologic problems, as can any contact lens material, fortunately these complications are usually easy to resolve. Certainly the improvements in material and manufacturing technology have resulted in a reduced incidence of these problems, with sight-threatening problems being especially rare. The purpose of this chapter is to provide both diagnostic and management information for several common problems or potentially problematic patients.

■ THE EVALUATION PROCESS

As discussed in Chapter 6, it is important for GP wearing patients to be evaluated at 1 week, 1 month, 3 months, and every 6 months thereafter. At each visit, it is recommended for practitioners to perform the procedures provided in Table 8.1.

Case History

A comprehensive case history is important, especially at the 1-week visit.[1] The four key areas to explore with the patient pertain to wearing time, comfort, vision, and compliance.[2] If wearing the lenses on a daily-wear schedule, patients should be able to wear their lenses 8 to 16 hours per day to maintain comfort.[3] Patients should be asked about their care and handling of the lenses; if handling problems are still present, this is an excellent time to solve the problem. These visits are good opportunities to ensure that patients are still using the prescribed care regimen. In addition, they can be asked about their comfort, vision, and overall level of satisfaction.

Procedures Before Lens Removal

Before lens removal, several procedures should be performed. Visual acuity should be assessed and compared with patients' baseline values. A quick spherocylindrical over-refraction via retinoscopy is important for several reasons, including to assess if any residual astigmatism is present and to confirm problems such as corneal distortion or lens warpage. A spherical over-refraction will ensure that the patient is not over- or underminused. Loose trial lenses can be used as well to better simulate the real-world environment. If minus power is indicated, it can be added in the office if modification capabilities are present.

A biomicroscopic evaluation can assess such factors as lens centration and movement with the blink. The surface quality can also be assessed to evaluate such factors as deposits and scratches. The fluorescein pattern can be evaluated to ensure that there is an absence of excessive apical bearing or clearance and likewise peripherally. If flexure is suspected, keratometry should be performed over the lenses.

TABLE 8.1 PROGRESS EVALUATION PROCEDURES (GAS-PERMEABLE LENS WEARERS)

Before Lens Removal

1. Case history: symptoms, wearing time, level of satisfaction, care system, review handling (if necessary)

2. Visual acuity

3. Retinoscopy for spherocylindrical over-refraction

4. Best sphere over-refraction

5. Biomicroscopic evaluation (before removal):
   a. Surface quality (deposits, scratches)
   b. Centration and movement with the blink
   c. Fluorescein pattern

6. Overkeratometry[a]

After Lens Removal

1. Biomicroscopic evaluation (after lens removal)
   a. Corneal staining
   b. Vascularization
   c. Edema
   d. Papillary hypertrophy

2. Manifest refraction[a]

3. Keratometry/corneal topography[a]

4. Verification (base curve radius, surface, edge)[a]

[a]Unnecessary at every visit.

Procedures After Lens Removal

After lens removal, the cornea should be evaluated for signs of vascularization (360-degree evaluation) and staining. Central corneal clouding (CCC), which is rare with the current generation of GP lens materials, can be evaluated by using sclerotic scatter of split limbal illumination and viewing the presence of any haze against the black pupil background. The lids should be everted to observe any possible changes in papillary hypertrophy.

Although not mandatory at every visit, it is always recommended to check the patient's manifest refraction and corneal curvature values at progress evaluation visits. Corneal topography instrumentation, if available, can assist in detecting if there are any regions of corneal distortion or large curvature change (i.e., inferior steepening via a superiorly decentered lens). Lens inspection procedures such as radiuscopy (warpage) or edge inspection (discomfort) should be performed as needed.

■ REDUCED VISION

A reduction in vision as compared to the best spectacle-corrected visual acuity is typically the result of one of the following five causes: (a) flexure, (b) warpage, (c) decentration, (d) poor surface wettability, or (e) power change.

Flexure

Flexure of a GP lens results from the bending force of the upper lid during the blink process. This bending force induces a certain amount of toricity within the lens. For example, on a high, with-the-rule astigmatic patient, this induced toricity will reduce the amount of astigmatic correction provided by the lens. There are several causes for this problem, including a steep fitting relationship, reduced center thickness, large optical zone diameter, and material flexibility.[4–6] Flexure can be diagnosed by performing keratometry over the patient's lenses (preferably during the diagnostic fitting process). The values obtained should be spherical; the presence of any toricity in this measurement is typically the result of flexure. If undiagnosed, patients will typically report asthenopic complaints indicative of inadequate astigmatic correction.

Flexure can be managed by changing the lens design. The most important design change would be to flatten the base curve radius (BCR) by, at minimum, 0.50 D, assuming this modification does not compromise the lens-to-cornea fitting relationship.[4] Increasing the center thickness by 0.02 mm per diopter of corneal astigmatism has also been recommended[7]; however, this change should only be considered if option one is not possible, since the increased lens mass may compromise the fitting relationship. Other secondary, but effective, management options include reducing the optical zone diameter of the lens by, at minimum, 0.3 mm or changing materials [typically from a higher to a lower oxygen permeability (Dk)].

Warpage

Another common GP-induced problem is warpage or permanently induced toricity within the lens. This problem differs from flexure in several ways:

1. It is diagnosed by verifying the base curve radius and will verify as toric with the radiuscope, whereas in flexure-related decreased visual acuity the warpage will verify as spherical.
2. This problem is acquired over time, whereas flexure-induced problems can be evident immediately.
3. The induced toricity is permanent.

The primary cause of warpage is the application of excessive digital pressure during the cleaning process. In fact, it has been determined that cleaning the lenses between the fingers will result in over three and one-half times more warpage than cleaning in the palm of the hand.[8] In addition, the incidence of warpage is higher in former polymethylmethacrylate (PMMA) wearers[9] (primarily a result of customary use of the digital cleaning method) and is proportional to the oxygen permeability of the material.[10] Finally, warpage and possibly an inverted lens may result from placing the lens upside down in a smooth-welled case.[6]

Warpage can be minimized by adherence to the following recommendations:

1. Routinely verify the base curve radius at all patient progress evaluation visits; therefore, if a small increase in toricity is detected, the patient can be properly educated before further change and possible dissatisfaction with rigid lenses result.
2. Educate all patients and especially former PMMA wearers to clean the lenses carefully in the palm of the hand.
3. Always provide patients with a case having ridges or holes within the wells.
4. If warpage persists (and some patients are truly "warpers" as a result of possessing thick, rough fingers and/or an inability to clean the lenses gently), changing to a lower-Dk material and to a multipurpose system that has surfactant cleaning agents is recommended as well.

Decentration

GP lens decentration can result in numerous problems, including corneal desiccation,[9] corneal warpage,[11] poor corneal alignment,[12] and reduced vision. The poor alignment results in a space underneath the lens as it rests on the flatter, more peripheral region of the cornea; therefore, poor tear exchange and even adherence can result.[13] Likewise, some region under the lens will exhibit excessive clearance, with a nonstaining dimple veil pattern possible with fluorescein (Fig. 8.1). However, the vision changes, including fluctuating visual acuity and flare, are typically the most frustrating to both patient and practitioner. Any form of decentration can result

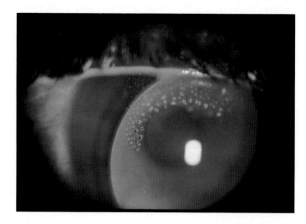

■ **FIGURE 8.1** Dimple veiling.

from a decentered corneal apex, an unusual corneal topography, lid characteristics, a less than optimum lens design, or the specific lens material. Ideally, as much of the corneal topography should be evaluated as possible. As keratometry is often the only option, lens design and, particularly, fluorescein pattern evaluation become very important. Inferior, superior, and lateral decentration will be discussed.

Inferior

Lens design plays an important role in reducing the incidence of a rigid lens decentering inferiorly. An "on K" to "flatter than K" fitting relationship appears to be preferable to steep fitting designs, especially in minus powers.[4] Center thickness should be maintained to a minimum; in fact, recommended center thickness values for any given material should be available from the manufacturer. This parameter should be routinely verified; however, verification of center thickness only occurs in approximately one-half of practices fitting contact lenses.[14] It has been found that increasing center thickness typically has only a slight effect on oxygen transmission but can have a large effect on lens mass and, therefore, centration characteristics.[15,16] The use of ultrathin lens designs, recommended for all patients with <2 D of corneal cylinder, should assist with centration.[17,18]

Perhaps the most important parameter affecting centration is lens edge. The effect of using a minus lenticular to "lift up" a lens of plus or low minus power is very dramatic.[16] Likewise, the use of a plus lenticular on high minus lenses minimizes the likelihood of inferior decentration resulting from the increase in lens mass and the effect of the upper lid on the thick lens edge. The anterior optic cap is generally designed 0.1 to 0.2 mm larger than the back optic zone diameter. The larger the anterior cap, the thicker the center thickness of the lens for a given lens overall diameter. In addition, the use of a "lid attachment" lens design with an anteriorly positioned edge[19] is also beneficial in cases of inferior decentration. However, if excessive edge clearance is present, either via an excessively flat base curve radius, a flat peripheral curve radius, a wide peripheral curve width, or a combination of these factors, the resulting lid interaction could result in an inferiorly positioned lens.[20]

It has also been found that specific gravity may also play a role. Materials of high specific gravity have greater lens mass than do equal volumes of materials with lower specific gravities.[21] Material-specific gravities range from approximately 1.05 to 1.27. It has been found that, for inferior positioning lenses, changing to a lower specific gravity material resulted in a greater effect on centration than reducing center thickness.[22]

Therefore, to minimize inferior decentration:

1. Consider a flatter base curve radius for myopic patients.
2. Keep center thickness to a minimum without inducing flexure.

3. Use a lenticular design when indicated (typically with all plus and < -1.50 D lens powers for a minus lenticular and > -5 D for a plus lenticular).
4. Consider use of a lid attachment design.
5. If options 1 to 4 are unsuccessful, changing to a lower specific gravity material, if possible, may be of benefit.

Superior

If slight superior decentration is present, this can be beneficial for both vision and comfort as a result of a "tucked under the lid" fitting relationship. However, if the decentration is excessive, lens adherence can result. In addition, the use of corneal topography instrumentation has confirmed that corneal distortion is possible in the region of bearing superiorly.[11,23–25] Therefore, these patients need to be carefully monitored. For lenses that decenter superiorly, the opposite types of changes are indicated, including the use of a thinner edge design, a greater center thickness, and a steeper base curve radius. Changing center thickness, in particular, has been found to be more effective than changing to a higher specific gravity material.[21]

Lateral

Lenses decentering laterally can be especially frustrating. This often results from either a decentered corneal apex or an against-the-rule astigmatic patient. In the latter case, the lens tends to move more in a lateral motion after the blink with a tendency (as in with-the-rule astigmatism) to transverse the steeper corneal meridian. Some options have enjoyed limited success, including selecting a larger overall diameter or a steeper base curve radius. However, a viable alternative is to fit an aspheric lens design in an effort to provide better alignment and possibly improve centration. If these options fail, a soft toric lens may be indicated.

Poor Surface Wettability

The importance of good GP lens surface wettability or the ability of the blink to spread tear film mucin across the anterior contact lens surface cannot be underestimated. In fact, good surface wettability may be the most desirable rigid lens property. Poor wettability can be divided into two separate categories: initial and acquired.[26]

Initial

Poor initial wettability is almost always a manufacturing problem and could result from the following:

1. Too much heat buildup during the manufacturing process.
2. Poor polishing techniques.
3. Improper or old diamond used for cutting.
4. Residual pitch polish left on the lens surface.

This problem is typically diagnosed by the appearance not of a film, but of a breakup of the tear film on the lens surface during biomicroscopic evaluation (Fig. 8.2). This is an especially frustrating problem to the patient who expected excellent visual acuity but instead is experiencing fluctuations in vision.

Many GP lenses are shipped from the laboratory dry in a flat pack. If dispensed directly from the pack, the lens often exhibits poor initial wetting and hazy vision. This problem can often be prevented by presoaking the lenses for a minimum of 24 hours prior to dispensing in the recommended soaking solution. This solution typically contains wetting agents that can condition the surface to be initially compatible with the tear film. If the wettability is still not optimum, a compatible laboratory cleaner (e.g., The Boston Laboratory Cleaner, Polymer

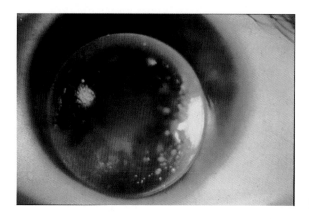

■ FIGURE 8.2 Poor initial surface wettability.

Technology Corporation) or solvent (e.g., FluoroSolve, Paragon Vision Sciences) can be used. After laboratory cleaning, the lens should be conditioned by rubbing wetting solution onto the surface using the same technique as when cleaning the lens. As a final procedure, light surface polishing of the lens can be performed, although this is rarely necessary and only if the lens is not plasma treated.

Many GP lenses today are available with wet shipping. This should usually allow for better and more consistent initial wettability. As discussed in Chapter 3, new plasma treatments are available for Boston, Paragon, Contamac, and Menicon lens materials. The treating of GP lenses with plasma is an effective method to remove any remaining lens-manufacturing residues. An outcome of this treatment process is a dramatic reduction in wetting angle, maximizing initial lens wettability and possibly increasing initial lens comfort. Plasma coating may also repel protein, cell, and bacterial adhesion.[27] Plasma-treated lenses should be shipped wet. The treatment effects will diminish over weeks to months but aid in initial GP lens wettability and patient adaptation.

Acquired

The more commonly experienced problem is acquired mucoprotein film or haze on the anterior lens surface. Typically, this occurs over a period of several weeks to several months. The thick, filmlike appearance is easily diagnosed by biomicroscopy (Fig. 8.3). There are several

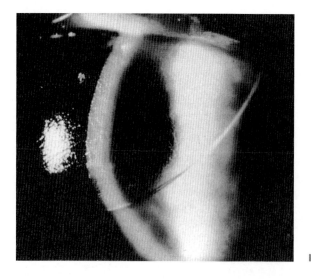

■ FIGURE 8.3 Mucoprotein film.

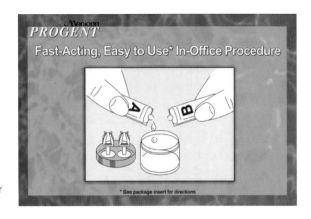

■ **FIGURE 8.4** The Menicon Progent Cleaner (Menicon).

causes of this film, including poor tear quality, improper blinking, inadequate compliance, use of improper solutions, foreign contaminants, and surface scratches.

Patients having a borderline tear quality should be placed on an aggressive care regimen, including daily use of either an abrasive cleaner or a surfactant cleaning/disinfecting regimen supplemented by both daily liquid enzymatic cleaning and rewetting drops several times each day. Patients should be educated about the importance of cleaning the lenses thoroughly immediately after lens removal followed by placement in the appropriate soaking solution; otherwise, any fresh deposits in contact with the tear film while on the eye will dry out and become more difficult to remove. Patients should also be advised to wash their hands thoroughly with a non–lanolin-containing hand soap (i.e., most bar soaps and all optical hand soaps) before handling their lenses because hand creams and other substances on the hand can adhere to the lens surface and compromise wettability. In addition, patient compliance with the proper care regimen can be evaluated by having a space on the progress evaluation form for listing the solutions; therefore, this can be asked at every patient visit. To clean a heavily deposited lens in the office, the aforementioned laboratory cleaners or solvents should be used. In cases of heavy lens deposits, even in the presence of plasma-treated lenses, the Menicon Progent (Menicon Inc.) system is valuable. Lenses are placed in a sodium hypochlorite–potassium bromide mixture for 30 minutes, then cleaned and rinsed. This is approved in the United States for in-office use only at this time (Fig. 8.4).

If scratches and/or deposits are present on the posterior surface of the lens, a light polish should be beneficial. Finally, if all else fails, a change in lens material is recommended. Changing from a silicone/acrylate (S/A) to a fluoro-silicone/acrylate (F-S/A) material or from a high-Dk to a lower (i.e., 25–50)-Dk F-S/A material should provide an improvement in deposit resistance as a result of a higher over-the-lens tear breakup time (TBUT).[28] To summarize, acquired surface wettability can be minimized by the following steps:

1. Use an aggressive cleaning regimen for the heavily depositing patients.
2. Proper patient cleaning should be supplemented by frequent monitoring of the care regimen; lanolin-containing products should be avoided.
3. In-office cleaning with a laboratory cleaner or solvent is often indicated in these cases; a light polish may be necessary in some cases.
4. Changing to a low-Dk fluoro-silicone/acrylate lens material will maintain the tear film in contact with the lens surface for a longer period.

Power Change

Another problem pertains to an increase in minus power over time accompanied by a decrease in center thickness in some GP lens wearers using an abrasive cleaner.[29–33] This change has been reported to be as much as −2.00 D.[30] The use of an abrasive cleaner, in combination with forceful digital cleaning in a circular manner, has been implicated as the cause of these changes. In particular, former PMMA wearers have been implicated in these reports. One study found that the greatest changes were exhibited by the Boston Cleaner (Bausch & Lomb), less change with a milder abrasive cleaner [Opticlean II (Alcon)], and the least change with a nonabrasive cleaner [Resolve (Allergan Optical)] in a three-cleaner comparison study.[8] This problem can be minimized by complying with the following recommendations:

1. Patients should clean the lenses gently in the palm of the hand.
2. For patients prone to warpage, the use of a mild abrasive cleaner or a hands-off regimen is recommended.
3. Practitioners should consider verifying lens power, center thickness, and base curve radius at follow-up visits, particularly when the patient is symptomatic.

■ REDUCED COMFORT

Initial

Methods of minimizing initial awareness are discussed in Chapter 5. These include how lenses are presented to the patient, the use of a topical anesthetic, and having the patient's first experience with GP lenses be a positive one (whenever possible) via providing lenses in his or her correct power. In addition, if the patient is especially apprehensive about wearing contact lenses in general (i.e., reacted negatively to such tests as lid eversion, tonometry, and dilation), a slow build-up schedule would be indicated to gradually adapt the patient's lids to the sensation of the lens edge.

Although as a result of improvements in manufacturing quality a defective edge is only an occasional problem, every lens should be inspected before dispensing to the patient. Decentration, as discussed in the previous section, may also impact initial comfort and should be managed accordingly. One design change that does appear to improve comfort, in addition to changes to improve centration (i.e., ultrathin design, lenticular use), would be to increase the overall diameter,[34] although a minimum change of 0.4 mm is recommended to have a significant effect.[35] Patients should also be warned that they may occasionally have a foreign body trapped behind the lens, causing momentary discomfort until the blink washes it away (Fig. 8.5).

Acquired

Lens awareness can be acquired, either from dryness-related causes such as corneal desiccation and vascularized limbal keratitis (to be discussed), from papillary hypertrophy, or from

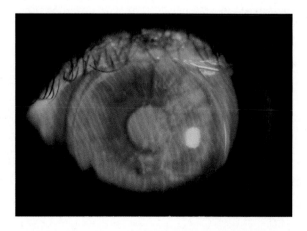

■ FIGURE 8.5 Foreign body tracks.

damage to the lens edge. As mentioned earlier, if papillary hypertrophy is problematic, lens wear should be discontinued, often up to several weeks while the prescribed mast cell stabilizer/anti-inflammatory medications are being used. If the edge would happen to become abraded or mildly chipped, in-office modification is invaluable. As discussed in Chapter 9, modification tools are available from many of the Contact Lens Manufacturers Association (CLMA) member laboratories.

▓ DRYNESS

Corneal Desiccation

Corneal desiccation, or "3- and 9-o'clock" staining, refers to the drying or dehydration of the peripheral cornea. The staining results from a disruption in the tear film, adjacent to the lens edge.[36-38] This is a very common lens-induced complication, occurring in over 40% to 90% of patients wearing GP contact lenses.[9,39-41] Initially, and in most cases, the desiccation consists of isolated punctate stains (Fig. 8.6). However, in certain cases the staining can coalesce with engorgement of the adjacent conjunctival blood vessels. It has been found to be clinically significant in 10% to 15% of cases.[20,39,42] Extended-wear GP wearers have greater than two times the incidence of corneal desiccation than daily wearers.[43] In most severe cases, peripheral corneal thinning occurs with ulceration, neovascularization, and scarring.[6,44] The term *dellen* has been ascribed to a well-circumscribed oval area of peripheral thinning occasionally resulting from desiccation in this region.[45] If symptoms are present, they are typically dryness and redness, with the latter often representing the first subjective symptom.[46,47] The following scale has been used to classify corneal desiccation[48]:

0 = No staining.
1 = Diffuse, superficial, noncoalesced staining.
2 = Superficial coalesced staining.
3 = Marked coalescence with some deep epithelial penetration.
4 = Complete coalescence with extensive loss of epithelial cells.

Factors to consider in the management of corneal desiccation include the lens material, lens centration, edge clearance, and tear film stability.

Lens Material

As mentioned previously, the most successful lens materials for minimizing the incidence of corneal desiccation are those that can maintain the tear film on the lens surface for the longest period. Therefore, the evaporation of the tear film peripheral to the lens edge may not occur during the interblink period. A low-Dk F-S/A material may be optimum for accomplishing this

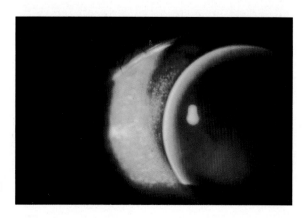

▓ **FIGURE 8.6** A corneal desiccation (3- and 9-o'clock) staining.

goal, although newer hyper-Dk lens materials such as the Menicon Z have appeared to demonstrate excellent short-term surface wettability.[49] If severe desiccation persists, a soft lens material may be necessary.

Lens Centration

A superior lens-to-cornea fitting relationship, with the lens tucked underneath the upper lid, is important in minimizing the incidence of moderate to severe cases of corneal desiccation. This position allows the lid and lens edge interaction to be at a minimum; therefore, interference with the normal blinking pattern is reduced.[26] Intrapalpebral and, especially, inferiorly positioned lenses encourage lens edge interaction with the upper lid, resulting in irritation and alteration of the normal blink reflex. This was confirmed in a 12-month GP extended-wear study in which the incidence of corneal desiccation was almost twice as high with inferiorly positioned versus superiorly positioned lenses.[9] To minimize this problem, the same design principles mentioned in the decentration section of this chapter apply here, namely, the use of an "on K" to "flatter than K" base curve radius (a steeper BCR may be necessary for plus power lens designs to obtain centration); center thickness at a minimum; a thin, rolled, tapered edge design (a thick, sharp, or chipped edge may increase desiccation by inducing a partial blink response); and the use of a minus lenticular edge design in all plus and low minus lens powers and a plus lenticular design for all high minus (≥ -5.00 D) power designs. Diameter is a controversial parameter. It's safe to assume that increasing the overall diameter will decrease the area of staining because of the greater amount of corneal coverage; however, this increase in diameter will also increase the overall mass, and the possibility of a more inferiorly decentered lens should be evaluated.

Edge Clearance

Edge clearance is another controversial parameter. It is important to avoid excessively high edge lift designs to reduce the peripheral tear volume, to decrease the gap in the periphery between the lid and the cornea, and to minimize the potentially compromising effect on the blink caused by the interaction between the upper lid and the lens edge[4,19,50–53] (Fig. 8.7).

This can be achieved by using a tricurve or tetracurve design with a peripheral curve width no greater than 0.3 mm and a peripheral curve radius no flatter than 11.0 mm. In addition, an aspheric design may be advantageous because of better alignment of the posterior surface with the cornea.[54] However, insufficient edge clearance can also result in corneal desiccation because of insufficient tear exchange and peripheral seal-off.[55] Therefore, the most effective method of determining if the edge clearance is appropriate is via fluorescein application and pattern evaluation. The peripheral band of fluorescein should be slightly greater or more dense than centrally.[56]

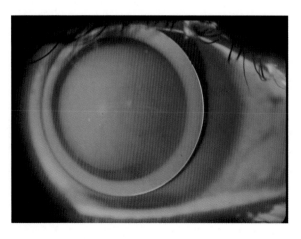

■ **FIGURE 8.7** A high edge clearance design, which often ultimately results in corneal desiccation.

Tear Film Stability

As the interblink interval is typically 4 to 6 seconds, patients should have a TBUT equal to, at minimum, 5 seconds to be fit with contact lenses. Patients with low to borderline tear quality (i.e., TBUT of 5–9 seconds) fit with GP lenses typically will have subjective symptoms of dryness accompanied by corneal desiccation caused by evaporation of the peripheral tear pool. The use of rewetting drops, as often as every hour, accompanied by a highly wettable lens material will help somewhat in increasing the number of hours of daily lens wear.

A summary management nomogram is provided in Figure 8.8.

Vascularized Limbal Keratitis

Associated with limbal desiccation is the presence of a more acute complication of the peripheral cornea in the 3- or 9-o'clock regions termed *vascularized limbal keratitis*.[57] With this condition, a raised translucent inflamed area is present that is accompanied by vascularization and adjacent bulbar conjunctival injection[58] (Fig. 8.9). It is more common in, but not limited to, GP extended wear. Patients typically report increasing lens awareness over the previous few weeks and often notice the "white spot" on their eye. It is often present in long-term rigid lens wearers—notably silicone/acrylate lens materials—with a steep lens-to-cornea fitting relationship and peripheral seal-off. It is best managed by having the patient discontinue lens wear until the affected region is no longer elevated and the vessels have receded. A combination antibiotic–steroid should be prescribed (i.e., Tobradex OS q.i.d.) and the patient should be evaluated after 24 hours. Typically, after 4 to 5 days this region is no longer elevated and the patient can taper the medication (Fig. 8.10).

If the patient is wearing a silicone/acrylate lens material, refitting into a fluoro-silicone/acrylate lens material would be recommended to provide enhanced surface wettability and, therefore, improved peripheral corneal lubrication. A new lens should be ordered with a flatter peripheral curve system to allow better tear exchange or the present lens modified to achieve the same result. In addition, reducing the patient to a flexible-wear or even a daily-wear schedule would be recommended. Table 8.2 shows GP-induced problems and their management.

■ REFITTING INTO GAS-PERMEABLE LENSES

There are numerous cases in which patients can benefit by refitting from another lens material into GP lenses. This includes PMMA, very-low- and high-DK GPs, and soft lens wearers.

Polymethylmethacrylate/Very-low-oxygen Permeability Gas-permeable Lens Into Higher-oxygen Permeability Gas-permeable Lens Materials

Why Refit Polymethylmethacrylate/Very-Low-Oxygen Permeability Gas-Permeable Lens Wearers?

There are, at minimum, three important considerations when refitting PMMA wearers into GP lenses. The first pertains to PMMA-induced complications. The philosophy often associated with allowing patients to continue wearing their PMMA lenses is "if it ain't broke, don't fix it." In other words, if no symptoms and clinical signs exist, then the PMMA or very-low-Dk (<25 Dk) GP lens wearer should not be refit into a higher-Dk lens material. However, the cornea needs an oxygen level of approximately 10% (equivalent to an oxygen transmission value of 24 Dk/t) to avoid corneal swelling in the daily-wear situation.[59] Therefore, with a comprehensive evaluation, it is very likely that any one or a combination of the following hypoxia-related complications will be present.[60]

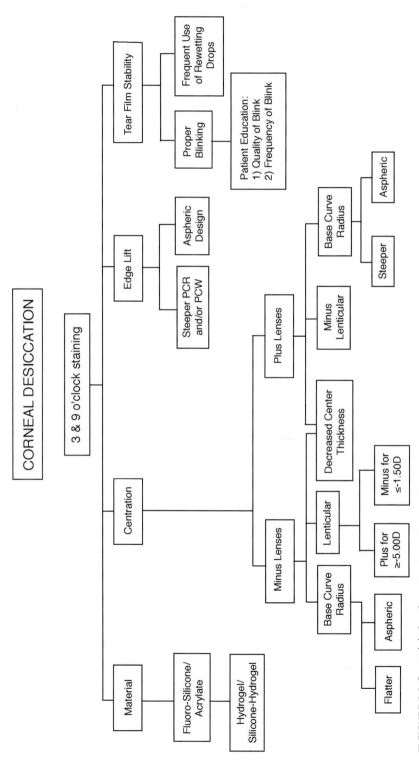

■ FIGURE 8.8 Corneal desiccation management nomogram.

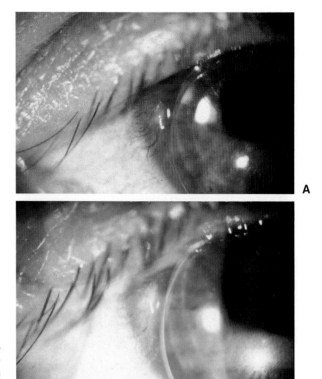

A

B

■ **FIGURE 8.9 (A)** Vascularized limbal keratitis showing the elevated, opacified, raised peripheral region. **(B)** This same area exhibits staining with fluorescein.

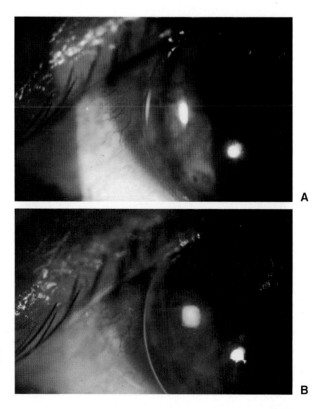

A

B

■ **FIGURE 8.10 (A)** The same patient in Figure 8.9 after 7 days of lens discontinuation. Notice the reduction in elevation of this region. **(B)** Reduced corneal staining.

TABLE 8.2 GAS-PERMEABLE PROBLEM SOLVING BASED UPON CONDITION

CONDITION	SYMPTOMS	CAUSES	DIAGNOSIS	MANAGEMENT
Flexure	Poor initial and variable vision	High (often ≥2 D) corneal cyl, steep BCR, Thin design, steep BCR	Toric over-K's Sph-Cyl OR	Flatter BCR, CT, Decr OZD Lower Dk
Warpage	Vision gradually decreases	High/hyper-Dk Digital cleaning	Toric radiuscope values Sph-Cyl OR	Clean in palm "Hands-off" care system
Power change	Vision reduced @ near (pre-presbyopic); may be asymptomatic	Abrasive cleaner Digital cleaning	Minus power with lensometer	Clean in palm Nonabrasive cleaner
Decentration				
1) Inferior	Variable vision with blink Lens awareness	Thick lens High WTR cyl Inferior apex Plus power lenses Loose lid tension	Inferior decentration Excessive movement	Ultrathin design +Lent ≥ −5.00 D −Lent for all + & low − (≤ −1.50D) Bitoric: ≥ 2.50 D cyl
2) Superior	Flare around lights Lens awareness	Flat BCR Ultrathin design	Superior position Possible adherence	Steepen BCR CT[a] +Lent if high − power
3) Lateral	Flare around lights Lens awareness	ATR cyl Lateral apex	Lateral decentration Movement along horizontal meridian	Steeper BCR OAD Aspheric design Soft toric design
Reduced Surface Wettability				
1) Initial	Poor initial/ fluctuating vision	Manufacturing problems (pitch, residues) Use of lanolin	Beading up of tear film/haze	Use plasma treatment lab cleaner/solvent Presoak lens
2) Acquired	Gradual reduction in vision	Noncompliance with cleaning Use of lanolin creams/soaps Poor tear quality/ volume Use of medications	Mucoprotein haze/film Papillary hypertrophy	Re-educate on care & avoid lanolin soaps before insertion Use liquid enzyme
Discomfort				
1) Initial	Lens awareness	Defective edge Decentration	Edge inspection Biomicroscopy	Polish edge/ new lens As noted above
2) Acquired	Lens awareness	Chipped edge GPC Staining	Edge inspection Lid eversion Biomicroscope	Polish edge/ reorder lens D/C lens wear & anti-inflammatory meds If 3- & 9-o'clock staining or VLK, treat as indicated below

TABLE 8.2 *(Continued)* GAS-PERMEABLE PROBLEM SOLVING BASED UPON CONDITION

CONDITION	SYMPTOMS	CAUSES	DIAGNOSIS	MANAGEMENT
Dryness				
1) Corneal desiccation	Dryness Redness Low-grade awareness	Poor tear quality Inferior decentration Thick edge/CT High edge lift Poor lid hygiene Poor blink quality	3- & 9-o'clock staining Injection Possible vascularization/ opacification	Ignore if diffuse only Decr center/edge thickness, add lent Decr edge lift, steepen PCR/decr PCW) Lid hygiene; if MGD, warm compresses/lid massage Frequent use of rewetting drops
2) Vascularized limbal keratitis	Acute awareness Reduced wearing time Red eye Observable opaque area at corneal periphery	Prolonged dryness S/A material Low edge lift Steep BCR EW schedule	Opaque, elevated vascularized region @ 3- & 9-o'clock region	D/C lens wear: 5–7 d Ab/steroid combination F-S/A material Daily wear only Flatter/wider periphery Flatter BCR Reduce diameter

Ab, antibiotic; BCR, base curve radius; CT, center thickness; cyl, cylindrical; D/C, discontinue; decr, decreased; Dk, oxygen permeability; EW, extended wear; F-S/A, fluoro-silicone/acrylate; GPC, giant papillary conjunctivitis; Lent, lenticular; MGD, meibomian gland dysfunction; OAD, overall diameter; OR, over-refraction; OZD, overall zone diameter; PCR, peripheral curve radius; PCW, peripheral curve width; S/A, silicone/acrylate; sph-cyl, spherocylindrical; VLK, vascularized limbal keratitis.

Central Corneal Clouding: Central corneal clouding (CCC) is a circumscribed region of epithelial edema that appears as a grayish haze against the dark background of the pupil when sclerotic scatter/split limbal illumination with biomicroscopy is used. Although the patient ordinarily experiences acceptable visual acuity with contact lens wear, vision is usually unsatisfactory through spectacles. In addition, an increase in myopia and steepening of the keratometer readings are also associated with CCC. This condition has been observed in almost every PMMA wearer.[61]

Edematous Corneal Formations: Edematous corneal formations (ECFs) are subepithelial arborized or dendritic-appearing formations located in the central cornea. ECFs reflect low-grade edema and develop gradually in the long-term wearer.[62] They are difficult to detect; using indirect illumination is recommended.

Polymegethism: Alteration or variation in the endothelial cell area is termed *polymegethism*. Since the endothelium controls corneal hydration, any disruption of this layer of cells may encourage edema or swelling. This is best observed during biomicroscopy with a parallelepiped using high magnification and illumination. It has been determined that a significant variation in the endothelial cell area occurs with long-term PMMA wear.[63] It has also been demonstrated in low- to medium-Dk GP lens wear as well.[64]

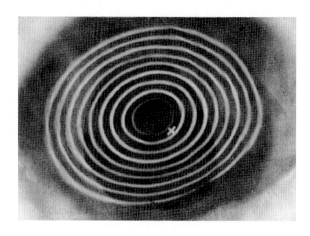

■ **FIGURE 8.11** Corneal distortion present in a patient with corneal warpage syndrome.

Corneal Warpage Syndrome: Prolonged corneal edema can result in corneal distortion and unpredictable keratometric and refractive changes in as many as 30% of long-term PMMA wearers.[65] Refitting this corneal warpage syndrome patient can be extremely difficult since the cornea tends to exhibit keratoconus-like changes (although often reversible) with the development of irregular astigmatism and reduced vision through the best spectacle correction (Fig. 8.11).

Corneal warpage syndrome is most likely caused by a sequence of events resulting from a combination of corneal hypoxia, leading to typically central corneal steepening and irregular astigmatism, and the mechanical effects of a rigid lens on the cornea. Eventually a change in the lens-to-cornea fitting relationship can occur, resulting in decentration. Studies by Wilson have concluded that once decentration has occurred, significant changes in corneal topography typically result.[11,24,25,66] The topographic abnormalities that result correlate with the decentered resting position of the contact lens on the cornea. For example, superior decentered lenses produced superior flattening with a relatively steeper contour inferiorly, simulating the topography of early keratoconus. In one study, 21 eyes of 12 predominantly PMMA-wearing patients with contact lens–induced warpage were followed with topography.[24] The corneal topography of these patients was characterized by central irregular astigmatism, loss of radial symmetry, and frequent reversal of the normal topographic pattern of progressive corneal flattening from center to periphery. Detection of the presence of corneal warpage that persisted for months was attributable to the increased sensitivity of computer-assisted topographic analysis relative to keratometry and other previous techniques.

Another important consideration pertains to convincing the asymptomatic PMMA or very-low-GP lens wearer—who may only desire a new spectacle prescription—about the need to be refit into higher-Dk GP lenses. With few exceptions, patients will accept this change if a comprehensive explanation is provided of why a refit is necessary and what they should expect during the rehabilitation period.[67]

Refitting Strategy

It is important to perform a comprehensive evaluation of the patient while the patient is still wearing his or her lenses, preferably for several hours. This will allow observation of the amount and types of corneal edema and the level of difficulty in determining the refractive and keratometric values. A good case history should be performed, including questions pertaining to length of rigid lens wear per day, years of lens wear, and incidence of corneal abrasion. Patients who have worn their lenses all their waking hours for more than 15 years and are prone to overwear abrasions are prime candidates for corneal warpage or corneal exhaustion syndrome.[68,69]

The most effective strategy is to immediately refit the patient into higher-Dk GP lenses without loss of wearing time. This has the benefits of limiting excessive refractive change and enhancing patient satisfaction.[70] When refitting a patient immediately, the procedure used will depend on the effects of hypoxia on the cornea. If there is minimal or no compromise, the patient can be refit with no change in wearing time. If corneal distortion is present, the patient should be advised to reduce the wearing time to the minimum number of hours possible. Typically, this equals 8 to 12 hours per day. The patient should be advised to return for a visit in 1 week. At this time much improvement in mire quality, post-refraction visual acuity, and corneal integrity is usually present, and the patient can be refit. Although uncommon, if the corneal compromise continues to make it difficult to have usable keratometric and refractive information, either the patient can maintain a reduced wearing schedule for a longer period or fluorescein pattern analysis can be used for determining the optimum base curve radius of the lenses to be ordered. In all cases, spectacles can be prescribed once refractive stability in the new GP lenses has been achieved.

Material, Lens Design, and Fitting

The first fitting decision is choosing which lens material is preferable. Although the initial temptation is to select the highest-Dk material available, especially for corneal warpage syndrome patients, low- to medium-Dk (i.e., 25–50) lens materials would provide greater rigidity. This results in less corneal sensitivity and refractive change during the stabilization period when compared to higher-Dk materials. In addition, former PMMA wearers appear to experience warpage-related problems with high-Dk GP lenses.[9] If clinical signs of hypoxia continue with GP lens wear, the patient can later be refit into a higher-Dk material. If the patient has an optimum lens-to-cornea fitting relationship, the parameters can typically be duplicated in a GP lens material, although it is not unusual to refit into a larger overall diameter and lower edge clearance design.

Soft Into Gas-permeable Lenses

Why Refit into Gas-Permeable Lenses?

There are many reasons why soft lens wearers would benefit by being refit into GP lenses. This need is confirmed by a study that evaluated the results of 200 consecutive refits from one material to another at the Park-Nicollet Medical Center in Minneapolis, perhaps the largest contact lens practice in the United States at that time.[71] The largest number of refits were in the category of being refit from hydrogel into GP lenses (92 patients, or 46%), whereas only 9% were refit from GP into hydrogel lenses. The most common reasons cited for refitting into GP lenses were reduced vision and giant papillary conjunctivitis (GPC), and a 98% success rate was present after 6 months of GP lens wear. Reduced vision can result from several causes, including uncorrected refractive astigmatism, surface deposits, corneal edema, and a poorly fitting, soft toric lens. Other reasons for considering refitting a patient from soft into GP lenses include persistent edema, infiltrative keratitis, neovascularization, and difficulty in handling the larger-diameter lenses.

   Soft lens wearers deserve a comprehensive explanation of why GP lenses will be more beneficial for them. In addition, they should be provided with a realistic idea of the adaptation period associated with GP lenses. Some individuals believe they are "semi-soft" lenses and will necessitate a similar adaptation schedule as soft lenses. It is essential to indicate that GP lenses do not feel the same as soft lenses at first, but that over time, they should reach a point where they are very comfortable. As indicated in Chapter 5, terms such as *discomfort* and *pain* should be avoided. If the soft lens wearer is not experiencing any symptoms or clinical signs but is simply inquiring about GP lenses (e.g., a friend may be wearing them successfully or perhaps he or she is simply interested in what's new), realistic expectations about the initial lens sensation and adaptation period need to be provided. In most cases, these patients should not be refit unless motivation is high.

Refitting Procedure

Unless severe corneal compromise or lid inflammation is present necessitating soft lens removal, these patients can be refit and can gradually increase GP lens wear while simultaneously decreasing soft lens wear. The refitting is similar to a new patient with the exception that even more encouragement than usual is necessary during the adaptation (i.e., "awareness") phase. If, for example, the patient is an "excessive reactor" and tears for a lengthy period and becomes disillusioned, it would be preferable to maintain this patient in soft lenses, if possible. If GPC is the cause for refitting into GP lenses, the symptoms must be eliminated and the clinical signs markedly reduced (i.e., grade 1 papillary hypertrophy) before refitting into the new material.[72] In all cases, topical anesthetic use is important during the initial fit process. Patients are often apprehensive about making the transition into "hard" lenses. However, this transition is often quite easy if the first few minutes of lens wear are comfortable ones.

Patients also need to be educated about properly caring for these lenses. Each patient must be aware of the differences in lens handling and care and must demonstrate a knowledge and competence in these procedures before leaving the office.

■ SUMMARY

The types of problems described in this chapter are typically minor in nature, often necessitating a change in lens design or material. In most cases, these changes result in the lessening, if not elimination, of the indicated problem. With advances in material, design, and manufacturing technology, these problems should become fewer in the years to come.

■ CLINICAL CASES

CASE 1

A new GP patient has the following refractive information at the time of examination:

Keratometry: 42.25 @ 180; 44.25 @ 090 OU
Spectacle Rx: −4.00 − 1.75 × 180 OU

As it was a hectic day in the office, the lenses were ordered empirically in the following parameters:

OU: overall diameter (OAD)/optic zone diameter (OZD) = 9.2 mm/7.8 mm
BCR = 7.85 mm
Secondary curve radius/width (SCR/W) = 9.0 mm/0.4 mm
Peripheral curve radius/width (PCR/W) = 11.0 mm/0.3 mm
Power = −4.50 D
Center thickness (CT) = 0.14 mm
Material: Fluoroperm 60

Upon dispensing, the visual acuities were 20/25−1 (fluctuating) OU with an overrefraction equal to +0.25 − 0.75 × 180. Overkeratometry also resulted in some toricity: 42.75/43.50. Slit-lamp evaluation (SLE) revealed good surface wettability, and no toricity was verified with the radiuscope.

SOLUTION: This is a flexure-induced problem that can be managed by changing lens design—preferably by selection of a flatter base curve radius, for example, 7.94 mm (42.50 D)—and re-evaluating visual acuity and over-keratometry. This problem could have been prevented by diagnostically fitting lenses of similar design and material. It is important to rule out warpage and poor surface wettability in making the diagnosis, which can then be confirmed by the presence of toric over-keratometric readings. Additional management alternatives to consider if the change in base curve radius does not solve the problem include increasing center thickness 0.02 to 0.03 mm minimum, reducing optical zone diameter, and changing to a lower-Dk material.

CASE 2

The following GP lenses were ordered for a new patient:

OAD/OZD = 9.4 mm/7.8 mm
BCR = 7.89 mm
SCR/W = 8.7 mm/0.3 mm
Intermediate curve radius/width (ICR/W) = 9.8 mm/0.3 mm
PCR/W = 11.2 mm/0.2 mm
Power = −4.00 D
CT = Minimum
Material: Fluoroperm 30

On dispensing, the lenses decentered inferiorly. The patient was advised to gradually increase wearing time. However, after the 1-week and 1-month visits, the patient was still unable to achieve full-time wear, complaining of poor vision and lens awareness. Verification of the lens at that time resulted in a center thickness equal to 0.15 mm, and the lenses were still decentered in an inferior position.

SOLUTION: Reorder the lenses in a thinner design (i.e., always make the change a significant one; therefore, a thickness of 0.11 mm can be ordered). If the original diagnostic lens was available, what was the center thickness of that lens? Do not ever assume that merely indicating "minimum" on the order form will provide you with the thinnest possible design; some laboratories are able to make a particular lens material in a thinner design than others. As mentioned previously, it is beneficial to obtain the manufacturer's recommended center thickness values and confirm that your laboratory can make the lenses to those specifications. It is important to always verify center thickness of all incoming lenses; in addition, this information should be provided on all of the diagnostic lenses.

CASE 3

This case is identical to Case 2 with the exception that the lens power is equal to +4.00 D OU. The lens was verified as ordered; however, after 1 month the patient was still symptomatic, and the lenses were decentered inferiorly.

SOLUTION: A minus lenticular (or similarly designed) edge design should be ordered with these lenses. The center of gravity of a plus lens is decentered anteriorly, and this factor, in combination with a thin edge, often results in an inferiorly decentered lens. The addition of a lenticular will often have a dramatic effect on improving lens centration and should always be ordered with all plus (and low minus) lens powers. Never assume the laboratory will automatically manufacture a lenticulated lens design; this typically involves a slightly higher fee, and the laboratory may have the opinion that you would prefer not to have this particular type of design. Secondary alternatives would include a steeper base curve radius and/or a smaller overall diameter (to decrease lens mass).

CASE 4

A patient has the following refractive information:

OD: −2.00 − 1.25 × 085
42.50 @ 085; 44.00 @ 175

The following three diagnostic lenses attempted on this eye all decentered nasally, all of which positioned such that reduced visual acuity and flare would be likely if ordered:

Dx Lens No. 1	Dx Lens No. 2	Dx Lens No. 3
BCR = 42.75 D	BCR = 42.25 D	BCR = 42.25 D
OAD/OZD = 9.0 /7.8 mm	OAD/OZD = 9.2/7.8 mm	OAD/OZD = 8.8/7.4 mm

All of these lenses were of tricurve construction, with the SCR 1 mm flatter than the BCR and the PCR 3 mm flatter than the BCR.

SOLUTION: Against-the-rule astigmatism of any amount is a great challenge to the contact lens practitioner. Often the trial-and-error process can be exhausted in attempting to achieve an optimum fitting relationship; in fact, we often have to be satisfied with some amount of displacement. A good alternative in this situation would be an aspheric design. However, since visual compromise can be even greater when an aspheric design decenters, other design options should be considered if this option fails—for example, the use of a steeper base curve radius or a larger overall diameter. The use of a bitoric lens can be used in slightly greater astigmatic cases (i.e., ≥2D).

CASE 5

A former PMMA wearer had been refit into the Paragon HDS100 lens material (Paragon Vision Sciences) over 1 year previously. He was not provided with any instructions pertaining to caring for the new lenses since he has been a hard lens wearer. In addition, he was provided with the Boston care regimen (Bausch & Lomb). He was in the office for the first time in 9 months complaining of blurred vision and eyestrain, especially after prolonged near work (he is a 39-year-old attorney). The lenses, originally ordered in a −5.25 D power OU, now verified as −6.50 D. In addition, the lenses exhibited 0.50 D of toricity with the radiuscope. Since the lenses had never previously been verified, an apology is given to the patient and the lenses are reordered and eventually dispensed. However, 6 months later he has the same complaints.

SOLUTION: This is a typical case of a patient who has unintentionally added minus power to the lenses by forceful cleaning with an abrasive cleaner on a high-Dk GP lens material. In addition, if asked, it is likely he is cleaning the lenses between the fingers ("digitally"), not in the palm of the hand. Obviously, the most important factor is to be aware that this problem can occur. The management approach is essentially threefold:

1. Educate all GP patients to clean the lenses gently in the palm of the hand; if the patient cleans very forcefully in the palm of the hand or, similarly, if the lenses are cleaned between the fingers, minus power can be added. These harsh cleaning methods, especially when a circular motion is applied, are similar to adding minus power and can result in both a power change and a reduction in center thickness. These changes are enhanced by the use of an abrasive cleaner on the softer, high-Dk materials. Former PMMA wearers are especially prone to this problem, and they need to be educated about the differences in care and handling between this material and their previous hard lenses.
2. Always verify GP lens parameters after arrival of the lenses from the laboratory (after soaking in the recommended soaking solution for, at minimum, 24 hours).
3. Verify these lens parameters at progress evaluation visits—especially BCR, power, and CT.

As a secondary option, the patient can be switched to a multipurpose solution or a separate, nonabrasive cleaner.

CASE 6

On dispensing the patient's new Optimum Extra (Contamac) lenses, poor surface wettability is present. In addition, the patient's visual acuity is two lines worse than at the diagnostic fitting. The lenses had just arrived from the laboratory and were stored in the dry state.

SOLUTION: GP lenses should be soaked, at minimum, 24 hours prior to dispensing as a preventative measure. To manage this case, some wetting/conditioning solution should be rubbed onto the surfaces of the lenses, and they should be reinserted by the patient. If poor wettability persists, it is most likely a manufacturing problem and the lenses should be cleaned with a laboratory cleaner or approved solvent followed by conditioning with the wetting solution. As a final resort, a light surface polishing can be performed.

CASE 7

A patient was dispensed Boston XO (Polymer Technology Corporation) lenses and was quite satisfied. At the 1-month visit, however, the tears are "beading" up on the lens surface. After extensive questioning, the patient mentions her frequent use of a hand lotion before lens insertion in the morning.

SOLUTION: Obviously, this is an example of either poor patient compliance or inadequate patient education since lanolin-based soaps, hand lotions, and even facial tissues with lanolin added can coat contact lenses, resulting in a reduction in surface wettability. Use of a laboratory cleaner, an approved solvent, or Menicon Progent will most likely remove the residue. The patient should then be instructed not to use any lanolin-based soaps or hand creams when handling the lenses. Liquid soaps often contain lanolin; therefore, it is necessary for the patient to examine labels and use a bar soap or special optical hand soap. Hand lotions should be used after lens insertion and then thoroughly washed off before handling the lenses.

CASE 8

The patient has been wearing Boston XO (Bausch & Lomb) lenses on a daily-wear basis for 6 months and is complaining of blurred vision, mild redness, and reduced wearing time. On biomicroscopic evaluation, the lenses have decreased surface wettability resulting from a thick adherent mucoprotein film. When the patient is asked about his lens care routine, it is evident that he does not adequately care for his lenses. He is cleaning the lenses, at most, two times per week with the prescribed cleaner and is not using an enzymatic cleaner.

SOLUTION: The same steps for in-office cleaning as recommended in Case 7 should be performed (i.e., laboratory cleaner or approved solvent and possibly a light surface polish). The patient needs to be re-educated about the importance of cleaning the lenses upon removal every night before placement in the recommended soaking solution. A secondary option would be to switch the patient into either the Boston Simplus solution system (Bausch & Lomb) or Optimum (Lobob) such that the lenses would soak in the cleaning/disinfecting solution. In addition, daily enzymatic cleaning should be performed. Frequent use of rewetting drops to both rinse off debris from the lens surface and rewet the lens surface should be recommended. Finally, this patient may need a brief lecture on how noncompliance can eventually result in, at minimum, a temporary discontinuation of lens wear. Upper lid eversion, not performed in this particular case, should be routinely performed on contact lens patients. It may have revealed mild to moderate papillary hypertrophy, commonly associated with lens surface contamination, which may have necessitated a reduction or discontinuation in lens wear.

CASE 9

The patient is returning for a 12-month follow-up visit wearing Boston IV silicone/acrylate contact lenses on a daily-wear basis. He is complaining of dryness and redness, especially toward the end of the day. SLE reveals a good lens-to-cornea fitting relationship with mild surface deposit formation. With lens removal, a grade 2 (mild coalescence) peripheral corneal staining is present.

SOLUTION: In this case simply changing to a fluoro-silicone/acrylate material should provide an improvement in over-the-lens tear breakup time; therefore, the peripheral tear film would not break up as quickly, and the probability of desiccation-induced symptoms and clinical signs would be minimized. Neither a reduction in wearing time nor a change in lens design is warranted since the fitting relationship is good and the staining is not severe. The patient's cleaning regimen should be reviewed. Are the lenses being cleaned in the palm of the hand every night upon removal? Is the appropriate cleaning regimen being used?

CASE 10

A patient presented with symptoms of a gradual reduction in lens comfort in the left eye over the last 3 weeks. In addition, her eyes were red, and she noticed a small white area on that eye. She had been a 10-year Boston IV lens wearer who had been refit first into Paraperm EW for extended wear 13 years previously and then, 7 years ago, into Fluoroperm 92. She is currently wearing the lenses about 8 hours per day. SLE revealed vascularized limbal keratitis (VLK). A raised area was present in the peripheral cornea at the 3-o'clock position. This area was translucent and was accompanied by vascularization. The adjacent bulbar conjunctiva was very injected. The left lens exhibited good centration, although peripheral seal-off was observed.

SOLUTION: This patient should be discontinued from lens wear until the affected region is no longer elevated and the vessels have receded. A combination antibiotic–steroid should be prescribed (i.e., Tobradex OS q.i.d.) and the patient should be evaluated after 24 hours. Typically, after 4 to 5 days this region is no longer elevated and the patient can taper the medication. A new lens should be ordered with a flatter peripheral curve system to allow better tear exchange. In addition, reducing the patient to a flexible-wear or even a daily-wear schedule would be recommended.

CASE 11

A 23-year PMMA wearer is in your office to obtain an updated spectacle prescription. The patient is very satisfied with the vision, comfort, and wearing time obtained with his hard lenses. He has not "had a doctor who could give him glasses he could see out of in many years." He is also concerned about the fees for an examination and new spectacles. The following information was obtained during the examination (the patient had been advised to wear his rigid lenses before the examination):

Visual acuity: OD: 20/20−1   OS: 20/20−2 (with contact lenses):
SLE (OU): inferior decentration, 1-mm lag, CCC grade 2+
Refraction: OD: −3.50 − 1.25 × 022 20/40−2
OS: −3.25 − 1.00 × 155 20/50+1
Keratometry: OD: 42.25 @ 020; 43.75 @ 110 (distorted mires)
OS: 41.75 @ 160; 43.00 @ 070 (distorted mires)
Lens parameters:

	OD	OS
BCR:	7.85 mm/43 D	7.94 mm/42.50 D
OAD/OZD:	8.8 mm/7.0 mm OU	
Power:	−3.25 D	−3.00 D
CT:	0.13 mm	0.13 mm

SOLUTION: This is a typical corneal warpage syndrome case in which the patient is a long-term PMMA wearer who has worn the lenses during all waking hours. Although he may have been told in the past that his eyes are not receiving sufficient oxygen, he is not motivated for change because, in his opinion, the contact lenses are performing very well.

The examination reveals good visual acuity through the contact lenses, but as a result of the severe edema, the best spectacle-corrected visual acuity is reduced by several lines; in addition, this is accompanied by an increase in myopic refractive error, since the patient tends to accept minus power to compensate for the edema-compromised cornea. Although small overall/optical zone diameters (typical of a 1970s PMMA design that minimizes the amount of corneal area covered by a non–oxygen-transmitting lens material) were employed, the lenses were also fit steep to enhance centration while at the same time minimizing lens movement and transfer of oxygenated tears. The end result was long-term chronic hypoxia resulting in irregular astigmatism and corneal distortion, which, in turn, compromised the lens-to-cornea fitting relationship. Cornea topography showed mild central and paracentral regions of corneal distortion. The patient should be refit into a low- to medium-Dk GP material; however, as a result of the corneal distortion, the following "loaner" lenses were provided to the patient:

Material: Boston ES
BCR: OD 7.94 mm (42.50 D)   OS 8.04 mm (42.00 D)

Power: OD −2.75 D   OS −2.50 D
OAD/OZD: 9.4 mm/7.8 mm OU
CT: 0.14 mm OU

The patient was advised to initiate full-time wear of these lenses and to return for a progress evaluation in 1 week. The corneas should rehabilitate underneath the GP lenses, and the patient should be monitored on a weekly basis until the corneas have stabilized and distortion is absent or minimal. If it is not possible to provide loaner lenses, the patient should be instructed to reduce the number of hours of PMMA lens wear and to return for an evaluation in 1 week. The corneal health may have improved sufficiently to refit at that time, using lens parameters similar to the loaner lenses recommended above.

The most difficult task, however, may be convincing the patient of the need to be refit into a GP material. The effects of insufficient oxygen to the eyes must be thoroughly explained, and the possibility of eventual loss of contact lens tolerance and reduction in vision should be mentioned. Usually, mentioning the condition (i.e., "corneal warpage syndrome") has a startling effect on the patient's concern about the health of the eyes. The use of audio-visuals to illustrate the PMMA-induced complications would be invaluable. Why they are unable to see out of spectacles and how this problem can be corrected with GP lenses (although no time frame should be provided) can be explained. If the patient still refuses to be refit because of such factors as fees and/or satisfaction with his present lenses, his reasons for refusal and your recommendations should be thoroughly documented in the record.

CASE 12

This patient is a 5-year daily-wear hydrogel lens wearer who is complaining of redness, itching, and a reduction in wearing time. She had been in a 55%-water-content, hydrogel lens material for 4 years, and these lenses had to be replaced frequently because of lens deposits. She was then diagnosed as having giant papillary conjunctivitis, and after the condition had lessened, she was placed on a 1-month planned replacement program with a low-water-content, hydrogel lens material. Initially, this was successful, but after 12 months she is symptomatic once again. The examination reveals the following (all results OU):

Visual acuity: 20/25−1 (fluctuates)
Overrefraction: plano − 0.25 × 180
SLE (lenses on): good centration, 0.5-mm lag
                 Heavy mucoprotein film
SLE (lenses off): diffuse staining
TBUT = 6 seconds
Grade 3 papillary hypertrophy

SOLUTION: The first step would be to discontinue contact lens wear until the papillary hypertrophy has greatly reduced (grade 1+ or better). The patient should be monitored on a regular basis (i.e., every 1–2 weeks) until recovery has occurred. The patient should be provided realistic expectations of when a refit can occur (typically, this could be a range of anywhere from 2 weeks to 3 months). At that time the patient should be refit into GP lenses, which should result in fewer complications in the borderline dry-eye patient as a result of the more wettable surface. This type of patient is usually motivated because of the hydrogel-induced problems; nevertheless, the adaptation schedule should be thoroughly explained. In addition, a topical anesthetic should be used at the refitting visit.

CASE 13

This patient has been a soft lens wearer for over 1 year and has been quite satisfied with the comfort and wearing time provided by these lenses. However, he has never been satisfied with his vision through the lenses. He is an accountant who obviously performs an immense amount of near work. He was originally fit with spherical soft lenses at a local optical establishment, and as a result of vision-related complaints, he was eventually fit into soft torics. At the time he visits your office, he has been in soft torics for 3 months and thinks his vision is no better than he achieved with his previous soft lenses and desires a change. You find the following information:

Visual acuity: OD: 20/25   OS: 20/25−2
SLE: both lenses are rotating excessively with the blink
Refraction: OD: −1.50 − 0.75 × 172 20/20+2
OS: −1.75 − 1.00 × 010 20/15−1

SOLUTION: This patient is an excellent candidate for GP lenses because of his need for critical vision, which has not been possible with soft lenses. He is actually a challenging soft lens patient as a result of the low ametropia in combination with a small but significant amount of refractive astigmatism for someone who performs many near-work tasks. Since he is very satisfied with the comfort of soft lenses, both the benefits of GP lenses—especially vision—and the lens awareness present during adaptation should be strongly emphasized. As in Case 13, a topical anesthetic should be used at the refitting visit.

CLINICAL PROFICIENCY CHECKLIST

■ Causes of reduced vision in GP lens-wearing patients include flexure, warpage, lens decentration, poor surface wettability, and power change.

■ Flexure-related reduced visual acuity can be minimized by selecting a flatter base curve radius (by an amount equal to, at minimum, 0.50 D flatter) and, secondly, by selecting a greater center thickness.

■ An improvement in fitting relationship with inferior decentering lenses can often be obtained by decreasing center thickness and, when indicated, by the use of a lenticular edge design.

■ Poor initial surface wettability can be minimized by presoaking the lenses for a minimum of 24 hours and by rubbing wetting solution into the lens surface. Ordering lenses that have been plasma treated will also minimize the incidence of this problem.

■ Poor acquired surface wettability can be managed by the use of a laboratory cleaner or approved solvent. Patients should be educated to clean the lenses regularly immediately upon removal and to avoid lens contact with lanolin-containing substances.

■ Minus power change over time can be minimized by educating patients to clean the lenses gently in the palm of the hand, supplemented by frequent verification of the lens parameters by the practitioner.

■ Corneal desiccation can be minimized by obtaining a lid attachment fitting relationship (if possible), selecting an F-S/A lens material, avoiding excessively high edge clearance designs, and keeping center thickness to a minimum.

■ PMMA and very-low-Dk GP patients with corneal edema—but no distortion—can be refit immediately into higher-Dk GP lenses without loss of wearing time. A low- to medium-Dk (i.e., 25−50) material is recommended.

■ The most common reasons why soft lens-wearing patients are refit into GP lenses are poor vision and giant papillary conjunctivitis. It is important for these patients to understand both the benefits of GP lenses and the need for a gradual adaptation period.

REFERENCES

1. Bennett ES. Problem solving. In: Bennett ES, Hom MM, eds. Manual of Gas Permeable Contact Lenses, 2nd ed. St. Louis: Elsevier Science, 2004:190–222.
2. Fonn D, Sorbara L. Progress evaluation procedures. In: Bennett ES, Weissman BA, eds. Clinical Contact Lens Practice. Philadelphia: Lippincott Williams & Wilkins, 2005:325–339.

3. Gasson A. Aspects of hard lens aftercare. Contact Lens J 1979;8:4–11.
4. Bennett ES. Silicone/acrylate lens design. Int Contact Lens Clin 1985;12(1):45.
5. Herman JP. Flexure. In: Bennett ES, Grohe RM, eds. Rigid gas-permeable contact lenses. New York: Professional Press, 1986:137–150.
6. Bennett ES, Egan DJ. Rigid gas-permeable lens problem-solving. J Am Optom Assoc 1986;57(7):504–512.
7. Egan DJ, Bennett ES. Trouble-shooting rigid contact lens flexure—a case report. Int Contact Lens Clin 1985; 12(2):147.
8. Carrell BA, Bennett ES, Henry VA, et al. The effect of rigid gas permeable lens cleaners on lens parameter stability. J Am Optom Assoc 1992;63(3):193–198.
9. Henry VA, Bennett ES, Forrest JF. Clinical investigation of the Paraperm EW rigid gas-permeable contact lens. Am J Optom Physiol Opt 1987;64(3):313–320.
10. Ghormley NR. Rigid EW lenses: complications. Int Contact Lens Clin 1987;14(6):219.
11. Wilson SE, Lin DTC, Klyce SD, et al. Rigid contact lens decentration: a risk factor for corneal warpage. CLAO J 1990;16(3):177–182.
12. Kikkawa Y, Salmon TO. Rigid lens tear exchange and the tear mucous layer. Contact Lens Forum 1990;15(12): 17–24.
13. Schnider CM, Bennett ES, Grohe RM. Rigid extended wear. In: Bennett ES, Weissman BA, eds. Clinical Contact Lens Practice. Philadelphia: JB Lippincott, 1991;56:1–14.
14. Bennett ES, Grohe RM. RGP quality control: The results of a national survey. J Am Optom Assoc 1995;66(3): 147–153.
15. Hill RM, Brezinski SD. The center thickness factor. Contact Lens Spectrum 1987;2(10):52–54.
16. Bennett ES, Gibbons G. Clinical grand rounds. Video-aided presentation given at RGP Lens Practice Today and Tomorrow, St. Louis, July 1990.
17. Bennett ES. Be flexible about rigid lenses. Rev Cornea Contact Lenses 2007;May:38–40.
18. Quinn TG. Avoiding the low riding lens. Contact Lens Spectrum 2000;15(7):21.
19. Korb DR, Korb JE. A new concept in contact lens design. I and II. J Am Optom Assoc 1970;40(12):1–12.
20. Fonn D, Sorbara L. Rigid gas-permeable lens problem solving. In: Bennett ES, Weissman BA, eds. Clinical Contact Lens Practice. Philadelphia: Lippincott Williams & Wilkins, 2005:341–354.
21. Levitt A. Specific gravity and RGP performance. Contact Lens Spectrum 1996;11(10):43–45.
22. Carney L, Mainstone J, Quinn T, et al. Rigid lens centration: effects of lens design and material density. Int Contact Lens Clin 1996;23(1):6–11.
23. Kalin NS, Maeda N, Klyce SD, et al. Automated topographic screening for keratoconus in refractive surgery candidates. CLAO J 1996;22(3):164–167.
24. Wilson SE, Lin DTC, Klyce SD, et al. Topographic changes in contact lens-induced corneal warpage. Ophthalmology 1990;16:177–182.
25. Ruiz-Montenegro J, Mafra CH, Wilson SE, et al. Corneal topographic alterations in normal contact lens wearers. Ophthalmology 1993;100:128–134.
26. Grohe RM, Caroline PJ. RGP non-wetting syndrome. Contact Lens Spectrum 1989;4(3):32–44.
27. Brown M. Gas permeable lens options continue to expand. Primary Care Optom News 2007;July:25–26.
28. Doane M, Gleason W. Tear film interaction with RGP contact lenses. Presented at the First International Material Science Symposium, St. Louis, March 1988.
29. Friedman DM. Too much lens cleaning can also be destructive. Contact Lens Forum 1989;14(9):80.
30. Boltz KD. The overzealous contact lens cleaner. Contact Lens Spectrum 1989;4(12):53–54.
31. Bennett ES, Henry VA. RGP lens power change with abrasive cleaner use. Int Contact Lens Clin 1990;17(3): 152–153.
32. Caroline PJ, Andre MP. Inadvertent patient modification of RGP lenses. Contact Lens Spectrum 1999;14(1):56.
33. O'Donnell JJ. Patient-induced power changes in rigid gas permeable contact lenses: a case report and literature review. J Am Optom Assoc 1994;65(11):772–773.
34. Williams-Lyn D, MacNeill K, Fonn D. The effect of rigid lens back optic zone radius and diameter changes on comfort. Int Contact Lens Clin 1993;20:223–229.
35. Szczotka LB. RGP parameter changes: how much change is significant? Contact Lens Spectrum 2001;16(4):18.
36. Andrasko G. Peripheral corneal staining: incidence and time course. Contact Lens Spectrum 1990;5(7):59–62.
37. Businger U, Treiber A, Flury C. The etiology and management of three and nine o'clock staining. Int Contact Lens Clin 1989;16(50):136–139.
38. Scheid T, Bennett E. 3&9 o'clock staining/peripheral corneal desiccation. Cornea and Contact Lens Living Library. http://www.aocle.org/livlib/3–9stain.htm. Accessed June 20, 2008.
39. Solomon J. Causes and treatments of peripheral corneal desiccation. Contact Lens Forum 1986;11:30–36.
40. Edrington TB, Barr JT. Peripheral corneal desiccation. Contact Lens Spectrum 2002;17(1):46.
41. Bennett ES. Lens design and troubleshooting. In: Bennett ES, Grohe RM, eds. Rigid Gas-Permeable Contact Lenses. New York: Professional Press, 1986:189–224.
42. Ghormley N, Bennett E, Schnider C. Corneal desiccation – clinical management. Int Contact Lens Clin 1990; 17:5–8.

43. Schnider CM, Terry RL, Holden BA. Effect of patient and lens performance characteristics on peripheral corneal desiccation. J Am Optom Assoc 1996;67:144–150.
44. Bennett ES. How to manage the rigid lens wearer. Rev Optom 1986;123(10):102–110.
45. Fonn D, Gauthier C. Aftercare of RGP lens wearers. Contact Lens Spectrum 1990;5(9):71–81.
46. van der Worp E, de Brabander J, Swarbrick H, et al. Corneal desiccation in rigid contact lens wear: 3- and 9-o'-clock staining. Optom Vis Sci 2003;80(4):280–290.
47. Lowther GE. Dryness, Tears, and Contact Lens Wear: Clinical Practice in Contact Lenses. Boston: Butterworth-Heinemann, 1997:84–90.
48. Schnider C. Rigid gas permeable extended wear. Contact Lens Spectrum 1990;5(9):101–106.
49. Ghormley NR. New guy on the block. Int Contact Lens Clin 1995;9&10:22.
50. Edrington T, Barr JT. We have edge lift. Contact Lens Spectrum 2002;17(10):49.
51. Musset A, Stone J. Contact Lens Design Tables. London: Butterworths, 1981:1–12.
52. Bennett ES. The effect of varying axial edge lift on silicone/acrylate lens performance. Contact Lens J 1986;14(4):3–7.
53. Lowther GE. Review of rigid contact lens design and effects of design on lens fit. Int Contact Lens Clin 1988;15(12):378–389.
54. Ames KS, Erickson P. Optimizing aspheric and spherical rigid lens performance. CLAO J 1987;13(2):165–169.
55. Schnider CM, Terry RB, Holden BA. Effects of lens design on peripheral corneal desiccation. J Am Optom Assoc 1997;68(3):163–170.
56. Bennett ES. Corneal desiccation: how to manage the most common GP problem. Rev Cornea Contact Lenses 2005;Sept:10.
57. Grohe RM, Lebow KA. Vascularized limbal keratitis. Int Contact Lens Clin 1989;16(7&8):197–209.
58. Edwards K, Hough T. Contact lens related case studies: vascularized limbal keratitis. Optician 1998;216(5680):36–37.
59. Holden BA, Mertz GW. Critical oxygen levels to avoid corneal edema for daily and extended wear contact lenses. Invest Ophthalmol Vis Sci 1984;25:1161.
60. Bennett ES. Refitting PMMA and hydrogel lens wearers into RGPs. In: Harris MG, ed. Contact Lens Problem-Solving, vol. 2. Special Contact Lens Procedures. Philadelphia: JB Lippincott, 1990:201–209.
61. Finnemore VM, Korb JE. Corneal edema with polymethacrylate versus gas permeable rigid polymer contact lenses of identical design. J Am Optom Assoc 1980;51(3):271–274.
62. Kame RT. Clinical management of edematous corneal formations. Rev Optom 1979;116(4):69–71.
63. Stocker E, Schoessler JP. Corneal endothelial polymegathism induced by PMMA contact lens wear. Invest Ophthalmol Vis Sci 1985;26:857–863.
64. Bourne WM, Holtan SB, Hodge DO. Morphologic changes in corneal endothelial cells during three years of fluorocarbon contact lens wear. Cornea 1999;18(1):29–33.
65. Rengstorff RH. The Fort Dix report: longitudinal study of the effects of contact lenses. Am J Optom Arch Am Acad Optom 1965;42(3):153–163.
66. Wilson SE, Klyce SD. Advances in the analysis of corneal topography. Surv Ophthalmol 1991;35:269–277.
67. Henry VA, Campbell RC, Connelly S, et al. How to refit contact lens patients. Contact Lens Forum 1991;16(2):19–30.
68. Holden BA, Sweeney DF. Corneal exhaustion syndrome (CES) in long-term contact lens wearers: a consequence of contact lens-induced polymegethism? Am J Optom Physiol Opt 1988;65:95P.
69. Sweeney DF. Corneal exhaustion syndrome with long-term wear of contact lenses. Optom Vis Sci 1992;69(8):601–608.
70. Bennett ES. Immediate refitting of gas permeable lenses. J Am Optom Assoc 1983;54(3):239–242.
71. Connelly S. Why do patients want to be refit. Contact Lens Spectrum 1992;7(5):39–41.
72. Henry VA, Bennett ES, Sevigny J. Rigid extended wear problem solving. Int Contact Lens Clin 1990;17(3):121–133.

CHAPTER 9

Modification

Edward S. Bennett and Keith Parker

The in-office modification of gas-permeable (GP) lenses is a well-established art that has existed for many decades. The ability to change the lens design to result in an immediate improvement in the fitting relationship, vision, or comfort is quite integral to the long-term success of all GP lens wearers and, as with verification, should be performed in any office where GP lenses are being fit.

■ WHY MODIFY?

Modification of gas-permeable lenses is essential for long-term patient satisfaction. The procedures are easy to perform, require little time or expense, and result in both patient satisfaction and a lower dropout rate.

In-office modification of rigid lenses enables any contact lens practice to increase its efficiency and provides a valuable service to the patient. Every student, assistant, and practitioner should be proficient at performing the modifications discussed in this chapter. Almost any material can be modified, including the superpermeables, if the modifier exercises care in the procedures. These valuable skills are acquired easily through practice and the benefits derived easily will justify the effort.[1]

If a patient's lenses need modification, the inconvenience of sending the lenses to the laboratory and interrupting the patient's wearing schedule can result in a very dissatisfied patient. Patients place a high value on their time and appreciate receiving personalized custom services. It also reduces practice expenditures incurred by purchasing additional lenses. The returned lenses may not be satisfactory to the practitioner or the patient, which leads to further delays and the need for readaptation. In-office modification not only provides for uninterrupted lens wear, but also allows the practitioner to correlate the applied lens modifications with the desired fitting results and, therefore, to develop techniques that allow the best lens-to-cornea fitting relationship. This gives the practitioner optimum control over the fit of the lenses, and saves time for patient and practitioner by reducing the number of patient visits.

The ability to modify GP lenses is a powerful in-office problem-solver. GP quality is improving because of technological advancements in manufacturing. Nevertheless, there will be that occasional defective edge, or poorly wettable lens. For example, a patient experiencing symptoms of lens awareness can often be managed by a simple edge polish.[2] Dryness and/or fluctuating vision can be managed by surface polishing. A lens that feels dry and exhibits very little movement with the blink can be managed by blending and/or flattening the peripheral curves. If the addition of a slight amount of power will provide the patient with better vision and eliminate the need for reordering the lens, this can be performed in the office as well. Solving these problems in the office will not only result in a much more satisfied patient, but will also minimize the resulting negative effects of a dissatisfied patient who may communicate his or her feelings to other people and, as a result of frustration, give up on contact lens wear in general.

Modifying rigid lenses is simple and requires little time. The procedures discussed in this chapter all take no more than a few minutes to perform. As will be discussed, there are several ways for practitioners to gain proficiency in performing common modification procedures. In addition, technicians in the office can easily be trained to perform these procedures. The expense for equipment is, at most, a few hundred dollars; this is not much to ask to keep patients satisfied while enhancing the lens performance. Some modifications, such as a clean and polish, can be provided as an annual service to patients who have a service agreement.

▒ THE MODIFICATION UNIT

Modification of gas-permeable contact lenses begins with the modification unit. Cost is not a factor since most units are very reasonably priced and pay for themselves over a short period. The basic modification unit consists of a small, electric, motor-driven spindle mounted below a steel or plastic bowl. Some units also have multiple spindles and a variable spindle speed. The latter option has become a very desirable feature with the introduction of newer, softer materials. Many units have fixed spindle speeds in the range of 1,200 to 1,600 rpm, whereas the new materials require speeds of only 1,000 rpm or less.[3] High spindle speed causes polish to be removed very quickly, which results in a dry tool. As the tool dries, excess heat is built up, resulting in lens surface defects that will affect surface wettability.[4,5] A variable speed modification unit would be preferable, although the spindle speed of a unit can be monitored with a rheostat system purchased at a local hardware store. Caution is needed when using variable speed units. These units are easily inadvertently set to the fastest speed, greatly increasing the risk of lens damage.

The spindle base may be encased in a wood, plastic, or metal protective covering or may be built directly into a table (Fig. 9.1). The splash bowl prevents water and polish from splashing onto the operator and gives the operator room to place his or her hands and tools near the spindle. A plastic bowl is less likely to scratch or chip a lens that may be thrown from the spindle and is therefore a safer option.[6] A table-mounted bowl is a desirable feature because it provides

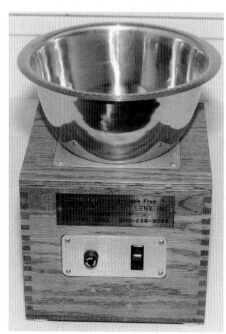
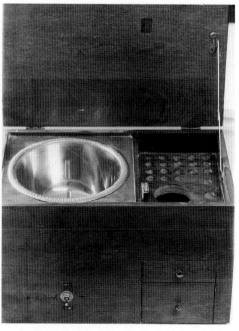

A **B**

▒ **FIGURE 9.1 (A)** Free-standing bowl modification unit. **(B)** Duffens modification unit.

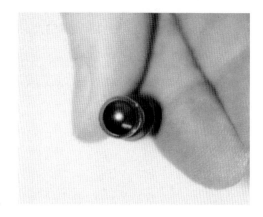

■ **FIGURE 9.2** Centered lens on a suction cup.

a place for the operator to rest his or her elbows and steady his or her hand during modification procedures.

■ **LENS ATTACHMENT DEVICES**

Holding the contact lens firmly with good centration without altering the lens parameters is crucial for all modification procedures. The most common types of lens holders include the suction cup, concave and convex tools incorporating double-sided tape, and spinners.

Most modification procedures involve the use of a suction cup as a lens holder. It is very helpful to use a suction cup that has interchangeable ends, such as the R & F Stronghold suction cup (DMV Corporation), so that both the concave and convex surfaces of the lens may be attached. It is suggested that though the concave and convex ends can be reversed, two separate holders are used to allow easy conversion from one to another. DMV now offers larger-headed suction cup tips for both convex and concave surfaces, providing more stability of holding increasingly more common larger GP lenses. The suction cup should be wet when the lens is attached, and special care should be taken to ensure lens centration (Fig. 9.2). Failure to center the lens will result in an oval optical zone diameter and uneven edge or surface polishing and will possibly compromise the lens optics.[4] Minimum pressure should be used during application to prevent lens warpage. The suction cup should be held by the operator as close to the lens as possible to impart maximum control during the modification process.

Spinner tools are very beneficial for certain procedures requiring care in maintaining optical quality, such as front surface polishing and power changes. The exact style of spinner may vary, but all types work similarly. Most utilize a suction cup for lens attachment, which is preferable over one requiring double-sided tape. Double-sided tape often leaves a residue on the surface of the lens that must be removed by a compatible solvent. Once the lens is attached to the spinner, it is free to spin along with the spindle while the handle is held stationary. This allows power changes or polishing to be performed slowly and evenly, resulting in little or no optical distortion.

■ **OTHER EQUIPMENT**

Several accessories are required in addition to the modification unit and lens attachment devices, including radius tools, polishing sponges, and polish (Table 9.1). The radius tools used for polishing and grinding are often included with the unit and commonly attach to the spindle by a form fit. The tool contains a tapered hole drilled along its axis that matches the tapering of the spindle. Friction then holds the tool in place as it is spinning. Although some tools are interchangeable with other units, taper size may vary for both units and tools. It is

TABLE 9.1 IN-OFFICE MODIFICATION EQUIPMENT

Required

Modification unit (variable speed or low single speed)

Edge and surface sponge polishing tools

Suction cups

Polish

Strongly Recommended

7× or 10× magnifying loupe

CLEPA or projection magnifying device

Recommended

Suction cup spinner

Radius tools

90-degree anterior bevel cone tool

CLEPA, contact lens edge profile analyzer.

important to keep in mind that the tapers must match exactly. Incorrect taper size can result in tool wobble and improper modification. Some Contact Lens Manufacturers Association (CLMA) Laboratories where you can obtain modification equipment are listed in Table 9.2.[7]

The amount of cost for modification equipment varies depending on the number of procedures that are performed. For basic edge and surface polish procedures, many laboratories have economical packages ranging from $225 to $350.[8] This typically includes a single-speed modification unit in addition to sponge and/or velveteen tools for polishing procedures. Suction cups and polish are also typically provided. A deluxe package (often $300–$500) allows the practitioner and/or staff to perform peripheral curve procedures such as blending and flattening, in addition to changing the power of the lens. This package typically includes a suction cup spinner for polishing and repowering, radius tools for peripheral curve procedures, a 90-degree anterior bevel cone tool for thinning the edge, and possibly a 7× magnifying loupe and/or a diameter gauge. As most CLMA laboratories either manufacture or distribute modification equipment, it is recommended to contact a local laboratory to determine if it provides modification equipment and, if so, what types of packages are available.

TABLE 9.2 WHERE TO OBTAIN MODIFICATION EQUIPMENT

MANUFACTURER	HOW TO CONTACT	EQUIPMENT/SUPPLIES
Advanced Vision Technologies	kdpcl@aol.com	Units and all tools
Boston/Bausch & Lomb	www.bausch.com	Polish
Conforma Contact Lenses	info@conforma.com	Units and all tools
DMV Corporation	www.dmvcorp.com	Suction cups
Lamba Polytech	ChrisJ@lambapolytech.co.uk	Units and all tools
Larsen Equipment Design	www.larsenequipment.com	Units and all tools
Polychem	PolychmUSA@aol.com	Units, tools, and polish
Valley Contax	(800) 547–8815	Units and all tools; polish

Modified from DeKinder J, Bennett ES. Equip yourself for modifying GP lenses. Contact Lens Spectrum 2005;20(2):48.

■ POLISHING COMPOUNDS

The importance of polishing compounds used for modification should not be overlooked. *Liberal* use of polish specifically designed for GP lenses is necessary for all modification procedures. These solutions contain a mild abrasive—typically a grit aluminum base—that erodes lens material along with surfactants and detergents to lubricate and cool the lens during modification. They all appear to be successful in modifying GP lens materials. One study evaluated the effectiveness of seven commonly used polishes in repowering GP lenses.[9] The polishes used included the following premixed liquid solutions: Boston White Finishing Polish (Polymer Technology Corporation, Wilmington, MA), Evergreen (R & F Products, Denver, CO), Mirapolish (ABBA Optical, Stone Mountain, GA), Nu-Care 2000 (Polychem, Gaithersburg, MD), and Sil-O2-Care (Polychem, Gaithersburg, MD). Two dry powder polishes were used (which can be mixed with water or saline): Al-Ox 721 (Transelco Ferro, Cleveland, OH) and X-Pal (Davison Chemical, Chattanooga, TN). It was found that all seven polishes were effective in adding 0.50 D of power to a 92-oxygen permeable (Dk) GP lens material. The powder forms were faster, taking 35 to 40 seconds, whereas the premixed solutions took up to 2½ minutes to add the desired amount of power. Therefore, it is advisable to practice with a particular polishing compound to ensure predictable results with future modifications. Products containing ammonia are not suitable for use with GP lenses since they can adversely affect surface wettability. Silvo was a popular polish with polymethylmethacrylate (PMMA) lenses, but it contains ammonia and therefore is not recommended for GP lenses.

■ MODIFICATION PROCEDURES

Introduction

It is important to obtain some baseline parameter information on the lenses before performing any modification procedure. An educated decision about how to modify a lens can only be made after first knowing what the specifications are. Be sure to record all verifications of the optical and structural quality of the lens before beginning *any* procedure since modification of one parameter can often affect another.

Obtaining the original specifications of the lens is very beneficial. It is, therefore, important to verify parameters of all new lenses from the laboratory before they are dispensed to the patient. This information becomes quite pertinent should the lens need modifying in the future. Note that some laboratories still measure front vertex power instead of back vertex. It becomes critical to know which was used when working with aphakic contact lenses, where the power can vary up to 2 D depending on the method.

Blending/Flattening Peripheral Curves

In-office blending and/or flattening of the peripheral curve radii allows the practitioner to adjust the fit of the lens and immediately observe an improved lens-to-cornea fitting relationship and, more than likely, an improvement in lens performance. If limited lens movement is present with the blink accompanied by tear stagnation, blending the junctions between peripheral curve radii should result in increased movement and better tear exchange. In addition, blending the peripheral curve junctions can also increase patient comfort.[10] If peripheral and/or midperipheral bearing is present, seal-off and possibly lens adherence—more common in GP extended wear—can result. Once again, only limited, if any, tear exchange will result. Flattening the peripheral curve radius should resolve the problem and result in greater clearance peripherally. If these problems are not promptly managed, edema and dryness-related problems can result.[11]

The radius tools used to apply peripheral curves are customarily made of brass, plastic, or Delrin (Conforma). Some brass tools may or may not be impregnated with an abrasive, such as diamond dust (Fig. 9.3). These diamond-coated tools are used to abruptly change the existing

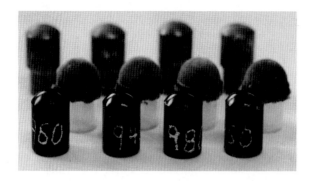

■ **FIGURE 9.3** Radius tools.

curve to re-establish a desired radius of peripheral alignment. The radius blending tools are normally available in 0.10- to 0.25-mm steps, with a minimum set consisting of the following radii: 7.50, 8.0, 8.5, 9.0, 10.50, and 12.00 mm. A more complete set for advanced modification could possibly include 7.6, 7.8, 8.0, 8.2, 8.4, 8.6, 8.8, 9.0, 9.3, 9.6, 10.0, 10.5, 11.2, 12.0, 12.5 and 13.0 mm.[4] Steeper tools such as 6.0, 6.25, 6.5, and 6.75 mm may be required and prove very useful in modifying steeper keratoconus designs. Radius diamond-coated tools are fairly expensive and are usually intended in grinding the outer peripheral curve. Hard-pad radius tools, though slower to change radii than a diamond radius tool, are recommended when establishing a change in the secondary or intermediate radii.

A peripheral curve is applied to a lens modified by first attaching the lens to a suction cup or spinner tool, concave side out. The appropriate radius tool is chosen, and either a square of waterproof adhesive tape or a precut velveteen soft pad or cotton hard pad is attached smoothly over its surface. Some practitioners prefer the softer velveteen pads for obtaining a more gradual peripheral curve or for blending. The soft pad will create a smoother blending area, whereas the hard pad will create a more abrupt change where contacted with the contact lens. The velveteen pad is approximately 0.4 mm thick, and the adhesive tape is 0.2 mm; therefore, either pad on a radius tool will actually be a flatter radius than the actual tool radius. Note: It is recommended to never use a radius blending tool with a soft or hard pad no less than 0.50 mm flatter than the central base curve of the contact lens to avoid pad marks in the optical surface area of the base curve. If a 9.0-mm curve is needed, an 8.6-mm tool should be used with velveteen and an 8.8-mm tool with adhesive tape.[6]

The soft pad on the radius tool is first thoroughly made wet with fresh clean water, and then the tool is placed on the spindle, the motor is turned on, and polish is applied to the tool surface.[4] Note that the appropriate polishing compound must be applied to the tool *before* use and throughout the modification procedure. In addition, the tool surface and polish must be kept free from all dirt and other abrasive materials, or scratches will appear on the posterior peripheral lens surface (Fig. 9.4A). Once the spindle is spinning, the lens is held lightly against the tool with the concave surface facing the tool (Fig. 9.4B). If a suction cup is used, the lens should be held at a 30-degree angle to the vertical, and entire outer edge should be in contact with the covered tool at all times. The suction cup is rotated smoothly and evenly with the fingers in the opposite direction of the spindle rotation. Since the spindle rotates clockwise in most units, the suction cup should be turned counterclockwise. Alternatively, rather than holding the suction cup at a 30-degree angle, the lens may be held vertically to the radius tool and rotated in a figure-eight design (Fig. 9.4C). The lens should be lifted from the tool every 5 to 10 seconds and a drop of polish added to the surface every time the lens is touched to the tool. Insufficient polish, as well as excessive pressure, can lead to heat build-up and lens damage.

This procedure may also be performed utilizing a spinner tool. The lens is centered on the spinner, again with the concave surface facing the tool. The spinner is held at a 45- to 60-degree angle off the center of the radius tool. The lens must be spinning at all times during the procedure and polish continually applied as previously discussed.

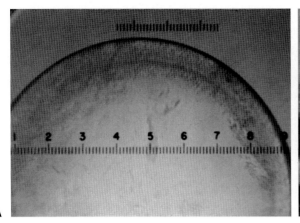

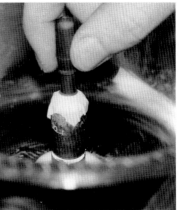

A

B

C

■ **FIGURE 9.4 (A)** "Bull's eye" effect from scratches on the posterior lens surface caused by excessive pressure or dirty polish. **(B)** Peripheral curve application with lens and suction cup. **(C)** Figure-eight design is used to apply peripheral curve.

Practice and experience are necessary to obtain confidence in producing consistent results with peripheral curves. The amount of bevel obtained depends on numerous factors, including spindle speed, pressure of the lens against the pad, consistency of the polish, and flatness of the radius tool (in relation to the base curve of the lens). After a little experience, the operator will be able to determine quickly the length of time needed to produce a peripheral curve of desired radius and width. It is recommended that records should be made of all adjustments made to the lenses, including peripheral curves applied, spindle speed, and time for each curve.[12] These records will enable the operator to duplicate a lens adjustment, if necessary, in the future.

The width and quality of the peripheral curve should be monitored periodically during the procedure. The lens is removed from the lens holder, cleaned thoroughly, and viewed through a magnified reticule graduated in 0.10-mm divisions. A projection magnifier can also be used to verify peripheral curves.

Blending

Following peripheral curve application, the junction between curves consists of a significant ridge of material that can inhibit tear exchange and cause discomfort to the patient. Blending of this transition zone is necessary to remove this ridge and, therefore, increase lens movement and promote tear exchange.[6] The tear exchange is accompanied by increased oxygen, as well as flushing of debris that may deposit on the back surface of the lens.

The tool selected for blending typically has a radius approximately halfway between the radii of the two adjacent curves. Again, the thickness of the tape or pad must be taken into consideration. Generally, only the peripheral curves are blended, but the optical zone junction also may be blended if it is unusually sharp or if the clinician desires to lower a high-fitting lens. The tool used to blend the optical zone junction, however, should never be less than the base curve radius of the lens. Otherwise, the base curve radius could be flattened or warped quickly.

The following is an example of how to determine the radius tool necessary for blending. All figures are in millimeters.

Base curve radius: 7.80 mm
Secondary curve radius: 9.00 mm
Peripheral curve radius: 12.00 mm

First blend:
$$7.80 + 9.00$$
$$16.80/2 = 8.40$$
8.40 blend radius
$-$ .40 pad thickness
_____
8.00-mm tool

Second blend:
$$9.00 + 12.00$$
$$21.00/2 = 10.50$$
10.50 blend radius
$-$ .40 pad thickness
_____
10.10-mm tool

In many cases the exact radius tool needed to create a blend is not available. The tool most approximating the desired one should be used in these instances. In the above example, a 10.00-mm radius tool would be used for the second blend. Whether the desire is to blend the junction toward the base curve or more toward the lens edge will determine if a tool slightly steeper or flatter than the best designated tool is used.

The methods for blending are the same as those discussed for peripheral curve fabrication. However, the ridge of plastic is removed easily, and therefore only a gentle touch for a short time is necessary to obtain the desired blend. There are three types of blends most commonly used. A light or *touch* blend is achieved with only a few seconds of blending, and the transition zone is still readily observable with a measuring magnifier. In a medium blend, the junction between curves is less distinct and measurement of the curves is more difficult. A heavy blend blurs but does not remove the transition zone completely. However, the measurement of curve widths can only be estimated (Table 9.3).

Excessive pressure should be avoided when creating or blending peripheral curves. The GP materials, particularly the newer ones, are relatively flexible, and increased pressure will likely produce steeper or slightly more distorted curves than desired. In addition, excessive pressure may produce a *bulls-eye* effect in the lens periphery, which appears as concentric scratches or scorch marks (see Fig. 9.4A). Fine scratches may also result from material particles contaminating the polish during the procedure. The finish of the peripheral curves should be examined with a projection magnifier or biomicroscope to confirm the optical quality of the lens surface.

TABLE 9.3 BLENDING GUIDELINES

BLEND	TIME	APPEARANCE
Light	5 s	Transition easily seen
Medium	10 s	Transition seen, but shadows begin forming at peripheral junction
Heavy	15–20 s	Very difficult to read accurately; nothing is observed but shadows

From Tracy D, Sanford M. Modification Procedures, Guidelines and Tips. Norfolk, VA: Conforma Laboratories.

Edge Shaping and Polishing

Arguably the most important component of a comfortable and well-centered GP lens fit is the shape and quality of the lens edge.[13] Modification of the lens edge has become a common procedure as a result of the difficulty in consistently fabricating the newer, softer materials, although recent advances in manufacturing technology has resulted in more consistency in edge quality.

Both the anterior and posterior edges should be rolled and tapered, since the posterior edge is in near alignment with the cornea and the anterior edge is often in contact with the upper lid. A poor edge will most often result in the patient complaining of persistent lens awareness or discomfort (usually monocular). Even if the edge appears acceptable on inspection, it should be polished to rule out the possibility of a defect.

Verification of the lens edge is essential before initially dispensing the lens to the patient. One simple initial method of determining if a lens edge is defective is using the palm test.[13] The lens, concave side down, is placed in the palm of the hand and then pushed across the palm by the forefinger of the other hand. If it fails to glide easily across the palm (i.e., does not tend to move or, if movement is present, the lens feels rough), the edge is defective. The edge should then be observed both frontally and in profile with some type of projection magnifier. It cannot be assumed that a replacement lens will have the same edge as the original or that the left lens will have the same edge as the right. Initial discomfort is very detrimental to the success of future lens wear, especially in the case of a first-time GP wearer. However, in recent years, edge quality has been consistently high. Most GP laboratories now use computerized lathes that generate a consistent edge thickness, and some lathes will generate a uniform apex on the lens. However, the lens edge should always be inspected whenever discomfort is suspected to be problematic.

There are several methods for shaping and polishing the lens edge. To thin the edge, or create an anterior bevel, a cone tool is most commonly used. Slight shaping and polishing of the edge may be performed with a sponge tool containing a central hole or with a flat sponge and the aid of a spinner tool.

Finger Polishing

A simple edge polishing technique using two fingers and a drop of polish will improve the polished edge quality of any GP lens. This procedure is quick and simple and will not affect any other parameters of the lens. A special tool holder is needed to hold the suction cup, or inserting the holder end of the suction cup holder through a hole in a sponge tool will work to hold the suction cup holder as it spins on the polisher spindle.

Cone Tool

A 90-degree cone tool is usually used to add an anterior or CN bevel to the lens edge. Alternatively, a 60-degree tool may be used to create a narrower bevel or a 120-degree tool for a wider bevel.[6] The CN bevel serves to decrease the edge thickness in an attempt to align the edge most comfortably with the cornea posteriorly and with the lid anteriorly. This procedure also is beneficial in lowering a high-fitting lens. To begin the procedure, the lens is mounted to a suction cup so that the convex surface faces the cone tool (Fig. 9.5A). A pellon or velveteen pad with a one-quarter section cut out is placed within the tool so that it conforms to the cone surface. The lens is then placed within the cone while it rotates and is gently rocked forward and backward and left and right to a slight degree. This rocking motion enables the modifier to apply a bevel with a smoother transition zone. The rocking should not be excessive, since this can alter the peripheral lens surface quality. The appropriate polish must be continually applied throughout the procedure. The lens should be examined approximately every 10 seconds until the desired edge thickness is reached (Fig. 9.5B). After the application of an anterior bevel, the edge will be quite sharp and somewhat rough. Therefore, it will be necessary to accompany this procedure with a thorough edge polish.

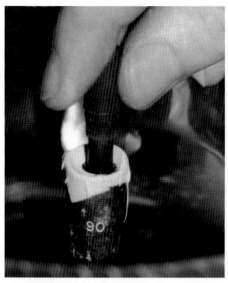 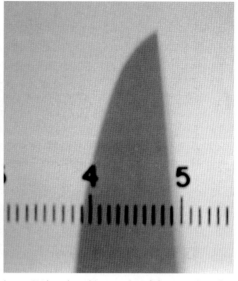

A   B

■ **FIGURE 9.5 (A)** Ninety-degree tool used in creating a CN bevel or thinner edge. **(B)** Lens edge after being thinned with a 90-degree tool (CN bevel).

Sponge Tool (Central Hole)

A small, flat sponge tool containing a central hole is very effective for routine polishing and minor edge shaping. The lens is positioned on a suction cup with the concave surface out. The sponge should be thoroughly moistened with water and placed on the spindle. As the sponge rotates, polish is applied and the suction cup is held vertically to the tool. The lens is then pushed into the central hole of the sponge and moved up and down in the sponge for 30 to 60 seconds (Fig. 9.6). Polish is again applied throughout the procedure. It is important to maintain good suction on the lens during this procedure because a large-diameter lens may become lodged in the sponge.

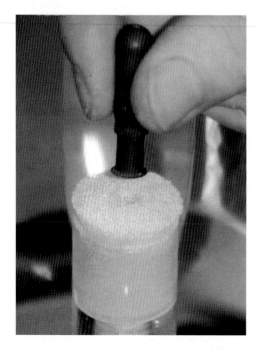

■ **FIGURE 9.6** Sponge tool with central hole used for edge polishing.

Flat Sponge

Alternatively, a large, flat sponge tool may be used to gently shape and polish the lens edge.[14,15] In this case, the lens is mounted on a spinner tool concave side out. The sponge is moistened with water and placed on the spindle. The spinner is then held at an approximately 30-degree angle to the rotating tool with the lens in contact with the sponge approximately halfway between the center and the edge of the sponge (Fig. 9.7A). The lens is then traversed back and forth across the sponge tool from approximately the 4 o'clock position to the 8 o'clock position for 30 to 60 seconds (Fig. 9.7B,C). Polish is continuously applied, and the lens should be spinning at all times while in contact with the tool. The edge is preferentially polished posteriorly while the lens is on the left side of the 6 o'clock position of the sponge tool and anteriorly on the right side of 6 o'clock. This allows the clinician to concentrate the effort more on the anterior or posterior surface of the edge as needed.

Surface Polishing

Surface polishing is one of the most commonly performed in-office modification procedures. The new, higher-Dk materials are more susceptible to surface scratches and accumulate more deposits, which necessitates, in many cases, polishing these lenses at least once a year.[16] Surface scratches will often interfere with the wetting performance of a GP lens. The patient will report "foggy" vision when the accumulation of debris in the crevices of the scratches and the subsequent surface filming occur. Unfortunately, to remove all the scratches completely could render the surface quality poor. The objective of polishing the surface of a GP lens is to remove the burrs of the scratches to decrease the awareness of a rough surface because of heavy scratches. These scratches are polished easily from the lens with the use of various sponge tools on the modification unit without risk of damaging the optical quality. The only exception for polishing—or adding power to—the front surface would pertain to plasma-treated lenses, as the surface wettability may be degraded if this surface is altered.

If a lens exhibits poor initial wettability, it is important to first use a laboratory cleaner or solvent to clean the lens, followed by rubbing in wetting solution to help condition the lens before reinsertion. Polishing the front surface should be a last resort because of the possibility of the poor initial wettability being caused by residual pitch polish left on the lens during the manufacturing process. If so, the pitch may just simply be further distributed on the lens surface and the problem is not alleviated. If the problem is an acquired mucoprotein film, which has become plaquelike and resistant to normal cleaning, once again a laboratory cleaner or solvent approved for use with GP lens materials should be used initially. If the deposits are not totally removed, a mild front surface polish should then be considered. Only occasionally does the posterior surface attract sufficient debris/deposits to warrant polishing.

Convex Surface

As previously mentioned, for removing thick adherent mucoprotein deposits and very light scratches, a hand polishing pad such as the Cleaner Accessory Pad (Eaton Medical Corp.) can be used.[16] The pad is wetted with preservative-free saline followed by six to eight drops of a rigid daily cleaning solution. The lens is placed on the tip of the thumb or index finger and gently rubbed into the pad for approximately 20 seconds. The lens power should be verified and noted before and after any front surface polishing to ensure optical quality and proper prescription.

More thorough polishing of the convex surface of the lens requires the use of a flat sponge tool and the modification unit. Many sponge tools allow for a small piece of velveteen or silk cloth to be placed over the sponge surface. This tool is referred to as a *drum tool*. The cloth will hold the polish better than a sponge, lessening the burning effect to the surface of the lens. A spinner tool with a suction cup lens holder is preferred for this method. The lens is centered on a suction cup of the spinner tool, convex side out. The sponge tool is wetted thoroughly and

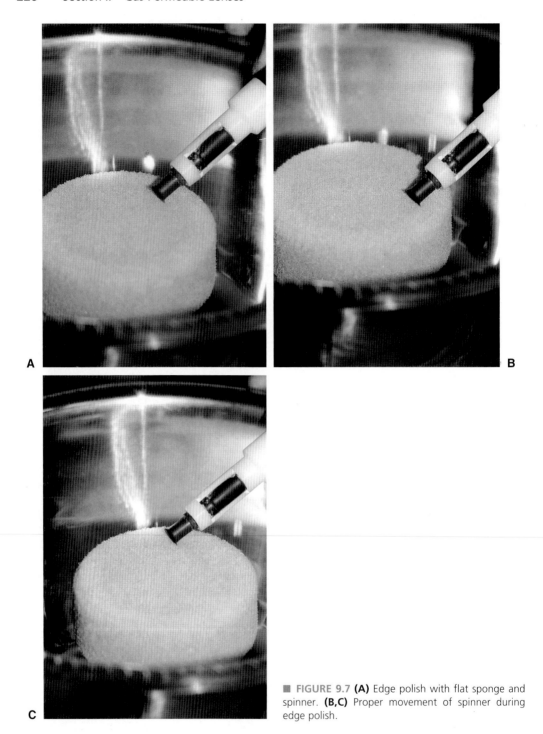

■ **FIGURE 9.7 (A)** Edge polish with flat sponge and spinner. **(B,C)** Proper movement of spinner during edge polish.

placed on the spindle. Once the tool is rotating, polish is continually applied to the center of the tool and the lens is placed halfway between the center and the edge of the sponge. The spinner tool should be slightly oscillated back and forth about 30 degrees while the lens stays in the center of the drum tool or flat sponge tool. A uniform polishing of the convex surface of the lens is desired. If too much polishing occurs either in the center or peripheral area of the convex surface, the power of the lens will be distorted and changed. The lens should only stay in contact with the polishing tool surface for 1 to 2 seconds at a time to minimize burning. Polish should be applied in between touches to the tool. Remember to apply the polish in the center of the polishing tool because the polish applied will spin away from the center of any spinning tool surface. Usually only three or four touches of the lens to the polishing tool are needed to remove the burrs from the scratches and debris built up on the lens surface. The lens surface should be examined after this process for remaining scratches with a projection magnifier and the power verified with a lensometer (Fig. 9.8). Frequent polish application and minimal pressure will ensure good lens optical quality following surface polishing.

Another method would pertain to using a suction cup held at a 45-degree angle and rotated in a direction opposite the rotation of a flat sponge tool (Fig. 9.9). This rotation of the lens may be accomplished with the manipulation of the fingers or by the use of a spinner tool, which requires less dexterity. The lens is depressed into the sponge about one-eighth of an inch during the procedure and continued for 10 to 15 seconds. The very center of the lens is polished by holding the suction cup perpendicular to the sponge and depressing the lens in and out of the center of the sponge 10 to 12 times. During this step, the lens should be in contact with the sponge for only 1 second at a time to prevent optical distortion or power changes.

An alternative method would be to use a spinner in combination with a rounded sponge tool. In this method, the spinner rolls the lens from edge to center and back until the desired surface quality has been obtained. As long as the spinner continues to rotate, the optical quality should not change. This will be discussed further during the section on repowering.

The lens surface should be examined every 20 to 30 seconds for remaining scratches with a projection magnifier and the power verified with a lensometer. Low spindle speed (1,000 rpm or less), frequent polish application, and minimal pressure will ensure good lens optical quality following surface polishing. In addition, it is not recommended to attempt to totally polish out deep scratches, as the optical quality could be compromised from frequent polishing.

Concave Surface

It is necessary to polish the concave surface of a lens primarily to remove deposits resulting from trapped tear debris behind the lens. These deposits may inhibit lens movement and centration, particularly in extended wear.

A cone-shaped sponge is used to polish the concave lens surface. The cone is ideal for forming a convex surface to match the concave surface of the lens during this procedure. The lens is mounted on a suction cup concave side out, and the cone sponge is moistened and placed on the spindle. After the spindle is rotating, polishing compound is added and the suction cup is tilted slightly, with the lens placed just off the center of the sponge (Fig. 9.10). The lens is depressed into the sponge about one-eighth of an inch and rotated opposite the spindle rotation for 10 to 15 seconds. This may be repeated, if necessary, after inspection. A circular sponge tool may be substituted using the same technique; however, the suction cup should be held at a 30-degree angle from the vertical.

Nonpolishing Alternatives

Menicon PROGENT Contact Lens Cleaner and Protein Remover is an excellent product for thoroughly cleaning a GP lens surface. This new product is intended for in-office use only. It is a very strong "bleaching" type of solution and needs to be handled correctly for maximum results. It is not intended for patient use. Make sure the instructions are followed to avoid exposure to the eye.[17]

Repowering

A significant advantage to fitting GP contact lenses is the ability to modify the power of the lens in the office to provide an immediate improvement in the patient's visual acuity. As a new lens would otherwise need to be ordered, repowering proves to be a very cost-effective procedure.

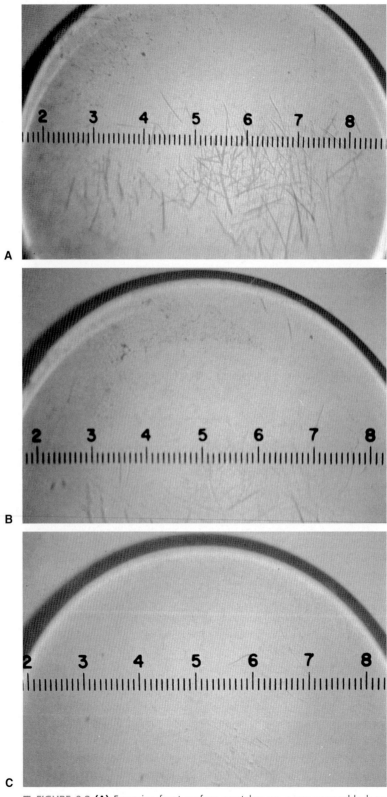

■ FIGURE 9.8 **(A)** Excessive front surface scratches on a gas-permeable lens. **(B)** Thinned scratches following initial front surface polishing (30 seconds). **(C)** Scratches remaining following 1 minute of front surface polishing.

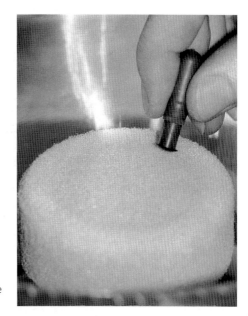

■ **FIGURE 9.9** Demonstration of front surface polish with the use of a flat sponge tool.

A change in power may be necessary—particularly with lenses ordered empirically—as factors such as the corneal curvature, refraction, and lens design may result in a slightly inaccurate power. Normal refractive changes in a young patient and changes in the lens-to-cornea fitting relationship also may necessitate repowering.

Adding Minus

The addition of minus power is more often necessary than the addition of plus power because of patients' visual symptoms. Fortunately, adding minus is the easier of the two procedures to perform. Although many techniques are used to add minus power, a very effective method involves the use of either a rounded sponge tool or the cone sponge tool in combination with a spinner. The sponge tool is mounted vertically on the spindle and wetted thoroughly with water and polish. The lens is mounted convex side out and well centered on a spinner tool that enables the lens

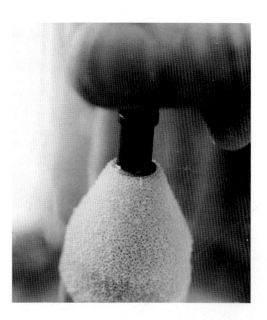

■ **FIGURE 9.10** Polishing the concave surface of a gas-permeable lens with a cone-shaped sponge tool.

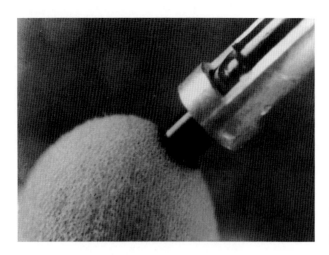

■ **FIGURE 9.11** The use of a rounded sponge pad and spinner for the addition of minus power.

to spin freely and rapidly. As the sponge tool rotates, the lens is first held with the edge adjacent to the side of the pad to begin the spinning action. Once the lens is spinning freely, the spinner is rotated so that the lens is perpendicular to the sponge pad, approximately 1 to 1.5 cm from its apex (Fig. 9.11). The lens should be turning freely on the spinner at all times when in contact with the sponge tool, and as the position and pressure are held constant, polishing compound is liberally applied. Proper position allows the center of the lens to be in direct contact with the pad while the periphery receives less friction. This, in turn, creates a flatter front curvature, resulting in increased minus power. The amount of minus power added with this technique depends on the amount of pressure, time, and polishing compound used. The power should be monitored every 10 to 15 seconds and as much as 1 D can be added without causing optical distortion.

An alternate method to add minus involves the use of a large, flat sponge tool. The lens is mounted convex side out on a suction cup with special care to ensure centration. With the flat sponge spinning on the spindle and thoroughly wetted, the lens is placed approximately 1 inch from the peripheral edge. The lens must be held perpendicular to the tool surface at all times. With very slight pressure, the lens is revolved around the tool counterclockwise (if the spindle turns clockwise). The lens should not be twisted about the axis of the suction cup.[14] Polish should be added throughout the procedure to the center of the tool (centrifugal force will spread polish out to the edge). Again, the power must be checked every 10 to 15 seconds to prevent overcorrection and to ensure that the lens is rotated to a different position on the suction cup, which will help to minimize optical distortion. The limit of minus power addition with this method is approximately −0.75 D.

Adding Plus

Adding plus power to GP lenses is more difficult and presents a greater chance of optical distortion compared to adding minus. The rounded sponge tool and spinner may be utilized to add plus power by initiating spinning of the lens, as with adding minus, but then rotating the spinner out of vertical alignment with the sponge pad so that only the periphery of the lens is in contact with the tool (Fig. 9.12). Plus power is now being added as the front surface curvature increases by material being removed from the periphery of the lens and not the center. The rate of power change is much slower for plus power than it is for minus power with the sponge pad.

An alternative method of adding plus power is to use a flat drum tool in combination with a suction cup. The drum tool is typically covered with velveteen or suede cloth.[14] With the motor running, a small amount of polish is added to the tool. The lens, convex side out on the suction cup, is brought in contact with the center of the drum tool with a perpendicular orientation. With mild pressure, the lens is rotated both clockwise and counterclockwise. As with

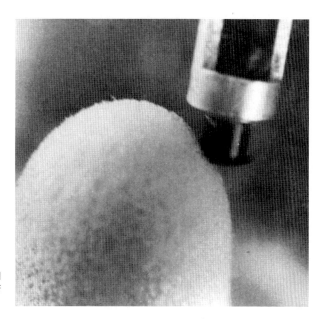

■ **FIGURE 9.12** The use of a rounded sponge pad and spinner for the addition of plus power.

all other methods, polish should be applied liberally. Only about 0.5 D of plus power can be added with these procedures.

The type of lens material should always be considered whenever power changes are indicated. The time required to change the power of a high-Dk material is less than that for a low-Dk material or PMMA.[2] Failure to allow for different lens materials can lead to improper amounts of power change or distortion of optics.

A summary of commonly performed modification procedures is provided in Table 9.4.[8]

■ MODIFYING SPECIAL DESIGNS

It is apparent that modification procedures can be the difference between success and failure in bifocal/multifocal patients as well as with keratoconic lens designs. In keratoconus, it is not uncommon to need to reduce the optic zone diameter and/or flatten the peripheral curve radii to reduce adherence and increase tear flow. Blending the peripheral curves can likewise have a dramatic effect. As a result of the high minus powers often required for keratoconus correction, edge polishing and thinning are not uncommon procedures.[1] The application of an anterior bevel, followed by an edge polish, is very beneficial in thinning a high minus edge.

As many bifocal designs are prism ballasted and truncated and are designed to rest on the lower lid, thinning the upper edge to minimize the lifting effects of the upper lid is a beneficial procedure. To accomplish this, all but the upper edge can be covered by velveteen or a similar material. The edge can be rolled against a sponge using a suction cup spinner. Polishing the occasional sharp thin edge of a plus-powered bifocal/multifocal design can be beneficial, and although we have not done so, some practitioners have found it useful to modify the truncation angle of translating bifocal designs.

■ SHOULD HIGH-OXYGEN PERMEABILITY LENS MATERIALS BE MODIFIED?

In recent years the concern over in-office modification of the newer high-Dk materials has increased. Some in-office procedures have been demonstrated to cause microcracks and scorching of the lens surface.[5] These surface defects are clinically unobservable but may affect wettability and long-term integrity of the lens.

TABLE 9.4 GAS-PERMEABLE LENS MODIFICATION PROCEDURES

PROCEDURE	INDICATION(S)	TOOLS	PRECAUTIONS
1. Edge polish	Patient experiences unilateral discomfort. Upon inspection, lens is abraded, sharp, blunt, or chipped	1. 1″ centerhole sponge with suction cup or spinner 2. Inspect with an edge profile analyzer or comparator	Use polish liberally
2. Surface polish	1. Patient has transient blurred vision 2. Patient reports redness and/or reduced wearing time. Scratches and mucoprotein film on front surface and/or back surface	1. 3″ flat sponge tool 2. 3″ polishing disc or drum tool in combination with velveteen or Delrin 3. Cone or convex sponge tool to polish back surface 4. All of the above in combination with spinner or suction cup	1. <1,200 rpm 2. Use polish liberally 3. Check optical quality with lensometer after 20–30 s
3. Repower	1. Patient has blurred vision that is managed by a change in lens power	1. 3″ polishing disc or drum tool in combination with velveteen or Delrin with suction cup or spinner 2. Cone or convex sponge tool with spinner	1. <1,200 rpm 2. Use polish liberally 3. Check optical quality with lensometer after 20–30 s
4. Blend/flatten peripheral curves	1. Tear stagnation under lens because of midperipheral or peripheral bearing 2. Insufficient lens lag with the blink	1. Approx. 10 tools ranging from 7.5–13 mm in radius 2. Diamond-coated tools preferable; brass tools most often used because of reduced cost 3. ¼″ velveteen or Delrin pad to cover tool 4. All procedures performed with either suction cup or spinner	1. <1,200 rpm 2. Use polish liberally 3. Be careful with high-Dk materials

Dk, oxygen permeability.

One procedure that should not be performed on contemporary GP lens materials is diameter reduction. As these materials are softer and are more likely to chip or break, it is not worth the time and effort to reduce the diameter and then reshape the edge and reapply peripheral curves. Likewise, prolonged surface polishing (i.e., several minutes) is not recommended, especially with high-Dk and hyper-Dk lens materials. Some of the defects that result are not evident with biomicroscopy. The effect of front surface polishing was evaluated on 20 GP lenses.[5] The modified lenses were then evaluated under high-magnification (100–500+) scanning electron microscopy. Several microscopic surface abnormalities were observed, including microcracks, splitting, scorching, and bleaching. It was concluded that prolonged polishing, diameter reduction, and repowering would be unacceptable in-office modification procedures for high-Dk GP lens materials. Walker[18] found similar results. If fluoro-silicone/acrylate lenses were surface polished for longer than 2 minutes, poor surface wettability resulting in patient awareness of the lens over time often resulted.

Repowering appears to be rather controversial. Whereas Grohe et al[5] contraindicated it with high-Dk lens materials, the studies by Reeder et al[9] and Morgan et al[3] appear to support it, although some precautions may be necessary depending on the polish used and the specific

TABLE 9.5 MODIFICATION "DO'S" AND "DON'TS"

A. Procedures

DO	DON'T
Edge polish	Diameter reduction
Surface polish	Prolonged surface polish
Peripheral curve blending/flattening (low/high Dk)	Blending/flattening (hyper-Dk)
Repowering	Repowering (velveteen pad/suction cup with high/hyper-Dk); consider proper polish

B. Techniques

DO	DON'T
Keep lens cool	Allow heat to build
1. Add polish frequently	Dispense lens immediately after procedure
2. Dip lens in water	
3. Keep sponge tools saturated with water	
4. Low spindle speed	
Optimize surface wettability	
1. Clean lens after procedure	
2. Condition surface before dispensing	

Dk, oxygen permeability.

procedure. It has been found that repowering, even at a high (1,600 RPM) spindle speed with a high-Dk lens material, did not result in optical distortion or reduced quality of vision if a spinner tool was used in combination with a rounded sponge tool.[3] Likewise, under scanning electron microscopy, the lens surface was free of defects. However, use of a velveteen-covered tool resulted in significant optical distortion and reduced vision of the high-Dk lens material, even with the use of a low (550 rpm) spindle speed. Numerous surface defects were typically present under scanning electron microscopy.

Overall, it appears that the use of low spindle speeds (≤1,000 rpm), sponge tools, and minimal pressure are safest when polishing the front surface, modifying the edge, or repowering GP lenses in the office. A summary of the do's and don'ts of modifying GP lenses is given in Table 9.5.[1]

■ OBTAINING PROFICIENCY AT MODIFICATION

Anyone can modify, and staff members can be of tremendous assistance in performing these procedures. Numerous organizations (GP Lens Institute, Contact Lens Association of Ophthalmologists, Contact Lens Society of America, Heart of America Contact Lens Society, to name a few) provide modification workshops, as do many CLMA member laboratories. Lenses to practice with should not be difficult to obtain, and GP contact lens laboratories are excellent about assisting in these activities.

■ SUMMARY

A summary nomogram of modification of GP lenses is given in Figure 9.13. The ability to modify GP lenses is of great benefit to both patient and practice. It takes little time and can solve a problem without losing a patient. In a time when managed care and disposable lenses put a premium on efficiency, it makes good sense to be able to perform in-office modification procedures.

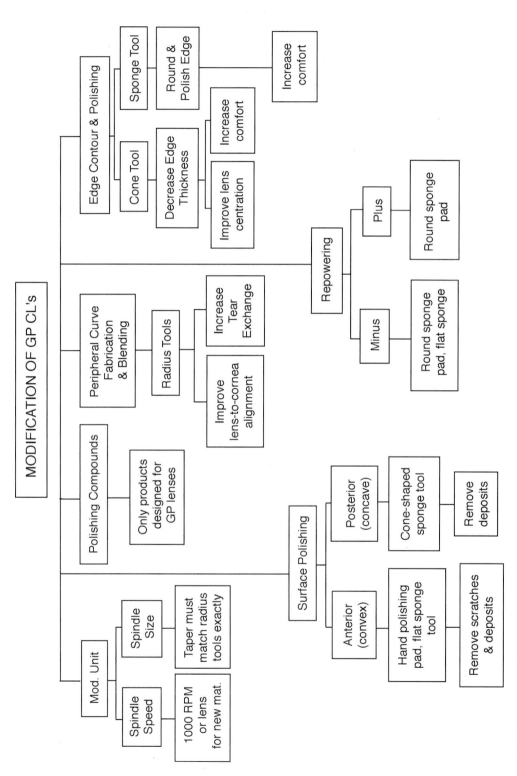

■ FIGURE 9.13 Modification summary nomogram.

■ CLINICAL CASES

CASE 1

A 14-year-old patient currently wearing daily-wear GP contact lenses returns for a 6-month follow-up visit complaining of slightly blurred vision in both eyes. Examination reveals a visual acuity of 20/30 OD and OS correctable to 20/20 with an overrefraction of −0.50 DS OU. A postrefraction of −3.75 DS OU to 20/20 was found, compared to −3.25 OU 6 months ago. Lens fit, fluorescein pattern, keratometry, and ocular health were unremarkable and unchanged from the previous visit.

SOLUTION: Progressive myopia in a young patient has increased the refractive error. The lenses should be repowered in the office utilizing a minus power addition technique (i.e., rounded sponge pad and spinner). The addition of −0.50 D to the lenses in the office will improve the patient's visual acuity to 20/20 in a matter of minutes and prevent an interruption of the patient's wearing schedule.

CASE 2

A patient is dispensed replacement lenses with the same parameters as the previous pair. The patient returns in 1 week complaining of discomfort in the left eye only. Examination reveals a good lens fit and 20/15 vision OU, unchanged from previous examinations.

SOLUTION: Monocular discomfort is a sign of a possible edge problem. Verification of the left lens with a projection magnifier reveals a slightly blunt edge. Therefore, a routine edge polish (i.e., sponge tool with central hole) is indicated for the left lens, to create a smoother, more rounded edge for greater comfort.

CASE 3

A patient wearing GP lenses for approximately 1 year returns to the office complaining of slightly blurred vision and dryness. Visual acuity measures 20/25 OD and OS with no improvement with overrefraction. The ocular health is normal, and the lens fit is adequate and unchanged from the previous visit. However, fine surface scratches and a quick surface haze after the blink are observed.

SOLUTION: Current GP materials often need routine surface polishing every 6 months to 1 year, and this procedure is indicated in this case. A front surface polish will not only remove the scratches, but will also most likely increase wettability by creating a smoother surface for the tear film and decreasing the affinity for deposit formation. The patient's cleaning regimen should also be reviewed to rule out inappropriate procedures that may be causing excessive front surface scratching.

CASE 4

A patient is dispensed a pair of daily-wear GP lenses. At the 1-month visit the patient reports that everything is well; however, the lenses occasionally feel "stuck" to the eye, and they are sometimes difficult to remove. Visual acuity has remained stable. The fluorescein pattern shows minimal edge clearance, and the lag after the blink is 1 mm.

SOLUTION: It is not uncommon for the lens-to-cornea fitting relationship to change slightly over the first few weeks of rigid lens wear. The lens fit has apparently tightened with this patient after 1 month of wear, and steps need to be taken to increase edge lift and increase movement. Flattening the peripheral curve should indeed achieve these goals and may be performed in the office in just a few minutes with the proper radius tool.

CLINICAL PROFICIENCY CHECKLIST

■ When considering modification units, keep in mind that 1,000 rpm is recommended for safe modification of newer materials.

■ It is essential that the taper size of the modification tools exactly matches the spindle size to prevent wobble during modification.

■ Remember to use only polish that is specifically designed for use with GP lenses.

■ Good centration is absolutely imperative when attaching a contact lens to a lens holder (i.e., suction cup) for modification.

■ Spinner tools are very beneficial for certain procedures requiring care in monitoring optical quality, such as power changes and front surface polishing.

■ It is important to obtain baseline parameter data on the lenses before performing any modification procedure.

■ When applying peripheral curves or blending, be sure to allow for the thickness of the adhesive tape or velveteen when selecting the radius tool (0.2 mm for adhesive tape, 0.4 mm for velveteen).

■ When using sponge tools, always moisten the sponge with water before beginning the procedure.

■ The use of a rounded sponge tool and spinner is most effective in repowering the newer materials.

■ Frequent polish, minimal pressure, and low spindle speed provide the best results with any modification procedure.

REFERENCES

1. Bennett ES. Successfully modifying contemporary RGP materials. Optom Today 1997;5(10):27–34.
2. Bennett ES, Clompus DJ, Hansen DW. A hands-on approach to RGP modification. Rev Optom 1998;135(1):88–103.
3. Morgan BW, Henry VA, Bennett ES, et al. The effect of modification procedures on silicone/acrylate versus fluoro-silicone/acrylate lens materials. J Am Optom Assoc 1992;63(3):193–198.
4. Mandell RB. Modification procedures. In: Mandell RB, ed. Contact Lens Practice, 4th ed. Springfield, IL: Charles C. Thomas, 1988:475–501.
5. Grohe RM, Caroline PJ, Norman C. The role of in-office modification for RGP surface defects. Contact Lens Spectrum 1988;3(10):52–60.
6. Bennett ES, Egan DJ. Modification. In: Bennett ES, Grohe RM, eds. Rigid Gas-Permeable Contact Lenses. New York: Professional Press, 1986:247–273.
7. DeKinder J, Bennett ES. Equip yourself for modifying GP lenses. Contact Lens Spectrum 2005;20(2):48.
8. Bennett ES. Offer added value with in-office RGP modification. Contact Lens Spectrum 1996;11(10):18–19.
9. Reeder RE, Pate JR, Snyder C. Effectiveness and efficiency of rigid gas permeable lens power modification with various polishes. Int Contact Lens Clin 1996;23(3/4):67–70.
10. Picciano S, Andrasko GJ. Which factors influence RGP lens comfort? Contact Lens Spectrum 1989;4(5):31–33.
11. Meszaros GK. Simplifying lens modification. Contact Lens Forum 1986;11(11):42–49.
12. Gordon Contact Lens. Contact Lens Adjusting Manual. Rochester, NY: Division of UCO Optics.
13. Morgan BW, Bennett ES. Modification of RGP lenses. Contact Lens Forum 1990;15(7):33–50.
14. Tracy D, Sanford M. Modification Procedures, Guidelines and Tips. Conforma Laboratories.
15. Jurkus JM. Modifying RGPs: a straightforward approach. Optom Management 1996;31(9):54–58.
16. Morgan BW, Bennett ES. Modification. In: Bennett ES, Weissman BA, eds. Clinical Contact Lens Practice, 2nd ed. Philadelphia: JB Lippincott, 1991;307–324.
17. Campbell R, Caroline P. New cleaning system for heavy depositors. Contact Lens Spectrum 1997;12(10):56.
18. Walker J. Overpolishing fluoro-silicone/acrylates: the consequence and the cure. Trans Br Contact Lens Assoc 1989;6:29 (Annual Clinical Conference at Birmingham, U.K.).

Soft Lenses

CHAPTER 10

Soft Material Selection/Fitting and Evaluation

Vinita Allee Henry and Julie Ott DeKinder

Soft contact lenses were introduced in the 1970s. The soft lenses were essentially hydrogel lenses, which were dependent on the water content of the lens to provide oxygen to the cornea. In the late 1990s and early 2000s, a revolutionary new soft lens material, silicone hydrogel, was introduced. This new material incorporated the high oxygen permeability (Dk) of silicone with the benefits of conventional hydrogel lenses.[1] Both types of soft contact lens materials are flexible and made of a plastic that is able to absorb or bind water. Although many similarities exist between hydrogel and silicone hydrogel materials, there are distinct differences between their material properties. When placed on the eye, both forms will conform to the shape of the cornea. Soft lenses have excellent memory; therefore, the lenses can be folded with the edges touching and, when released, will return to the normal shape. The lenses may be inverted and returned to right side out without damaging the optics. Increased water content in the lens, surface treatments, wetting agents, or hydrophilic monomers are used to make this lens surface wettable. This increased wettability also increases the adherence of environmental contaminants (i.e., bacteria, tear lipids and proteins, dust) when the lens is placed in contact with these substances. The purpose of this chapter is to discuss soft lens materials, their similarities and differences, and their properties.

■ MATERIAL PROPERTIES

Hydrogel contact lens materials are made with a stable, solid polymer component that can absorb or bind with water. Spaces exist in the crossed-linked polymer and are called pores. These pores allow fluid (water) to enter the lens material, thus making it hydrated and soft.

The polymers consist of small building blocks called monomers. Therefore, a sequence of repeating units is created. When more than one monomer is used, the term *copolymer* is more appropriate. Most soft contact lens materials are copolymers. A chemical is added to the monomers to create polymerization. Thus, the backbone of the lens has a series of repeating units that can be arranged, either in a random or nonrandom manner, depending on how the polymerization was initiated.[2] These repeating units are then cross-linked to each other. By varying the amount of cross-linking agents, the copolymer will vary in its ability to absorb fluid, in this case, water.

By polymerizing different combinations of monomers, the physical and chemical properties of the lens material can be created, such as water content, refractive index, hardness, mechanical strength, and oxygen permeability. The following monomers are those that are most commonly used to create hydrogel contact lenses[3]:

- 2-Hydroxyethyl methacrylate (HEMA) is the monomer that was used to create the first commercial hydrogel contact lens, and it continues to be the monomer most often utilized. By itself, it will allow a water content of about 38%. When it is combined with other monomers (such as N-vinyl pyrrolidone or methacrylic acid), the water content can be increased to 55%

to 70%.[2] HEMA is an extremely stable material, and variations in temperature, pH, or tonicity have relatively little effect on its water content. It also offers good wettability.

- Ethylene glycol dimethacrylate (EGDMA) is used primarily as a cross-linking agent. Its primary function is to increase the dimensional stability of the material.[3] Increased use of EGDMA will tend to make the material stiffer, lower in water content, and less stretchable.
- Methacrylic acid (MAA) is used to increase the water content of the lens material. It is extremely hydrophilic because of the presence of a free carboxylic acid group that bonds water. It therefore also tends to impart ionic (charged) properties to a material.
- Methyl methacrylate (MMA) is sometimes used to lower water content or to increase the material hardness or strength of a material. It offers excellent optical clarity and is completely inert and very stable, but does not offer any permeability to oxygen.
- N-vinyl pyrrolidone (NVP) is very hydrophilic and is used to increase water content; it offers excellent wettability, and its high water uptake allows for increased oxygen permeability. It generally imparts an ionic property to the material.
- Glyceryl methacrylate (GMA) offers good wettability and helps to increase deposit resistance because it creates smaller pore sizes.[4] Because it also lowers the water content of the material, it imparts a lower Dk.
- Polyvinyl alcohol (PVA) is very hydrophilic, thereby increasing the water content and the Dk of the lens material. It is highly biocompatible and extremely resistant to deposits. It also imparts increased hardness and strength, along with excellent optical clarity. It is completely inert and very stable.

The characteristics of these polymers are summarized in Table 10.1.[5]

Silicone hydrogel lenses were the result of years of research to find a way to combine silicone with conventional hydrogel monomers. Before the introduction of silicone hydrogels, lenses made of silicone elastomers had exceptional oxygen transmission, yet demonstrated poor

TABLE 10.1 COMMON MATERIAL MONOMERS AND THEIR CHARACTERISTICS

MONOMER	ABBREVIATION	ADVANTAGES	DISADVANTAGES
Hydroxyethyl methacrylate	HEMA	• Hydrophilic • Flexible • Softness • Good wettability	• Low oxygen permeability
Ethylene glycol dimethacrylate	EGDMA	• Stability	• Low oxygen permeability
Methacrylic acid	MAA	• Hydrophilic	• pH sensitive
Methyl methacrylate	MMA	• Hardness • Machinable • Optical clarity • Stability; inert	• No oxygen permeability
N-vinyl pyrrolidone	NVP	• Hydrophilic • Good wettability • High water uptake • High oxygen permeability	• pH sensitive
Glyceryl methacrylate	GMA	• Good wettability • Good deposit resistance	• Low oxygen permeability
Polyvinyl alcohol	PVA	• Hydrophilic • High water uptake • Deposit resistance	• May be more difficult to manufacture

wettability, poor comfort, manufacturing difficulties, corneal adherence, and were prone to deposits.[1] Silicone has the ability to link carbon, hydrogen, and oxygen. Silicone-based polymers are composed of long chains of polymers. It is this make-up of long chains and small relative diameter that gives these polymers their elasticity and strength.[6] The properties of silicone have already been observed in gas-permeable (GP) lenses, where silicone was added to increase oxygen transmission in high-Dk GP lens materials. Discovering the method of combining hydrogel properties with silicone allowed for the manufacture of a high-Dk, comfortable, wettable lens with optical clarity and deposit resistance.

Whether a hydrogel or silicone hydrogel material, ideally, material properties are chosen to create a contact lens material that has the following characteristics:

- Safe
- Inert
- Nontoxic
- Biocompatible
- Chemically and physically stable
- Good wettability
- Deposit resistant
- Durable
- Easy to formulate and manufacture
- Good optical clarity

In reality, tradeoffs between some of these characteristics must be made. The final lens material can then be evaluated in terms of the following properties:

Transparency

Transparency refers to the clearness (clarity) of a material. Among other factors, it is a function of the chemistry, purity, and hydration of the material. No material is completely transparent, as some light will always be reflected, absorbed, and scattered. Transparency is often expressed as a percentage of incident light of a certain wavelength that passes through a sample of the material. Values for most clear (nontinted) contact lens materials range from 92% to 98%.

Hardness and Stiffness

The hardness of a lens material is an important quality affecting its ability to be used for the manufacture of contact lenses and its durability. Generally, hardness is an attribute that is more relevant to rigid lens materials than soft materials. Stiffness is the degree of flexibility of a material, and this can be an important factor when a lens material is selected for a patient. More flexible materials usually result in better initial comfort but do not mask or correct corneal astigmatism, as they tend to drape over the cornea and conform to its shape. Stiffer materials retain their shape during handling and will make insertion and removal of the lens easier.

Tensile Strength

The tensile strength of a material is a value that expresses how much stretching force can be applied before it breaks. Materials with a high tensile strength tend to be more durable, as they are better able to withstand the forces applied during lens handling procedures (i.e., cleaning, inserting) without tearing.

Modulus of Elasticity

The modulus of elasticity is a constant value that expresses a material's ability to keep its shape when subjected to stress and to resist deformation. Materials with a high modulus are stiffer, resist deformation, hold their shape better, are easier to handle, and may provide better visual acu-

TABLE 10.2 LENS MODULUS VALUES

MATERIAL NAME	HYDROGEL OR SILICONE HYDROGEL	MODULUS (MPA)
pHEMA	Hydrogel	0.50
lotrafilcon A (Focus N & D)	Silicone hydrogel	1.4–1.52
balafilcon A (PureVision)	Silicone hydrogel	1.1–1.25
lotrafilcon B (O$_2$Optix)	Silicone hydrogel	1.0–1.2
asmofilcon A (PremiO)	Silicone hydrogel	0.90
comfilcon A (Biofinity)	Silicone hydrogel	0.75–0.8
senofilcon A (AV Oasys)	Silicone hydrogel	0.6–0.72
enfilcon A (Avaira)	Silicone hydrogel	0.5
galyfilcon A (AV Advance)	Silicone hydrogel	0.4–0.43

ity. Many silicone hydrogel materials have a lens modulus much greater than hydrogel materials. The stiffer lens may have the benefits mentioned previously, or it may adversely affect the lens performance by causing edge lift or fluting, superior epithelial arcuate lesions (SEALs), mucin balls, or giant papillary conjunctivitis [GPC, also called contact lens papillary conjunctivitis (CLPC)].[7–9] Materials with a low modulus of elasticity are less resistant to stress. Most hydrogel materials fall in the low-modulus category. Modulus values can be found in Table 10.2.[1,7,9,10]

Refractive Index

Refractive index of a lens material is the ratio of the speed of light in air to the speed of light in the material. Materials with higher refractive indices cause more refraction of incident light. For soft lens materials, the index of refraction is related to water content. Generally, increasing the water content lowers the refractive index. A hydrogel lens material with a water content of 80% has a refractive index of about 1.37, and one with a water content of 42% has a refractive index of about 1.44, compared to silicone hydrogel materials (lotrafilcon A and balafilcon A), which have a refractive index of 1.43.[11,12]

Wettability

The surface wettability of a soft lens is an important property. The wettability aids in the closure of the lid over the lens, thereby improving comfort and preventing changes to the papillary surface on the internal surface of the lid.[13] The very wettable surface creates a stable, even tear film. This assists with optimizing comfort, visual acuity, and deposit resistance. As silicone is naturally hydrophobic, its use in soft lenses created a dilemma until the ability to increase the wettability of silicone was discovered.

Early silicone hydrogel materials used a surface treatment to cover up the hydrophobic properties of silicone. Ciba Vision uses a gas plasma technique to apply a uniform plasma coating, approximately 25 nm thick with a high refractive index, on the surface of its silicone hydrogel lenses (lotrafilcon A and B) (Fig. 10.1). The gas plasma technique is also used by Bausch & Lomb to apply a plasma oxidation surface treatment to its silicone hydrogel lens (balafilcon A). This surface treatment results in glassy silicate islands on the surface of the lens. The islands leave small areas of exposed hydrophobic regions; however, the wettability of the silicate appears to create a bridge over these areas to produce a net hydrophilic surface.[6] Menicon combines the benefits of plasma coating and plasma oxidation for a plasma surface treatment on its lens (asmofilcon A) called Nanogloss surface modification. The manufacturer reports that this creates a smooth surface with a low contact angle.[10] Silicone hydrogel materials have also used

Surface Modifications

All photos 5 x 5 micron resolution

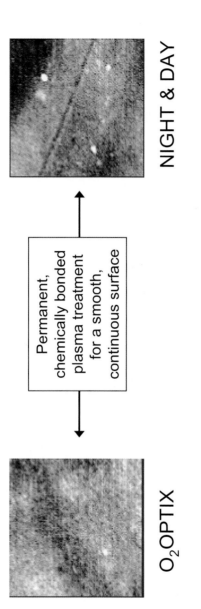

O₂OPTIX

Permanent, chemically bonded plasma treatment for a smooth, continuous surface

NIGHT & DAY

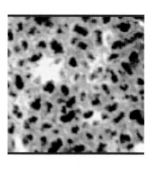

ACUVUE OASYS

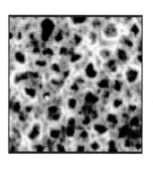

ACUVUE Advance

No permanent plasma treatment

PureVision

Surface made up of silicate islands that do not completely cover the surface

■ FIGURE 10.1 Silicone hydrogel surface modifications. (Courtesy of Ciba Vision.)

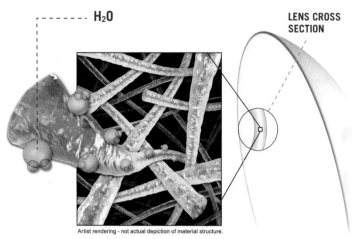

Artist rendering - not actual depiction of material structure.

■ **FIGURE 10.2** Biofinity: Siloxane molecules attract and bond to surrounding water molecules, continuously wetting and lubricating the material. (Courtesy of CooperVision.)

an internal wetting agent, polyvinyl pyrrolidone (PVP), to create wettability (Vistakon, galyfilcon A, and senofilcon A).[1] CooperVision reports that its silicone hydrogel lens (comfilcon A) has no surface treatment or wetting agent. Instead, the lens material contains two silicone-based macromers (a large monomer preassembled to transfer advantageous properties to the final polymer).[6] These macromers, when incorporated into the material with hydrophilic monomers, result in a naturally wettable lens (Fig. 10.2).

Another factor that has changed the wettability of soft contact lenses is the incorporation of PVA or PVP, moisturizing agents, into daily disposable hydrogel lens materials. Potentially, adding these agents to the lens material will result in increased wettability, increased comfort, and enhanced tear film stability. Early results indicate that this may be beneficial to dry-eye patients and provide increased comfort throughout the day, including end-of-the-day comfort.[14,15]

Ionic Charge

Contact lens materials may possess an electric charge, or they may be electrically neutral. This attribute is especially important in soft lens materials, as it affects factors such as solution compatibility and deposit formation. Materials that have an electric charge are said to be ionic. The charge results from the presence of electrically charged groups in their chemical formulation. In most cases, this is an overall negative charge. The presence of a negative ionic charge causes the material to be more reactive, especially in solutions that are acidic. This, in turn, can cause dimensional changes and even material degradation.

An ionic charge may also cause a material to be more prone to deposit formation. Most deposits are positively charged substances from tears that are attracted to the negative ionic charge of the lens material. Materials that are electrically neutral are said to be nonionic. These materials tend to be more inert and less reactive with tear constituents, so they also tend to be more deposit resistant.

Hydration (Water Content)

Most contact lens materials, both GP and soft, absorb some water. The amount absorbed is usually expressed as a percentage of the total weight. When a material absorbs water, it swells, a fact that must be considered during the manufacturing process to achieve precise specifications. Materials that absorb <4% of water by weight are referred to as *hydrophobic materials*; those that absorb ≥4% water are termed *hydrophilic polymers*. With hydrophilic polymers (hydrogels), increasing the water content generally increases Dk. However, this often increases lens fragility and may make the material more prone to deposit formation. Even if it were possible to create a 100% water content lens material, the Dk of water is 80; therefore, this lens would still be unable to meet the Holden-Mertz criterion for extended wear (87×10^{-9}).[1] Silicone hydrogel materials have low water contents, because the material is dependent on silicone, not water, to transmit oxygen.

Oxygen Permeability/Oxygen Transmission

Oxygen permeability usually depends on the water content of the hydrogel lens and is a property of the material.[3,16] Generally, the Dk of a lens increases logarithmically with an increase in water content.[17] Oxygen transmission (Dk/t) is defined as the Dk of the lens divided by its thickness (t). Lens power indirectly affects Dk/t. As center thickness (CT) varies considerably in higher powers (both plus and minus), average thickness is typically used for the determination of Dk/t. The highest Dk value obtainable with a HEMA-based hydrogel lens is approximately 40.[18] It is not unusual for a low-water-content, ultrathin hydrogel lens to have a similar Dk/t value as a high-water-content hydrogel lens, which typically has to be manufactured in a greater CT. Decreasing the CT or increasing the water content increases the Dk/t of the lens; however, it also results in a more fragile lens material.

Silicone hydrogel materials have been successful in breaking the dependence on water content for Dk (Fig. 10.3).[19,20] Silicone hydrogel materials tend to have an inverse relationship between Dk and water content; the lower the water content, generally the higher the Dk.[6] Silicone hydrogel materials offer Dk/t values in the range of approximately 86 to 175. Many of these lenses meet the Holden-Mertz criterion for extended wear of 87×10^{-9} (cm $\times$ mL O_2)/s $\times$ mL $\times$ mm Hg) and Harvitt and Bonanno's suggested Dk/t of 125×10^{-9} (cm $\times$ mL O_2)/s $\times$ mL $\times$ mm Hg) to avoid stromal anoxia. These materials make it possible for contact lens patients to wear lenses on a continuous basis overnight for up to 30 days, as silicone hydrogel materials provide up to eight times the Dk/t of conventional hydrogel lenses.[1] Although the estimated value of Dk necessary for daily wear (24–35)[21] is much lower than the values of silicone hydrogels (60–175), these materials are beneficial to the ocular health of patients who wear their lenses daily and remove them each night by reducing both epithelial thinning and chronic limbal inflammation (Fig. 10.4).[16] A summary of silicone hydrogel material characteristics can be found in Table 10.3.[1,7,16,22]

Classification of Lens Groups

The U.S. Food and Drug Administration (FDA) has classified soft lens materials according to their water content and ionic charge. This classification has become widely accepted internationally.

This classification simplifies the large number of possible soft lens materials into four groups. This helps to predict the performance of the various lens materials both on and off of the eye. The rationale for this classification is that water content and ionic charge will determine how a soft lens material will interact with contact lens solutions. Additionally, many properties of the material, such as strength, refractive index, deposit resistance, and, generally, Dk, depend on its water content. Lens strength, deposit resistance, and refractive index all decrease as the water content of the material increases. Generally, pore size and oxygen permeability will increase as water content increases.

In the FDA classification, low water content is defined as <50% water; high water content is defined as >50% water.[8] The four classification groups are:

Group 1: low water content, nonionic polymers.
Group 2: high water content, nonionic polymers.
Group 3: low water content, ionic polymers.
Group 4: high water content, ionic polymers.

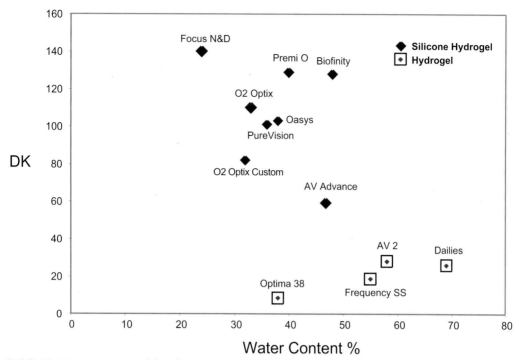

■ **FIGURE 10.3** Oxygen permeability relationship with water content for silicone hydrogel and some hydrogel lenses.

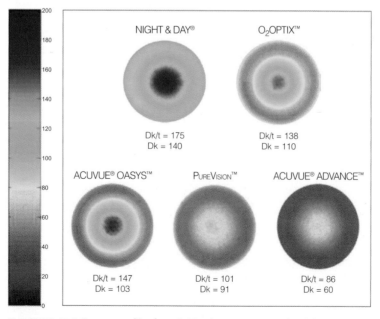

■ **FIGURE 10.4** Oxygen profiles for −3.00 sphere; oxygen permeability values are as reported by the manufacturers. (Courtesy of Ciba Vision.)

TABLE 10.3 SILICONE HYDROGEL LENSES

Brand Name	Focus Night & Day	O$_2$ Optix/Air Optix Aqua	PureVision	Acuvue Advance	Acuvue Oasys	Biofinity	Avaira	O$_2$ Optix Custom	PremiO
Manufacturer	Ciba Vision	Ciba Vision	Bausch & Lomb	Vistakon	Vistakon	Cooper Vision	Cooper Vision	Ciba Vision	Menicon
Material	lotrafilcon A	lotrafilcon B	balafilcon A	galyfilcon A	senofilcon A	comfilcon A	enfilcon A	sifilcon A	asmofilcon A
Dk	140	110	101	60	103	128	100	82	129
Dk/t	175	138	110	86	147	160	125	117	161
Water content	24%	33%	36%	47%	38%	48%	46%	32%	40%
Modulus (MPa)	1.4–1.52	1–1.2	1.1–1.5	0.4–0.43	0.6–0.72	0.75	0.5	1.1	0.90
Surface modification	Plasma coating	Plasma coating	Plasma oxidation	Internal wetting agent	Internal wetting agent	None	None	Plasma coating	Nanogloss
Recommended replacement	Monthly	2 wk	Monthly	2 wk	2 wk	Monthly	2 wk	3 mo	2 wk
FDA group	1	1	3	1	1	1	1	1	1
Wear schedule	DW, EW, or CW	DW or EW	DW, EW, or CW	DW	DW or EW	DW	DW	DW	DW or EW
Additional lens modalities		Toric	Toric & multifocal	Toric	Toric				

CW, continuous wear; Dk, oxygen permeability; Dk/t, oxygen transmission; DW, daily wear; EW, extended wear; FDA, Food and Drug Administration.

Group 1

This group consists of the low-water-content, nonionic polymers. This includes such materials as HEMA and hydrophobic monomers. No lenses with MAA are included in this group. These materials exhibit lower protein deposition because of the lower water content and nonionic nature.[23]

Group 2

This group consists of high-water-content, nonionic polymers. As these lenses have a high water content, they have a potential for greater protein attraction. However, they have the advantage of a nonionic polymer matrix that prevents additional interaction between protein and the lens. Heat disinfection should not be used with these lenses because of the high water content. The preservatives sorbic acid and potassium sorbate should also be avoided with these lenses because of discoloration problems.[23]

Group 3

This group of lenses consists of low-water-content, ionic polymers. The negatively charged surfaces of these lenses show greater attraction for the positively charged tear proteins and lipids. Therefore, they tend to exhibit more deposits than materials in the nonionic groups.[23]

Group 4

This group consists of the high-water-content, ionic polymers. Lenses in this group tend to attract more protein than do those in any other lens group. The high water content and ionic properties cause greater absorption of proteins into the lens matrix. Heat disinfection should be avoided in this group of lenses because of the high water content. Sorbic acid and potassium sorbate-preserved solutions should also be avoided. Ionic polymers are more sensitive to change in lens care product composition because added ions in the matrix can change the water content. Changes in pH may alter the lens parameters.[23]

Given the differences between hydrogel lens materials and silicone hydrogel materials, it would appear that silicone hydrogel materials would need their own classification. These materials react differently to deposits and solutions, because their basic characteristics (e.g., wettability, water content, Dk) differ from conventional hydrogel materials. A new group, group 5, has been proposed, which would classify silicone hydrogel materials.[24,25] The current FDA classification can be found in Table 10.4[22] and the group 5 classification can be found in Table 10.5.[24]

■ MANUFACTURING METHODS

Soft lenses can be spun-cast, lathe-cut, cast-molded, or manufactured via a combination of these procedures. The manufacturing of contact lenses involves many different procedures, steps, and technologies. The following section provides a brief overview of the major manufacturing methods. All contact lens-manufacturing methods begin with the formulation and preparation of the lens material. In this preparation stage, monomers are added in precise amounts, any impurities are removed, and in some cases the material is polymerized into rods, buttons, or sheets.

■ LATHE CUTTING

Lathe cutting is used to manufacture polymethylmethacrylate (PMMA), GP, and many soft contact lenses. This process begins with a long, plastic cylinder of material that is cut into lens buttons. The lathe cut process is composed of the following steps:

Lathing

In this procedure, the hard, dry "button" of the lens polymer is ground on a lathe. Computerized, automatic lathes are now available to cut the front and base curves onto the lens, along with any secondary curves and edge bevels.

TABLE 10.4 FOOD AND DRUG ADMINISTRATION (FDA) CLASSIFICATION OF SOFT LENSES

	GROUP 1	GROUP 2	GROUP 3	GROUP 4
	(low-water, nonionic polymers)	(high-water, nonionic polymers)	(low-water, ionic polymers)	(high-water, ionic polymers)
The FDA has created the four lens groups to clarify categories of similar polymers for investigating solutions approvals.	tefilcon (38%) tetrafilcon A (43%) crofilcon (39%) hefilcon A&B (45%) isofilcon (36%) polymacon (38%) mafilcon (33%) genfilcon A (48%) dimefilcon A (36%) hioxiflilcon B (49%) lotrafilcon A (24%) lotrafilcon B (33%) galyfilcon A (47%) senofilcon A (37%) sifilcon A (32%) comfilcon A (48%) asmofilcon A (40%)	acofilcon A (58%) omafilcon A (59%) alphafilcon A (66%) hioxifilcon A (59%) hioxifilcon D (54%) lidofilcon B (79%) lidofilcon A (70%) ofilcon A (74%) xylofilcon A (67%) scafilcon A (71%) vasurfilcon A (74%) surfilcon A (74%) netrafilcon A (65%) nelfilcon A (69%) atlafilcon A (64%) hefilcon C (57%) hilafilcon B (59%)	etafilcon A (43%) bufilcon A (45%) deltafilcon A (43%) droxifilcon A (47%) phemfilcon A (38%) ocufilcon A (44%) balafilcon A (36%)	bufilcon A (55%) epsilfilcon A (60%) perfilcon A (71%) etafilcon A (58%) ocufilcon B (53%) ocufilcon C (55%) ocufilcon D (55%) ocufilcon E (65%) ocufilcon F (60%) phemfilcon A (55%) methafilcon A,B (55%) vifilcon A (55%) focofilcon A (55%) tetrafilcon B (58%)

Polishing

The lenses are then removed from the lathe and polished to remove any lathing marks, improve the optics, and smooth the edges.

Hydration

For soft lenses, the brittle, dry lenses now undergo hydration, where they are immersed in saline until they absorb as much water as their formulation will allow. This is the step where the lens actually transforms from a dry, rigid material to the soft and flexible lens.

During the hydration stage, the lenses swell as they absorb water. For this reason, careful calculations are made regarding the size of the dry lens to achieve the exact dimensions of the fully hydrated lens.

Extraction

Lenses are then moved to the extraction stage. During extraction, lenses are processed to remove all unpolymerized chemicals or materials that may be present.

TABLE 10.5 CLASSIFICATION OF SILICONE HYDROGELS GROUP 5[a]

A	B	C	D
Nonlinear relationship of Dk to water content	Contains an ionic component	Plasma or bonded surface modification	Contains a "releasing" wetting agent
comfilcon A enfilcon A	balafilcon A	lotrafilcon A lotrafilcon B sifilcon A	galyfilcon A senofilcon A

[a]Asmofilcon A has not yet been classified.

Dk, oxygen permeability.

Tinting

If the lens is to be tinted, the tinting process normally occurs as the next stage in this process.

Finishing

Numerous quality assurance steps occur throughout the manufacturing process. A full quality inspection of the lens is then performed before the lens is finished and the final processing steps before it is distributed.

Sterilization

The lenses are now sterilized. Trays of lenses are loaded into an autoclave, in which a temperature of 121° to 124°C is maintained for at least 20 minutes. This step inactivates any microorganisms and spores that may be present and ensures the sterility of the packaged lens. Lathe cutting is a relatively labor-intensive and expensive process and is not generally as reproducible as spin casting or cast molding. However, it is a useful method for the manufacture of certain lenses, especially those made in low quantities or with custom parameters.

■ SPIN CASTING

Spin casting was the first method employed in the manufacture of soft contact lenses. It was invented by Otto Wichterle in 1951 and was further developed by Bausch & Lomb. The process is used to manufacture some hydrogel contact lenses.

Spin casting consists of a liquid form of the lens polymer being injected into a spinning mold. The final shape and power of the resulting lens is from the combination of temperature, gravity, centrifugal force, surface tension, amount of liquid in the mold, and rate of spin, which is computer controlled. Slower speeds produce flatter posterior curves, and faster speeds produce steeper curves.

The outer (front or anterior) surface of the lens is determined by the curvature of the mold. The inner (base curve) of the lens is determined by the factors listed above; because of these forces, the resultant base curves are aspheric.

After spinning for the proper time, the lens material is treated with heat and/or ultraviolet light. This treatment is called "curing," and causes the liquid polymer to solidify. The lens is then hydrated, extracted, and finished similar to lathe-cut lenses.

Spin casting is an inexpensive manufacturing method. The lenses produced are highly reproducible and have a very thin, comfortable edge. The primary problem when fitting spin-cast lenses is their tendency to decenter on the eye. They often position temporally or in a superior-temporal position.

■ CAST MOLDING

Cast molding is a more reproducible and less labor-intensive process. It is a cost-effective method of production for the high-volume manufacture of contact lenses. Many of the disposable and frequent replacement lenses are manufactured using this process.

The first step in cast molding is making the molds from which the lenses will be formed. Each different lens design (every possible combination of power, base curve, and diameter) requires a separate master mold. Thousands of plastic molds can be produced from a single metallic master mold.

Liquid polymer is poured into the concave half of the mold. The convex portion of the mold is then applied and clamped into place, and the material is cured with ultraviolet light.

After the lens is removed from the mold, it undergoes the hydration process. Stabilized Soft Molding (Vistakon), Lightstream Technology (CIBA Vision), and Aquaform Molded Science

(CooperVision) are proprietary methods of cast molding used to produce high-quality, inexpensive, reproducible soft contact lenses.

■ LENS TYPES

Wearing Schedules

The FDA approves lenses to be worn for either daily wear (DW) or extended wear (EW). In DW, the lenses are prescribed to be worn during the day and removed before sleep. EW lenses are currently approved for a maximum of 7 days and 6 nights of wear before removal or for 30 nights of continuous wear (CW) before removal. Some practitioners use the term "flexible wear" to describe the use of EW-approved lenses on an occasional EW basis (i.e., 2 or 3 nights of wear or an occasional nap with the lenses in place).

Generally, EW-approved lenses have a higher DK/t value than DW lenses. The higher DK/t value is generally achieved by using a higher-water-content material, a thinner lens, or both. This may make the lenses more difficult to handle or insert/remove, as well as more fragile. Currently, these conventional hydrogel lenses are discouraged for EW use as silicone hydrogel lens materials provide, as previously mentioned, up to eight times more oxygen to the cornea. Silicone hydrogel lens materials may be used for DW, EW, or CW depending on their FDA approval (see Chapter 16 for more information on EW). When selecting a wearing schedule for a patient, the practitioner must evaluate the patient's ocular health, desires, needs, and lifestyle to determine which schedule is most appropriate for that patient.

Replacement Schedule

The FDA does not directly approve replacement schedules. They classify devices as either disposable (intended for single use) or conventional (cleaned upon removal from the eye and then reused). The FDA does not specify how many times conventional lenses may be reused or how often they should be replaced.

Manufacturers, based on their knowledge of their own lens material's features and attributes, will specify a recommended replacement time. Although the lens may still be usable beyond the recommended replacement time specified by the manufacturer, generally its performance will begin to decline. This is manifested by decreased comfort, increased deposits, decreased vision, increased lens awareness, and increased lens tears or nicks.

In 1989, when the first disposable (true single use) lens was approved by the FDA, it was to be used once and thrown away upon removal from the eye, generally after 7 days of EW use. Because of a variety of factors, the disposable lenses then received approval for "reuse" on a DW basis for up to 2 weeks. Practitioners still referred to these lenses as "disposables," even though they were no longer being used once and then discarded. Currently, most practitioners term any lenses that are used for a month or less "disposable."

In an effort to reduce this confusion, terms such as "frequent replacement," "planned replacement," and "programmed replacement" developed. These terms indicate a lens that is replaced on a practitioner-specified schedule. This schedule may be 2 weeks, 1 month, 3 months, 6 months, or any period within this time frame. It is important to emphasize that this replacement schedule is not dictated or approved by the FDA. Rather, it is only a recommendation by the manufacturer to help maximize lens performance, patient comfort, and patient health. The lenses that most practitioners refer to as "disposable" are really more correctly termed as "frequent-replacement" lenses. Most lenses in vials, which most practitioners refer to as conventional lenses, are recommended to be used on a specified replacement schedule, usually 6 months to 1 year.

Practitioners and the industry have increased their use of disposable and frequent-replacement lenses, virtually eliminating conventional lenses replaced greater than every 6 months.

The benefits of this type of lens use are convenience, comfort, health, decreased need for enzyme or separate cleaners, fewer lens deposits, availability of spare lenses, and increased patient satisfaction.

With confusion surrounding replacement schedules, how should a practitioner determine what schedule is best for a patient? In general, two rules apply:

1. The more frequent the replacement, the fewer the number of ocular complications.
2. If deposits are ever observed on a patient's lenses, the lens replacement schedule needs to be reduced.

Daily disposable lenses are an affordable reality for most people. In a very large study[26] (almost 46,000 eyes), lenses disposed of on a daily basis had the lowest ocular complication rate at only 2.5%. As a comparison, GP lenses showed a complication rate of 10.5%, PMMA 15.8%, conventional HEMA lenses 8.5%, and weekly disposable extended-wear lenses 4.9%.

Other studies[27,28] have shown fewer unscheduled office visits with daily disposable lenses as well as improved visual acuity, comfort, and patient satisfaction. Additionally, daily disposable lenses require no lens care, and this is a tremendous convenience for many patients. Beyond daily disposable use, most lenses are recommended for 2-week, monthly, or quarterly replacement.

The recommended wearing schedule for silicone hydrogel lens materials is 2 to 4 weeks, depending on the material. Like daily disposable lenses, several studies have shown that silicone hydrogels have improved corneal health and decreased signs of corneal hypoxia[29–31] as compared to conventional hydrogel materials (for more information see Chapter 16).

Depending on the lens material, different replacement schedules should be recommended. Studies have shown that for group 4 lenses, monthly replacement produces better results, whereas group 2 lenses are able to be replaced quarterly without much change in the lens performance.[32] However, some studies suggest that monthly replacement is easier for patients to maintain and comply with as compared to quarterly replacement.[33,34]

The difference between 2-week and monthly replacement has not been adequately addressed, and the schedule chosen is currently determined more by manufacturer recommendations. Even though the great majority of "disposable" lenses are prescribed for 2-week use, it has been found that the average patient wears these lenses for approximately 1 month.[35]

Clinically, the only way to observe lens deposits is with a slit lamp. However, studies using scanning electron microscopy have found that by the time lens deposits are visible through the slit lamp, they are already heavy enough to begin to degrade the lens surface. Additionally, these deposits begin to decrease visual acuity long before they are able to be observed with a slit lamp at a clinically significant level.[36] This is why the replacement schedule should be reduced immediately if clinically detectable levels of deposits are ever observed. As with the wearing schedule, the practitioner must evaluate a large number of clinical, health, and patient factors when prescribing a replacement schedule. The schedule should then be monitored for both compliance and health reasons.

■ SUMMARY

This chapter has summarized the characteristics of hydrogel and silicone hydrogel lens materials. There are many options for the eye care practitioner to select from including material factors (i.e., Dk/t, modulus, water content, and wettability), wearing schedules (i.e., DW, EW, or CW), and replacement schedules (i.e., daily, weekly, monthly). Preliminary evaluation of the patient and the desires of the patient will aid the practitioner in finding the material that will provide good vision and ocular health as well as fit the patient's lifestyle.

■ CLINICAL CASES

CASE 1

A 28-year-old woman who has worn conventional EW hydrogel lenses (58% water content) for 5 years comes into your office. She wears the lenses for 4 to 6 nights before removing them. Although she does not have any major complaints, you notice limbal engorgement and vascularization, an increase in myopia, and corneal edema grade 1+.

SOLUTION: As the patient desires to stay in EW, she is fitted with a silicone hydrogel lens material approved for EW. She may keep her current wearing schedule of 4 to 6 nights EW. At the follow-up visit, the limbal vessels have emptied, her prescription has stabilized with less myopia, and her cornea is clear.

CASE 2

A patient with refraction and keratometry readings of $-3.00 - 1.00 \times 180$, 43.00 @ 180; 44.00 @ 090 OU is fitted with GP lenses and has a resulting visual acuity of 20/15 OU. The patient appears to be compliant and motivated to wear contact lenses. Two weeks after dispensing, the patient is experiencing difficulty adapting to GP lens wear. The importance of gradually increasing wearing time is emphasized to the patient. At 1 month, the patient is only able to wear the lenses for 2 to 4 hours and reports discomfort.

SOLUTION: Discomfort appears to be the primary factor that is preventing this patient from wearing contact lenses. The patient is fitted into a soft toric lens with a power of $-3.00 - 0.75 \times 180$ and an 8.6-mm base curve radius OU with a visual acuity equal to 20/15 OU. The patient is able to achieve full-day wear.

CASE 3

A patient has been a successful daily-wear GP patient with the exception of chronic lens adherence. The lens design has been changed and no improvements have been observed. Dry eyes and/or dirty lenses do not appear to be the cause as the patient is very careful and compliant with lens care. Rewetting drops also proved to be unsuccessful.

SOLUTION: Generally lens adherence in daily-wear GP lenses can be prevented by changing the lens design; however, there are some patients who are prone to lens adherence, and changes in the lens design are unsuccessful. In this case, the patient may be fitted into a soft lens to achieve contact lens wear. While the cornea is rehabilitating, it is possible that there may be a series of lens changes necessary before the lens power and base curve radius are finalized. Using disposable trial lenses, with regular follow-up examinations, will allow the practitioner to make the necessary lens changes before ordering the final lens parameters.

CASE 4

A 30-year-old man who has worn soft lenses for 15 years has been diagnosed as having GPC (or CLPC). After managing the GPC, the patient is provided with new, clean lenses. The patient notices that about every 9 months the symptoms of GPC recur as the lenses become deposited.

SOLUTION: There are several ways to manage this case: (a) The patient can be fitted with a daily disposable lens. (b) The patient can be placed on a frequent replacement program. As the deposits and symptoms begin to recur every 9 months, a monthly replacement program will provide him with new lenses before his symptoms recur. (c) The patient can be refitted into a disposable lens to be worn daily, removed at night and discarded at the end of 2 weeks.

CASE 5

A 20-year-old athlete complains of frequently tearing his contact lenses (high water content, group 4). He is in college and his parents want to know if there is a more durable lens than the one he is currently wearing.

SOLUTION: Re-education on soft lens care and handling should be performed with this patient. Secondly, he may need to be refitted into a more durable lens, such as a group 1 lens material that is a disposable or frequent-replacement lens (i.e., replacement every 2–4 weeks). This way he not only has a lens that is easier to handle and care for, but he also has spare lenses. Other options would be daily disposable or silicone hydrogel lenses.

CASE 6

A patient who was previously wearing conventional hydrogel lenses is refitted into a silicone hydrogel lens with a high modulus. The patient is educated that the lenses may require a couple of weeks to adapt to the feel of the lens. At the 3-week follow-up examination, the patient is still unhappy with the comfort despite wearing the lenses for 8 to 12 hours.

SOLUTION: The patient is refitted into a lower modulus silicone hydrogel lens. This time the patient is satisfied with the comfort. Other issues to address with this patient are the type of solution he is using and if there is any edge fluting. Poor comfort might be the result of not using a recommended care regimen or a preservative sensitivity. If the lens is demonstrating fluting of the edge, using a steeper base curve may solve his symptoms of discomfort.

CLINICAL PROFICIENCY CHECKLIST

- The strength, deposit resistance, and Dk of a hydrogel lens material are all components that generally depend on water content. The Dk of a hydrogel lens material increases logarithmically with an increase in water content.
- Silicone hydrogel lenses do not depend on water content to be permeable to oxygen; generally, the Dk of the material increases as the water content decreases.
- Hydrophilic monomers (i.e., NVP, MAA), copolymerized with HEMA, increase the water content of hydrogel lenses.
- Group 1 nonionic/low-water-content lenses demonstrate the lowest rate of protein formation, whereas group 4 ionic/high-water-content lenses tend to develop more protein deposition than the other groups.
- Silicone is hydrophobic; therefore, most silicone hydrogel lens materials require a surface treatment, internal wetting agent, or special design to make the lens hydrophilic.
- Wearing schedules and replacement frequencies must be determined for each patient. In general, more frequent replacement of lenses results in better ocular health and vision.
- Most silicone hydrogel materials have a higher modulus than hydrogel materials. Although this aids in handling and durability, it may result in edge fluting, SEALs, GPC, or lens awareness.
- Silicone hydrogel lenses provide up to eight times higher Dk/t than hydrogel lenses.

The authors would like to thank Sally Dillehay, O.D., for her contributions to the Material Selection chapter in the second edition of this textbook.

REFERENCES

1. Sweeney D, Fonn D, Evans K. Silicone hydrogels: the evolution of a revolution. Contact Lens Spectrum 2006;Special Edition:14–19.
2. White P. A complete guide to contact lens materials. Contact Lens Spectrum 1994;9(11):31–44.
3. Winterton LC, Su KC. Chemistry and processing of contact lens materials. In: Bennett ES, Weissman BA, eds. Clinical Contact Lens Practice. Philadelphia: Lippincott Williams & Wilkins, 2005:355–362.

4. Hom MH. An inside look at soft lens materials. Contact Lens Forum 1985;10(12):38–39.

5. Dillehay SM, Henry VA. Material selection. In: Bennett ES, Henry VA, eds. Clinical Manual of Contact Lenses. Philadelphia: Lippincott Williams & Wilkins, 2000:239–258.

6. Tighe B. Silicone hydrogels: structure, properties and behaviour. In: Sweeney DF, ed. Silicone Hydrogels Continuous-Wear Contact Lenses. Edinburgh: Butterworth Heinemann, 2004:1–27.

7. Young G. Exploring the relationship between materials and ocular health and comfort. Contact Lens Spectrum 2007;Special Edition:37–40.

8. Snyder C. Modulus and its effect on contact lens fit. Contact Lens Spectrum 2007;22(2):36–40.

9. French K. Why is modulus important? Editorial. October 2007. http://www.siliconehydrogels.org. Accessed January 8, 2008.

10. Jones L. A new silicone hydrogel lens comes to market. Contact Lens Spectrum 2007;22(10):23.

11. Fatt I, Chaston J. The effect of temperature on refractive index, water content and central thickness of hydrogel contact lenses. Int Contact Lens Clin 1980;7:37–42.

12. Yeung KK, Weissman BA. Soft contact lens application. In: Bennett ES, Weissman BA, eds. Clinical Contact Lens Practice. Philadelphia: Lippincott Williams & Wilkins, 2005:363–377.

13. Jones L. Understanding the link between wettability and lens comfort. Contact Lens Spectrum 2007;22(6):S4–S6.

14. Nichols JJ. A look at lubricating agents in daily disposables. Contact Lens Spectrum 2007;22(1):22.

15. Nick J, Winterton L, Lally J, Long B. Lubricating lens focuses on patient comfort. Contact Lens Spectrum 2006;21(1):40–41.

16. Holden BA, Stretton S, de la Jara PL, et al. The future of contact lenses: Dk really matters. Contact Lens Spectrum 2006;Special Edition:20–28.

17. Brennan N, Efron N, Weissman B, et al. Clinical application of the oxygen transmissibility of powered contact lenses. CLAO J 1991;17:169–172.

18. Mandell RB. Basic principles of hydrogel lenses. In: Mandell RB, ed. Contact Lens Practice, 4th ed. Springfield, IL: Charles C. Thomas Publisher, 1988:502–527.

19. Alvord L, Court J, Davis T, et al. Oxygen permeability of a new type of high Dk soft contact lens material. Optom Vis Sci 1998;75(1):30–36.

20. Lowther GE. Will high Dk hydrogel lenses become a reality? Int Contact Lens Clin 1998;251(2):39.

21. Fonn D, Bruce AS. A review of the Holden-Mertz criteria for critical oxygen transmission. Eye Cont Lens 2005;31:247–251.

22. Thompson TT. Tyler's Quarterly Soft Contact Lens Parameter Guide 2007;25(1):1–7.

23. Stone RP. Why contact lens groups? Contact Lens Spectrum 1988;3(12):38–41.

24. Stone RP. A new perspective for lens care - classifying silicone hydrogels. Editorial. June 2007. http://www.siliconehydrogels.org. Accessed January 8, 2008.

25. Hutter JC. FDA group V: is a single grouping sufficient to describe SiH performance? Editorial. November 2007. http://www.siliconehydrogels.org. Accessed January 8, 2008.

26. Hamano H, Watanabe K, Mitsunaga S, et al. A study of the complications induced by conventional and disposable contact lenses. CLAO J 1994;20(2):103–108.

27. Freeman M, Dubow B, Lopanik R, et al. A three-year study of the clinical performance of daily disposable contact lenses. Optician 1997;213:36–45.

28. Nason RJ, Boshnick EL, Cannon WN, et al. Multisite comparison of contact lens modalities. Daily disposable wear vs. conventional daily wear in successful contact lens wearers. J Am Optom Assoc 1994;65(11):774–780.

29. Dumbleton K, Richter D, Simpson T, et al. A comparison of the vascular response to extended wear of conventional lower Dk and experimental high Dk hydrogel contact lenses. Optom Vis Sci 1998;75(12):170.

30. Keay, L, Sweeney DF, Jalbert I, et al. Microcyst response to high Dk/t silicone hydrogel contact lenses. Optom Vis Sci 2000;77(11):582–585.

31. Doughty, MJ, Aakre BM, Ystenaes AE, et al. Short-term adaptation of the human corneal endothelium to continuous wear of silicone hydrogel (Lotrafilcon A) contact lenses after daily hydrogel lens wear. Optom Vis Sci 2005;82(6):473–480.

32. Bleshoy H, Guillon M, Shah D. Influence of contact lens materials surface characteristics on replacement frequency. Int Contact Lens Clin 1994;21(3):82–94.

33. Jones L, Franklin V, Evans K, et al. Spoilation and clinical performance of monthly vs. three monthly group II disposable contact lenses. Optom Vis Sci 1996;73(1):16–21.

34. Pritchard N, Fonn D, Weed K. Ocular and subjective responses to frequent replacement of daily wear soft contact lenses. CLAO J 1996;22(1):53–59.

35. Gerber GS. Power Practice Seminar, Hawthorne, New Jersey, 1998.

36. Gellatly KW, Brennan NA, Efron N. Visual decrement with deposit accumulation on HEMA contact lenses. Am J Optom Physiol Opt 1988;65(12):937–941.

CHAPTER 11

Soft Lens Fitting and Evaluation

Vinita Allee Henry

■ PATIENT SELECTION

Soft contact lenses, including conventional hydrogel and silicone hydrogel, are appealing to many patients as a result of both the immediate comfort provided by these materials and the availability of specialty lenses; however, soft lenses are not a viable option for all patients, and careful patient selection will help ensure a successful fit. A comprehensive preliminary evaluation will provide the practitioner with information that will be the key to selecting the type of contact lens suitable for each particular patient, whether it is gas permeable (GP), soft, extended wear, disposable, or no lens wear at all. Patients may have preconceived ideas about which type of lens they want to wear; however, their selection may not be a viable one. It will be necessary to explain the risks and benefits, advantages and disadvantages, and available options. Only after this has been performed is it possible to select a particular lens modality.

Indications and Contraindications

Some factors contraindicate contact lens wear of any type, such as inflammation or disease of the anterior segment, any systemic disease that can be complicated by contact lens wear, poor hygiene, poor compliance, and lack of motivation (Table 11.1). Factors that may contraindicate soft lens wear include irregular corneas (i.e., keratoconus, ocular trauma), autoimmune disease, immunocompromised patients, chronic allergies, chronic antihistamine use, and giant papillary conjunctivitis (GPC, also known as contact lens papillary conjunctivitis [CLPC]).

The initial comfort afforded by soft lenses makes this lens type particularly appealing to patients.[1,2] The initial comfort of soft lenses is due to the large diameter, thin edges, limited movement, and minimal resistance to lid closure.[3] Potential contact lens patients often do not want to tolerate the adaptation period that may be present with GP lenses. In addition, the decreased initial reflex tearing and lens awareness help to reduce the time required for the practitioner to fit the lens. Likewise, the practitioner benefits from the ability to dispense new and replacement lenses from inventory.

Patient information to further consider when selecting soft lenses include refractive error, occupation, hobbies, wearing schedule, hygiene, and compliance. Typically, individuals with spherical refractive errors, low astigmatism, and lenticular astigmatism will be the best candidates for soft lens wear. These patients will be able to achieve acceptable visual acuity with a spherical or toric soft lens. Obviously, occupations with tasks that include exposure to fine particles of dust or mist (e.g., sandblasting) are not suitable for contact lens wear unless the recommended protective eye wear, such as safety goggles, is worn. Many occupations and hobbies may be enhanced by contact lens wear (e.g., those of athletes, actors, models, or politicians). These groups benefit from improved cosmesis and elimination of spectacle wear, which may decrease the field of view, fog up with precipitation changes, slide down, or possibly break. Soft lenses are preferable for athletes and sports activities as they are more difficult to dislodge than GP lenses. The minimal movement present with a soft lens aids in initial comfort; provides more stable vision, which may not be present initially with GP lens wear as a result of increased

TABLE 11.1 SOFT LENS WEAR

INDICATIONS	CONTRAINDICATIONS
Good tear quality and quantity	Inflammation or disease of the anterior segment
Spherical refractive errors	Poor hygiene
Low astigmatism	Lack of motivation
Low lenticular astigmatism	Chronic allergies and antihistamine use
Athletes	Systemic diseases aggravated by contact lens wear
Unable to adapt to GP lenses	Autoimmune disease/immunocompromised
Occasional/flexible wear	Poor tear quality and quantity
Desires tint to enhance or change eye color	Irregular astigmatism
Previous GP adherence	Radial keratotomy
Previous 3 and 9 o'clock staining with GP lenses	Dry, dusty environments
High motivation	GPC

GP, gas permeable; GPC, giant papillary conjunctivitis.

lens movement; and reduces the likelihood of a trapped foreign body. Occasionally, patients desire lenses to wear strictly for sports, such as tennis or basketball, or just for social occasions to improve their appearance. Soft lenses are preferable for these part-time wearers. They are also advantageous for individuals desiring a change or enhancement of eye color as well as anyone benefiting from a disposable lens.

Soft lenses are more prone to deposits, and lens-wearing patients are more susceptible to infections than GP patients because of the characteristics of the lens. As a result, patients who exhibit poor hygiene, work in an environment that may be unsanitary or dirty (e.g., automobile mechanics, garbage collectors), or are noncompliant with their follow-up visits or care regimen are at risk to develop problems resulting from the contamination of their lenses. Extra caution is necessary for both the practitioner and the patient if these patients are to be fitted with any contact lens, in particular, a soft contact lens.

Other disadvantages of soft lenses are that some patients may experience reduced vision resulting from inadequate correction of refractive astigmatism, and the lenses are more fragile and more difficult to verify. Hydrogel lenses generally have lower oxygen transmission; however, silicone hydrogel lenses have higher or comparable oxygen transmission to GP lenses. Advantages and disadvantages are further summarized in Table 11.2.

■ PATIENT FACTORS AFFECTING MATERIAL SELECTION

Overall, most lens materials can be used for the majority of patients with excellent results. The following recommendations take into consideration certain patient factors when selecting a lens material that will maximize patient health, comfort, compliance and satisfaction.

Refractive Error

Soft spherical lenses are available in powers of ±20 D, but most commonly the lenses are available in powers of approximately −10.00 to +4.00 D. If in doubt, it is important to check the power availability before fitting the lens. A smaller number of stock lenses and custom lenses are available in high plus, aphakic, and high minus powers. Toric lenses to correct for astigmatism are available in cylinder powers up to −1.75 or −2.25 D. Several lens brands and custom lenses are available in cylinder powers of −5.75 D or higher. Generally, the higher corrections are not available in a variety of materials, tints, or lens designs (i.e., bifocal).

TABLE 11.2 SOFT LENS ADVANTAGES AND DISADVANTAGES

ADVANTAGES

Excellent initial comfort

Minimal adaptation time

Part-time wearing schedule possible

Risk of corneal distortion minimal

Minimal spectacle blur

Dislocation uncommon

Foreign-body sensation rare

Ability to fit and dispense from inventory

Low incidence of flare

Low incidence of discomfort caused by excessive lens lag

Ability to change or enhance eye color

Simplicity of fit

Rarely causes excessive tearing

Disposable/frequent replacement possible

Therapeutic use possible

DISADVANTAGES

Reduced visual acuity in uncorrected astigmatism

Limited durability

Oxygen transmission with hydrogels

Deposit formation/GPC possible

Greater chance of bacterial contamination/infection

Greater risks with noncompliance

More difficult to verify

Limitations of corrections

Quality of vision may be reduced

GPC, giant papillary conjunctivitis.

Aspheric lenses, offered by several companies, may be beneficial for patients with low amounts of astigmatism (i.e., ≤ −0.75D). The lenses appear to improve spherical aberration, not correct astigmatism. Studies have shown that there is little difference between the spherical and aspheric lenses, although patients have reported subjective preferences for aspheric lenses.[4,5]

Handling Issues

First-time wearers will generally benefit from a slightly thicker lens or one with an increased stiffness or modulus of elasticity. Both of these attributes help to make insertion, removal, and handling of the lens easier. Silicone hydrogel lens materials have a higher modulus than most soft contact lenses. Additionally, a handling tint will be beneficial for these patients.

Deposit-Prone Patients

Patients who experience frequent lens deposits, even when using a rigorous care routine, would be best fitted in a daily disposable lens. If this is not used, then a disposable or frequent-replacement lens should be used (i.e., weekly to monthly replacement). Certain lens materials (i.e., Proclear and Preference by CooperVision and CSI by Ciba Vision) are more resistant to deposits. With the availability of disposable lenses, deposit issues should not be a problem if the patient is following the recommended replacement schedule.

Marginal Dry Eye

Many contact lens wearers experience dry-eye symptoms with lens wear. As many as 50% of contact lens wearers have reported symptoms of dry eye.[6–8] Factors that affect dry-eye symptoms are wettability, dehydration, contact lens solutions, poor tear film quality, environmental temperature, time of day, humidity, wind, and blink rate.[6,9] In hydrogel lens materials, low-water-content and thicker lenses are thought to dehydrate less than high-water-content or thin lenses. This is thought to be the one of the reasons why patients are more comfortable in low-water-content, thick hydrogel lenses. However, a fixed relationship between initial water content and dehydration cannot always be demonstrated.[9] Additionally, some studies have shown that increasing the lens thickness has a greater effect on dry-eye symptoms than the water content.[10]

Recent advances have given practitioners more lens options to aid marginal dry-eye patients. Extreme H_2O (Hydrogel Vision Corp) is a hydrogel lens that the manufacturer claims retains its water saturation on the eye, thus exhibiting less dehydration and better end-of-the-day comfort. Proclear (CooperVision), mentioned previously, is deposit resistant and contains phosphorylcholine, which aids in hydration of the lens.[11] Focus Dailies with AquaRelease (Ciba Vision) and 1-Day Acuvue Moist (Vistakon) contain lubricating agents incorporated into the material, which reportedly make the lens more wettable and increase comfort, particularly end-of-the-day comfort. The lubricating agent in Focus Dailies with AquaRelease is polyvinyl alcohol (PVA), and the agent in 1-Day Acuvue Moist is polyvinyl pyrrolidone (PVP). In the Dailies lens, the lubricating agent is released from the lens during wear, whereas in the Acuvue lens, the agent is not released. Study data comparing these lenses to their predecessors and to each other are few and results appear variable regarding how much impact they have.[6] However, they do provide an option to the patient, and after a trial period, the patient may determine whether he or she detects improvement. Another benefit of daily disposable lenses is that no solutions are necessary, eliminating preservative sensitivities.

Silicone hydrogels have demonstrated increased comfort for dry-eye patients.[12,13] This may be because of increased oxygen transmission, decreased water content, and internal wetting agents and natural wettability of some of the lens materials.

Besides trying to find the best lens material for a marginal dry-eye patient, the choice of a care system is important. Hydrogen peroxide is beneficial, especially to patients sensitive to a preserved solution. With the newer preservatives, sensitivity symptoms are more subtle, manifesting in dryness, decreased wear, and superficial staining. Many dry-eye symptoms may be caused by one-bottle lens care symptoms or coated lenses.[14] A good first step is to use a nonpreserved hydrogen peroxide care regimen. In addition, there are some chemically preserved solutions that are reported to increase comfort and decrease dryness. If hydrogen peroxide is not beneficial to the patient, the use of one of these solutions should relieve dryness symptoms. In addition, lubricating drops can be used to rehydrate and rinse the lens in the eye.

Therapeutic Use

Only certain lenses are approved by the Food and Drug Administration (FDA) for therapeutic use (sometimes called bandage lenses). Close monitoring and frequent replacement are required. Silicone hydrogel lenses with high oxygen permeability (Dk) that are FDA approved for therapeutic use are Focus Night and Day (Ciba Vision), PureVision (Bausch & Lomb), and

Acuvue Oasys (Vistakon).[15] Conditions that warrant the use of a therapeutic contact lens include corneal erosions, chronic epithelial defects, bullous keratopathy, mechanical trauma, dry eyes, and filamentary keratitis. Therapeutic lenses are also used following ocular surgery, to aid in sealing a corneal wound, and for drug delivery. Therapeutic lenses should not be used in the presence of an active ocular infection, in filtering blebs, or for patients who will not return for follow-up evaluation.[16]

Ocular Disease

Obviously, a patient presenting with a serious ocular or systemic disease is not a good candidate for contact lenses, other than those approved for therapeutic use. For example, diabetic patients are at risk when fitted with soft or GP contact lenses because of a decreased wound-healing ability. However, studies have shown that diabetic patients can successfully wear daily-wear (DW) lenses if carefully monitored.[17] For those patients with some form of ocular compromise (i.e., staining, papillary hypertrophy, deficient tear quality), DW is indicated because prolonged lens wear, such as extended wear (EW), may increase these symptoms. Additionally, daily disposable lenses should be considered for these patients.

Age

Children fitted with a soft lens may experience difficulty inserting the large lens diameter. A few lenses are available in smaller diameters (i.e., 13 mm), and this may aid in lens insertion. Most children who are motivated to wear a soft contact lens will be able to learn to insert and remove the contact lens. If the contact lens is considered medically necessary (i.e., aphakia, anisometropia) and the child is too young to perform insertion and removal, the parents may be taught to insert, remove, and care for the lens. There are many contact lenses to use with children that have a 13.8-mm diameter. In addition, disposable lenses are a good modality for children to provide a cost-efficient lens, to be used as spare lenses, and to decrease the complications of lens care.

Presbyopes may have difficulty viewing the lens when inserting, removing, or caring for it. A visibility tint or a cosmetic tint is beneficial to these patients when handling the lens. Additionally, they may appreciate a slightly thicker or higher modulus lens, which is easier to handle.

Aphakia

A lens material with high oxygen transmission (Dk/t) is required for aphakic patients. Generally, these lenses are silicone based, available in limited parameters, and very expensive. O2 Optix Custom (Ciba Vision) is a quarterly replacement silicone hydrogel lens that is available in aphakic powers of +10 to +20 D. It has a Dk/t of 117 at −3.00 D. This lens is more affordable than most conventional specialty lenses and provides frequent replacement. (See Chapter 17 for more information.)

Occupation

There are a variety of occupational factors that can affect lens wear and comfort. Generally, a wearing and replacement schedule should be selected to fit the patient's lifestyle. For patients who work unusual hours or travel frequently, lenses that they can sleep in even for a couple of nights or daily disposable lenses may be beneficial. The ability to take spare lenses along when traveling is advantageous. With airline restrictions on liquids, daily disposable lenses eliminate the need for extra solution.

Pilots, airline attendants, and computer users are examples of occupations that will benefit from a lens that provides good wettability, such as those suggested for dry eyes noted previously. Occupations that require being outdoors or sports that are performed outdoors may benefit from a lens with an ultraviolet (UV) blocker. UV damage to the eye and surrounding tissue will not be eliminated by a contact lens with a UV blocker alone, but it can be one more barrier to UV radiation.

Part-Time Wearers

Patients who might not otherwise be a good contact lens candidate or have a desire to wear contact lenses for limited periods of time (i.e., golfing, tennis, social occasions) may be fitted with soft lenses. These patients are excellent candidates for daily disposable lenses. If daily disposable lenses are not used, caution should be taken by these patients in storing lenses for long periods of time. Lenses should be disinfected weekly and before wear, and the storage solution should be frequently changed to minimize contamination and dehydration. Likewise, caution should be taken not to overwear the lenses when they haven't been worn for a long period of time. Soft lens adaptation takes very little time, making this a good choice for part-time wear.

Refits

Typically, caution should be taken when refitting a long-term GP lens wearer into a soft material. There are occasions when a GP lens wearer may require refitting into a soft lens material, such as inability to adapt to GP lenses, chronic staining, or chronic adherence that will not improve with GP lens parameter changes.[18] In these cases, the patient should reduce lens-wearing time or completely de-adapt to determine if the cornea will change or remain stable. Disposable trial lenses are successful for these patients, as the trial lenses can easily be changed if the cornea fluctuates after discontinuing the GP lenses. When the corneal curvature and refractive error stabilize, the final soft lenses can be ordered.

Compliance

If a patient is noncompliant with lens care and disinfection of lenses, a daily disposable lens should be considered. Monthly replacement schedules may also help to improve compliance for certain patients. Patients who sleep occasionally in their lenses should be fitted in an EW lens material even if the intention is to wear the lens DW. Noncompliance creates a real dilemma for the eye care practitioner about whether to fit the patient into contact lenses or not. Patient education and information regarding adverse events that can occur as a result of noncompliance may aid in the patient's willingness to adhere to directions. Patients who refuse to follow proper wear, care, and handling steps should not be fitted into contact lenses.

■ LENS SELECTION AND FITTING

Once it has been determined that a patient is suitable for soft lenses, the lens selection process begins. Lens materials may be grouped into many different categories. Basically, patients will desire soft lenses that can be placed in one of the following categories: DW lenses, EW lenses, disposable/frequent-replacement lenses, tinted lenses to enhance or change the eye color, toric lenses, and multifocal lenses. Lenses are available in varying powers, base curve radii (BCR), diameters, thicknesses, water contents, and tints. To select a lens for the patient, it is important to first determine which one of the aforementioned categories of lens wear the patient is most interested in. Although lenses may be fitted empirically, the ability to fit diagnostic lenses is beneficial to both the patient and the practitioner by increasing patient confidence and compliance while also decreasing lens reorders.[19] In addition, if a large enough inventory of soft lenses is available, the patient can be dispensed lenses the same day.

Base Curve Radius

Soft contact lenses will typically be available in two to four different BCR. On average, the selected BCR is approximately 4 D flatter than K; however, a good guideline to follow is:

Flat K is >45.00 D	Fit the steeper BCR
Flat K is 41.00–45.00 D	Fit the median BCR
Flat K is <41.00 D	Fit the flatter BCR

If there are only two base curves, the flatter BCR can be used for flat K readings <45.00 D. For example, many soft contact lenses are available in 8.4, 8.7, and 9.0 mm BCR (or radii very close to these). A cornea with average keratometric readings should be diagnostically fitted with an 8.7 mm BCR. If the lens is too tight, a flatter BCR should be attempted, in this case 9.0 mm; if the lens is too loose, a steeper BCR can be fitted, in this case 8.4 mm. Likewise, if the keratometric readings are steeper than 45.00 D, the patient can be initially diagnostically fitted with the 8.4 mm or steeper BCR, and if the keratometric readings are flatter than 41.00 D, a 9.0 mm or flatter BCR can be selected. Corneas that are borderline values (e.g., 45.00 D) might be fitted with an 8.7 mm BCR on one eye and an 8.4 mm BCR on the other eye to determine which is the better fit. Some manufacturers recommend fitting the steep BCR on flatter corneas. It is helpful to verify fitting guidelines before fitting the lens.

A tight lens will exhibit <0.5 mm movement, often producing conjunctival drag, in which the conjunctiva moves with the lens and the lens movement, separate from the conjunctival movement, is little to none. When removed, the tight lens may leave an impression ring on the sclera at the position of the lens edge. A flat lens will move >1.5 to 2 mm, often moving partially off the cornea. On gazing straight ahead, the lens may be decentered inferiorly on the cornea, and on superior gaze, the lens will drop inferior (Fig. 11.1). In addition, edge lift may be observed inferiorly. If the edge is curling out, the lens will decenter superiorly when the patient views inferiorly. A properly fitting soft lens will center well over the cornea and exhibit approximately 0.5 to 1 mm movement (Fig. 11.2). In superior gaze the lens may move as much as 2 mm. Generally, lenses that are thinner will move less. A method called the "push-up test" may be used to judge if the lens is truly tight or just exhibiting minimal movement. This test is performed by gently pushing on the inferior edge of the lens with the lower lid; a tight lens resists movement, whereas an acceptable lens will move when nudged with the lower lid. In one study, the push-up test was found to be the most accurate single test of lens fit acceptability; therefore, it is an important yet simple tool to use in the fitting process.[20] The test is recorded as a positive push-up test when movement is observed and a negative push-up test when the lens shows no movement or difficulty in moving the lens with the lid.

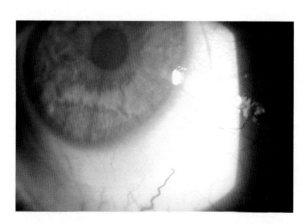

■ **FIGURE 11.1** Lens falling inferiorly when the patient is looking up because of a flat base curve. (Lens is dyed with fluorescein to enhance observation.)

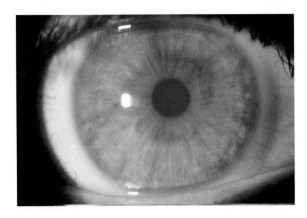

■ **FIGURE 11.2** Well-centered lens with good corneal coverage. (Lens is dyed with fluorescein to enhance observation.)

Lens Diameter

The overall diameter of the soft contact lens is selected to obtain 360 degrees of corneal coverage. Ideally, the lens will extend onto the sclera, at minimum, 0.5 mm in all directions (see Fig. 11.2). By measuring the horizontal visible iris diameter (the diameter across the iris from limbus to limbus) and adding 2 mm, the approximate diameter needed can be obtained (Fig. 11.3). If the lens decenters, a larger than predicted overall diameter may be needed to provide adequate coverage. Lenses are customarily available in diameters of 13.8 to 15.0 mm; however, there are a few manufacturers who produce stock lenses with smaller or larger diameters. Custom lenses with smaller diameters and various BCR (steep to flat) are available for those hard-to-fit patients who require parameters outside the normal ranges.

Power

The power of the lens is based on the predicted power and an overrefraction over the diagnostic lens. The predicted power of the lens is determined by the patient's spectacle prescription, which is vertexed back to the corneal plane if the prescription is $> \pm 4.00$ D (Appendix 2). If the patient has a spherocylindrical prescription with a low amount of astigmatism, it may be necessary to use the spherical equivalent to predict the patient's contact lens prescription. The final prescription should be equal to that achieved by the best sphere overrefraction plus the diagnostic lens power, or a close compromise between the predicted power and the overrefraction plus the diagnostic lens power. For example:

Patients 1 and 2
Spectacle Rx: −4.75 D

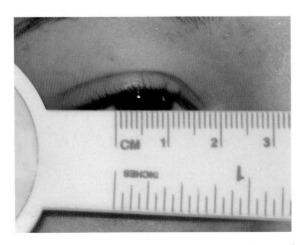

■ **FIGURE 11.3** Demonstration of how to obtain horizontal visible iris diameter.

Vertexed back to corneal plane: −4.50 D
Predicted contact lens (CL) Rx: −4.50 D
Diagnostic CL Rx: −4.00 D

Patient 1
Overrefraction: −0.50 D
Final CL Rx dispensed: −4.50 D

Patient 2
Overrefraction: −1.00 D
Final CL Rx dispensed: −4.75 D

Patient 1 has an overrefraction equal to the predicted Rx. In the case of patient 2, the over-refraction results in a power of −5.00 D; however, the lens dispensed (−4.75 D) is a compromise of the predicted Rx and the overrefraction. The final lens power ordered can be determined after the patient has worn the lens for 1 week and returned for a follow-up evaluation.

Center Thickness

Typically, a center thickness of a −3.00 D lens will be approximately 0.08 mm. Minus power lenses range from 0.04 to 0.18 mm in center thickness. Plus lenses range from 0.20 to 0.70mm in center thickness.[21] The greater the minus power, the thinner the lens; likewise, the greater the plus power, the thicker the lens. A thicker hydrogel lens (0.12 mm) is easier for the patient to handle, and thinner hydrogel lenses (0.035 mm) with low water contents may be approved for EW; however, many manufacturers currently provide their standard daily-wear lenses in 0.05 to 0.07 mm thicknesses for low-minus powers. With the introduction of silicone hydrogel materials, using a hydrogel lens for EW is not recommended. In addition, thicker hydrogel lenses are easier to handle; however, the silicone hydrogel lenses have a higher modulus, which is a benefit for patients who exhibit difficulty in handling a lens.

As a thinner lens tends to drape the cornea more, less lens movement with the blink is commonly experienced. Therefore, these individuals need to be monitored for clinical signs of a tight lens, including absence of lens lag, limbal engorgement, and trapped debris underneath the lens. Likewise, if a thicker, high-water-content lens is used, the patient should be monitored, even if good lens movement with the blink is present initially, as these lenses tend to dehydrate, which will steepen the BCR and reduce lens lag.

After selecting the soft diagnostic lens, the lens should be inserted and allowed to settle. It is debatable on how long it takes for a soft lens to settle. One study concluded that evaluating within the first 5 minutes was the optimal time.[22] Others have suggested that 10 to 15 minutes is best.[23] As this might vary with lens material, practitioners should evaluate the lens movement over the first 5 to 30 minutes and compare that with lens movement at follow-up examinations with greater wearing times (i.e., ≥4 hours). Toric and multifocal soft lenses may require more time than spherical lenses to stabilize on the eye. Visual acuity, overrefraction, lens movement, centration, and coverage should all be evaluated to assist in determining the final lens design. The parameters to specify when ordering a soft contact lens are BCR, overall lens diameter (OAD), power, name of lens, tint, and add if necessary. On lens dispensing, the lenses should be evaluated on the eye, and the patient should be educated on insertion, removal, wearing schedule, normal adaptive symptoms, and lens care (see Chapter 12).

Tinted Lenses

The decision to select a tinted lens depends on the patient's needs and desires (i.e., handling, enhancing, or opaque tints). An enhancing tint enhances the present color of the eye (i.e., a blue eye is made bluer). Opaque tints are used to change eye color. It is not unusual for patients who do not require a refractive correction to desire tinted lenses for the cosmetic effect.

Likewise, some patients who may not be best fitted in soft lenses may desire to wear cosmetic tinted lenses for social occasions (e.g., a presbyope who has found presbyopic contact lens options not to be optimal or a successful GP lens wearer with corneal astigmatism). Disposable tinted lenses, especially daily disposable, make occasional social wear a convenient option. Many lenses are available with a handling or visibility tint to make the lens easier to locate.

Disposable/Frequent-Replacement Lenses

Today, it is rare for a patient to wear a conventional soft lens that does not have a predetermined replacement schedule, except for some specialty/custom lenses. Most soft contact lens patients can be fitted with—and will benefit from—a lens that is thrown away, either after a single use, weekly, every 2 weeks, monthly, or quarterly. Especially beneficial is a disposable, silicone hydrogel lens, which gives the patient the benefits of a clean lens with good oxygen transmission. More information on disposable and frequent-replacement modalities is presented in Chapter 10.

Silicone Hydrogel Lenses

Silicone hydrogel lenses provide greater amounts of oxygen than hydrogel lenses. The trend in soft lens materials is moving toward the silicone hydrogel materials to improve corneal health. Silicone hydrogel lenses are available in spheres, torics, and multifocals. Most patients will benefit from—and be satisfied with—silicone hydrogel lenses. Silicone hydrogel lenses depend on silicone, not water content, to increase oxygen transmission through the lens. Patient education will aid in the success of this type of lens. When educating a new silicone hydrogel wearer, it is important to discuss that a hypoxic or edematous cornea, resulting from conventional hydrogel lens wear, may be less sensitive. Upon improving oxygen transmission, the healthier cornea may become more sensitive or less "numb." This may result in a slight lens sensation after a few days of silicone hydrogel lens wear. If the patient continues to wear the lenses for 1 to 2 weeks, an adaptation to the new lens occurs. Additional ways to aid lens comfort include using a lower lens modulus and presoaking the lens in the recommended solution regimen before wear. More information on silicone hydrogel lens materials and care is presented in Chapters 10 and 12.

■ PROGRESS EVALUATIONS

Lens Evaluation

An optimum-fit soft lens will exhibit good centration, moving 0.5 to 1 mm with the blink. In addition, the lens should exhibit complete corneal coverage and extend, at minimum, 0.5 mm onto the sclera. Vision should be 20/25 or better and should be, at minimum, equal to spectacle visual acuity. However, depending on the use of the lens (such as social wear), slightly reduced visual acuity may be acceptable. The lens should be comfortable and should be worn 12 to 14 hours for daily wear, 3 to 7 days for extended wear, or 30 days for continuous wear, if not worn solely for sports or social occasions. After dispensing of the lenses, evaluations should be performed on a routine basis to ensure that an absence of compromise in corneal physiology is present. For example, follow-up visits for daily wear can be scheduled at 1 week, 1 month, and 6 months after dispensing and every 6 months thereafter. Follow-up visits for extended wear can be scheduled at 1 week, 1 month, 3 months, and 6 months after first wearing the lenses extended wear and every 3 months thereafter.

There are complications resulting from soft lens wear; however, with adequate follow-up and patient compliance, most complications can be prevented. A routine follow-up examination should include the following tests: visual acuity, overrefraction, biomicroscopy with and without lenses, keratometry, and subjective refraction (Table 11.3). When performing biomicroscopy, the

TABLE 11.3 TESTS TO PERFORM AT LENS EVALUATION VISITS

Visual acuity
Overrefraction
Overkeratometry
Too steep
Too flat
Clear and undistorted
Biomicroscopy with the lenses on
Lens centration
Lens position
Lens coverage
Lens movement
Condition of the lens (tears, surface deposition)
Biomicroscopy with the lenses off
Limbal vasculature
Fluorescein application
Lid evaluation
Cornea evaluation
Injection
Microcysts
Striae
Polymegethism
Limbal engorgement
Tarsal conjunctiva; follicles, papillae
Keratometry
Subjective refraction

lens should be evaluated for position, coverage, movement, and lens condition. Fingernail tears, edge tears, holes, rust spots, jelly bumps, and protein and lipid deposits can easily be viewed with the lens on the eye by carefully scanning the entire lens surface and the lens edges, including the inferior and superior edges, which may be hidden under the lids. Fingernail tears are generally characteristic slits with a hairlike or lintlike appearance in the central to midperipheral areas of the lens, which result from the lens being pinched off the cornea between the fingernails. Edge tears may appear as an absent wedge-shaped area of the lens or a diagonal slit. Rust spots are orange dots within the lens matrix, which should signal that the patient may be using tap water to rinse the lenses. These can also be caused by the environment or foreign bodies in the eye; however, the most common cause pertains to the use of tap water for rinsing the lenses. Jelly bumps and protein and lipid deposits are all forms of deposits that originate, in part, from the tear film chemistry. Adequate lens care will help prevent these deposits. When deposits are observed, the practitioner should determine whether the cause is lens age, poor patient compliance, or a tear film predisposed to deposits. Jelly bumps, which can be the result of changes in tear pH, appear as clear-to-white elevations of various sizes and quantities on the front surface of the lens, whereas lipid and protein deposits appear as a film with lipid deposits exhibiting a greasy film (Fig. 11.4) and protein as a semiopaque white haze.[24,25]

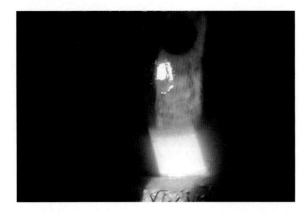

■ FIGURE 11.4 Lipid deposits on a lens.

Keratometry can be performed over the lenses to aid in determining if the fit is too flat or too steep. The mires observed when performing keratometry over the lens should be clear and undistorted. A steep fit will exhibit a clear mire image immediately after the blink that then becomes distorted and blurry, whereas a flat fit will exhibit mire distortion that becomes more distorted immediately after the blink.[26]

Ocular Examination

After removing the lens, the cornea and conjunctiva should be inspected for changes resulting from edema (i.e., striae, microcysts, polymegethism), neovascularization, limbal engorgement, and injection (Fig. 11.5A,B). Fluorescein will assist in the evaluation of numerous possible

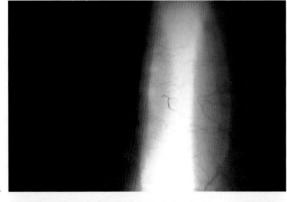

A

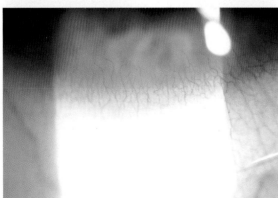

B

■ FIGURE 11.5 **(A,B)** Limbal vessel engorgement and encroachment.

forms of corneal staining, including inferior arcuate staining from lens dehydration,[27] diffuse staining from either an allergic reaction or trapped debris, or a foreign-body stain. In addition, it enables the practitioner to evaluate lid papillary hypertrophy upon eversion. It is important to evaluate the lids and the cornea with fluorescein at every visit to monitor any subtle changes that may occur with long-term soft lens wear such as GPC (also known as CLPC) or corneal staining. Care must be taken to rinse the fluorescein from the eye by repeated use of saline or have patients wear their spectacles for 2 to 4 hours afterward to prevent staining of the lens. There are high-molecular-weight fluorescein dyes that will not discolor the soft lens; however, fluorescence is reduced, affecting the ability to view staining. If the soft lens should be discolored by fluorescein, it should be replaced, or the lens may be bleached with repeated cycles of hydrogen peroxide.

■ SUMMARY

Soft contact lenses are relatively simple to fit. A well-fitted lens, thorough evaluation, and follow-up examinations will aid in successful lens wear. Soft lenses are popular with patients because of the initial comfort and the ability to fit and dispense lenses from inventory.

■ CLINICAL CASES

CASE 1

A 45-year-old attorney expresses a desire for contact lenses. In his spare time, he plays golf, basketball, and numerous other athletic activities. He recently began wearing bifocal spectacles while at work; however, he would like to wear contact lenses when involved in recreational activities. His refraction is $-3.00 - 0.50 \times 180$ with a $+1.25$ add OU, and his keratometry readings are 42.00 @180/42.37 @ 90 OU.

SOLUTION: Disposable lenses, especially daily disposable, would be beneficial to this patient since he desires lenses he can wear occasionally while participating in sports. Bifocal contact lenses or monovision might be desirable for this patient, but may not provide the optimum distance visual acuity and depth perception during recreational activities. However, successfully fitting this patient with good near and distance visual acuity may transform this patient from a part-time contact lens wearer to a full-time wearer. One multifocal soft lens that might work well for this patient is the Biomedics EP (CooperVision), which is a nice transition between spherical distance-only lenses and multifocals (see Chapter 15).

The benefits of soft lenses for a patient wanting recreational lenses include the opportunity for occasional wear and limited risk of decentration or loss; in addition, a near correction is unnecessary for recreational activities with the possible exception of golf, where he should be able to see well enough to complete his scorecard without a near correction. Most likely he will need the medium BCR available because his K readings are 42.00 D. The final lens power will depend on the overrefraction; typically, it will equal the spherical equivalent, -3.25 D.

CASE 2

A 12-year-old girl and her mother enter the office to be fitted with contact lenses. The girl appears to be highly motivated for contact lens wear. Her mother says she is very responsible. The girl is interested in making her gray eyes green. The patient's refractive error is OD -4.50 DS and OS -4.25 DS, and the keratometric readings are 42.00 DS OU.

SOLUTION: The patient is fitted with a medium BCR, such as 8.6 or 8.7 mm. The predicted lens powers are OD -4.25 D and OS -4.00 D vertexed back to the corneal plane. A green enhancing tint or a green opaque tint changes the color of the girl's gray eyes in addition to providing her with an automatic handling tint that is beneficial for first-time wearers. This type of patient is generally successful with contact lenses because visually she will think her sight is improved and cosmetically she will think her appearance is improved. As a result of peer pressure to maintain an attractive appearance, the probability of her being success-ful is quite good. This patient would be an excellent candidate for disposable or frequent-replacement tinted lenses, not only for the improved health, but also for spare lenses in case of lens loss or damage. In addition, using a daily disposable tinted lens would give her the option of wearing clear lenses, plus a variety of tinted opaque lenses that may be discarded after use.

CASE 3

A patient desires to be fitted in soft lenses. Her refraction is OD −5.00 DS, OS −3.00 − 1.00 × 180. The keratometric readings are OD 42.50 @ 180/42.75 @ 90 and OS 43.00@ 180/43.75 @ 90. The horizontal visible iris diameter (HVID) is 12 mm. All ocular findings, including tear quality and quantity, are normal.

SOLUTION: The BCR selected is 8.6 mm (or the medium base curve radius available if three base curve radii are available and the flatter base curve if two base curve radii are available). The diameter selected is 14.5 mm, which should provide adequate corneal coverage since the HVID + 2 would be 14 mm. Both diagnostic lenses have a power equal to −3.00 D. The pre-dicted powers are OD −4.75 D and OS −3.50 D (spherical equivalent). After evaluating the lenses on the eye, the BCR is changed to an 8.9 mm/−3.00 D OD as the lens appeared slightly tight on the push-up test and conjunctival drag was present with the blink. With good cen-tration present and movement of 1.0 mm OU, an overrefraction results in OD −1.75 D and OS −0.75 D with a visual acuity of 20/15 OU. With a −0.50 D overrefraction OS, the patient has a visual acuity equal to 20/20 + 2, and with the −0.75 D overrefraction she thinks the 20/15 line is much clearer and easier to read. The final lens parameters ordered are OD 8.9 mm BCR, −4.75 D power, and OS 8.6 mm BCR, −3.75 D power. The lenses come in a handling tint, which will assist in lens handling.

CASE 4

A 20-year-old woman is prone to jelly bumps and deposits. She replaces her lenses about every 2 to 3 weeks. Changing the care regimen does not appear to solve the problem.

SOLUTION: The patient is placed in a daily disposable lens. This provides clean, new lenses every day, ensuring good health and convenience. A care regimen is not necessary as the lenses are disposed daily; therefore, even though the lens fees are higher, the patient has reduced cost for solutions.

CASE 5

A 28-year-old man has worn contact lenses for 12 years. He has completed his training as a paramedic and has increased his wearing time to 17 to 20 hours. He states that his eyes become very red and irritated by the end of the wearing period. He is currently wearing a DW hydrogel lens material. Biomicroscopy reveals good centration and lens movement; however, upon lens removal microcystic edema, conjunctival injection, and incipient superior corneal neovascularization are present.

SOLUTION: This patient needs to be refitted into a silicone hydrogel lens material. Whether he wants to wear the lenses EW or DW, this material will increase the oxygen transmission six to eight times. Increasing the oxygen transmission will improve the signs of corneal hypoxia like edema and neovascularization. Educating the patient on some initial adaptation may be necessary, as the hypoxia he is experiencing causes his eyes to be less sensitive. As the health of his eye improves with silicone hydrogel wear, the sensitivity may increase. After 1 to 2 weeks, he should be over any adaptation symptoms.

CASE 6

A 26-year-old woman presents to the office to be fitted with soft contact lenses for the first time. The case history reveals that the patient is 3 months pregnant. All other findings make this patient a good soft contact lens candidate.

SOLUTION: She should be educated on what changes may occur during pregnancy (e.g., dry eyes caused by increased tear viscosity, changes in corneal curvature and vision). It may be beneficial for her to wait to be fitted (e.g., until 6 weeks postpartum or 6 weeks after discontinuation of breast-feeding); however, she should be reassured that she is a good contact lens candidate. Education is imperative, so as not to have her base future contact lens wear success on her current poor experiences from pregnancy-related ocular symptoms. Many contact lens wearers successfully continue lens wear during pregnancy with no ocular problems.

CASE 7

An 18-year-old man desires to be fitted with soft lenses. He wants to wear the lenses two to three times a week. He desires to provide little care and mentions his busy lifestyle. His demeanor, in addition to his comments, causes the practitioner some concern about potential patient noncompliance.

SOLUTION: The best option for this patient is a daily disposable lens. This type of lens would require no lens care as the lens would be thrown away daily after wear. In addition, concern about proper lens disinfection and storage would not be an issue with daily disposable lenses. Solution cost would be minimal as only the solution in the blister pack or saline to insert the lenses is needed. This patient *must* be educated on the complications that may occur with noncompliance. Photographs or videotapes may be used to demonstrate complications of noncompliance. If this patient appears to be very noncompliant, it may be necessary for the practitioner to refuse to fit him.

CASE 8

A patient is fitted in a soft lens, BCR of 8.4 mm, worn daily wear. The lenses are available in BCR of 8.4, 8.7, and 9.0mm. The patient returns in 2 weeks for a follow-up evaluation of the trial lenses. The patient has had the lenses on for 6 hours. Upon the return visit, engorged limbal vessels and conjunctival drag are observed.

SOLUTION: This lens is too tight. The BCR may be flattened to 8.7 mm and the lens movement should be increased. The use of trial lenses and a trial period of wear are helpful to determine lens fit, lens rotation of toric lenses, and visual acuity. Although many times the trial lenses are successful, occasionally a patient returns for follow-up evaluations with a subjective symptom or clinical sign that requires a change in the BCR, diameter, lens material, power change, etc.

CASE 9

A 55-year-old woman complains of her eyes feeling dry all of the time. She also thinks the lens will fall out of her eye with quick eye movements. She has used rewetting drops in the past but only experiences relief immediately after using them. She is wearing disposable lenses (medium water content) on a daily-wear basis. She would like to continue wearing disposable lenses. Biomicroscopy results in a tear breakup time of 5 seconds OD and 6 seconds OS.

SOLUTION: If the patient would like to continue with disposable lenses, she has several options. Disposable/frequent-replacement lenses that are recommended for marginal dry eyes are Proclear (CooperVision) and Extreme H_2O (Hydrogel Vision Corp). In addition, silicone hydrogel lens materials may be an alternative. Daily disposable lenses like Proclear 1 Day (CooperVision), Focus Dailies with AquaRelease (Ciba Vision), and 1 Day Acuvue Moist (Vistakon) (the latter two have lubricating agents) may be beneficial in making contact lens wear more successful and comfortable. Patient education about the composition of her tears and the problems associated with low tear breakup time should be reviewed.

CASE 10

A patient is wearing an extended-wear hydrogel lens EW for 7 to 10 days. She replaces the lenses about once a month. She is satisfied with her vision and comfort. Upon examination with the biomicroscope, neovascularization is observed 360 degrees around the limbus.

SOLUTION: The patient is educated that although her hydrogel lenses were approved for 7-day EW, there are new materials that provide up to eight times more oxygen to the cornea. A digital photo is taken of her cornea to demonstrate the hypoxic condition of the cornea. She is enthusiastic to try a silicone hydrogel lens that she can sleep in. She is refitted in a monthly silicone hydrogel approved for EW and she intends to take the lenses out once a week for overnight disinfection. At her 2-week follow-up examination, digital photos are taken to demonstrate that the increased oxygen has resulted in a whiter eye, with emptying of the limbal vessels.

CASE 11

A 10-year-old myope is brought for a contact lens fitting by her mother. She has a prescription of −1.50 D OU. The mother reports that the girl is a good student and very responsible. All testing is normal and the girl is motivated to wear contact lenses.

SOLUTION: This young girl is a good candidate for contact lenses. Because she plays soccer and basketball, it is decided that a soft lens would be the best option for her. The benefits of a silicone hydrogel lens are discussed with the girl and her mother. The girl is fitted with a 2-week silicone hydrogel lens to be worn DW. This girl is likely to be a long-time contact lens wearer; therefore, fitting her in a silicone hydrogel lens will be beneficial to her long-term ocular health. In addition, the increased modulus of a silicone hydrogel lenses may be easier for a young, first-time wearer to handle.

CLINICAL PROFICIENCY CHECKLIST

- Patient selection is as important to contact lens success as lens selection.
- In selecting patients for soft contact lenses, it is important to evaluate motivation, occupation, compliance, hygiene, and intended use.
- Soft lens advantages versus GP lenses include initial comfort, variable wearing schedule, the availability of daily disposables, and the ability to fit and replace lenses from an existing inventory.
- Lens selection includes selecting the following: BCR, power, overall diameter, material, tint, wearing schedule, and replacement schedule.
- BCR selection is generally the flattest lens that provides adequate but not excessive movement.
- An ideally fitted soft lens will center well, cover the cornea completely, and move 0.5 to 1 mm with the blink.
- The push-up test is a simple but accurate method of determining an optimal lens fit.
- The proper power of the initial lens is determined by calculating the spherical equivalent of the refraction at the corneal plane (i.e., effective power considerations will be necessary for $> \pm 4$ D). Any spherical overrefraction over this lens should then be added to the diagnostic lens power to achieve the final power.
- Adequate follow-up evaluations are important to reduce the risk of complications.
- Follow-up evaluations should include visual acuity, overrefraction, biomicroscopy with and without lenses, keratometry with and without lenses, lid eversion, and subjective refraction.
- Fluorescein evaluation, an often neglected step in evaluating eyes that wear soft lenses, is an important part of the follow-up evaluation.

REFERENCES

1. Edrington TB, Schornack JA. Initial evaluation. In: Bennett ES, Weissman BA, eds. Clinical Contact Lens Practice. Philadelphia: Lippincott Williams & Wilkins, 2005:197–213.
2. Yeung KK, Weissman BA. Soft contact lens application. In: Bennett ES, Weissman BA, eds. Clinical Contact Lens Practice. Philadelphia: Lippincott Williams & Wilkins, 2005:363–379.
3. Mandell RB. Basic principles of hydrogel lenses. In: Mandell RB, ed. Contact Lens Practice, 4th ed. Springfield, IL: Charles C. Thomas, 1988:502–528.
4. Kollbaum P, Bradley A. Aspheric contact lenses: fact or fiction. Contact Lens Spectrum 2005;20(3):34–38.
5. Vaz TC, Gundel RE. High- and low-contrast visual acuity measurements in spherical and aspheric soft contact lens wearers. Contact Lens Anterior Eye 2003;26(3):147–151.
6. Nichols JJ. Mechanism of contact lens-related dry eye. Contact Lens Spectrum 2007;Special Edition:14–20.
7. Doughty MJ, Fonn D, Richter D, et al. A patient questionnaire approach to estimating the prevalence of dry eye symptoms in patients presenting to optometric practices across Canada. Optom Vis Sci 1997;74(8):624–631.
8. Begley CG, Chalmers RL, Mitchell L, et al. Characterization of ocular surface symptoms from optometric practices in North America. Cornea 2001;20(6):610–618.
9. Brennan NA, Efron N. Hydrogel lens dehydration: a material-dependent phenomenon? Contact Lens Forum 1987;12(4):28–29.
10. Orsborn GN, Zantos SG. Corneal dessication staining with thin high water content contact lenses. CLAO J 1988; 14:81–85.
11. Landers RA, Rixon AJ. Contact lens materials update: options for most prescriptions. Contact Len Spectrum 2005;20(3):24–28.
12. Dillehay SM, Miller MB. Performance of Lotrafilcon B silicone hydrogel contact lenses in experienced low-Dk/t daily lens wearers. Eye Contact Lens 2007;33(6 Pt 1):272–277.
13. Schafer J, Mitchell GL, Chalmers RL, et al. The stability of dryness symptoms after refitting with silicone hydrogel contact lenses over 3 years. Eye Contact Lens 2007;33(5):247–252.
14. Caroline PJ, Andre MP. Profession still deciding between preservative free and preserved chemical disinfection. Primary Care Optometry News 1997;1(6):32.
15. Mack CJ. Contact lenses 2007. Contact Lens Spectrum 2008;23(1):26–34.
16. Chan WK, Weissman BA. Therapeutic contact lenses. In: Bennett ES, Weissman BA, eds. Clinical Contact Lens Practice. Philadelphia: Lippincott Williams & Wilkins, 2005:619–628.
17. O'Donnell C, Efron N. A prospective evaluation of contact lens wear in diabetes. Optom Vis Sci 1996;73(125):163.
18. Henry VA, Campbell RC, Connelly S, et al. How to refit contact lens patients. Contact Lens Forum 1991;16(2): 19–30.
19. Bennett ES, Henry VA, Davis LJ, et al. Comparing empirical and diagnostic fitting of daily wear fluoro-silicone/acrylate contact lenses. Contact Lens Forum 1989;14(3):38–44.
20. Young G. Evaluation of soft contact lens fitting characteristics. Optom Vis Sci 1996;73(4):247–254.
21. Harris MG, Gilman E. Consultation, examination and prognosis. In: Mandell RB, ed. Contact Lens Practice, 4th ed. Springfield, IL: Charles C. Thomas, 1988:352–387.
22. Schwallie JD, Bauman RE. Fitting characteristics of DailiesTM daily disposable hydrogel contact lenses. CLAO J 1998;24(2):102–106.
23. Davis RL, Becherer PD. Techniques for improved soft lens fitting. Contact Lens Spectrum 2005;20(8):24–27.
24. Kleist FD. Appearance and nature of hydrophilic contact lens deposits. I. Protein and other organic deposits. Int Contact Lens Clin 1979;6(3):49–58.
25. Kleist FD. Appearance and nature of hydrophilic contact lens deposits. II. Inorganic deposits. Int Contact Lens Clin 1979;6(4):177–186.
26. Mandell RB. Hydrogel lenses with spherical surfaces. In: Mandell RB, ed. Contact Lens Practice, 4th ed. Springfield, IL: Charles C. Thomas, 1988:540–553.
27. Zadnik K, Mutti D. Inferior arcuate staining in soft contact lens wearers. Int Contact Lens Clin 1984;12(1): 110–115.

CHAPTER 12

Soft Lens Care and Patient Education

Vinita Allee Henry

■ DISINFECTION

Many complications of soft lens wear develop after the lenses have been successfully fitted, when patients care for and handle their lenses. Problems arise in numerous ways, such as when patients delete steps in the care regimen, alter the care regimen, or care for and handle the lenses in a careless manner. Because of the nature of soft lens materials, these lenses are susceptible to contamination by bacteria and fungi. Routine lens care, including disinfection and cleaning, is necessary to prevent lens contamination. Soft lens care systems are changed and updated frequently, which makes it difficult for the practitioner to stay updated. This chapter addresses soft lens care and patient education to improve lens care and compliance.

There are three methods of disinfection used with soft lenses: chemical, oxidative (hydrogen peroxide), and thermal. Each has its own advantages and disadvantages. Becoming aware of these advantages and disadvantages will aid the practitioner in selecting the care regimen best suited for each patient and each lens. With a wide variety of care systems available, it is easiest for the practitioner to use only one care system; however, it is beneficial to select a care system appropriate for each individual patient, rather than provide all patients with the same care regimen.

Another issue involved in selecting care regimens is providing a lens that requires no care regimen at all. There are several daily disposable lenses available that allow the contact lens wearer the option to insert a clean, sterile lens each morning and throw it away each night. These wearers need only the solution that is available in the blister pack. If they find that they need to remove the lens during the day and reinsert it, saline or multipurpose solution to aid in inserting the lens may be helpful. This is a viable option for many soft wearers. Additionally, other single-use soft lenses worn for 1 week or 30 days continuously and disposed upon lens removal require only a solution for use with inserting the lens.

Chemical Disinfection

Chemical systems [also called multipurpose solutions (MPSs)] that combine cleaning, rinsing, and disinfection are extremely popular with patients and practitioners because of their simplicity. MPSs consist of a combination disinfecting/cleaning/rinsing solution containing one or more preservatives. A separate surfactant cleaner, enzymatic cleaner, or both may be added; however, with disposable/frequent replacement soft lenses, these additional solutions are rarely necessary. These one-bottle care systems are very popular and are especially beneficial for those patients who tend to be noncompliant when using multiple bottles or are confused by a complicated system.

The problem that originally became apparent with chemical disinfection systems was the use of preservatives, such as thimerosal and chlorhexidine. Although both of these preservatives exhibit excellent preservative action, many patients were sensitive to them. The preservatives currently used cause less patient sensitivity. Occasionally, some patients may still exhibit sensitivity, reporting symptoms of dryness, itching, burning, injection, decreased wearing time, and discomfort. A condition called multipurpose nonkeratitis has been reported.[1] The soft contact lens wearer using a multipurpose chemical solution presents with normal external findings, but complains of ocular dryness. Changing the patient to a preservative-free, hydrogen peroxide care regimen alleviates the dry-eye symptoms. A study with adolescents found that overall, patients on a hydrogen peroxide system show less staining and inflammatory response than those patients using a chemical care regimen.[2] The Andrasko Staining Grid and the Institute for Eye Research (IER) Matrix both pertained to solution-induced corneal staining. In the Staining Grid study, staining was assessed after 2 hours of wear and overnight soaking. The IER study investigators looked for the presence of staining three times over a 3-month period. Both studies found a hydrogen peroxide care regimen (ClearCare, Ciba Vision) to perform well with four silicone hydrogel materials (Acuvue Advance & Acuvue Oasys, Vistakon; O₂Optix, Ciba Vision; and PureVision, Bausch & Lomb). The three chemical care regimens resulted in inducing more corneal staining to a small extent in the Staining Grid study and even more in the IER Matrix study.[3] Although the sensitivity rate may be lower with the newer preservatives, the practitioner needs to be aware that symptoms of sensitivity to them may be delayed and somewhat vague. If in doubt, changing the patient to a nonpreserved care regimen or a daily disposable contact lens modality may eliminate the symptoms.

Additionally, the preservatives in chemical care regimens are not as effective against bacteria, fungi, and *Acanthamoeba* as hydrogen peroxide care regimens. Chemical care regimens have been removed from the market because of cases of *Fusarium* (ReNu MoistureLoc) and *Acanthamoeba* (Complete Moisture Plus) that were linked to the use of these solutions. Although patient noncompliance may be partially responsible in these two outbreaks, it is also believed that the disinfection efficacy of these two solutions was decreased, part of the formulation facilitated the pathogen growth, and the solution caused disruption to the corneal surface creating a portal for the infection to occur.[4] Extended wear, noncompliance, and poor lens hygiene increase the chances of a fungal infection.[5,6] The risk of *Acanthamoeba* keratitis is increased by tap water use, swimming, use of hot tubs and showering with contact lenses on, and improper care. Recent outbreaks of *Acanthamoeba* keratitis may be associated with changes in water purification.[7,8] Digital rubbing in these chemical regimens is important in removing *Acanthamoeba* from the lens.[9] Digital rubbing and rinsing have been found to remove up to 99% of *Acanthamoeba* found on a lens before chemical disinfection.[10] As would be expected, one study found that the care regimen (chemical or oxidative) is most effective when all steps are performed (i.e., rubbing, rinsing, and disinfecting).[11] The effects of chemical disinfection alone on *Acanthamoeba* and the human immunodeficiency virus (HIV) are minimal.[12] Other wearer tips to minimize the risk for *Acanthamoeba* keratitis include if lenses are worn during swimming, airtight goggles should be worn and, if not, the lenses should be disposed immediately after swimming.[13] For more information on diagnosis and treatment of *Fusarium* and *Acanthamoeba*, see Chapter 21.

Chemical disinfection may be used on all types of lenses and has little effect on lens life. At minimum, 5 minutes to 4 hours are required for a chemical disinfecting cycle; however, as most patients perform disinfection overnight, this is rarely a disadvantage. Although no-rub, rinsing-only multipurpose solutions have been promoted to lens wearers, rubbing the lens with the multipurpose solution *before* disinfection is an important step to prevent the preservatives from binding to deposits, thus decreasing the effectiveness of disinfection. In addition, cleaning alone has been found to remove >90% of a measured amount of bacteria placed on new and used contact lenses, thus enhancing disinfection.[14] The importance of rubbing and rinsing before disinfection cannot be overemphasized, as rubbing is often the first step noncompliant patients eliminate in their lens care systems. The microbial efficacy of these systems is based on the entire regimen (rubbing, rinsing, and disinfection), and when steps are omitted, the efficacy is thus reduced.[15]

Aquify (Ciba Vision) is the one chemical disinfection system that can be completed in 5 minutes. To disinfect a lens in 5 minutes, the lens should be rubbed on both sides for 10 seconds with three drops of Aquify, rinsed, and then soaked in Aquify for 5 minutes. This brief disinfection time is helpful if the patient must remove a lens during the day or for in-office disinfection (e.g., during the eye examination or a lens that has been dropped during insertion).

If a patient has a reaction to the preservatives in the solution, the preferable method would be to replace the lens. This is a simple process with a disposable lens. However, if the patient is wearing a conventional replacement, custom lens that needs to be salvaged, purging the lens may remove the offensive preservative. To purge a lens, place it in a vial of distilled water for 8 hours and repeat this for a total of three cycles. An 8-hour cycle in saline followed by disinfection in a nonpreserved system will complete the purging. Purging may also be used to remove fluorescein from a lens that has been stained with this dye.

A complete listing of available chemical disinfecting solutions is provided in Table 12.1.[16–18]

Oxidative Disinfection (Hydrogen Peroxide)

Another method of disinfection, oxidative, consists of a 3% hydrogen peroxide solution, neutralizing tablet or disc, case vial, and possibly a saline. Neutralization, by the disc or tablet, takes approximately 6 hours. The neutralizing tablet with Oxysept contains cyanocobalamin, which tints the solution pink to confirm that the tablet has been added to the hydrogen peroxide.[19] The case vial should be replaced every 3 months. Oxidative disinfection can be more complicated and confusing for patients; however, one-bottle oxidative systems have greatly reduced patient confusion over its use. Oxidative disinfection is safe, effective, and preservative free. Contact lens wearers who use oxidative disinfection typically are very loyal to their system. Patients, particularly those with solution sensitivities, find that oxidative disinfection can make the difference between comfortable, all-day wear and the inability to achieve comfortable wear.

Oxidative disinfection utilizes hydrogen peroxide, which, in addition to disinfection, provides a deep cleaning of the lens.[9] Hydrogen peroxide is hypotonic and has a pH of 4, which makes it effective at removing protein, lipid, and trapped debris.[20] Hydrogen peroxide has long been known for its antimicrobial characteristics. A longer exposure time has been recommended to be more effective against fungi and *Acanthamoeba*. This is accomplished by soaking the lenses 45 to 60 minutes in the hydrogen peroxide solution. Hydrogen peroxide is also effective against HIV and against fungal contamination by *Aspergillus* on soft contact lenses.[21]

TABLE 12.1 CHEMICAL DISINFECTION SOLUTIONS

BRAND NAME	MANUFACTURER	PRESERVATIVE	WETTING AGENT	LONG-TERM STORAGE
Complete Multi-Purpose	Advance Medical Optics (AMO)	Polyhexamethylene biguanide		30 d
Opti-Free Express	Alcon	Polyquad & Aldox	Tetronic 1304	30 d
Opti-Free RepleniSH	Alcon	Polyquad & Aldox	TearGlyde (Tetronic 1304 and C9-ED3A)	30 d
ReNu MultiPlus	Bausch & Lomb	Dymed		30 d
Aquify	Ciba Vision	Polyhexanide	Dexpant-5, sorbitol	30 d
Opti-One and Opti-Free	Alcon	Polyquad		

Hydrogen peroxide is very acidic and will produce a mild to moderate punctate keratitis if it comes in contact with the cornea. No severe damage results if the patient fails to neutralize the hydrogen peroxide before lens insertion or does not fully neutralize the hydrogen peroxide (e.g., old catalytic disc or too brief of a neutralization/dilution soak); however, the patient will experience stinging, moderate discomfort, and injection. Treatment for this keratitis requires proper neutralization or dilution of the residual hydrogen peroxide in the lens and discontinuing lens wear until the symptoms have disappeared (i.e., 2 to 12 hours). The use of an artificial tear drop will improve comfort and reduce symptoms for a patient with this type of keratitis. To assist in the prevention of hydrogen peroxide being used directly in the eye, the hydrogen peroxide solutions are currently packaged in bottles with red tips, and warning labels on the bottles direct the patient not to use this solution directly in the eye (Fig. 12.1).

Removing the hydrogen peroxide before lens insertion may be accomplished by one of three methods. Two of the three methods are based on a catalyst that is contained primarily in a tablet or platinum disc. Advanced Medical Optics (AMO) has a preservative-free tablet that is placed directly in the vial containing hydrogen peroxide. The neutralizing tablet is coated with a viscosity agent that prevents activation of the tablet for 20 to 30 minutes, thus allowing disinfection with hydrogen peroxide to occur before neutralization. This tablet is placed in the vial immediately with the hydrogen peroxide, Oxysept-Ultracare formula (AMO).

The AODisc (Ciba Vision) is a platinum disc attached to the lens cage that begins neutralizing ClearCare or AOSept (Ciba Vision) immediately on contact when the lens cage is placed in the vial. The entire vial with the disc should be replaced after approximately 3 months of daily use or 100 cycles if used weekly. When the disc is losing its effectiveness, it will not fully neutralize the hydrogen peroxide, resulting in a mild stinging sensation when the lenses are inserted. The vial also includes an opening in the lid, which should remain upright and unobstructed so oxygen may escape during the neutralizing step. Sauflon Pharmaceuticals also uses a neutralizing disc to neutralize its hydrogen peroxide solution (Sauflon One-Step Cleaning & Disinfection Solution).

The final method of removing hydrogen peroxide from the lens is dilution of hydrogen peroxide by osmosis with the use of saline solution. Although no commercially available care regimens utilize this method, it is still valuable for the practitioner to be aware of in cases in which the wearer may need an emergency backup method for the tablet or disc. The hydrogen peroxide is emptied from the vial after disinfection is completed. The lenses and vial are generally rinsed once with saline solution and allowed to stand in saline solution for a specified time period (e.g., 10 minutes). Studies have shown that there is no significant difference in the "sting factor" between this type of method and that of neutralization with a catalyst.[22,23]

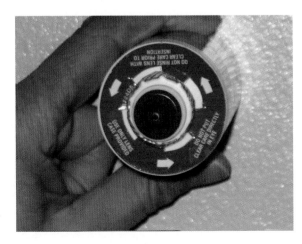

■ **FIGURE 12.1** Red-tipped warning on hydrogen peroxide solution bottle.

Oxidative disinfection systems were previously categorized as one-step or two-step disinfection systems. Currently, only one-step systems are available. Two-step systems have been discontinued, as one-step systems are useful in increasing patient compliance. However, in a one-step system, the concentration of hydrogen peroxide is much reduced and may not provide a long enough exposure time. For example, past studies found that only the two-step systems were effective against *Acanthamoeba*.[9,12,24] AOSept has been found to be significantly more effective against *Acanthamoeba* than chemical disinfection when cleaning and rubbing of the lens were not performed before disinfection.[11] Proper cleaning and rinsing before all types of disinfection will enhance the effects on *Acanthamoeba*. Likewise, hydrogen peroxide has been found to be more effective on *Pseudomonas* than a multipurpose solution when cleaning and rubbing were not performed.[25] New evidence shows that hydrogen peroxide is effective against the trophozoite forms of *Acanthamoeba*.[26] ClearCare and AOSept have been found to demonstrate antimicrobial activity against the cyst form of *Acanthamoeba* castellani after 6 hours.[27] In the same study, a multipurpose chemical disinfection solution was shown to have no antimicrobial activity against the cyst form after 6 hours. These findings show protective benefits of hydrogen peroxide for noncompliant contact lens wearers.[25]

MiraFlow Extra Strength Cleaner (Ciba Vision), added to the AOSept disinfection system, will enhance disinfection because it has disinfecting characteristics of its own. Caution should be taken to ensure that the patient thoroughly rinses MiraFlow from the lens before disinfection. A chemical reaction between AOSept and the catalytic disc will increase the sudsing action of any residual cleaner and may result in all of the AOSept pouring out of the opening in the vial, leaving the lenses in an empty vial with inadequate disinfection.

Three percent hydrogen peroxide is commercially available over the counter, typically in brown bottles for nonophthalmic use. The cost of this solution is much less than that of solutions used in contact lens disinfection. Although it is similar to that used for contact lens disinfection, it is not ophthalmically pure and may contain inexpensive stabilizers and/or heavy metals that may cause lens discoloration. In addition, contamination of the solution may easily occur in these wide-mouthed containers, whereas the narrow openings found in contact lens solution containers decrease the risk of contamination. Available oxidative disinfection systems are listed in Table 12.2.[16–19]

Silicone Hydrogel Disinfection and Care

Because of the differences in hydrogel versus silicone hydrogel materials, not all solutions may perform as well with silicone hydrogel lenses. The solutions currently indicated by the Food and Drug Administration (FDA) for use with silicone hydrogel lenses are ClearCare and Aquify (Ciba Vision) and Opti-Free RepleniSH and Opti-Free Express (Alcon Laboratories). In addition, silicone hydrogel materials are more prone to lipid deposits; therefore, rubbing the lens before disinfection is recommended. MiraFlow Extra Strength Cleaner (Ciba Vision) is useful for removing lipid deposits if rubbing and frequent replacement of the lenses is not sufficient. In the IER Matrix study, PureVision lenses were found to exhibit more solution-induced

TABLE 12.2 OXIDATIVE DISINFECTION SYSTEMS

BRAND NAME	MANUFACTURER	METHOD OF NEUTRALIZATION	RECOMMENDED LONG-TERM STORAGE TIME
Oxysept UltraCare	AMO	Tablet	7 d
AOSept	Ciba Vision	Platinum disc	30 d in Softwear saline
ClearCare	Ciba Vision	Platinum disc	7 d
Sauflon One Step	Sauflon USA	Neutralizing disc	24 hr

corneal staining with Aquify, Opti-Free RepleniSH, and Opti-Free Express than the other silicone hydrogel materials in the comparison. In the IER and Staining Grid studies, ClearCare performed well with the PureVision material.[3]

Thermal Disinfection

Thermal disinfection is the least expensive and most effective disinfection system in the short term; however, as the heat bakes on the deposits not cleaned off the lens, lens life is shortened and complications such as giant papillary conjunctivitis [GPC, also known as contact lens papillary conjunctivitis (CLPC)] or red-eye reactions may arise from the deposited lens. As a disinfectant, thermal disinfection is effective against all forms of bacteria, including *Pseudomonas*, both cyst and trophozoite forms of *Acanthamoeba*, and HIV. The solutions used with thermal disinfection can be preservative free for those patients sensitive to preserved solutions. Despite the advantages, the popularity of thermal disinfection has declined to the point where it is not used by contact lens wearers because of electrical requirements and the long-term problem of baked-on deposits. In addition, heat is contraindicated with lenses containing >55% water, and caution must be taken when switching a patient from another type of disinfection to thermal since it is not interchangeable with all systems. Manufacturers no longer support this type of disinfection with heat units for individual use. It is used for in-office disinfection of vial lenses.

Other alternative methods of disinfection that are available are ultrasonic disinfection (Lens Comfort, Best Health, Inc.) and UV subsonic disinfection (Purilens UV, Purilens/Lifestyle Co. Inc.).[17]

In-Office Disinfection

Most diagnostic soft lenses are used on a one-time basis and discarded. This is the most acceptable method of diagnostic lens use; there is no danger of ocular infection spread from one patient to the next because the lenses are packaged in sterile containers. At the present time, some diagnostic lenses are reused after being disinfected, which does not produce a sterile lens. There is no perfect method of disinfecting large numbers of lenses and keeping these large numbers of diagnostic lenses disinfected. Large thermal disinfection units are available to disinfect lenses in glass vials, which is an acceptable method of disinfection; however, some lens materials contraindicate thermal disinfection use, primarily those with >55% water content. Oxidative disinfection, although an excellent method of disinfection, is difficult to use for diagnostic lenses because of the necessity of disinfecting the lens in a special case and transferring the disinfected lens to a glass vial. The lens may become contaminated in the transfer process, or the vial may become contaminated. It is acceptable to store lenses in a glass vial in a chemical disinfecting solution; however, their effects on *Acanthamoeba* and HIV are questionable. In addition, it has been recommended, based on study results, that diagnostic lenses disinfected with oxidative or chemical disinfection be redisinfected at least once a month to prevent contamination.[28]

Possibly the best type of in-office disinfection, disregarding disposable diagnostic lenses, is the combination of two disinfection systems. In the past, chemical disinfection was not compatible with thermal; however, Opti-Free Express (Alcon Laboratories), as a result of both the preservative action and the omission of a surfactant, may be used and is approved for use in heat disinfection. The other chemical disinfection systems, conversely, contain a surfactant that, after repeated thermal disinfection cycles, may result in a cloudy lens. It is acceptable to fill a glass vial with Opti-Free Express and place the vial in an in-office thermal disinfecting unit. As with any lens worn by the patient, the lens should be thoroughly cleaned and rinsed before disinfection. Lenses of >55% water content may be stored in Opti-Free Express or other chemical disinfecting solution without thermal disinfection. The practitioner must keep in mind the limitations of the systems. Thermal disinfection is effective against *Acanthamoeba* and HIV; however, chemical disinfection systems are questionable. Any lens used on a known HIV-positive patient or a patient exposed to *Acanthamoeba* should be disposed of and not reused, even though at the present time it is thought that the risk of transmission via the tears is low.[29,30]

Another combination method is to clean the diagnostic lens with MiraFlow Extra Strength Cleaner (Ciba Vision); disinfect in one of the 3% hydrogen peroxide disinfecting solutions for 2 to 12 hours, followed by neutralization; and then store the lens in the glass vial in a chemical disinfection solution. As noted previously, the lenses should be redisinfected every month. Autoclaving will produce a lens that should be sterile for a year. A procedure for autoclaving is to clean the lens with MiraFlow cleaner, rinse with a nonpreserved saline, and put the lens in the glass vial with nonpreserved saline. The vial should be sealed and placed in an autoclave. This final method guarantees sterility of the lens.[31]

■ SALINE

Saline solutions have almost disappeared from the marketplace. Saline solution, which is not toxic to the eye, is a sterile solution used to rinse lenses free of foreign matter and cleaner. In addition, it is used as an in-office rinsing solution or to wet a fluorescein strip. Saline solution is not capable of disinfecting the lens when used alone. Although practitioners are aware of this, it is not always adequately communicated to the patient, and he or she may alter the care system to the use of saline solution alone with no disinfecting solution. The potentially devastating effects of this include vision-threatening complications that can be avoided if the patient is educated initially and the care system is carefully monitored at follow-up evaluations. A list of available salines is provided in Table 12.3.[17,18]

Saline is available in preserved and unpreserved forms. The first preserved salines were preserved with thimerosal; however, after the sensitivity reactions experienced with thimerosal, less toxic preservatives such as sorbic acid, potassium sorbate, and polyaminopropyl biguanide were used. Currently, the available saline solutions are nonthimerosal preserved or unpreserved. Unpreserved saline solutions are available in aerosol containers and 4 oz. bottles (to be used within 14 days). A benefit of aerosol saline is that the patient is provided with a sterile, nonpreserved solution, thus decreasing the risk of solution sensitivity. However, a frustrating problem with aerosol saline occurs when the propellant is depleted before the saline. This results in the inability to use the saline remaining in the container. A few simple tips will prevent this frustration: (a) the nozzle should be turned to match a red dot on the upper rim of the container, and (b) the container should not be tipped below a horizontal position. Both of these tips will help prevent the propellant from being used up before the saline solution.[9]

A unique method of preserving saline, yet preventing the sensitivities often found with preserved salines, is the use of an antimicrobial buffer system found in SoftWear Saline (Ciba

TABLE 12.3 SALINES

BRAND NAME	MANUFACTURER	PRESERVATIVE
Sensitive Eyes Saline Solution	Bausch & Lomb	Sorbic acid and edetate disodium
Sensitive Eyes Plus Saline Solution	Bausch & Lomb	Polyaminopropyl biguanide and edetate disodium
Softwear Saline	Ciba Vision	Trace hydrogen peroxide
Unisol 4	Alcon	None
PuriLens Solution	PuriLens Plus	None
Lens Plus Aerosol Saline	Exaeris	None

Vision). This antimicrobial buffer naturally protects the saline from pathogens. When the solution is opened, carbon dioxide from the atmosphere causes a shift in the pH that in turn causes sodium perborate to react with sodium borate and boric acid to create a physiologic balance of the pH. The further combination of the sodium perborate buffer with water yields trace amounts of hydrogen peroxide. The presence of trace amounts of hydrogen peroxide provides antimicrobial action, in addition to being nontoxic to the eye. Studies of this saline have demonstrated its effectiveness and patient comfort.[32,33]

The final type of saline to be discussed is homemade saline made from distilled water and salt tablets. Homemade saline was introduced with the introduction of soft lenses; however, *homemade saline should never be used today*. The sale of salt tablets has been banned by the FDA. There is no benefit to homemade saline and there are many risks, primarily the possible risk of *Acanthamoeba* keratitis. Sixty percent of reported cases of *Acanthamoeba* keratitis resulted from using homemade saline, swimming with lenses on, or using no disinfection system.[9] The risk presented by homemade saline use is the result of a nonsterile solution that is easily contaminated because the containers used to mix the solution and the large containers of distilled water used to dissolve the tablet may be contaminated.

■ DEPOSITS

Soft lens-induced complications are largely the result of corneal edema or deposits. The popularity of daily disposable, 1- to 2-week disposable, and frequent-replacement soft lenses aids in diminishing the complications found with deposits. When conventional replacement soft lenses are used, proper lens care will aid in maintaining a clean lens surface; however, lens care must be performed routinely as soft lenses are prone to deposits as a result of the hydrophilic surface, patient tear film, environment, and lens handling. A deposited lens will result in a reduction in the effectiveness of the preservatives, oxygen transmission, surface wettability, vision, and wearing time; in addition, the patient is at risk for GPC, red-eye reactions, and/or corneal ulcers. Silicone hydrogel lenses are more prone to lipid deposits than hydrogel lenses; therefore, rubbing the lens before disinfection is important to remove deposits from the lens.

There are several types of soft lens deposits, which may be identified by the color and appearance of the deposit and categorized as either organic or inorganic deposits.[34,35] The most common organic deposit is protein, which leaves a white opaque film on the lens surface. Other organic deposits include pigment deposits, which are a result of melanin polymers in the tears and are increased with the use of thermal disinfection; microorganism growth, which is a result of fungi/yeast appearing in various colors in a filamentary appearance; and finally, lipid deposits, which have a smeared, greasy appearance.

"Jelly bumps" are the most common type of inorganic deposit; they occur more frequently in extended wear (EW). Jelly bumps are named for their characteristic appearance of white to clear elevations on the anterior lens surface (Fig. 12.2). The primary composition is somewhat controversial; however, calcium, lipids, and cholesterol have been found to be a part of the composition.[36,37] Typically, calcium precipitates to form the white base of the deposit. It is then covered with an oily lipid layer and, finally, a mucoprotein outer layer. Jelly bumps become a part of the lens matrix and result in pits in the lens surface if removed. As jelly bumps increase in size and number, vision may be affected and discomfort may be experienced by the patient.

Another type of inorganic deposit is a rust spot. The rust spot is generally a circular orange deposit. When a rust spot is observed, the practitioner should immediately question the patient about possible tap water use. Comprehensive patient education and documentation are necessary when rust spots are found. The other possible causes of a rust spot are the environment or a metal foreign body. The concern in the latter case is that the foreign body may still be present in the eye, the lid, or the contact lens; therefore, a careful examination with the biomicroscope is required.

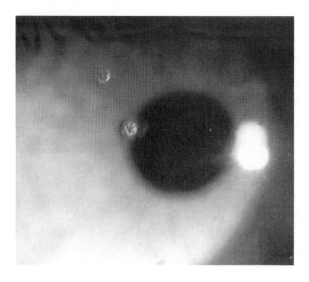

■ **FIGURE 12.2** Jelly bumps on a hydrogel lens.

The last type of inorganic deposit observed on soft lenses is the result of contamination with cosmetics, including mascara, hairspray, aftershave lotion, soaps, or suntan lotion. These deposits appear iridescent, filmy, or greasy. Comprehensive patient education will assist in the prevention of these deposits. Simple hand washing before lens handling will greatly reduce this type of contamination.

■ SURFACTANT CLEANERS

Thorough and routine cleaning will prevent buildup of lens deposition. Multipurpose solutions contain cleaning agents. If patients are wearing a conventional lens or are prone to deposits, they may require a separate surfactant cleaner; however, separate surfactant cleaners are becoming increasingly difficult to find on store shelves. The cleaner, whether used in combination with the solution or as a separate cleaner, acts as a soap to remove debris, unbound proteins, lipid deposits, and some microbial contamination. The lens should be placed in the palm of the hand with a few drops of solution or a separate surfactant cleaner and rubbed gently back and forth for 20 to 30 seconds. The back-and-forth motion is less likely to cause lens damage than a circular motion.

After careful cleaning, the lens should be thoroughly rinsed before lens disinfection. The reasons for instructing patients to care for their lenses in this sequence include the following: first, disinfection is greatly enhanced by cleaning and rinsing; second, residual cleaner left on the lens will be rinsed off further by the disinfection process, providing a more comfortable lens for the patient on insertion; and finally, deposits will be removed more easily on lens removal than later when the deposits become bound to the lens surface. In addition, the patient should not develop the bad habit of "left lens syndrome," in which the right lens is thoroughly cleaned initially and the patient then reduces the care time given to the left lens, resulting in more contamination of this lens.

Opti-Free Daily Cleaner (Alcon Laboratories) is an abrasive cleaner preserved with Polyquad. This cleaner has fewer abrasive beads than previous Alcon abrasive cleaners; therefore, rinsing is more effective in removing all the cleaner from the lens. Patients prone to deposits and wearing conventional replacement lenses may benefit from the use of an abrasive cleaner.

MiraFlow Extra Strength Cleaner (Ciba Vision) contains, among other cleaning ingredients, isopropyl alcohol. Isopropyl alcohol eliminates the need for a preservative because of its broad-spectrum antimicrobial effects. It is also an excellent cleaner, especially for patients with a tendency to lipid deposits, as it dissolves lipids.[9,38]

TABLE 12.4 ENZYMATIC CLEANERS AND DAILY PROTEIN REMOVERS

BRAND NAME	MANUFACTURER
Opti-Free Supraclens Daily Protein Remover	Alcon
Ultrazyme Enzymatic Cleaner	AMO
Unizyme Enzymatic Cleaner	Ciba Vision

▓ ENZYMATIC CLEANERS

The overwhelming number of contact lens wearers who are fitted in disposable or frequent-replacement soft lenses has almost eliminated the need for enzymatic cleaners. In addition, many multipurpose solutions contain ingredients to aid in protein removal. Typically, enzymatic cleaners are reserved for conventional replacement patients. For these patients, enzymatic cleaners are to be used once a week to break down peptide bonds, allowing protein to be rubbed off mechanically. The proper care sequence when enzymatically cleaning soft lenses is to clean and rub, rinse, enzymatically clean, and disinfect the lens. Enzyme cleaners are placed in the disinfecting solution and allowed to soak overnight during disinfection. Available enzymatic cleaners are listed in Table 12.4.[17,18]

SupraClens (Alcon Laboratories) is a daily protein remover. One drop is placed directly in Opti-Free Express, Opti-One, or Opti-Free RepleniSH solution in each side of the lens case. The advantages of this cleaner are the convenience it affords the patient, its daily use, and its effectiveness.[39]

▓ LENS LUBRICANTS/REWETTING

The use of lens lubricants or rewetting drops is optional; however, they may be beneficial in cases of dry eyes, foreign-body sensation, or irritations and for morning and evening use in overnight lens wear. Lens lubricants are used directly in the eye with or without the lenses. Patients should not substitute artificial tears, gas-permeable (GP) lens lubricants, or ophthalmic medications for soft lens lubricants because the preservatives are not necessarily compatible with the soft lens materials, the possible result being lens discoloration and toxic reactions. Lubricants that are beneficial to patients by helping clean the lens in the eye are Blink-N-Clean, Opti-Free RepleniSH Rewetting Drops, and Clerz Plus Lens Drops. Blink Contacts, Aquify Long-Lasting Comfort Drops, Refresh Contacts, and TheraTears Contact Lens Comfort Drops contain disappearing preservatives to decrease sensitivity reactions.

Contact lens wearers who suffer from symptoms of dryness are especially benefited by a lens lubricant. Lens lubricants initially amounted to little more than a solution similar to saline, but are now carefully formulated to produce solutions that protect and lubricate the eye. The use of disappearing preservatives prevents ocular sensitivities to preservatives (i.e., sodium perborate changes to oxygen and water, and the stabilized oxychloro complex changes to sodium chloride and water upon instillation). These preservatives break down when exposed to light, which leaves them preservative free upon instillation. Wetting agents bind water and aid in spreading the tears between blinks, in addition to retaining the tear film longer. Hyaluronic acid is a viscoelastic component found naturally in the body. Its use in lubricating drops has been found to increase tear breakup time, thus improving lens-wearing comfort. The potential of these new ingredients to combat dry-eye symptoms is highly useful in lubricating/rewetting drops.[40]

Available lens lubricants or rewetting drops and their manufacturers are listed in Table 12.5.[16–18]

TABLE 12.5 LENS LUBRICANTS/REWETTING DROPS

BRAND NAME	MANUFACTURER	PRESERVATIVE	SURFACTANT/WETTING AGENT
Clerz Plus and Opti-Free RepleniSH Rewetting Drops	Alcon	Polyquad	Tetronic 1304 and RLM-100
Complete Blink-N-Clean	AMO	Polyhexamethylene biguanide	Tromethamine, tyloxapol, HPMC
Blink	AMO	OcuPure	Sodium hyaluronate
Theratears CL Comfort Drops	Advanced Vision Research	Sodium perborate	Carboxymethyl cellulose
Refresh Contacts	Allergan	Purite or preservative free	Carboxymethyl cellulose
Sensitive Eyes, ReNu Multiplus, ReNu rewetting drops	Bausch & Lomb	Edetate disodium and sorbic acid	Povidone
Aquify Long-lasting Comfort Drops	Ciba Vision	Sodium perborate	Sodium hyaluronate

■ PATIENT EDUCATION AND HYGIENE

Educational Environment

Educating patients about the wearing, handling, and care of soft lenses should be considered as *serious* and *important* to the success of soft lens wear as the fit of the lenses. Patient noncompliance and absence of knowledge are primary causes of soft lens complications, which may be a result of the patient's lack of concern, the practitioner's lack of seriousness, or both. When patient education becomes secondary, taught by staff members who are less than knowledgeable and with little emphasis, a lack of importance is perceived by the patients that carries over into their routine for lens care. Typically, four practitioner factors contribute to patient noncompliance: poor instructions, no instructions, poor example, and overloading the patient with information at dispensing.[41] Every office should provide the patient with written information pertaining to insertion and removal, lens care, and lens handling. At minimum, preprinted material may be obtained from many contact lens manufacturers; however, an attractive booklet personalized for each individual office is recommended. Suggested topics for inclusion (in addition to methods of insertion and removal) are recommended wearing schedule, emergency phone numbers, and consequences of noncompliance. Also, a photo album or framed poster of soft lens complications (e.g., GPC, ulcers, deposited lenses, *Acanthamoeba* keratitis) that result from noncompliance may be placed in the examination room. These are not to scare the patient away from soft lens wear but to emphasize the seriousness of proper lens wear and care.

The office should provide a good example for the patient. An area should be provided for patient insertion and removal of lenses that has adequate lighting, capped unexpired solutions, large counter space, and a sink with a drain capable of being closed. A poor example in the office endorses a poor example at home. Likewise, staff and practitioners should set a good example when handling lenses. Even if the practitioner's or staff member's hands have been washed, washing the hands in the patient's presence before handling the lenses reinforces to the patient that this is proper lens care.

The final area where practitioners and staff can be responsible for confusing patients is overloading patients with information at the dispensing. Patient education should be an ongoing process in which the patient's routine is discussed at future visits and bad habits broken before they become routine. Obviously insertion and removal and lens care must be discussed before the patient takes the lenses home; however, some patients may need more than one visit to learn how to insert, remove, and care for their lenses. In addition, the patient can be taught how to disinfect and clean lenses at the dispensing visit and additional steps of surfactant or enzymatic cleaning (if necessary) may be taught at the 1-week progress visit; in this way, the patient is not overwhelmed with information. Comprehensive written instructions will reassure the patient by reinforcing important points, and patients should be encouraged to phone the office with questions they might have.

Optimum patient education is provided by a trained staff member in an area designed with patient education in mind. This area should include adequate mirrors for teaching insertion and removal, a large counter next to which the patient may be seated, and audio-visual aids. These are a valuable aid in educating both staff members and the patients. If staff members are going to instruct patients in lens care and handling, they should be well educated in lens care. A checklist of information to be discussed may be helpful to ensure that no information is omitted. An example of a checklist is shown in Table 12.6. In addition, the practitioner may wish

TABLE 12.6 PATIENT EDUCATION CHECKLIST

Was the patient taught the following tasks?

Washing hands before handling lenses ____

Lens insertion ____

Lens removal ____

Taco test or other method of determining lens inversion ____

How to open the blister pack ____

Was the patient instructed in the following lens care procedures?

How to clean a lens ____

How to disinfect a lens ____

When to use saline (optional) ____

When to use lens lubricating drops ____

Were the following topics discussed?

Hygiene ____

Swimming with lenses ____

Showering in lenses ____

Sleeping in lenses ____

Lens care products to use and not to use ____

Cosmetics ____

Case replacement and cleanliness ____

Lens replacement schedule ____

Normal and abnormal adaptive symptoms ____

Risks of noncompliance ____

Emergency numbers ____

Was the patient reminded to call the office with any questions regarding symptoms or lens care? ____

Was the patient reminded to wear the lenses to follow-up examinations? ____

to provide staff members with the opportunity to attend conferences that will train them in contact lens-related topics, such as patient education and lens care.

In addition to new wearers needing education on care and handling of contact lenses, practitioners should never assume that a current contact lens wearer is completing all the steps for proper lens care. The current wearer should be asked to verbally explain their current care regimen. The practitioner should discuss proper lens care with the patient. This should be ongoing at each visit to maintain proper lens care habits.[42] It is also important to review the lens replacement and wear schedule as some patient overwear issues may be patient noncompliance and others may be related to inadequate or inaccurate education in the past.

Patient Compliance

Even when patient education is optimum, various factors affect patient compliance. Some factors are related to the care system itself, which may be too complex, too time consuming, or too costly; therefore, a change in the type of lens care system may improve compliance. Manufacturers can assist in this area of noncompliance by a continued effort to develop lens care systems that are simple and inexpensive. Noncompliance may also occur if the patient takes shortcuts, forms sloppy habits, or is just generally lazy. This type of patient is potentially the most dangerous, and re-education as well as thorough documentation of noncompliance in the record will be required. It is possible that the patient is using solutions improperly or that substitutions have been made in the lens care regimen. Patients should be cautioned to consult with their practitioner before changing any solution in their regimen. In the local area, it may be desirable to provide pharmacists with information pertaining to soft lens care and an open invitation to call you if there should be any questions, as pharmacies will at times suggest improper solution substitutions to patients. At each progress visit, it is important to have patients restate their care routine to the practitioner or a staff member to ensure that the care regimen is still accurate. When substitutions have been made, patients may discontinue a step without even realizing it.

Noncompliance was most likely a contributing factor to the recent outbreaks of *Fusarium* and *Acanthamoeba* keratitis. The author has educated patients to disregard the "no rub" label on MPS solutions as patients have interpreted "no rub" as no rub and no rinse. One practitioner uses a permanent marker to mark out "no rub" on solution bottles, to emphasize the importance of rubbing the lens in the care process.[43] To aid in patient education of the importance of rubbing a lens, the author uses the illustration of a dirty dish that is rubbed and rinsed versus only rinsed. This illustration helps the patient understand the importance of rubbing the lens during the cleaning process.

Past studies evaluating solution cost to the consumer estimated that patients were spending <25% of the amount indicated if they were using the solutions according to directions.[44-46] This reduction in spending is a perfect example of patient noncompliance. The shortcuts that patients take are easily evident when they are asked about their lens care regimens. A study by Ciba Vision found that only 33% of soft contact lens wearers report that they follow the recommended lens replacement schedule, 30% report storing their lenses in saline or an eye drop overnight, and 23% report rinsing their lenses with tap water.[47]

Private-label solutions create another area of confusion and noncompliance for the lens wearer. In 2005, 30% of disinfection solution sales were private label. Contact lens wearers believe they are getting identical solutions at a lower price, which is inaccurate. Rather than being identical to the new generation of solutions, many times these solutions are formulations from several generations prior.[48] For example, for many years thimerosal had been eliminated from the major name-brand solutions, but it was still being used in private-label

TABLE 12.7 TEN COMMON RULES FOR PATIENT COMPLIANCE

1. Wash hands with soap and water, and dry thoroughly before handling contact lenses.
2. Store lenses in the recommended disinfecting solution and disinfect at every lens removal.
3. Rub and rinse lenses before disinfection.
4. Wear lenses according to the prescribed wearing schedule (i.e., dispose of lenses according to the recommended replacement schedule, do not sleep in lenses that are DW lenses, and do not sleep in EW lenses longer than the prescribed amount of time).
5. Always discard used solution and start with fresh solution (no topping off).
6. After inserting lenses, dump the solution from the case, rinse the case with disinfecting solution, and allow to air dry. The case should be replaced at least every 3 months.
7. Do not use tap water with lenses.
8. Do not swim or shower with lenses on, unless proper precautions are taken.
9. If dissatisfied with current solutions, discuss the care regimen with the doctor to avoid purchasing solutions that are incompatible or cause preservative sensitivities.
10. Solutions become contaminated when old, expired, or uncapped or by repackaging in nonsterile containers. [49,50]

DW, daily wear; EW, extended wear.

solutions. Great strides have been made to provide effective preservatives that are mild and compatible with the ocular surface. Another issue with private-label solutions is that it may be purchased in one formulation and be a totally different formulation 6 months later. The complications resulting from these issues with private-label solutions may result in lens wearers discontinuing wear, not realizing that the real problem is the solution they are using, not the lens or their eye. Ten common rules that aid in patient compliance are found in Table 12.7.

It is surprising that practitioners do not observe more complications related to these factors; however, patients often enjoy a period of success, even when they are being noncompliant, and this reinforces their thinking that it is acceptable to continue this noncompliance. Unfortunately, when problems do occur, they are often vision threatening and it is too late to manage the problem successfully by simply reinstating proper lens care. The answer to noncompliance is good, intensive patient education; reinforcement of education at each visit; and frequent evaluations to monitor lens wear. Vision is an invaluable sense, and patients must learn not to take it for granted.

Insertion and Removal

Insertion of a soft contact lens may be performed by either of two methods. The first method is to place the lens on the index finger. The index finger should be dry because the lens will stick to the finger instead of the eye if the finger is too wet. While the lids are held apart with the third finger of each hand, the lens is placed on the sclera as the patient looks up (Fig. 12.3A). The second method is performed the same way, except the lens is placed directly on the cornea as the patient looks straight ahead into a mirror (Fig. 12.3B). It is recommended that patients always insert and remove the same lens first; for example, the patient always inserts the right lens first and removes the right lens first.

A patient placing the lens on the index finger before insertion should be able to determine if the lens is right side or wrong side out. A lens that is right side out will appear bowl shaped (Fig. 12.4A), whereas one that is inverted will appear more like a saucer, with the edges flared

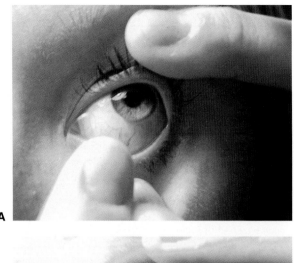

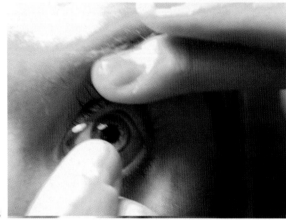

■ FIGURE 12.3 **(A)** Insertion of lens onto sclera. **(B)** Insertion of lens onto cornea.

out (Fig. 12.4B). If this method does not help the patient, the "taco test" is another method of determining if a lens is inverted. The lens edges are pushed together. If the edges curl toward each other, like the edges of a taco, the lens is correctly positioned (Fig. 12.5A). On the other hand, if the edges curl out, the lens is inverted (Fig. 12.5B). Typically, an inverted lens will result in mild discomfort, slightly reduced vision, excessive lens movement, or edges flared out from the sclera. If the patient observes any of these symptoms, an inverted lens may be suspected, and the patient should try to insert the lens in the other direction to determine if this corrects the symptoms. The patient may be assured that an inverted soft lens will not damage the eye. In addition, some manufacturers provide inversion indicators, which aid the patient in determining the correct position of the lens.

Soft lens removal is accomplished by holding the lids apart with the third finger of each hand, placing the index finger directly on the cornea, and sliding the lens off onto the sclera as the patient looks up. The lens is gently pinched off the sclera with the pads of the thumb and index finger (Fig. 12.6). Caution should be taken that the lens is not pinched directly off the cornea because this may result in a corneal abrasion. Likewise, the fingernails should not be used to pinch the lens because this may result in fingernail tears in the central portion of the lens. Generally, with practice, patients can learn to insert and remove their lenses without a mirror and without holding both lids open.

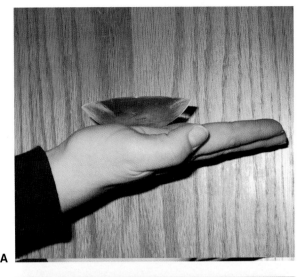

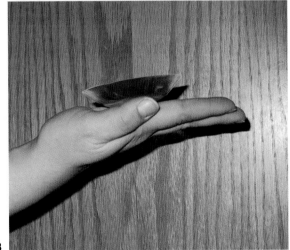

■ **FIGURE 12.4 (A)** Lens positioned correctly using large demonstration lens. **(B)** Lens inverted using large demonstration lens.

Hygiene

Hygiene would seem to be an area that would need little attention in today's society; however, even our cleanest, neatest patients will come to the office with dirty cases, dirty solution bottles, and lenses contaminated by substances on their hands. Simple hand washing before lens handling, with soaps that do not contain lanolin, creams, or oils, will prevent transfer of bacteria and environmental contamination (makeup, suntan lotion) of the lens. Any mild soap that does not have deodorants, creams, lanolin, or oils is compatible.

The second area of hygiene is the case in which the lenses are stored. For years, this component of lens care has been relatively ignored. It is important for cases not to be used for lengthy periods. Not only do they need occasional cleaning, but a biofilm also develops that remains in the wells of the case. This biofilm is difficult to remove and provides a perfect environment for microorganisms. One study found 27 different types of bacteria plus fungi in the contact lens cases of study subjects.[51] Other studies have shown an 80.95% rate of contamination of cases after 270 days of use[52] and 70% of cases contaminated by bacteria, fungi

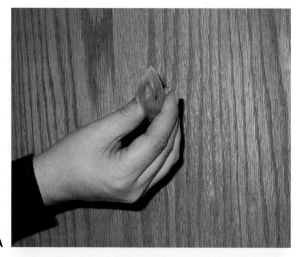

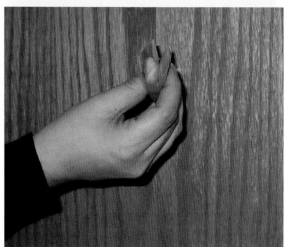

■ FIGURE 12.5 **(A)** Taco test demonstrating a proper lens orientation (using large demonstration lens). **(B)** Taco test demonstrating an inverted lens (using large demonstration lens).

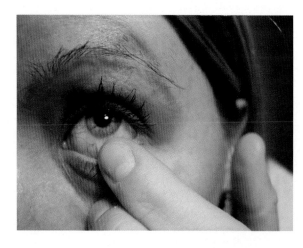

■ FIGURE 12.6 The lens has been pulled down on the sclera to remove the lens from the eye. The thumb is not yet positioned to pinch the lens.

yeasts, and amoebae.[53] A new case should be given to the patient, at minimum, every 3 months at follow-up evaluations, or manufacturers often package cases with solutions to encourage frequent case replacement.[54] Between periods of case replacement, the case should be emptied of solution each time the lenses are inserted, rinsed with disinfecting solution, and allowed to air dry. Once a week, the case should be thoroughly scrubbed to eliminate biofilm, which can develop within 7 days.[55] This can be achieved by digitally scrubbing with the disinfecting solution and allowing the case to air dry. Rinsing the case in tap water is not recommended, as the risk of *Acanthamoeba* in the cyst form is a possibility. Cases may be boiled in water periodically or microwaved for 3 minutes to sterilize.[13] Ciba Vision has produced a case called Pro-Guard, which incorporates silver, an inorganic antibacterial agent, into the case to decrease microbial contamination.[16,56]

Another area of microbial contamination is the solution bottles. The solution is provided initially sterile; however, microbial contamination may occur if the solution is left uncapped, the tip of the bottle comes in contact with the fingers or lens, the solution is old and expired, or the solution is transferred to another container.

Cosmetics

Cosmetics are associated with women; however, cosmetics may also include suntan lotions, aftershave lotions, acne medications, shampoo, and deodorants.[57] When cosmetics are thought of in this broader sense, all patients, including men, women, and teenagers, are using cosmetics. This is an important area to mention during routine patient education. Washing the hands before handling the lenses will prevent contaminating the contact lens surface with, for example, oils and creams. Water-soluble cosmetics are preferable for contact lens patients because they can be cleaned from the surface of the lens. Hypoallergenic cosmetics are often suggested for contact lens wearers; however, there are cosmetics that are made to be compatible with contact lenses. Cosmetics will become contaminated with time; thus, it is recommended that cosmetics be replaced every 3 to 6 months. In addition, cosmetics, especially eye makeup, should not be shared as this increases the risk of spreading ocular infections. Cosmetics should be applied around the eyes with caution to avoid blocking the openings to the glands, introducing them into the eye, or producing an abrasion from the application wand or cosmetic particles. Cosmetics should be applied after the lenses are inserted to prevent contamination of the lens surface. Hairspray, however, should be used before the insertion of contact lenses, or if the lenses are in, the eyes should be kept closed until the patient moves to another room away from the place where the hairspray was applied. Likewise, spray deodorants should be avoided.[58,59]

Miscellaneous Tips

Soft lens durability is generally 6 months to 1 year for conventional replacement lenses. The older the lenses, the more likely the lenses are to be deposited, which, in turn, results in decreased oxygen supply to the cornea, reduced vision, and ocular complications. Replacement of lenses on a frequent basis (daily, every 1–2 weeks, monthly, or quarterly) obviously reduces the number of complications that result from old, dirty lenses. *This option is the preferred method of lens wear.* Patients tend to extend the wear of the soft lenses dispensed beyond the time the practitioner recommends; therefore, emphasis should be placed on educating the patient thoroughly about the replacement schedule. Generally, daily or monthly replacement is easiest for the patient to remember.

It is permissible to take occasional short naps (1–2 hours) while wearing daily-wear soft lenses; however, there is always the risk the patient may sleep much longer than intended. Silicone hydrogel lenses provide greater oxygen to the eye, especially for those who may sleep or nap in their lenses. When a patient awakens, the lenses will likely have dehydrated to some extent, and a few drops of rewetting solution in the eye before lens removal are suggested to prevent a corneal abrasion. Likewise, anytime a soft lens becomes dehydrated, the lens should be soaked in solution to restore the lens to its hydrated state. Disinfection before wearing the lens is also recommended. Lenses that have been dehydrated for a lengthy period may not be fully restored to their previous condition. Soft lenses become very brittle when dehydrated and may break.

If, for some reason, the patient discontinues lens wear for a period (2 weeks or more), the wearing time should gradually be increased when lenses are worn again. The lenses should be disinfected within 24 hours of lens wear. This is also true of spare lenses. Spare lenses may be stored in a deep-welled case with frequent replacement of the solution; however, these lenses also should be disinfected within 24 hours before lens wear. Long-term storage of soft lenses depends on the solution used (see Tables 12.1 and 12.2).

Some very definite areas of potential noncompliance that should be avoided with soft lens wear are tap water, GP lens solutions, use of ophthalmic medications while wearing lenses, shallow lens cases, and swimming with the lenses on. Tap water and swimming place the patient at risk for *Acanthamoeba* keratitis. Ophthalmic medications and GP solutions contain preservatives and ingredients that may discolor the lens or cause a toxic reaction as a result of absorption into the lens. Soft lenses are often damaged by closure of the lens case, particularly lens cases that are shallow and intended for shipping GP lenses.

Patients should always *read* the labels on contact lens solution bottles. Some GP solutions look very similar to soft solutions. In addition, the person stocking the store shelves may not be educated regarding ophthalmic solutions; thus, tear substitutes may be mixed in with rewetting drops, GP solutions may be mixed in with soft solutions, or hydrogen peroxide solutions may be mixed in with saline solutions. The bottles are clearly marked regarding their purpose; however, it may be necessary to read the label. Of course, if patients are purchasing the same solutions given to them by their contact lens practitioner, they should be familiar enough with the solutions to be able to obtain the same ones every time. This makes a case for practitioners providing solutions for purchase directly from their office.

■ SUMMARY

Patient education and care of soft lenses are an important part of successful lens wear. Emphasis on education and lens care by the practitioner will aid in producing a serious patient attitude toward this aspect of lens wear. A summary nomogram on lens care and patient education is provided in Figure 12.7.

■ CLINICAL CASES

CASE 1

A patient who was a previous wearer received a replacement pair of lenses. Visual acuity was OD 20/15 and OS 20/15 on dispensing. Two days later, she calls to report hazy vision through her contact lenses that does not clear up on the blink. Slit-lamp examination reveals a filmy coating on the lenses. The patient admits to using hairspray after lens insertion.

SOLUTION: The patient needs to be re-educated on lens handling. She must be cautious about contaminating her lenses with cosmetic products that are on her hands or in the air. She should use hairspray before lens insertion or cover her eyes when using hairspray. After the use of hairspray, she should leave the room where the hairspray was used while it is still in the air.

CASE 2

A patient has monthly replacement lenses that are 4 months old (OD) and 1 month old on the OS. He wears the lenses on a daily-wear basis. He made an appointment for his annual examination. He admits that he is overdue for his visit, but as he had extra left lenses he had

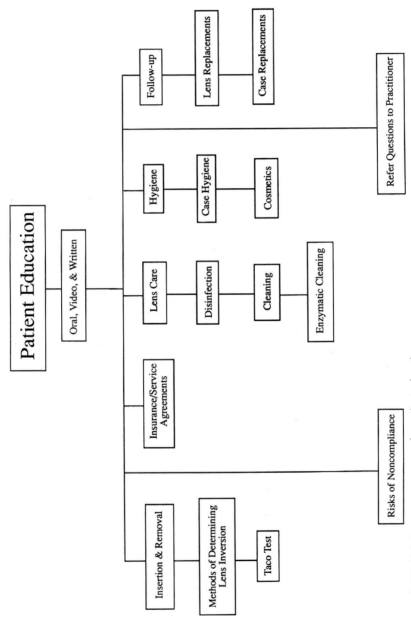

■ FIGURE 12.7 Summary nomogram for patient education

procrastinated about coming in. He reports that the right lens feels like it has sand or something under it. Lens removal and cleaning does not improve the condition.

SOLUTION: Upon examination with the biomicroscope, three jelly bumps are noted on the right lens. New lenses are ordered for the patient and the patient is educated on the importance of maintaining the recommended replacement schedule of disposing of his lenses every month.

CASE 3

A first-time soft lens wearer returns to the office for her 1-month follow-up visit. She thinks the lenses and visual acuity are good; however, she admits that her allergies seem to be bothering her slightly because her lenses, primarily her left lens, have been mildly irritating. Slit-lamp examination reveals two superficial slits in the midperiphery of the left lens. On lens removal and fluorescein evaluation, there is mild superficial corneal staining in the region where the slits were visible.

SOLUTION: The patient has fingernail tears in the lens that have penetrated the lens and resulted in irritation to the cornea in that region. Demonstration of the patient's removal technique reveals that she is using her fingernails to remove the lens. Re-education of soft lens removal with the pads of the fingers is demonstrated to her. If her nails are too long, she should be warned that it would be best to cut them to prevent a reoccurrence of the problem. Treatment for the corneal staining depends on the severity. In most cases where the patient is able to wear the lens and the staining is superficial, the patient only needs to discontinue lens wear for 12 to 24 hours and use a lubricating drop to improve comfort and healing during lens discontinuation.

CASE 4

A patient returns to the clinic for a follow-up visit. He has worn soft lenses for 8 years. His present lenses are 3 months old. Inspection of the lens reveals a small, round orange mark.

SOLUTION: This patient has a rust spot on the lens. The first thought of the practitioner should be that the patient is using tap water on the lenses and should be questioned about this. The rust spot may be the result of frequent tap water use (e.g., rinsing the cleaner from the lens). The patient should be cautioned about the dangers of tap water use and educated to never use tap water on the lenses. This should be documented in the patient's file. If the patient has not used tap water on the lens, the eye and lid should be examined for a metal foreign body that may be embedded. The lens should be replaced.

CASE 5

A patient is wearing a daily disposable soft lens. She reports that some days one lens or the other is mildly uncomfortable. Other than this, she is happy with the lenses.

SOLUTION: Most likely she is wearing an inverted lens. Soft lenses, especially some daily disposable lenses, are very thin and many are difficult to determine if they are inverted. The patient denies checking to see if the lens is inverted. The patient is re-educated on how to determine if the lens is wrong side out (e.g., the "taco test" and/or if the lens looks like a bowl or a saucer). If she is unsure if the lens is inverted and she notices mild lens awareness, she should remove the lens and try inserting it the other direction to see if this makes the lens more comfortable.

CASE 6

A patient is asked at the follow-up evaluation about the solutions she is using. She is not sure of the names but she knows the disinfecting solution she uses is in a green bottle.

SOLUTION: A patient will sometimes be unsure of the names of her solutions; however, she will be able to describe the bottle to her practitioner. This indicates two important points:

(a) if she is unsure of the name of the solution, then the practitioner must make sure she is purchasing the proper solution at the store, and (b) it will be helpful if the practitioner and staff are up to date on the solutions that are commercially available and have samples of these in the office to enable them to determine which solution the patient is using, either by description or by having the patient determine which of the samples she is using. In this case, she is using either Opti-Free Express or Opti-Free RepleniSH (both manufactured by Alcon Laboratories). Re-education of lens care solutions would be appropriate for this patient. In addition, the practitioner may find that patient compliance can be enhanced by dispensing solutions directly from his or her office, eliminating the patient's need to try to find appropriate solutions at the store or to price-shop.

CASE 7

A patient comes to your office with mildly irritated eyes. The patient has no discharge of any kind. She complains of dryness. Her wearing time is reduced because of the discomfort. She left her lenses out for 2 days, which seemed to help; however, on wearing lenses again the irritation returned. Tear breakup time was previously recorded as 12 seconds OU. Mild diffuse punctate staining is noted.

SOLUTION: This patient is likely experiencing a preservative sensitivity. She should be questioned about the solutions she is presently using. The lenses may need to be replaced. She should be given a new solution system, possibly one that is preservative free, or refit into a modality such as daily disposable lenses, which require no care regimen.

CASE 8

A 35-year-old woman desires replacement soft lenses. The patient has worn soft lenses for 2 years, dispensed from another office. The present pair of lenses is 6 months old. The patient wears substantial amounts of eyeliner, mascara, and eyeshadow. Biomicroscopy reveals much debris in the tear layer in addition to surface deposits and pigment spots on the lenses. The patient's eyeliner is present on the lid margins, and it is evident that this is flaking off into the eye. The patient admits to separating her eyelashes with a straight pin, keeping cosmetics for a year or more, and frequent sensations of burning and discomfort as if something is behind the lens.

SOLUTION: Caution should be taken in fitting this patient. Patient education is necessary to avoid serious complications. Abrasions are often caused by trapped debris such as mascara behind the lens. Cosmetics can become contaminated, and it is wise to have patients replace their cosmetics every 3 months. An eye infection or corneal ulcer may occur if this contamination occurs and is introduced to the eye. This patient needs to be cautious that her hands are washed thoroughly before handling the lenses, that lenses are inserted before applying makeup, that eyeliner is never placed on the lid margin closest to the eye, and that lenses are properly cleaned and disinfected to clean off any makeup that adheres to the lenses. This patient should benefit from a comprehensive education program and disposable/frequent lens replacement.

CASE 9

A long-time patient comes to the office complaining of decreased wearing time and lens awareness. The patient has been lost to follow-up for 2 years. During that period of time, he admits to extending his lenses to a period of 4 to 6 months. When asked about the care regimen he uses, he pulls out a plastic bag containing an assortment of private-label solutions.

SOLUTION: Lens replacement schedules are discussed with the patient and he agrees to a monthly replacement lens. The patient is given a new care regimen. Both the care regimen and the replacement schedule are thoroughly discussed and the importance of adhering to both is noted. The patient seems somewhat skeptical that the solutions and replacement schedule are the issue, but agrees to closely follow this recommended plan for the next couple of months. At his 2-month visit, he is pleased with his lens comfort and wearing time. He admits that replacing the lenses monthly and the new care regimen have made the difference.

CASE 10

A patient comes to the office for the first time for an emergency visit. He is experiencing irritation and injection in the left eye. The patient reports sleeping in his lenses for 7 to 10 days. The brand he is using is not approved for extended wear. When asked about his care regimen, he reports that he is using purified water and sea salt. He does not like to use chemicals in his eyes. He reports that the practitioner at the previous establishment where he purchased lenses was aware of his sleeping in the lenses and his care regimen.

SOLUTION: First the patient's immediate problem must be addressed. This patient is at risk for *Acanthamoeba* keratitis because of the homemade saline use. This patient may never be a good candidate for contact lenses, depending on the diagnosis of his left eye and his ability to be compliant to a proper lens-wearing and care regimen. If he is ever to wear lenses again, thorough education about daily-wear and extended-wear lenses, following recommended guidelines, and use of proper solutions must be discussed. Some patients are willingly noncompliant and some have been given poor instructions from another source. Differentiating the cause of the noncompliance will be the difference between fitting this patient again in lenses and refusing to fit on the basis that he is a poor candidate. Of course, all this is based on the diagnosis and recovery of the left eye.

CASE 11

A young college student comes to see you and is concerned with irritation and dryness with her contact lenses. She has been wearing lenses since she was 12 years old and had been successful until the last few months. She is using an MPS chemical disinfection system, which she has used for several years, and has worn the same lens brand for the last 2 years.

SOLUTION: Upon examination with the biomicroscope, mild diffuse punctate staining is noted OU. The patient reports using "Visine" drops during the day if her lenses feel dry and look red. The patient is given a new pair of lenses and contact lens rewetting drops. She is advised to continue the use of her current MPS care regimen. She is asked to not use any rewetting solutions except the one prescribed to her. When the patient returns for her follow-up examination, she reports good comfort with her lenses. No corneal staining is evident with the biomicroscope. The patient is educated on using only solutions that are specified for contact lens use, and that if she is unsure to call the office to verify that she may alter her care regimen. Eye drops that are not recommended for soft contact lenses may have incompatible preservatives or build up preservatives within the matrix, resulting in corneal staining.

CLINICAL PROFICIENCY CHECKLIST

- Chemical disinfection generally provides one-bottle systems that encourage patient compliance; however, rubbing and rinsing the lenses before disinfection is still the best method to fight bacteria, fungi, and *Acanthamoeba* and to maintain lens cleanliness.
- Oxidative disinfection is an effective method of disinfection and is especially beneficial for patients prone to preservative sensitivities.
- Thorough cleaning and rinsing should be performed before lens disinfection.
- The value of patient education should not be underestimated. Patients should be taught insertion, removal, lens care and handling, and risks of noncompliance.
- Patients should be told to contact their eye care practitioner with any questions.

(Continued)

- The best type of in-office disinfection of diagnostic lenses is disposable diagnostic lenses.

- Patients should be taught simple hygiene; they should wash their hands with soap and water, and dry them before handling lenses.

- Frequent case replacement will aid in prevention of biofilm and case contamination.

- Frequent lens replacement prevents soft lens deposits such as jelly bumps, lipid and mucoprotein deposits, and the complications that may result.

- Tap water should never be used on soft lenses because of the risk of *Acanthamoeba* keratitis.

- Many complications with soft lenses are a result of noncompliance, which may be caused by poor education on the part of the practitioner.

REFERENCES

1. Campbell R, Caroline P. Multipurpose non-keratitis. Contact Lens Spectrum 1997;12:56.
2. Soni PS, Horner DG, Ross J. Ocular response to lens care systems in adolescent soft contact lens wearers. Optom Vis Sci 1996;73:70–85.
3. Mack CJ. Contact lenses 2007. Contact Lens Spectrum 2008;23(1):26–34.
4. Epstein AB. How products fail: déjà vu solution and lens material incompatibilities once again appear on the radar, but this time with more serious consequences. Rev Optom Supplement 2007;144(10):11–14.
5. Chang DC, Grant GB, O'Donnell K, et al. Fusarium Keratitis Investigation Team. Multistate outbreak of Fusarium Keratitis associated with use of a contact lens solution. JAMA 2006;296(8):953–963.
6. Ward MA. Mycotic keratitis and lens care. Contact Lens Spectrum 2006;21(7):27.
7. Joslin CE, Tu EY, McMahon TT, et al. Epidemiological characteristics of a Chicago-area Acanthamoeba keratitis outbreak. Am J Ophthalmol 2006;142(2):212–217.
8. Gutman C. Acanthamoeba keratitis increasing at alarming rate. Ophthalmol Times 2006;Jan. 1.
9. Weisbarth RE, Henderson BA. Hydrogel lens care regimens and patient education. In: Bennett ES, Weissman BA, eds. Clinical Contact Lens Practice. Philadelphia: Lippincott Williams & Wilkins, 2005:381–419.
10. Penley CA, Willis SW, Sickler SG. Comparative antimicrobial efficacy of soft and rigid gas permeable contact lens solutions against *Acanthamoeba*. CLAO J 1989;15(7–9):257–260.
11. Liedel KK, Begley CG. The effectiveness of soft contact lens disinfection systems against Acanthamoeba on the lens surface. J Am Optom Assoc 1996;67:135–142.
12. Zadnik K. *Acanthamoeba* and bacterial keratitis in hydrogel lens wearers. Presented at the Twenty-ninth Annual Contact Lens and Primary Care Congress of the Heart of America Contact Lens Society. Kansas City, MO, February 1990.
13. Bennett ES. *Acanthamoeba* keratitis in 2007: stay informed but calm. Contact Lens Spectrum 2007; 22(7):50–52.
14. Klein P, Solomon J, Snyder RP. Cleaning: the key to contact lens care. Rev Optom 1990;127(4):42–44.
15. Sakuma S, Reeh B, Dang D, et al. Comparative efficacies of four soft contact lens disinfection solutions. Int Contact Lens Clin 1996;23:234–239.
16. Watanabe RK. Contact lens solution update 2006. Contact Lens Spectrum 2006;21(8):26–31.
17. Thompson TT. Tyler's Quarterly Soft Contact Lens Parameter Guide 2007;25(1):1–7.
18. White P, Scott C. 2007 Contact Lenses & Solutions Summary Supplement to Contact Lens Spectrum 2007;22(7).
19. Gromacki SJ. Taking a closer look at hydrogen peroxide products. Contact Lens Spectrum 2007;22(2):26.
20. Gromacki SJ. Hydrogen peroxide disinfection. Contact Lens Spectrum 2006;21(12):19.
21. Connor CG, Presley L, Finchum SM, et al. The effectiveness of several current soft contact lens care regimens against Aspergillus. CLAO J 1998;24:82–84.
22. Sibley MJ. Hydrogen peroxide residues: a comparison between chemical and osmotic extraction. Contact Lens Spectrum 1988;3(8):39–43.
23. Melton JW, Phillips JH. Patient comfort comparison of hydrogen peroxide systems. Contact Lens Spectrum 1988;3(9):48–51.
24. Anger CB, Ambrus K, Stoecker J, et al. Antimicrobial efficacy of hydrogen peroxide for contact lens disinfection. Contact Lens Spectrum 1990;5(11):46–51.
25. Key JE, Monnat K. Comparative disinfectant efficacy of two disinfecting solutions against *Pseudomonas aeruginosa*. CLAO J 1996;22:118–121.
26. Hughes R, Kilvington S. Comparison of hydrogen peroxide contact lens disinfection systems and solutions against *Acanthamoeba polyphaga*. Antimicrob Agents Chemother 2001;45(7):2038–2043.
27. Mowrey-McKee M, George M. Contact lens solution efficacy against *Acanthamoeba castellani*. Eye Contact Lens Sci Clin Pract 2007;33(5):211–215.

28. Simmons PA, Edrington TB, Lao KF, et al. The efficacy of disinfection systems for in-office storage of hydrogel contact lenses. Int Contact Lens Clin 1996;23:94–97.

29. Mandell RB. Symptomatology and aftercare. In: Mandell RB, ed. Contact Lens Practice, 4th ed. Springfield, IL: Charles C. Thomas, 1988:598–643.

30. Friedberg DN, Stenson SM. AIDS and your eye exam. CLAO Patient information pamphlet 1994–2004.

31. Ward M. In-office hydrogel contact lens disinfection. Contact Lens Spectrum 2005;20(7):27.

32. Christensen B, Janes JA. Clinical investigation of the new SoftWear saline. Contact Lens Spectrum 1990;5(11): 37–40.

33. Zigler LG. SoftWear saline and the sensitive patient. Contact Lens Spectrum 1990;5(12):50–51.

34. Kleist FD. Appearance and nature of hydrophilic contact lens deposits. I. Protein and other organic deposits. Int Contact Lens Clin 1979;6(3):49–58.

35. Kleist FD. Appearance and nature of hydrophilic contact lens deposits. II. Inorganic deposits. Int Contact Lens Clin 1979;6(4):177–186.

36. Begley CG, Waggoner PJ. An analysis of nodular deposits on soft contact lenses. J Am Optom Assoc 1991;62(3): 208–214.

37. Caroline PJ, Robin JB, Gindi JJ. Microscopic and elemental analysis of deposits on extended wear soft contact lenses. CLAO J 1985;11(4):311–316.

38. Ward M. Soft lens daily cleaners: what's available. Contact Lens Spectrum 2006;21(11):21.

39. Thomas E, Stein H, Cox D, et al. A new standard in lens hygiene. Contact Lens Spectrum 1996;11:32–36.

40. Szczotka-Flynn LB. Chemical properties of contact lens rewetters: a review of hyaluronic acid as a contemporary ingredient in contact lens rewetters. Contact Lens Spectrum 2006;21(4):40–45.

41. Harris MG. Lens care systems—pros and cons. Presented at the Twenty-eighth Annual Contact Lens and Primary Care Congress of the Heart of America Contact Lens Society. Kansas City, MO, February 1989.

42. Schafer J. Improving compliance with patient education. Contact Lens Spectrum 2007;22(10):50.

43. Lanier JC. Ensuring compliance and patient satisfaction. Contact Lens Spectrum 2007;22(6):50–51.

44. Lens-care systems: what they cost. Consumer Reports 1989;June:416–420.

45. O'Connor M (A. C. Nielson, Inc.). The "real" cost of soft contact lens care: a Nielson report. Presented at the Eighteenth Annual National Research Symposium, Toronto, Canada, August 1991.

46. Schornack JA, Watanabe R, Dillehay SM, et al. Annual soft contact lens solution usage and costs. Contact Lens Spectrum 1998;13:43–48.

47. Quinn TG. Help your patients be compliant. Contact Lens Spectrum 2006;21(11):47.

48. Ward MA. How private-label solutions affect your practice. Contact Lens Spectrum 2006;21(3):25.

49. Lowther GE. Patient compliance. Int Contact Lens Clin 1988;15(5):142.

50. "Horror stories" fail to stir compliance. Rev Optom 1987;124(11):10.

51. Willcox MDP, Power KN, Stapleton F, et al. Potential sources of bacteria that are isolated from contact lenses during wear. Optom Vis Sci 1997;74:1030–1038.

52. Velasco J, Bermudez J. Comparative study of the microbial flora on contact lenses, in lens cases and in maintenance liquids. Int Contact Lens Clin 1996;23:55–58.

53. Lakkis C, Harding AS, Brennan NA. Case contamination with hydrogel lens wear. Clin Exp Optom 1997; May–June:111.

54. Snyder C. Planned replacement of contact lens cases: rationale and practical approaches. Presented at the Eighteenth Annual National Research Symposium, Toronto, Canada, August 1991.

55. Smythe JL. The forgotten lens care step. Contact Lens Spectrum 2003;18(9):21.

56. Gromacki SJ. Making a case for clean cases. Contact Lens Spectrum 2006;Special Edition:12–13.

57. Tlachac CA. Cosmetics for contact lens wearers. Contact Lens Spectrum 1988;3(8):65–70.

58. Ghormley NR. Contact lens solutions and materials: cosmetics and contact lenses. Int Eyecare 1986;1(3):218.

59. Coopersmith L, Weinstock FJ. Current recommendations and practice regarding soft lens replacement and disinfection. CLAO J 1997;23:172–176.

CHAPTER 13

Soft Lens Problem Solving

J. Bart Campbell, Vinita Allee Henry, and John W. Marohn

Two significant developments in the field of soft lenses have enormously enhanced the clinician's available tools for soft lens problem solving: the development of modern disposable lenses and the development of silicone hydrogel lenses. During the 1990s, disposable contact lenses rapidly became the modality of choice for most wearers being fitted for the first time or being refitted with hydrogel lenses. This resulted in changes in the way contact lenses are perceived and cared for by the public, and in the way practitioners manage fittings and many complications.

However, most disposable contact lenses are manufactured with the same hydrogel materials initially used for conventional replacement lenses. Consequently, there is no inherent difference in the interaction between the eye and the lens. That said, hydrogel disposable contact lenses do provide substantial benefits in managing deposition-related complications. In fact, such complications should be eliminated when disposable lenses are used properly.

Disposable lenses have also encouraged manufacturers to develop a generation of care systems that emphasize convenience through the utilization of multipurpose solutions. Although these systems should enhance compliance, they may not accomplish the task of disinfection and cleaning when patients do not follow instructions.[1,2]

The emergence of silicone hydrogel lenses in the late 1990s addressed a major problem not solved by the initial generation of hydrogel disposable lenses: oxygen transmissibility (Dk/t). Lenses manufactured from silicone hydrogel materials have vastly improved Dk/t values compared to conventional hydrogel materials. This characteristic, combined with the existing disposable modality, has enabled the clinician to address two of the biggest causes of soft lens problems: lens deposition and corneal hypoxia. However, patient compliance remains a key issue in avoiding complications. This fact, combined with a demand for 30-day continuous wear (CW) of silicone hydrogel lenses, has resulted in the conclusion that even these lenses are not without complications.[3]

It must also be noted that there are still conventional replacement contact lens wearers in existence. Patients who have extremely high refractive errors, high amounts of astigmatism, and other special conditions often have not been fitted in disposable lenses because there are fewer lenses available in the required parameters. These patients, as well as the wearers of disposable lenses who do not replace their lenses or who experience non–deposition-related complications, continue to provide the practitioner with ample justification to be concerned with soft lens problem solving.

■ TERMINOLOGY

Most lenses that practitioners refer to as "disposable" do not actually meet the criteria for disposable lenses that have been defined by the Food and Drug Administration (FDA). To meet the FDA criteria, a device must be used only once and then discarded. Only the so-called "1-day" or "daily disposable" lenses are routinely used in this fashion. Typically, practitioners prescribe "disposable" lenses to be replaced every 7 to 14 days. Further complicating the terminology issue are lenses prescribed as "planned-replacement," "frequent-replacement," or

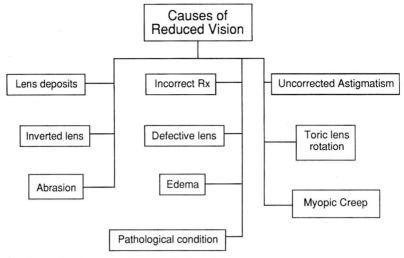

■ **FIGURE 13.1** Summary of causes of reduced vision.

"programmed-replacement" lenses. In this replacement schedule, the lenses are usually replaced every 1 to 3 months.

▓ SYMPTOMS

Reduced Vision

Visual reduction as a result of contact lens wear may be attributed to a number of causes (Fig. 13.1). A problem-oriented case history is often invaluable in disclosing the factor(s) instrumental in contact lens-induced reduction of visual acuity. The clinician should determine onset and duration, and whether the reduced visual acuity is present when spectacles are worn. Reasons for contact lens-related visual acuity reduction may include lens contamination, uncorrected refractive error, defective lens material, improper lens-to-cornea fitting relationship, and excessive tearing. The use of pinhole visual acuity measurement may assist in determining if the cause of decreased visual acuity is uncorrected refractive error. Visual acuity reduction, noted with both contact lens and spectacle correction, may be attributed to corneal abnormalities, including edema, abrasions, punctate keratitis, and infectious keratitis. The presence of intraocular abnormalities as a source of visual acuity reduction must also be recognized, and all contact lens wearers should undergo regularly scheduled comprehensive visual examinations.

Lens Deposits

Surface deposits are most often attributed to inadequate lens hygiene. A mucoproteinaceous film, primarily composed of lysozyme, is frequently the major factor in causing reduced vision.[4] Complaints of "foggy" or "hazy" vision with distortion, especially when bright lights are viewed, are often expressed by affected patients. This symptom will not be noted after the lens is removed. If it is, the possibility of corneal edema must be considered. Lipid deposits and calcium–lipid complexes (e.g., "jelly bumps"), in addition to other organic and inorganic debris, may cause visual reduction, but their principal effect is on lens comfort.[5] Diagnosis is achieved by examining the lens in vivo with the biomicroscope; excessive deposition may be noted without the use of magnification.

Treatment of lens deposition often depends on the type of deposit. Protein coatings, if observed before extensive accumulation is present, may be removed with enzymatic cleaning because of their superficial nature. If the lens is moderately coated, a series of two to three successive enzymatic cleanings may be necessary to remove the protein adequately; a weekly enzymatic cleaning should be sufficient for most patients. Utilization of a daily protein remover, either one incorporated into a multipurpose solution or a separate solution like SupraClens (Alcon Laboratories), may be helpful. Rubbing of the lens following enzyme soaking with either saline solution or cleaner, in addition to the recommended daily cleaning, may be beneficial in removing any remaining protein. The presence of jelly bumps on the lens surface necessitates replacement of the lens because of their penetrating nature into the lens matrix. Removal of the jelly bumps results in subsequent holes or pits, rendering the lens inadequate for continued wear. Nevertheless, the current practice is to refit the patient in disposable contact lenses if possible. This precludes the need for "heroic" measures to save a contaminated lens.

Incorrect Prescription

Reduction in Snellen visual acuity will be observed if the patient is wearing an incorrect lens prescription. Verification of soft lens power is difficult to perform because of the nature of the material but may be necessary if inadequate visual acuity is noted. If possible, it is desirable to evaluate new lenses on the patient's eyes at the time of dispensing. This can easily detect incorrect prescriptions, visible lens defects, and uncomfortable lenses. Unfortunately, such evaluations may not be possible in every case and are never possible with every disposable lens. In these situations, patients must be thoroughly educated to be aware of symptoms that indicate defective lenses and to discontinue wear of the affected lens. In addition to manufacturer error, the possibility of such problems as lens reversal by the patient or practitioner or an incorrect refraction must be considered. An expedient method of determining whether the reduction in visual acuity is refractive or possibly pathologic in nature is a pinhole visual acuity measurement. An overrefraction is also definitive in indicating whether the patient is wearing an incorrect prescription or whether the lenses may be switched. If the difference in the refractive error between the two eyes is relatively equal, the patient may not notice that the lenses are switched. New lenses must be ordered with the correct prescription or, if switched, each lens should be placed in the appropriate eye.

Uncorrected Refractive Astigmatism

Another source of reduced visual acuity in soft lens wearers is uncorrected refractive astigmatism. The inherent flexibility of these lenses limits their ability to correct effectively for astigmatism generated by the corneal surface. Approximately 16% of the refractive astigmatism is compensated for by the lens–cornea interface, reflecting the inability of the soft lens to conform totally to the corneal surface.[6] Patients with 0.75 D to 1.00 D of refractive astigmatism may begin to experience symptoms of decreased visual acuity while wearing spherical soft lenses.[7] Some aspheric soft contact lens designs have been found to provide good vision in patients with small amounts of astigmatism (i.e., 0.50–1.00 D). Aspheric soft contact lens designs do not correct astigmatism, but enhance the optics by reducing the spherical aberration; thus, the patient may perceive enhanced vision.[8,9] The ability to tolerate small amounts of blur depends primarily on the visual awareness and activities performed by the contact lens wearer. Persons who perform extensive near tasks involving small detail may require a toric lens correction. Overrefraction with placement of the appropriate cylinder in the phoropter will improve visual acuity, allowing the patient to determine the acceptability of the compromised vision. Astigmatic correction may be obtained with the use of either a soft toric or rigid gas-permeable (GP) contact lens.

Toric Lens Rotation

Soft toric lens rotation, either subsequent to each blink or as a result of persistent mislocation, is a principal cause of reduced visual acuity in astigmatic patients. Patients who exhibit astigmatism on an oblique axis are more prone to lens rotation than are those exhibiting with-the-rule and against-the-rule astigmatism. An oblique cross-cylinder effect, generated as a result of misalignment between the refractive cylinder axis and the toric lens, results in disturbances in visual acuity. Near tasks may be compromised by toric lens rotation with eye convergence, resulting from encyclo-rotation of the globe. A nasal and upward rotation of soft lenses has been noted and may need to be compensated for in axis selection, especially for presbyopic and esotropic patients.[7] This problem is even more pronounced for presbyopic patients wearing toric contact lenses with one eye corrected for distance vision and the other corrected for near vision (i.e., monovision). Slit-lamp examination of the toric lens will determine whether the lens is stable with adequate centration and movement or whether excessive "rocking" occurs after each blink. Refraction performed over the patient's current contact lenses or diagnostic lenses may be beneficial in determining the appropriate power and axis to order for the patient. This is especially apparent in persons with refractive astigmatism >3.00 D, in whom small amounts of rotation that can have a significant impact on visual acuity may be difficult to assess.[10] Excessive lens movement may require a steeper base curve to reduce rotation and improve visual acuity. Changing to a different design (e.g., slab off, thin zone designs) may also be beneficial. The option of refitting into spherical GP lenses may also be considered in a challenging case, especially when corneal toricity accounts for most of the patient's refractive astigmatism.

Defective Lenses

Characteristics of a defective lens include either abrasions (scratches, tears, nicks, holes) or poor optics. Both may contribute to irritation, discomfort, and reduced visual acuity. During initial wear, lenses with abrasions are the most common cause of lens replacement. Although the actual defect may not always cause reduced vision, deposit accumulation in the area of a scratch or tear may affect visual acuity. Poor lens manufacturing may result in inadequate optics, resulting in the need for lens exchange. Increased tearing and mucous production secondary to irritation of the palpebral conjunctiva from an elevated lens defect may also degrade vision. Biomicroscopy will elicit the source of the problem if a lens abrasion exists. Careful examination of the lens edge may be necessary to locate a nick or small tear, many of which may not be detected by the practitioner. The absence of improvement in visual acuity with an overrefraction may be indicative of poor optics, necessitating lens replacement. A small peripheral tear, if not irritating to the patient, may be clinically tolerable but will undoubtedly increase in size with continued lens manipulation. Lens replacement is undoubtedly the most effective method of handling defective lenses.

Patients may report discomfort or heightened lens awareness when there are no observable lens defects. If the symptoms are present in only one eye, briefly switching the lenses can determine if the discomfort follows the lens or remains in the initially affected eye. If it follows the lens, then the most expedient solution is simply to replace the lens. If the discomfort remains only in the initially affected eye, closer examination of the eye itself is warranted. Replacement of the lens may still be the only way to alleviate the patient's concerns, even when no clinically observable cause for the discomfort is present.

Lens Inversion

A common complaint, especially with new soft lens wearers, is difficulty with lens inversion. Patients wearing thin lenses often exhibit frustration in determining whether the lens is properly oriented before insertion (i.e., "right side out"). Mild irritation may be observed as a result of increased movement of the lens. Examination of the lens edge with the biomicroscope will reveal standoff from the bulbar conjunctiva and excessive movement. Some lens manufacturers print their name or a symbol at the periphery of the lens to facilitate determining the presence of lens inversion. Familiarity with each design is essential, as there is no consistency between manufacturers. The "taco test" may assist patients in placing the lens correctly on the eye (Chapter 12). Removal of the lens, accompanied by correct orientation, will resolve any decrease in visual acuity or irritation noted by the patient. Patients should be counseled that an inverted lens will not damage their eye and that if they are unsure whether the lens is inverted, it is acceptable simply to remove it and try wearing it with the other side toward the eye.

Reduction of Visual Acuity with Contact Lenses and Spectacles

A reduction in visual acuity, apparent with both contact lens and spectacle correction, may be indicative of a more serious complication. Removal of the contact lenses and inspection of the cornea and conjunctiva are imperative in determining the cause of the decreased visual acuity. Some physiologic factors that may influence vision with soft contact lens wear include the following:

1. An abrasion secondary to insertion and removal, poor lens fit, surface defects, or a foreign body.
2. Edema related to the physical fit, water content, prescription, or lens deposition.
3. Central punctate staining secondary to poor lens fit, solution sensitivity, surface defects, inadequate wetting, poor tear exchange, or trapped debris.
4. Increased mucous production as a result of giant papillary conjunctivitis.
5. "Myopic creep" resulting from corneal edema.
6. Irregular astigmatism or corneal distortion secondary to keratoconus or other causes.
7. A pathologic condition affecting the anterior or posterior segment that is unrelated to contact lens wear.

Discomfort

When a soft contact lens wearer experiences discomfort, the lens should be removed immediately. If the discomfort persists, the patient should be educated to contact the practitioner immediately. A comprehensive case history will be very important in determining the cause of the pain (Fig. 13.2). A differential diagnosis is possible by classifying the discomfort into one of four categories. It is important to determine if the discomfort occurs on insertion or after lens removal and if the onset is immediate or delayed. Duration of the discomfort (e.g., transient, constant, or intermittent) should be determined. Further biomicroscopic evaluation of the cornea, both with lens wear and on removal, will aid in determination of the source of the discomfort. In addition, evaluation of corneal staining with fluorescein application is important.

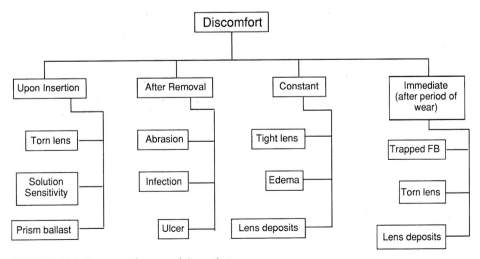

■ **FIGURE 13.2** Summary of causes of discomfort.

Discomfort on Lens Insertion

If discomfort occurs on insertion, the source is most likely either a torn lens, a sensitivity to the solutions used, or (if applicable) the prism ballast of a toric lens. A torn lens can be detected by carefully examining both the entire lens surface and the lens edge with the biomicroscope. The upper lid should be raised to evaluate the superior lens edge. Lens tears may be difficult to observe. The lens should be carefully observed on the blink, which will make the tear more evident. The tear may actually be a hole or nick in the lens or have the appearance of a scratch or adhered debris. Apparent trapped debris that cannot be cleaned off and remains on the lens with a blink is most likely a lens defect. A torn lens should be replaced immediately.

If a patient uses an improper solution in the eye or on the soft lens (i.e., hydrogen peroxide or a GP lens solution) or has acquired a sensitivity to the preservative in a solution, an immediate burning and stinging sensation will be experienced. Lens removal should improve the discomfort; however, a mild to moderate superficial punctate keratitis will remain; thus, mild discomfort and injection may still be present. By questioning the patient about the solutions used with the lenses and evaluating the cornea and conjunctiva with a biomicroscope, the practitioner will be able to determine if the source of the discomfort is preservative sensitivity. If the practitioner is still unsure, another care system can be prescribed for the patient. Replacing the lens with a fresh, sterile lens is optimal. If the discomfort is eliminated by a change in the solution system, sensitivity to the solution was most likely the cause. In severe cases, lens wear may have to be discontinued until the subjective discomfort has been alleviated. This may occur after a few hours or take up to several days.

A rare cause of discomfort is the prism ballast of a toric lens. Occasionally, a patient will complain of lens sensation caused by the thickness of the lens in the area of the prism ballast. If no other source of discomfort is found, a change in the type of toric lens design (i.e., use of eccentric lenticulation, thin zones) may alleviate the lens sensation.

Discomfort with a previously unworn lens versus discomfort with a worn but previously comfortable lens may be approached differently. If the lens is new and the patient experiences discomfort from a design that has previously been satisfactory, the cause may be debris trapped under the lens on insertion. Simply removing the lens and rinsing it may provide relief from the discomfort. If the discomfort persists and the cause is not visible, the lens itself may be defective in a way that is not visible with conventional inspection techniques. The most expedient course of action is to replace the lens. If the discomfort occurs with a lens that has been previously worn with no discomfort, the most likely cause is a torn lens. The lens should be removed and inspected. If no damage is found, the lens may be rinsed and inserted again to determine if the discomfort persists.

Discomfort after Lens Removal

When pain or discomfort is present after lens removal, the origin of the problem is typically the cornea. Pain that continues after lens removal is an ocular emergency, and the patient should be evaluated in the office as soon as possible. Corneal abrasions, ocular infections, corneal ulcers, or other ocular problems may be causing the pain. Fluorescein evaluation is important in determining the extent of the corneal disturbance. Discomfort and pain that remain after the removal of soft lenses should be taken seriously until a differential diagnosis is made.

Constant Discomfort during Lens Wear

When the discomfort of soft lenses is constant, the source of the discomfort may be a poorly fitting lens, corneal edema and edema-related symptoms (i.e., microcysts), or lens deposits. Biomicroscopy and fluorescein evaluation will aid in determination of the cause. A compression ring around the limbal area after lens removal is indicative of a tight lens. Higher-modulus silicone hydrogel lenses that are fitted too flat may exhibit edge lift and cause discomfort. After alteration of the lens parameters, either by changing the base curve radius (BCR) or the lens diameter, the symptoms should disappear. For a patient experiencing edema-related symptoms, a change to a higher-Dk/t silicone hydrogel lens will be beneficial.

Another cause of constant discomfort with a soft lens is a deposited lens. These deposits will be evident when the lens is viewed with the biomicroscope. The deposits may be a result of poor lens care, old lenses, or lenses that have been contaminated with substances such as hair spray or lotion. Silicone hydrogel lenses are more prone to lipid deposits than conventional hydrogel lenses. Despite the claims of "no rub" solutions, silicone hydrogel lenses should be rubbed upon removal to aid in the removal of lipid deposits. The authors recommend educating all soft lens patients to rub and rinse their lenses to provide the cleanest and most comfortable lenses. Replacing the deposited lens with a clean, new lens will alleviate the symptoms.

Sudden Discomfort after a Period of Lens Wear

Patients may experience sudden discomfort after the lens has been worn for several hours. The most frequent cause of sudden discomfort is a trapped foreign body, such as dust or cosmetic particles. Removing the lens and rinsing it with solution should eliminate this discomfort. A large foreign body may cause a corneal abrasion; therefore, if the pain continues, it is important for the patient to be evaluated in the office. A deposited lens, especially one with jelly bumps, or a contaminated lens may result in discomfort that increases as the period of lens wear increases. Finally, a torn lens may also cause immediate discomfort; however, typically the discomfort is noticed on lens insertion. Obviously, the treatment for a foreign body is its removal. If the lens is not damaged, deposited, or torn, the lens may be worn again. Conversely, a damaged lens will require replacement. In the case of a foreign body, the cornea, conjunctiva, and lids should be examined to make sure the foreign body has not become embedded.

Burning or Stinging Sensation

Burning and stinging are most often related to contact lens solution sensitivity. Reinforcement of appropriate lens hygiene at each visit is beneficial in maintaining patient compliance and avoiding unnecessary irritation. Irritation with continued use of a chemical disinfecting system may indicate a possible hypersensitivity or toxic reaction to the preservative and/or an added surfactant. Discomfort noted by patients is typically minimal because of the low concentration of preservatives in the solution. Often the complaint is a feeling of dryness, rather than burning. A generalized stippling is indicative of a toxic or hypersensitivity reaction, and, if severe enough, may elicit tearing and photophobia as well as decreased visual acuity. Patients who exhibit this problem may achieve success with the use of a preservative-free, hydrogen peroxide disinfecting system. Incomplete neutralization of hydrogen peroxide can result in the symptoms of burning and stinging; a low pH (4.0) after disinfection and the buffer system to control pH may also contribute to irritation. A typical scenario with systems that use a catalytic disc for neutralization is a gradually increasing burning sensation each morning on lens insertion. Although most patients no longer use a separate daily cleaner or enzyme cleaner with their soft lenses, the use of a daily cleaner before insertion or inadequate rinsing of the lens after cleaning may elicit a burning sensation. Any residual cleaner remaining on the lens after enzyme cleaning may also cause discomfort. A comprehensive case history may be extremely beneficial in determining the cause of the ocular irritation. Reviewing cleaning and disinfection procedures at each visit can assist in alleviating solution-related discomfort associated with the use of inappropriate technique. Instructions and diagrams may help in maintaining patient compliance with acceptable cleaning and disinfecting procedures. The emergence of multipurpose solutions may make it difficult to determine the offending component, as many of these products contain surfactants and other compounds in the disinfecting solution (Fig. 13.3).

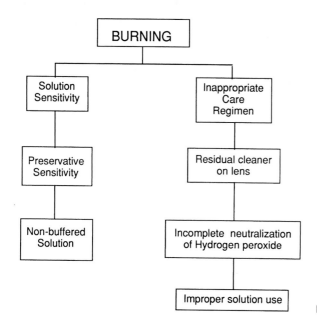

■ **FIGURE 13.3** Summary of causes of burning.

Photophobia

Definition

The term *photophobia* is often used loosely in describing irritation and discomfort as a result of contact lens wear. When the term is used appropriately, photophobia is typically considered a pathologic condition that occurs when light entering the eye causes pain. Photophobia may be contrasted with dazzle, a sensation of discomfort as a result of excessive light that is usually not associated with pain. A temporary sensation of dazzle is experienced with inadequate adaptation of the eye from dark to lighted conditions. Also, dazzle, unlike photophobia, is not accompanied by blepharospasm and lacrimation. Pathologic conditions affecting the anterior segment of the eye are often accompanied by photophobia. Typically, the more superficial the corneal defect, the more severe the photophobia because of the arrangement of the innervation of the epithelium.[11] It is important to remember that photophobia is a *symptom* of an ocular problem and that the logical method to address this symptom is to determine and then treat the condition causing the photophobia.

Causes

Epithelial abrasions may be observed in contact lens wearers and, in severe cases, may induce photophobia. Superficial corneal abrasions may occur as a result of contact lens defects (including tears and nicks), moderate lens "overwear," mild trauma, trapped debris, and an uneven surface. Often, superficial defects go unnoticed by the patient but may result in mild discomfort and irritation. Deeper abrasions typically result in more severe pain, including lacrimation, blepharospasm, and photophobia. Removal of the entire thickness of the epithelium occurs most commonly as a result of blunt trauma (e.g., hand, thumb, or ball in the eye), improper insertion or removal of the contact lens, or a foreign body under the lens.[12]

In addition to abrasions, photophobia has been attributed to other factors.[5,11,13] Initial adaptation to contact lens wear may initiate photophobia, and this is considered normal unless the symptom continues longer than a few weeks. Uncorrected refractive error and residual astigmatism may also contribute to a photophobic response.[11]

Determining the Cause of Photophobia

A thorough case history may be extremely beneficial in eliciting the cause of photophobia. Biomicroscopic examination of both the contact lens and the cornea will eliminate any gross defects contributing to the symptoms. The presence of discharge, in conjunction with lacrimation and blepharospasm, may indicate the possibility of infection. The type of discharge (e.g., mucopurulent, watery, stringy) should be elicited in determining the possible etiology. Fluorescein staining is beneficial in determining the presence, location, and depth of an abrasion. The configuration of the staining pattern may allude to a causative factor (e.g., tear, nick, foreign body, deposited lens). Examination of the lens under magnification may further assist in locating any lens defects.

Treatment of the Causes of Photophobia

Conservative treatment of superficial abrasions includes contact lens removal to ensure proper healing. Epithelial cell coverage of the abrasion usually is complete within 24 hours. Although antibiotic therapy is typically not warranted, consideration may be necessary in patients exhibiting poor lid hygiene, coated lenses, or poor compliance. Deeper corneal abrasions require more aggressive therapy, including lens removal and antibiotic use if the threat of infection is present; however, preservatives found in medications may slow down the healing process.[12]

Infections require discontinuation of contact lens wear and appropriate antibiotic treatment (Chapter 21). Microbial keratitis (MK) is a serious infection found primarily in overnight wear of contact lenses. More information on MK is provided in Chapter 16. Lens wear should not be resumed until the clinician is comfortable that the infection has resolved.

Dryness

Dry-eye symptoms are very common among hydrogel lens wearers.[14–17] These symptoms may be a result of the patient's poor tear quality or quantity or the effect of the contact lens itself on the tear film.[18] Historically, the tear film was described as composed of three layers: aqueous, lipid, and mucin. More recent theories have described the tear film as a gel-like structure with several layers derived from these components.[19] If a deficit occurs in any component, contact lens wear may be affected. A complete blink approximately every 5 seconds is required to spread the tear film over the cornea. Incomplete or partial blinks will result in dryness of the inferior region of the cornea. Blinking exercises may alleviate dryness in these cases. Other factors that can contribute to dry-eye symptoms with soft contact lenses are the environment, medications, computer use, and pregnancy.

Patient and Environmental Factors

A thorough case history will be important to elicit possible causes of dryness. Additionally, the patient should be questioned about any medical conditions, such as Stevens-Johnson syndrome (mucin deficiency), pregnancy (increase in tear viscosity), or Sjögren syndrome (aqueous deficiency). Medications that can alter the tear film are antihistamines, anticholinergics, antianxiety agents, phenothiazines, and oral contraceptives.[20]

The occupational environment (e.g., working near heating and air conditioning vents) may exacerbate dryness symptoms. Circulating air from automobile vents may also cause discomfort. The use of vent covers to redirect the air away from the wearer or changing the angle of the automobile vents should relieve dryness. Long-term computer use may cause a decreased blink rate, resulting in symptoms of dryness. This may be alleviated by having the wearer take blink breaks, such as at the end of each page of material. The same technique may be useful for others, such as students, who spend significant amounts of time reading. Airline passengers

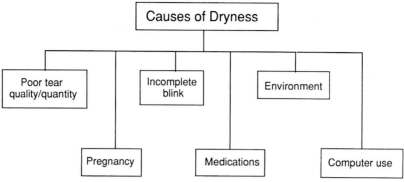

■ **FIGURE 13.4** Summary of causes of dryness.

may also experience dryness, particularly on long trips, because of the low relative humidity in airplane cabins at high altitude (Fig. 13.4).

Refitting the patient into a different material may be beneficial in reducing symptoms of dryness. Lenses containing phosphorylcholine have been reported to provide improved comfort.[21,22] Additionally, some manufacturers incorporate compounds such as polyvinyl pyrrolidone and polyvinyl alcohol into lenses during the manufacturing process in an effort to provide comfort and lens hydration.[23-25]

Silicone hydrogel lenses have also been reported to provide increased comfort.[26] This may be due in part to the low water content of silicone hydrogel lenses, which results in less lens dehydration. There is additional evidence that the increased oxygen provided by silicone hydrogel materials may decrease the ocular inflammatory response that may be found in hydrogel materials with low oxygen permeability (Dk). This inflammatory response may be responsible for ocular surface and lacrimal gland damage, which may cause ocular dryness; therefore, silicone hydrogel materials eliminate this damage and the dryness that results.[27]

Excessive Lens Movement

Deposited Lens

Surface deposits have been found to occur less frequently on disposable contact lenses than on conventional replacement lenses.[28] Conventional replacement soft lenses or those that are used beyond their recommended replacement schedule may become very deposited and exhibit excessive movement. The patient may present with symptoms of decentration of the lens during eye movement or with complaints that the lens is easily dislodged from the eye. On observation with the biomicroscope, it will be apparent that the soft lens has become deposited. These deposits may be filmy coatings or elevated deposits. The most common and effective treatment for lens deposition is to fit the patient in disposable lenses. If the patient is already wearing disposable lenses, then education on compliance with replacement instructions is recommended.[29]

In addition, a patient exhibiting clinical signs and symptoms of a dry eye may also experience lens decentration or lenses that dislodge as a result of dehydration of the lens. Use of a soft lens that is recommended for dry eyes or the use of lens lubricants may alleviate dryness.

Inverted Lens

Another cause of a lens that moves excessively or that dislodges from the eye easily is an inverted lens. Patients should be educated on how to determine lens inversion at the dispensing visit; however, this is more difficult to distinguish with certain types of lenses and some patients. Methods of determining lens inversion by visual inspection have been described

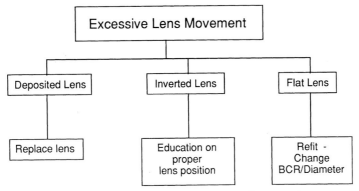

■ **FIGURE 13.5** Summary of causes and management of excessive lens movement.

previously (see Chapter 12). Repeated demonstration of these two methods may aid the patient in determining lens inversion. Graphics and photographs demonstrating lens inversion may be of additional help. When the lens is observed with the biomicroscope, it may exhibit excessive movement and edge lift. In addition, visual acuity may be reduced. If the patient finds visual inspection of lens inversion difficult and is experiencing decreased visual acuity, excessive lens movement, minor discomfort, or a lens that dislodges, the patient should suspect lens inversion and attempt to insert the lens in the other direction.

Flat Lens

Excessive lens movement is also observed in soft lenses with a BCR that is too flat. Biomicroscopic evaluation of a soft lens that is too flat may reveal any of the following clinical signs or combination of signs: inferior lens decentration with the patient gazing straight ahead, corneal exposure on lens movement, edge lift, superior decentration on downward gaze, or lens movement >1.5 mm with the blink. A change to a steeper base curve or larger lens diameter should improve the soft lens-to-cornea fitting relationship (Fig. 13.5).

Foggy/Hazy Vision

Diagnosis

Foggy or hazy vision through a soft contact lens may result from a coated lens or corneal edema. A common symptom elicited from patients may be the appearance of halos around or distortion of bright point sources of light. Clinical signs of either a contaminated lens or corneal edema may be observed with a biomicroscope. To assist in determining the cause of the reduced vision, the patient may be questioned about the frequency of cleaning, method of disinfection (chemical, hydrogen peroxide), use of a daily cleaner and weekly enzyme, cleanliness of hands before lens handling, use of hand lotions or soaps containing moisturizers, and age of lenses. Patients in whom corneal edema is suspected should be questioned about their wearing time. The presence of epithelial edema as a result of "overwear" is infrequently noted in hydrogel lens wearers but may be observed in wearers of thick, low-water-content hydrogel lenses.[12] Symptoms may be more prevalent after long periods of lens wear.

Treatment

In cases of a contaminated or coated lens, visual acuity will improve with the placement of a new lens on the eye. If the patient's lens modality is only available in a conventional lens, they may need to utilize an abrasive cleaner, increase the number of enzymatic cleanings per week, replace the contact lenses more frequently, or switch to a GP material. Patient education on proper cleaning and disinfecting techniques will help prolong the viability of the contact lens.

Removal of the contact lens and exposure of the cornea to air will result in a reduction of epithelial edema.[12] Hypertonic solutions may be beneficial in severe cases of edema, although their use may be unnecessary with the level of epithelial edema found in hydrogel contact lens wearers.[30] Switching patients to a lens material with a higher Dk/t (e.g., silicone hydrogel) and maintaining the patient on a daily-wear (DW) schedule will help reduce or eliminate the edema.[12] Likewise, those patients who were fitted in lower-water-content lenses for comfort (e.g., dry-eye patients) may be refitted in silicone hydrogel lenses to alleviate epithelial edema.

■ CLINICAL SIGNS

The practitioner will detect clinical signs during biomicroscopic evaluation of the patient's anterior segment. The use of grading scales and diagrams is beneficial to monitor and evaluate changes in the various conditions discussed in this section. The individual practitioner may develop the grading scale, or a currently published scale may be used. Regardless, the scale is typically based on numeric grades, as follows[5]:

0 = not present
1 = minimal
2 = mild
3 = moderate
4 = severe

This scale may be more descriptive when applied to a specific clinical sign (e.g., edema, injection). Assignment of a grade to the clinical sign will aid in accurate record keeping and further evaluation of the condition. In addition, drawings of the findings (infiltrates, staining, vessel growth) will enable the practitioner to compare the findings at each visit to determine if any changes have occurred.

Staining

The use of fluorescein can be an effective method of monitoring alterations in corneal integrity secondary to contact lens wear. Practitioners often choose not to use fluorescein during routine examination because of its inconvenience for patients wearing soft lenses (e.g., discoloring the lens). Following the application of fluorescein, either the eye should be rinsed with saline solution or the patient should be instructed not to reinsert the lenses for approximately 2 hours after insertion of the dye. A hand-held ultraviolet lamp is useful in checking for the presence of residual fluorescein. The introduction of high-molecular-weight fluorescein (fluorexon) and its ability to be used with the soft lens in the eye have helped to increase the use of fluorescein as a diagnostic tool in the evaluation of the corneal response to soft contact lens wear; however, it should be noted that this type of fluorescein exhibits reduced fluorescence in comparison with fluorescein strips.

The configuration of corneal punctate staining may be used to identify its cause (Fig. 13.6). Infection, mechanical trauma, trapped debris, desiccation, oxygen deprivation, inappropriate corneal bearing, and solution hypersensitivity are some of the more common causes of decreased corneal integrity.[12] Because of its serious nature, the presence of infectious keratitis must be considered in patients presenting with corneal staining. A comprehensive case history and evaluation of patient symptoms may be beneficial in determining the possibility of infection.

Mechanical trauma can arise from excessive pressure on the cornea from the contact lens. The center and edge of the lens represent the most common areas of bearing. A ring-shaped pattern of staining may result from contact between the peripheral edge of the central bearing

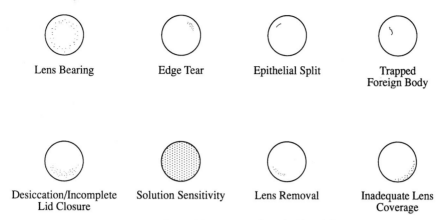

Lens Bearing   Edge Tear   Epithelial Split   Trapped Foreign Body

Desiccation/Incomplete Lid Closure   Solution Sensitivity   Lens Removal   Inadequate Lens Coverage

■ **FIGURE 13.6** Diagram representing staining patterns found with soft lenses.

area of the lens and the cornea.[5] More isolated areas of staining can occur as a result of lens tears or nicks. Evaluation of the lens for damage is often easiest with the use of the biomicroscope while the lens is on the eye. Fluorescein pooling will be evident within the epithelial break and may mimic the pattern of damage to the contact lens.

Lifting the upper lid may reveal an arc-shaped pattern of staining secondary to epithelial splitting, also known as superior epithelial arcuate lesions (SEALs). The cause of this phenomenon is thought to be mechanical in nature. Patients are typically asymptomatic; therefore, appropriate evaluation of the superior cornea is necessary to detect this condition. Treatment consists of removal of the lenses until healing occurs. Higher-modulus silicone hydrogel lenses have been associated with this finding.[31] Switching to a different design usually alleviates the problem (Chapter 16).[32–34]

Linear corneal staining may be secondary to a foreign body trapped under the lens. The appearance of "tracking" may occur as a result of lens movement during the blink. Removal of the lens in combination with appropriate cleaning of the lens and flushing of the eye will assist in removing any foreign particles. Lens deposits, as well as trapped epithelial debris, may result in scattered punctate staining. Appropriate lid and lens hygiene may help in alleviating this source of staining. If the patient is not wearing a disposable lens, daily surfactant or weekly enzyme cleaning may be necessary to remove lens deposits. Conventional lens replacement (>6 months) is not recommended; however, some specialty designs are not available for frequent replacement.

Lens dehydration may also be a source of punctate staining in hydrogel lens patients. Silicone hydrogel lenses have a lower water content, so are not as prone to dehydration. Typically, drying occurs in the region of the cornea where the lids meet as a result of minimal wiping of the cornea with tears in this area. Incomplete lid closure on blinking may also result in inferior punctate staining. Patients who have a tendency to this type of staining and are wearing thin, high-water-content hydrogel lenses may benefit from switching to a lower-water-content, thicker hydrogel or a silicone hydrogel lens. Frequent use of rewetting drops may also help alleviate corneal desiccation.

A generalized form of superficial punctate staining may develop following a solution hypersensitivity to a chemical preservative. This condition is most often bilateral and disappears following removal of the offending substance. The patient may also experience a foreign-body sensation and photophobia in severe cases. Replacing the lens and switching the patient to a different preservative or to preservative-free solutions will help prevent further reaction. Cold compresses may help alleviate discomfort in severe cases.

Diffuse punctate staining has been found in silicone hydrogel lens materials in combination with a multipurpose care system.[35] Treatment of this type of staining requires switching to a different multipurpose solution or a hydrogen peroxide care system, or changing the silicone hydrogel material.

Trauma to the cornea secondary to lens removal may be found in soft lens wearers who remove the lens directly from the cornea rather than sliding the lens down onto the bulbar conjunctiva before removal. The use of the fingernails, instead of the pads of the fingers, will result in a midperipheral staining pattern at the area corresponding to the pinching of the lens. This area of staining is typically arcuate or V-shaped. If the area of staining arouses suspicion, the practitioner may observe the patient's lens removal technique to confirm the cause.

Inadequate soft lens coverage or lens decentration may result in fluorescein staining near the corneal–scleral junction. Typically, this area will also be injected. Refitting with a larger-diameter lens or one that achieves better centration and coverage will alleviate this problem.

Corneal Edema

Clinical Evaluation

Clinical signs of corneal edema secondary to conventional hydrogel lens wear are typically apparent only in severe cases (Table 13.1). Alterations in the corneal structure may be clinically apparent initially with the presence of approximately 6% edema.[5] The absence of significant changes in the radius of curvature and spectacle blur in hydrogel lens wearers can be attributed to the symmetry of the edema throughout the epithelium.[36,37] The presence of a generalized epithelial edema is noted in hydrogel lens wearers and may be partially responsible for a progressive increase in myopia (myopic "creep" or myopic shift).[38] Silicone hydrogel lens materials have increased the oxygen transmission to the cornea by as much as eight times the amount of transmission of conventional hydrogel lenses.[39] Edema and symptoms related to corneal hypoxia are reduced with these materials (Chapter 16).

In evaluating corneal structural changes as a result of edema, the biomicroscope and pachometer are both acceptable clinical instruments, although the biomicroscope is used far more frequently in clinical practice. Striae and epithelial edema may initially be visible with 4% to 6% corneal thickening. Mild folds of Descemet membrane become apparent with approximately 7% edema, whereas major folds become apparent with swelling in excess of 15%.[38]

Primary changes are typically apparent within the epithelium and may be observed with the microscope focused on the corneal surface and the illumination source directed toward the limbus. Magnification of, at minimum, 25× must be used to visualize these changes. Vertical striae may also be present in conjunction with epithelial edema and are typically much easier to identify. They may be observed within the deep stroma and are detected by using a narrow parallelepiped. During assessment of the presence of striae, a differentiation must be made from

TABLE 13.1 SIGNS AND SYMPTOMS OF CORNEAL EDEMA

Reduced visual acuity
Foggy/hazy vision
Increase in myopia
Generalized loss of corneal transparency
Striae
Microcysts
Folds of Descemet membrane
Endothelial changes
Possible steepening of keratometry readings

corneal nerves. Striae appear as white lines and usually occur within the pupillary region of the cornea. They are typically 1 to 6 mm in length and rarely bifurcate. Corneal nerves bifurcate and extend to the peripheral limbus. When striae do bifurcate, the angle formed is much smaller than the angle observed with corneal nerves.[5]

Corneal Swelling

Placement of a hydrogel lens on the eye results in a decrease in the amount of oxygen available to the cornea. Lid closure further decreases the oxygen tension at the anterior surface of the contact lens in comparison with the open-eye condition. Indirect endothelial function studies of the corneal swelling response to the overnight use of conventional hydrogel contact lenses confirm corneal swelling between 8% and 15% after overnight wear, in comparison with a swelling rate of 4% in a control, non–lens-wearing group.[40] Variation in the level of swelling is evident as a result of differences in individual responses to decreased oxygen availability.[41] The presence of clinically observable edema secondary to hydrogel lens wear indicates a significant level of swelling, necessitating appropriate alterations in current contact lens management.

In contrast to conventional hydrogels, silicone hydrogels have been found to demonstrate overnight corneal swelling similar to that of a closed eye with no contact lens.[42] The use of silicone hydrogel lenses for daily wear or overnight wear has virtually eliminated corneal hypoxia in most patients.[43]

Epithelial Edema

A principal cause of epithelial edema may be exposure of the cornea to a hypotonic solution. Intercellular penetration of fluid results in an increase in the fragility of the cornea caused by the increased separation between the epithelial cells and loosening of the junctional complexes. As a result of the vulnerability of the cornea in this state, there is a dramatic increase in its susceptibility to an abrasion.[44] Removal of the corneal barriers to fluid penetration may also be compromised by trauma. A "roughening" of the epithelial surface will allow pooling of tears within the abraded area, as well as edema of the surrounding cells.[12]

The use of fluorescein will significantly enhance the appearance of edema adjacent to the abrasion. A central area of green will appear as a result of pooling of tears within the abraded area, and the edges will appear gray as a result of "heaping" of the epithelium surrounding the lesion. Therefore, a green haze will demarcate the surrounding edema. Generalized edema may best be viewed by retroillumination, whereas the addition of fluorescein may elicit a green, mottled appearance. Because of the difference in refractive indices between the epithelium and water, epithelial edema will also generate a "sparkly" appearance when viewed with white light.[12]

Microcysts

Epithelial microcysts, a complication found with both DW and extended wear (EW) of hydrogel lenses, can be observed biomicroscopically. Microcysts typically are found in the midperipheral cornea and become apparent between 3 weeks and 6 months after EW is initiated with conventional hydrogel lenses.[45] They may vary from 15 to 50 μm in diameter and appear as spheres scattered throughout all layers of the epithelium. These cysts, thought to be composed of disorganized epithelial growths rather than fluid, result from abnormal metabolism during conditions of corneal hypoxia. Discontinuance of contact lens wear is typically unnecessary if fewer than 50 microcysts are present, although there should be some concern if more than 10 are observed. With the presence of more than 50, conventional hydrogel contact lens wear should be discontinued and the patient refitted in a silicone hydrogel lens. Reduction of wearing time has not been found successful in reducing the number of microcysts.[41] Lens removal will often result in an increase in the number of microcysts during the first week, but a gradual reduction will occur within a 5- to 10-week period.[46,47] Surfacing of the microcysts will produce punctate staining with fluorescein.

Management

A number of viable contact lens management options may be considered in cases of hydrogel lens-induced edema. The current standard of care for managing patients in this situation is to refit them in a silicone hydrogel lens. For those patients for whom this is not an option, thin, higher-water-content lenses will maximize the level of oxygen reaching the cornea. In conventional hydrogel lenses, a combination of both water content and lens thickness determines the level of Dk/t to the cornea. Average lens thickness is a more accurate determinant of central corneal edema than is center thickness. Higher-power lenses with the same center thickness as lower-power lenses of the same material cause a higher degree of central corneal swelling.[40]

"Tight-Lens" Syndrome

Corneal edema may or may not arise secondary to a lens that is clinically deemed to be "too tight." A soft lens that exhibits no movement under magnification is typically considered to be a "tight lens." The significant exchange of new tears under a soft lens is minimal compared with that under a GP contact lens. Therefore, a variation in the lens-to-cornea fitting relationship has little to do with preventing corneal edematous changes by altering the flow of tears under the lens. The thickness of a hydrogel lens appears to be the parameter that determines the amount of corneal edema.[48] Silicone hydrogel lenses have a high Dk value. Even when the thickness is taken into consideration, the Dk/t is high, allowing, in most of the materials, for the oxygen transmission to exceed the recommended Dk/t of 125×10^{-9} (cm $\times$ mL O$_2$)/(sec $\times$ mL $\times$ mm Hg)[39] (see Chapters 10 and 16).

The presence of minimal or no lens movement on the cornea may result in conjunctival injection caused by impingement of the limbal vasculature. Limbal vascular compression results from a "suctioning" of the lens to the eye subsequent to a steep fitting relationship. Biomicroscopic examination of the limbus may reveal congestion of the limbal blood flow posterior to the lens edge with blanching of the vessels just anterior to the lens edge. Conjunctival movement with the blink may also be observed; this is termed *conjunctival drag*. If conjunctival compression occurs with an inadequately fit lens, either the base curve should be flattened or the diameter reduced to provide better movement. The presence of corneal edema may or may not accompany this condition. Its resolution may be accomplished by changing to a silicone hydrogel lens material. Additional edema-related conditions found primarily in EW or continuous wear (CW) are addressed in Chapter 16.

Injection

Generalized Injection

A symptom and clinical sign found with both soft and GP lens wear is conjunctival injection (typically expressed as "redness" by patients). There are many causes of generalized injection found in soft contact lens wearers that may or may not be related to contact lens wear (Table 13.2). Typically, if the soft lens is the cause, the injection results from corneal hypoxia, a tight lens, solution sensitivity, trapped foreign body, deposits, lens defects, inflammatory reaction to overnight wear (i.e., Contact Lens Acute Red Eye), or ocular complications of these conditions. The injection may also be a result of conditions not related to the lens, such as allergic, viral, or bacterial conjunctivitis or other ocular and systemic conditions. To identify the cause of injection, a thorough case history should include questions such as the following: When was the injection initially observed? Does it continue after the lenses are removed? Is the injection of recent onset or is it chronic? Are the eyes irritated,

TABLE 13.2 FACTORS RESULTING IN INJECTION

RELATED TO CONTACT LENSES	NOT NECESSARILY RELATED TO CONTACT LENS WEAR
Damaged lens	Foreign body
Edema	Conjunctivitis
Solution sensitivity	Ocular pathology
Tight lens	Trauma
Deposited lens	Cigarette smoke
Contaminated lens	Swimming in chlorinated pools
Trapped foreign body	Lack of sleep
Poor-fitting lens	Excessive alcoholic beverages
Improper use of solutions	Allergies
CLARE	Dryness

CLARE, contact lens acute red eye.

burning, or itching? Is there any discharge and, if so, of what type—mucous, watery, or stringy? Was there an occurrence that preceded the injection, such as change in solutions, swimming, lack of sleep, illness, traumatic injury, or foreign body? Based on the case history, the elimination of causative factors, and a thorough evaluation with the biomicroscope, the diagnosis can be made.

Lens-Related Generalized Injection: Narrowing a diagnosis of injection to contact lens-related causes is based on symptoms, lens-to-cornea fitting relationship, lens condition, and wearing time. Moderate to severe injection of the eye at any time should be treated as an ocular emergency because of the risk of corneal ulcers and infection. It is not unusual for some patients to present with mild injection caused by a variety of factors (e.g., environment, dryness); however, if the injection is acute with no known cause, a thorough evaluation is necessary to rule out serious conditions.

Symptoms: Lens-related injection will typically occur upon insertion or after lens wear and will improve as lens wear is discontinued. Immediate injection with burning on insertion will most likely be related to solution sensitivity. The use of preservatives such as thimerosal, chlorhexidine, and benzalkonium chloride in increased concentrations or for a prolonged period of time have resulted in patient sensitivity.[49] Newer preservatives found in multipurpose solution regimens are more subtle in sensitivity symptoms. Symptoms may be dryness, loss of wearing time, or minor discomfort. Immediate discomfort and injection may also be the result of improper use of the soft lens solutions, which includes use of a daily cleaner before insertion without a thorough rinsing, inadequate neutralization of hydrogen peroxide disinfecting solutions, and use of incompatible solutions. Management of injection resulting from preservatives requires changing to a care regimen with a different preservative, to a nonpreserved system (such as hydrogen peroxide disinfection with nonpreserved solutions), or to a solution-free lens (i.e., daily disposable contact lenses).

As the wearing time increases over the period of a day with DW or over a period of days with EW, corneal hypoxia, a tight lens, or a deposited or damaged lens may result in a generalized injection. By evaluating the lens and eye with the biomicroscope, the cause of the injection may be determined. Eliminating the injection requires either replacing the lens with a new lens or refitting to improve the fitting relationship or Dk/t of the lens.

Lens fitting relationship: As noted previously, a tight-fitting lens may impinge on the limbal vasculature, resulting in injection. When the lens movement is evaluated, no movement will be observed, even with the use of the "push-up test," which consists of manipulating the soft lens with the lower lid in an attempt to push the lens upward. A tightly fitting lens will resist movement when pushed up with the lower lid, whereas a lens that is not adherent will exhibit movement with this test. In addition, the lens should adequately cover the cornea and extend onto the sclera. A lens that is too small may result in injection in the area not adequately covered or in the area of the limbus on which the lens impinges. Altering the soft lens parameters to achieve better movement and coverage will eliminate this form of injection.

Lens condition: An old, deposited, contaminated, or damaged soft lens may result in a generalized injection. When the lens is removed from the eye, the injection should resolve unless further corneal insult has occurred. Evaluation with the biomicroscope will reveal the condition of the lens. The cornea should be evaluated after lens removal to ensure that the cornea is not affected. Simple replacement of the soft lens with a fresh, clean lens will alleviate the symptoms. In addition, re-educating the patient on the proper care and handling and recommended replacement schedule for the lens may be necessary. Refitting the patient in a more frequently replaced lens, if possible, may preclude recurrence of the problem.

Wearing time: An acute red eye associated with excessive or overnight wear should be treated with extreme caution. One large-scale study found that conventional hydrogel EW patients who wore their lenses overnight had a 10 to 15 times greater risk of ulcerative keratitis than did DW patients who did not wear their lenses overnight.[50] Fortunately, the use of conventional hydrogel materials for EW has been primarily replaced with silicone hydrogel materials, which provide more oxygen to the cornea for overnight wear.

Contact lens acute red eye (CLARE), characterized by an EW patient awakening with a red, watery eye, is an inflammatory reaction that occurs with overnight wear of soft contact lenses. This inflammatory reaction is observed in both hydrogel and silicone hydrogel lenses. More information on CLARE and other complications (i.e., contact lens peripheral ulcer, infiltrates) found primarily in overnight wear are discussed in Chapter 16.

For the acute red eye, the cornea should be examined with and without fluorescein for signs of edema, ulceration, or other compromise. If the corneal epithelium is intact, discontinuing lens wear, use of an ocular lubricant, and frequent monitoring until the injection disappears may be all that is necessary. Returning to overnight wear depends largely on the patient's compliance with wearing instructions. Wearing contact lenses for longer than the recommended wearing schedule is likely to result in corneal compromise. A compliant patient may be fitted into a silicone hydrogel lens with a higher Dk/t. The wearing time may be reduced as needed. A CW or EW soft lens worn on a flexible wear (FW) or DW basis or a GP lens may also improve the patient's success at lens wear. In any case, the patient should be educated about why the injection is occurring and about the importance of following directions pertaining to wearing schedule.

Injection Not Related to Contact Lens Wear: It may be difficult for the practitioner to determine if the injection is not lens related. If the soft lens is fitting properly, nonpreserved solutions are used, the lens is clean and new, and the injection continues after lens wear is discontinued, the assumption would be to evaluate the eye for other causative factors. A simple case history may elicit the cause, such as allergies, dryness, lack of sleep, trauma, or cigarette smoke. Further evaluation with the biomicroscope with and without fluorescein will aid in diagnosing the problem. Some patients present with mild injection on a consistent basis that may be improved with the use of lens lubricants to rinse the lens off, to rinse and relieve the eye exposed to chlorine in swimming pools and cigarette smoke, and to rewet the lens and dry eye.

Sectorial Injection

Injection located in a specific area of the eye typically signals an irritation in that specific area. With soft contact lenses, this is generally the result of a lens tear or deposit that is located in the same area as the injection. Any damaged lens should be replaced, and the injection will disappear.

Another form of sectorial injection sometimes occurs when a lens impinges on a pinguecula. If the lens is observed to be irritating a pinguecula, the lens should be refitted with a larger or smaller diameter that either covers the pinguecula to a greater extent or does not contact the pinguecula. A GP lens may need to be fitted to eliminate contact between the contact lens and the pinguecula.

Episcleritis, a condition that is not contact lens related, often presents as a form of sectorial injection. It is usually unilateral and recurrent, and it may be accompanied by variable levels of discomfort. It is a self-limiting disease that can be treated with topical steroids.[51]

Corneal Vascularization

Introduction

Vascularization of the normally avascular cornea is a serious complication of hydrogel contact lens wear. Severe cases involving visual reduction and corneal translucency typically occur after surgery or as a result of a pathologic incident. The presence of a vascular response to contact lens wear, whether involving limbal capillary filling or "true" corneal vascularization, is indicative of contact lens intolerance. This intolerance is generally a result of a tight lens fit, limbal compression, corneal edema, or excessive wear by the patient.[52] Corneal vascularization occurs more commonly in EW than in DW hydrogel patients. Filling of pre-existing limbal capillaries is a common vascular response noted in daily wearers of hydrogel lenses, with the possibility of prolonged engorgement leading to new vessel growth. Silicone hydrogel materials have been shown to reduce limbal hyperemia and corneal vascularization for previous lens wearers in DW or overnight wear, and not to cause vascularization in new wearers.[53]

Normal versus Abnormal

Variation in the anatomic configuration of the corneolimbal junction can lead to difficulty in defining actual new vessel growth from capillary engorgement. Difficulty may arise in defining an anatomic reference point at the limbus to be used to measure the vascular response.[44] A vascularized translucent overlay, composed of conjunctival and subconjunctival tissue, may extend onto the cornea and varies in width depending on the peripheral limit of the Bowman membrane.[54,55] The extension of the overlay is greatest at the superior limbus (up to 2.5 mm) and is least nasally and temporally.[56] The vascular nature of this region may be misleading when an attempt is made to determine the presence of abnormal vessel growth or looping. Penetration of the limbal vasculature beyond the leading edge of the overlay should be considered indicative of contact lens intolerance, but it may be difficult to assess because of leakage of exudate into the surrounding tissue causing translucency of the normally transparent cornea.[52] The narrow separation between stromal collagen fibrils normally inhibits the advancement of vessels beyond 1 mm from the limbus. Edematous changes to the stroma may result in an increase in the separation between the collagen fibrils, facilitating extension of the limbal vasculature into the visual axis and resulting in reduced vision.[57]

Appearance

The appearance of the vascular response will vary depending on the duration of corneal irritation and type of pathology. Decompensation of the highly organized architecture of the corneal stroma will result in tortuosity of the penetrating vasculature, whereas maintenance of stromal uniformity and compactness will render a straighter course.[58] Peripheral corneal edema secondary to hydrogel contact lens wear may predispose the tissue to vascular penetration.[59] High minus and prism ballast lenses that have thick edges are more likely to cause such a response. Superficial vascularization is typically nonuniform and irregular and may consist of individual "spikes" that on greater resolution may be connected to a venous return. The loop formed between the vessels is much narrower than the anastomoses seen in normal limbal arcades.[52]

Initiating Factors

A variety of factors may be necessary for the initiation of a corneal vascular response. It is apparent that a single mechanism is not entirely responsible for the initiation of this event. Predisposing factors most important in promoting contact lens-induced vascularization include anaerobic metabolism, inflammatory cells within the cornea, and damaged or disturbed epithelial cells. Hypoxic conditions resulting in the buildup of lactic acid, the inability to remove metabolic waste and debris caused by impingement of the conjunctival venous return, and irritation or damage to the corneal epithelium may all initiate the release of vasostimulator substances, resulting in vascularization.[52] Inflammatory cells that migrate to the cornea in response to an inadequate contact lens fit may also elicit a vascular response.[60,61]

Stages

Three stages occur in the process of corneal vascularization secondary to contact lens wear. The first stage encompasses the filling of a pre-existing limbal capillary plexus. The second stage involves new vessel growth in the form of endothelial "spikes" or "sprouts" that extend from limbal arcades toward the central cornea. Thirdly, these sprouts form canaliculi and then "true" vessels that may be at any depth within the cornea. This network of abnormal vessel growth may form new arcades.[62] Removal of the contact lens from the eye will result in the emptying of blood from the patent vessels. Actual vascular regression may occur but appears to depend on the length of time the vessels are present, resulting in a critical period of growth beyond which regression may not occur. Remaining empty blood vessels, or "ghost vessels," appear as fine white lines extending in a nonbranching linear pattern toward the central cornea.[52]

Management and Treatment

The management of corneal vascularization is initiated by removal of the causative source of ocular irritation. Isolation of any obvious source of vascularization may be easily addressed, but often the presence of a variety of contributing factors may hinder successful management. It is necessary in each situation to identify the most prominent causative factors in an attempt to eliminate any potential source for vascular growth. Other pathologic conditions, including dry eye, blepharitis, acne rosacea, seasonal allergies, and sensitivity to a solution preservative, may contribute to the vascular response and must be eliminated. Detection of vascularization while the vessels are in their immature state may allow for total regression of the capillary "spikes" and emptying of the filled limbal vascular arcades.[52]

One of the most effective means of controlling vascularization is through refitting the patient in a silicone hydrogel lens material, which, as previously noted, provides up to eight times more oxygen to the cornea than hydrogel lens materials.[39] If this is not effective, a reduction of wearing time, such as reducing the number of nights the lens is worn overnight or wearing the lens DW only, should manage vascularization with a silicone hydrogel lens material. In situations in which contact lens wear must be discontinued, a pair of current spectacles is essential. The patient may be more likely to wear spectacles if they are attractive and use an up-to-date prescription.

Silicone hydrogel lenses are becoming increasingly available in toric, multifocal, and custom designs to meet the needs of all patients. This availability provides high oxygen transmission to patients who require high minus, high plus, or prism ballast toric lenses, which in the past might have contributed to corneal vascularization.

A tight lens-to-cornea fitting relationship, causing a constriction in venous return, may need to be loosened. Peripheral constriction, appearing as a distinct ring circumscribing the limbus on lens removal, may be observed with the use of fluorescein.

The presence of corneal vascularization is often considered innocuous by the patient but can be a primary indicator to the practitioner of contact lens intolerance. Typically, changing a patient's wearing schedule or lens design to afford more adequate lens tolerance will help to diminish the vascular response and allow the patient to maintain successful contact lens wear. This is an excellent opportunity to educate the patient on the advantages of a silicone hydrogel over a hydrogel lens and make the switch to a healthier modality.

Giant Papillary Conjunctivitis (Contact Lens-Induced Papillary Conjunctivitis)

Clinical Signs and Symptoms

Giant papillary conjunctivitis, also termed contact lens-induced papillary conjunctivitis, is a complication affecting both soft and rigid contact lens wearers. The condition, first described in 1974 by Spring[63] in an attempt to differentiate the entity from other forms of allergic conjunctival disease, was further described by Allansmith et al.[64]

GPC is most often associated with contact lens wear, although irritation from ocular prosthetics and exposed suture ends after penetrating keratoplasty and cataract extraction have also contributed to its development.[56,63,65–67] Clinical signs commonly accompanying this condition include conjunctival hyperemia, excess mucus, giant papillae on the upper tarsal conjunctiva, and increased contact lens movement. The development of GPC has been noted in both rigid and soft contact lens wearers, with earlier initiation occurring in soft lens wearers.[65] This is a complication in which the symptoms do not appear to be improved via refitting into silicone hydrogel lens materials. Silicone is naturally hydrophobic and prone to deposits; in addition, silicone hydrogel materials tend to have an increased lens modulus, all of which may contribute to GPC (Chapter 16). Newer designs with a lower modulus appear to be decreasing the mechanical irritation that may increase the risk of GPC.

Because of size and material differences, the papillary appearance may vary between soft and rigid lens wearers. In documenting papillary response location, the upper tarsal conjunctiva may be divided into three zones: zone 1 represents the superior one-third of the tarsus, zone 2 the middle one-third, and zone 3 the lower one-third near the lid margin. Papillae in soft lens wearers are typically noted to occur in zone 1 initially, progressing inferiorly with advancement of the condition (Fig. 13.7).

Mild hyperemia of the upper tarsal conjunctiva is often the initial clinical sign observed in GPC and may be accompanied by small strands of mucus.[57] Lid eversion, accompanied by fluorescein staining, is essential in the early diagnosis of GPC and should be performed on all contact lens patients before fitting and at each subsequent visit. Initial signs of mild lens coating,

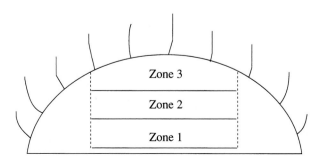

■ **FIGURE 13.7** Diagram representing zones of upper tarsal conjunctiva.

TABLE 13.3 STAGES OF GIANT PAPILLARY CONJUNCTIVITIS

SYMPTOMS	SIGNS
STAGE 1	
Few strands of mucus	None
Mild itching	
STAGE 2	
Minimal mucus	Mild lens coating
Moderate itching	Elevation of normal papillae
Slight lens awareness	Beginning of underlying giant papillae
Slight decrease in vision through lens	Mild hyperemia
	Mild sheets over papillae
STAGE 3	
Moderate to severe mucus	Moderate to severe lens coating
Moderate to severe itching	Increase in the number, size, and elevation of papillae
Increased blinking with intermittent blurring of vision	Variable hyperemia and edema
Slight lens movement	Heavy mucus
STAGE 4	
Severe mucus with adhesion of eyelids	Excessive mucus
Moderate to severe itching	Giant papillae with flat apices
Extreme lens awareness, pain	Marked hyperemia and edema
Blurring of vision	Heavy lens coating
Excessive lens movement	

formation of giant papillae, and increased mucous production (stage 1) may progress to the formation of excessive mucus, the presence of giant papillae and erythema, and heavy lens coating (stage 4) (Table 13.3).[65] A distinction has been made between the papillae found in persons who do not wear contact lenses and those in patients with GPC. To assist in this distinction, the appearance of the upper tarsal conjunctiva has been divided into four types: a satin-textured conjunctiva with a smooth surface devoid of papillae, a uniform papillary response (four to eight per millimeter), a nonuniform papillary response (approximately 0.4–0.8 mm in size), and a giant papillary appearance with papillae, at minimum, 1 mm in diameter.

Although papillae are the most common inflammatory sign in GPC, follicles may also be observed with active inflammation of the conjunctiva. The practitioner often experiences confusion in differentiating these two signs. Follicles, or lymphoid elevations, are typically located in the inferior conjunctiva and fornix. They appear translucent and exhibit a superficial vascular pattern. Papillae are composed of a central vascular tuft or stalk of vessels and may in later stages exhibit white "tops" as a result of collagen scarring. They are more commonly noted to occur in the upper tarsal conjunctiva.[57]

Patient symptoms often precede objective signs in GPC. The presence of mucus in the nasal corners of the eye in the morning and itching following lens removal (stage 1) may often be noted in lieu of objective signs, including giant papillae, conjunctival thickening, and erythema. Symptoms may progress in later stages (stage 4) to extreme contact lens intolerance, marked hyperemia, moderate to severe itching, and excessive mucous production leading to eyelid adherence on awakening. With the progression of the papillary response, contact lens movement becomes more excessive, resulting in discomfort to the patient and a reduction in wearing time. Pseudoptosis has also been reported in some patients.[57]

The papillary reaction of the upper tarsal conjunctiva in GPC has been most often attributed to both an immunologic response to and a mechanical irritation from surface deposits on the contact lens. A cutaneous basophil hypersensitivity reaction (including both a type 1, IgE-mediated reaction and a variety of type 4 delayed reactions) has been implicated.[57] The allergic reaction results from the presence of antigens (e.g., proteins, lipids) on the surface of the lens. Omission of proper and frequent cleaning and infrequent replacement of the contact lens contribute to the initiation and exacerbation of the disease process.

Treatment

Many cases of GPC can be alleviated by early intervention. Contact lens removal will cause the disease process to subside and eventually cease. Most patients, however, are dissatisfied with discontinuing lens wear for long periods. The goal of therapy is to control the clinical signs and symptoms of GPC while allowing contact lens wear to continue with minimal disturbance to the patient.

Patients presenting with GPC should be replacing lenses on a recommended replacement schedule, ideally monthly replacement or more frequently. Altering the replacement schedule to a more frequent replacement will aid in eliminating the symptoms of GPC. Most refractive errors can now be corrected, at maximum, with a quarterly replacement lens. The patient should be educated about the necessity of replacing the lenses on schedule. The emergence of disposable lenses as the primary choice for fitting soft lens wearers has accomplished more than anything else to decrease the incidence of GPC in contact lens wearers.

The following recommendations are provided for those patients whose refractive errors can only be corrected with a conventional replacement (6–12 months) lens material. In the early stages of GPC, regular surfactant and enzymatic cleaning should alleviate most symptoms. Surfactant cleaning is essential for the removal of deposits, especially lipids, and should be performed daily or on lens removal and disinfection. If symptoms persist with daily cleaning, an abrasive cleaner or more frequent cleanings are recommended. Weekly enzymatic cleaning to remove denatured proteins (predominantly lysozyme) is essential in maintaining a relatively deposit-free surface; the possibility of biweekly or even more frequent cleaning may be beneficial in cases of GPC. The use of hydrogen peroxide disinfection systems, accompanied by preservative-free saline solution, will assist in reducing the number of possible antigens exposed to the ocular surface.[49]

Replacement of conventional replacement lenses on a more frequent basis, 3 or 6 months, will minimize the incidence of GPC. Low-water-content, nonionic materials are advantageous in these cases because of their greater resistance to deposits in comparison with high-water-content, ionic materials. Changing the lens material or lens design or switching to a GP lens are all alternatives that may increase the likelihood of continued lens wear.

Discontinuing lens wear, exclusive of the severity of the condition, will result in the disappearance of symptoms within approximately 5 days following lens removal. In patients with severe GPC (stages 3 or 4), discontinuing lens wear is usually necessary to terminate progression of the condition.[65] Lenses may be reinserted following the resolution of hyperemia, excessive mucous production, and itching, although the presence of giant papillae may persist for several months to years.[49]

The most effective way to treat moderate to severe GPC is the use of a combination antihistamine/mast cell stabilizer once or twice a day before lens insertion and after lens removal, depending on the dosage (Chapter 21). This, in combination with clean, new lenses, will be effective in most cases. Severe cases of GPC may warrant discontinuing lens wear and use of topical steroids. The use of short-term applications of 0.10% fluorometholone (one drop in each eye four times daily for 1 week, tapered by one drop each week for 3 weeks) is effective in reducing both clinical signs and symptoms of the condition.[49] Once the patient is stabilized, the use of a mast cell stabilizer while tapering the steroid can be used. A conservative approach to topical steroid use is necessary in avoiding complications, including glaucoma and cataracts. The use of disposable lenses and mast cell stabilizers has been reported as successful treatment of 93% of patients presenting with GPC.[68]

■ SUMMARY

Thorough, ongoing patient care may prevent future complications associated with soft contact lens wear. Symptoms elicited from the patient during the case history and clinical signs observed with the biomicroscope signal contact lens-related conditions that should be eliminated or monitored before severe complications develop. Disposable/frequent-replacement soft lenses and silicone hydrogel lens materials are beneficial to the patient and have played a role in reduction of soft contact lens complications. Frequent follow-up evaluations, every 6 months for DW patients and every 3 months for EW/CW patients, are recommended for monitoring. Contact lenses are not a cosmetic device but a medical device and therefore require evaluation by an eye care practitioner to ensure successful wear.

■ CLINICAL CASES

CASE 1

A first-time lens wearer presents with the inability to wear soft lenses because of poor comfort and dryness. He has discontinued lenses fitted at another office after not being able to achieve any substantial wearing time and having "dry eyes." During the case history, the patient reported wearing 2-week replacement contact lenses for about 2 to 3 months with wear time not greater than 8 hours per day because of dryness and slight burning. He reports to being compliant with the care regimen and replacement schedule. The patient had previously used two multipurpose solution care regimens. His tear breakup time is 10 seconds and all findings appear normal.

SOLUTION: Preservative sensitivity is suspected. The patient is fit with daily disposable lenses and is instructed to use nonpreserved saline solution if necessary. The patient is able to achieve all-day wear and has good comfort.

CASE 2

A patient presents with reduced vision and a mild burning sensation in the left eye only. She is a long-term soft lens wearer. She reports that she had something "stuck" behind her left lens that morning and that she was not able to remove the lens for a period of time. She notices that her vision is still reduced with spectacles after the contact lenses are removed. On examination, best-corrected visual acuity is OD 20/20 and OS 20/80. Evaluation with the biomicroscope reveals a central coalesced area of staining.

SOLUTION: This patient has a central corneal abrasion. Treatment of the abrasion depends on its severity. The current lens wear should be discontinued until the abraded area has healed. A mild abrasion might be monitored only. In more severe cases, a broad-spectrum antibiotic may be used prophylactically. In addition, a cycloplegic agent might be administered. Patching a contact lens-induced abrasion is *contraindicated* because the lens may have introduced bacteria to the eye that will thrive in the warm, moist environment that results from patching. The patient should be monitored frequently (e.g., 24 hours, 3 days, and 1 week after the abrasion) until the area has healed completely. The cause of the abrasion should be confirmed so the condition will not occur again. For example, the abrasion might be the result of a damaged lens, a tight lens, solution misuse, removal with the fingernails, or a foreign body. This may require that the lens be refitted or the patient re-educated regarding care and handling.

CASE 3

A patient has EW hydrogel lenses. He wears the lenses for 5 days before removal. He complains of hazy vision. What should you think of and look for?

SOLUTION: The cornea should be evaluated for signs of edema (striae, microcysts). Keratometry and subjective refraction should also be performed to detect changes resulting from edema (e.g., steepening of the keratometric readings, increase in myopia). If the presence of edema is verified, the patient should be fitted into a lens with a higher Dk/t (e.g., silicone hydrogel). If refitting is not an option, a daily wear schedule should be recommended.

CASE 4

A contact lens patient is fitted in Focus Dailies (daily disposable contact lenses). The patient remarks that at times one or both lenses are mildly uncomfortable and can become annoying as the day progresses. What is the probable cause?

SOLUTION: This lens is most likely inverted. Soft lenses have become very thin and it may be quite difficult to determine if the lens is inverted. At times, an inverted lens may result in less comfort, reduced vision, and more movement than a lens that is not inverted, but with newer designs, vision can be good despite lens inversion. By removing the lens, checking to see if it is in the proper position, and reinserting it, the patient should notice that the symptoms have disappeared.

CASE 5

The patient has been refitted with silicone hydrogel lenses for 30-day CW. The patient has been wearing hydrogel lenses for 7 days and 6 nights for about 2 years. When the patient returns at the 1-week follow-up visit, she has discontinued the silicone hydrogel lenses as she thinks they are not as comfortable as her previous lenses.

SOLUTION: Most likely this patient has had corneal edema with her previous hydrogel contact lenses. As her cornea rehabilitated with the silicone hydrogel lenses, it has become more sensitive (or less numb). The higher modulus of the 30-day lens, in addition to the healthier cornea, has resulted in more lens sensation. Typically, if the patient is educated on this and asked to wear the silicone hydrogel lenses, at minimum, for 2 weeks (DW or CW), she will be comfortable in the new lenses. If this does not improve the lens comfort, fitting with a lower modulus silicone hydrogel lens material can be attempted. Most patients will adapt well to the silicone hydrogel lenses with education and patience with the adaptation process.

CASE 6

A patient comes to the office complaining of reduced vision in the right eye. Overrefraction is OD −0.50 D and OS +0.50 D. The patient was dispensed the following parameters:

OD: BCR 8.6 mm, overall diameter 14.5 mm, Rx −3.75 D
OS: BCR 8.6 mm, overall diameter 14.5 mm, Rx −3.00 D

What is the problem?

SOLUTION: This patient has switched the lenses. The lenses should be switched back to the proper eye and the patient re-educated about removing the right lens first and the left lens second to avoid confusing the two lenses. Patients will typically refuse to believe, sometimes adamantly, that they have switched their lenses until it is demonstrated to them.

CASE 7

A patient has corneal vascularization of 2 mm superiorly and 1.5 mm inferiorly. He has not returned for follow-up evaluation for more than a year. What might be the cause of the vascularization?

SOLUTION: This patient should be questioned about his wearing schedule. He is very likely overwearing his contact lenses or, less likely, the patient's corneal oxygen requirement may be greater than what the current lenses provide. The patient should be educated about the importance of both a proper wearing schedule and routine follow-up evaluations. A refit into a silicone hydrogel lens material that provides more oxygen to the cornea would be beneficial.

CASE 8

A long-term soft lens wearer comes to your office for her annual examination. She sleeps in her hydrogel lenses about two times a week. The fit of the lenses is good and the patient is content with her current lens brand, but upon slit-lamp examination, limbal hyperemia and neovascularization inferiorly are noted.

SOLUTION: The patient is refitted into a silicone hydrogel lens material that can be worn for 7 days and 6 nights extended wear. The patient intends to continue her current wearing schedule of about 2 nights per week of overnight wear. At the 2-week follow-up examination, the limbal region is white and clear, and the neovascularization has regressed. The new lenses provide more oxygen to the cornea, thus improving ocular health.

CASE 9

A patient has had soft lenses for 3 months. She complains of discomfort immediately on insertion. Fluorescein evaluation with the lenses off reveals a superficial staining pattern in the nasal periphery. What might be wrong?

SOLUTION: When the lens is evaluated on the eye, it is likely that there will be an edge tear. The lens should be replaced and the patient educated about the care and handling of soft lenses. The patient should be reminded not to wear lenses that cause discomfort. Depending on the severity of the staining, the patient may have to discontinue lens wear until the cornea heals.

CASE 10

A patient complains of dry eyes and increased lens intolerance. She received her lenses in April, and it is now November. Her solution regimen has remained the same. She finds the symptoms to be worse at work. What might be the problem?

SOLUTION: The two most likely causes are a dry environment at work, caused by the heating system, and antihistamine use. Seasonal allergies and sinus conditions often occur in the spring and fall, and antihistamines are taken. The heat may have recently been turned on at the patient's workplace, creating a dry environment. She should check vents in her work area to prevent air from being directed toward her, especially her head. The use of lens lubricants or perhaps even discontinuation of lens wear while on antihistamines may be helpful. Another factor with a female patient is pregnancy. If the patient has recently become pregnant, this may result in dryness of the eyes not noticed previously. In addition, this patient might benefit from a lens material better suited for dry eyes (i.e., Proclear, CooperVision; 1 Day Acuvue Moist, Acuvue Advance, or Acuvue Oasys, Vistakon; Focus Dailies, Ciba Vision; Extreme H2O, Hydrogel Vision Corp.; or other silicone hydrogel lens not listed).

CASE 11

A patient has worn soft lenses for 1 year. He admits failing to replace his disposable lenses as scheduled and cannot remember the last time he did so. He experiences mild itching and increased mucous discharge on awakening. Biomicroscopic evaluation reveals grade 2 papillae, and the lenses are moderately coated.

SOLUTION: This patient has GPC. His lenses should be replaced and the patient re-educated about the proper care of the soft lenses. If the GPC does not resolve with new lenses and increased cleaning, the patient may need to discontinue lens wear until the GPC improves. Daily disposable lenses would be beneficial for this patient.

CLINICAL PROFICIENCY CHECKLIST

■ Daily disposable, disposable, and frequent-replacement lenses may aid in providing the patient with relatively problem-free wear.

■ Two of the most valuable tools used to diagnose complications associated with soft contact lens wear are the case history and the biomicroscope.

■ Frequent evaluations, every 6 months for DW patients and every 3 months for EW patients, will aid in reducing serious complications that may result from soft lens wear.

■ Reduced vision with contact lenses *and* spectacles may be attributed to corneal abnormalities that require immediate attention.

■ Discomfort with a soft lens is not normal and requires evaluation of the patient and the lens. Generally, the lens is found to be damaged or deposited; however, abnormalities of the cornea such as abrasions or ulcers may be observed.

■ A recent onset of dryness with lens wear is often found to be the result of antihistamine use, a dry environment, solution sensitivity, or pregnancy.

■ The symptom of burning is often related to solution sensitivity or improper solution use.

■ Fluorescein evaluation of the cornea after lens removal should be a routine part of any soft lens evaluation.

■ Striae and epithelial edema may be visible with 4% to 6% corneal thickening.

■ A tight lens may be associated with conjunctival "drag," in which the conjunctiva is seen to move with the soft lens on the blink.

■ Silicone hydrogel lenses have reduced complications due to hypoxia by providing greater oxygen transmission to the cornea.

■ GPC may be prevented by compliance with disposable lens replacement schedules and rubbing the lens with solution upon removal. For the treatment of GPC, the use of disposable soft lenses and an antihistamine/mast cell stabilizer are beneficial.

REFERENCES

1. Connor CG, Presley L, Finchum SM, et al. The effectiveness of several current soft contact lens care systems against *Aspergillus*. CLAO J 1998;24:82–84.
2. Sakuma S, Reeh B, Dang D, et al. Comparative efficacies of four soft contact lens disinfection solutions. Int Contact Lens Clin 1996;23:234–239.
3. Szczotka-Flynn L, Diaz M. Risk of corneal inflammatory events with silicone hydrogel and low Dk hydrogel extended contact lens wear: a meta-analysis. Optom Vis Sci 2007;84:247–256.
4. Benjamin WJ, Hill RM. Surface coating: the fatal facade. Contact Lens Forum 1979;4:107–109.
5. Mandell RB. Symptomatology and aftercare. In: Mandell RB, ed. Contact Lens Practice, 4th ed. Springfield, IL: Charles C Thomas Publisher, 1988:598–643.
6. Sarver MD. Vision with hydrophilic contact lenses. J Am Optom Assoc 1972;43:316–320.
7. Mandell RB. Hydrogel lenses for astigmatism. In: Mandell RB, ed. Contact Lens Practice, 4th ed. Springfield, IL: Charles C Thomas Publisher, 1988:659–680.
8. Snyder C. Aspheric hydrogels "correct" minimal astigmatism? Contact Lens Spectrum 2000;15 (12):15.
9. Edrington TB, Barr JT. Creating better locus of focus. Contact Lens Spectrum 2002;17(6):44.

10. Blaze P. Refining toric soft lens correction. Contact Lens Forum 1988;13:53–58.

11. Mandell RB. Symptomatology and refitting. In: Mandell RB, ed. Contact Lens Practice, 4th ed. Springfield, IL: Charles C Thomas Publisher, 1988:388–439.

12. Bergmanson JPG. Contact lens-induced epithelial pathology. In: Bennett ES, Weissman BA, eds. Clinical Contact Lens Practice. Philadelphia: JB Lippincott Co, 1991:60-1–60-16.

13. Mandell RB. Clinical procedures. In: Mandell RB, ed. Contact Lens Practice, 4th ed. Springfield, IL: Charles C Thomas Publisher, 1988:310–325.

14. Doughty MJ, Fonn D, Richter D, et al. A patient questionnaire approach to estimating the prevalence of dry eye symptoms in patients presenting to optometric practices across Canada. Optom Vis Sci 1997;74:624–631.

15. Chalmers RL, Begley CG, Edrington T, et al. The agreement between self-assessment and clinician assessment of dry eye severity. Cornea 2005;24:804–810.

16. Nichols JJ, Mitchell GL, Nichols KK, et al. The performance of the contact lens dry eye questionnaire as a screening survey for contact lens-related dry eye. Cornea 2002;21:469–475.

17. Nichols JJ, Ziegler C, Mitchell GL, et al. Self-reported dry eye disease across refractive modalities. Invest Ophthalmol Vis Sci 2005;46:1911–1914.

18. Nichols JJ, Sinnott LT. Tear film, contact lens, and patient-related factors associated with contact lens-related dry eye. Invest Ophthalmol Vis Sci 2006;47:1319–1328.

19. Lorentz H, Jones, L. Lipid deposition on hydrogel contact lenses: how history can help us today. Optom Vis Sci 2007;84:286–295.

20. Bennett ES, Gordon JM. The borderline dry-eye patient and contact lens wear. Contact Lens Forum 1989;14:52–74.

21. Young G, Bowers R, Hall B, et al. Clinical comparison of Omafilcon A with four control materials. CLAO J 1997;23:249–258.

22. Lemp MA, Caffery B, Lebow K, et al. Omafilcon A (Proclear) soft contact lenses in a dry eye population. CLAO J 1999;25:40–47.

23. Peterson RC, Wolffsohn JS, Nick J, et al. Clinical performance of daily disposable soft contact lenses using sustained release technology. Contact Lens Anterior Eye 2006;29:127–134.

24. Nick J, Winterton L, Lally J. Enhancing comfort with a lubricating daily disposable. Optician 2005;229:30–32.

25. Osborn K, Veys J. A new silicone hydrogel lens for contact lens-related dryness, part 1: material properties. Optician 2005;229:39–41.

26. Dumbleton K, Keir N, Moezzi A, et al. Objective and subjective responses in patients refitted to daily-wear silicone hydrogel contact lenses. Optom Vis Sci 2006;83:758–768.

27. Dillehay SM. Does the level of available oxygen impact comfort in contact lens wear?: review of literature. Eye Contact Lens Sci Clin Pract 2007;33(3):1448–1155.

28. Ilhan B, Irkec M, Orhan M, et al. Surface deposits on frequent replacement and conventional daily wear soft contact lenses. CLAO J 1998;24:232–235.

29. Coopersmith L, Weinstock FJ. Current recommendations and practice regarding soft lens replacement and disinfection. CLAO J 1997;23:172–176.

30. Luxenberg MN, Green K. Reduction of corneal edema with topical hypertonic agents. Am J Ophthalmol 1971;71:847–853.

31. Jalbert I, Sweeney DF, Holden BA. Epithelial split associated with wear of a silicone hydrogel contact lens CLAO J 2001;27(4):231–233.

32. Pole JJ, Malinovsky VE, Pence NA, et al. Epithelial splits of the superior cornea in hydrogel contact lens patients. Int Contact Lens Clin 1989;16:252–255.

33. Dumbleton K. Noninflammatory silicone hydrogel contact lens complications. Eye Contact Lens 2003;29(1 Suppl):S186–S189; discussion S190–S191, S192–S194.

34. Dumbleton K. Adverse events with silicone hydrogel continuous wear. Contact Lens Anterior Eye 2002;25:137–146.

35. Carnt N, Wilcox MDP, Evans V, et al. Corneal staining: the IER matrix study 2007;22(9):38–43.

36. Benjamin WJ, Hill RM. Ultra-thins: the case for continuous care. J Am Optom Assoc 1980;51:277–279.

37. Hill JF. Changes in corneal curvature and refractive error upon refitting with flatter hydrophilic contact lenses. J Am Optom Assoc 1976;47:1214–1216.

38. Kame RT, Hayashida JK. Lens evaluation procedures and problem solving. In: Bennett ES, Weissman BA, eds. Clinical Contact Lens Practice, vol. 38. Philadelphia: JB Lippincott Co, 1991:1–10.

39. Sweeney D, Fonn D, Evans K. Silicone hydrogels: the evolution of a revolution. Contact Lens Spectrum 2006;Special Edition:14–19.

40. Holden BA, Mertz GW, McNally JJ. Corneal swelling response to contact lenses worn under extended wear conditions. Invest Ophthalmol Vis Sci 1983;24:218–226.

41. Mandell RB. Extended wear. In: Mandell RB, ed. Contact Lens Practice, 4th ed. Springfield, IL: Charles C Thomas Publisher, 1988:683–717.

42. Steffen RB, Schnider CM. The impact of silicone hydrogel materials on overnight corneal swelling. Eye Contact Lens 2007;33(3):115–120.

43. Fonn D, Dumbleton K, Jalbert I, et al. Benefits of silicone hydrogel lenses. Contact Lens Spectrum 2006;Special Edition:38–44.
44. Bergmanson JPG. Histopathological analysis of the corneal epithelium after contact lens wear. J Am Optom Assoc 1987;58:812–818.
45. Zantos SG. Cystic formations in the corneal epithelium during extended wear of contact lenses. Int Contact Lens Clin 1983;10:128–143.
46. Madigan MC, Holden BA, Kwok LS. Extended wear of hydrogel contact lenses can compromise the corneal epithelium. Invest Ophthalmol Vis Sci Suppl 1986;27:140.
47. Humphreys JA, Larke JR, Parrish ST. Microepithelial cysts observed in extended contact lens-wearing subjects. Br J Ophthalmol 1980;64:888–895.
48. Mandell RB. The "tight" soft contact lens. Contact Lens Forum 1979;4:21–32.
49. Silbert JA. Contact lens-related inflammatory reactions. In: Bennett ES, Weissman BA, eds. Clinical Contact Lens Practice. Philadelphia: JB Lippincott Co, 1991:65-1–65-9.
50. Schein OD, Glynn RJ, Poggio EC, et al. The relative risk of ulcerative keratitis between extended and daily wear soft contact lens wearers: a case-control study. N Engl J Med 1989;321:773–778.
51. Jones WL. Diseases of the sclera. In: Bartlett JD, Jaanus SD, eds. Clinical Ocular Pharmacology. Boston: Butterworth–Heinemann, 1995:763–765.
52. McMonnies CW. Corneal vascularization. In: Bennett ES, Weissman BA, eds. Clinical contact lens practice. Philadelphia: JB Lippincott Co, 1991:61-1–61-9.
53. Papas E, Willcox M. Reducing the consequences of hypoxia: the ocular redness response. Contact Lens Spectrum 2006;Special Edition:32–37.
54. Wolff E. The Anatomy of the Eye and Orbit. London: HK Lewis, 1958:30–180.
55. Duke-Elder S, Leigh AG. Diseases of the outer eye. In: System of Ophthalmology, vol. 8. London: Henry Kimpton, 1977:676.
56. Sugar A, Meyer RF. Giant papillary conjunctivitis after keratoplasty. Am J Ophthalmol 1981; 91:239–242.
57. Allansmith MR. Giant papillary conjunctivitis. J Am Optom Assoc 1990;61(Suppl):S42–S46.
58. McMonnies CW. Contact lens-induced corneal vascularization. Int Contact Lens Clin 1983;10:12–21.
59. Larke JR, Humphreys JA, Holmes R. Apparent corneal neovascularization in soft lens wearers. J Br Contact Lens Assoc 1981;4:105.
60. McMonnies CW. Risk factors in the aetiology of contact lens-induced corneal vascularization. Int Contact Lens Clin 1984;11:286–293.
61. Arentsen JJ. Corneal neovascularization in contact lens wearers. In: Cohen EJ, ed. International Ophthalmology Clinics, vol. 26. Boston: Little, Brown, 1986:15–23.
62. Allansmith MR. Palpebral conjunctiva: factors associated with papillary response and contact lens wear. J Am Optom Assoc 1984;55:199–200.
63. Spring TF. Reaction to hydrophilic lenses. Med J Aust 1974;1:499–503.
64. Allansmith MR, Korb DR, Greiner JV, et al. Giant papillary conjunctivitis in contact lens wearers. Am J Ophthalmol 1977;83:697–708.
65. Stenson S. Superior limbic keratoconjunctivitis associated with soft contact lens wear. Arch Ophthalmol 1983; 101:402–404.
66. Srinivasan BD, Jakobiec FD, Iwamoto T, et al. Giant papillary conjunctivitis with ocular prosthesis. Arch Ophthalmol 1979;97:892–895.
67. Donshik PC, Ballow M, Luistro A, et al. Treatment of contact lens induced giant papillary conjunctivitis. CLAO J 1984;10:346–350.
68. Ehlers WH, Donshik PC. Allergic diseases of the lids, conjunctiva, and cornea. Curr Opin Ophthalmol 1994;5: 31–38.

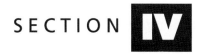

Challenging Cases

CHAPTER 14

Correction of Astigmatism

Edward S. Bennett, Kimberly A. Layfield, and P. Douglas Becherer

The purpose of this chapter is to discuss methods of managing the astigmatic contact lens patient. These patients can often be challenging to the eye care practitioner; however, it is the ability to fit these people successfully that makes practice both enjoyable and profitable. The principles of residual and high astigmatic correction with gas-permeable (GP) lenses and astigmatic correction with soft toric lenses are reviewed.

■ GAS-PERMEABLE CONTACT LENS APPLICATIONS

Residual Astigmatism

Residual astigmatism can be defined as the astigmatic refractive error present when a contact lens is placed on the eye to correct an existing ametropia. When a spherical lens is applied, the residual astigmatism is approximately equal to the difference between the corneal astigmatism and the refractive or total astigmatic error of the eye.

Residual astigmatism can be classified as either induced or physiologic. *Induced* residual astigmatism is associated with lens application and can be caused by lens warpage, flexure, decentration, or a toric anterior or posterior lens surface. This section of the chapter primarily addresses *physiologic* residual astigmatism, which commonly results from curvature refractive index differences of the posterior cornea and crystalline lens.

Calculated and Actual Residual Astigmatism

The calculated (or predicted) residual astigmatism (CRA) can be defined as the amount of astigmatism one would predict to result when a spherical GP lens is placed on the eye. It can be obtained directly by subtracting the patient's central anterior corneal toricity (as measured by keratometry) from the total astigmatism of the eye at the plane of the cornea. The following examples illustrate the determination of CRA. In these examples, TRA refers to the total refractive astigmatism and ΔK refers to the difference between the keratometric readings of the two corneal meridians.

EXAMPLE 1

Given: Spectacle Rx $= -1.00 - 2.00 \times 090$

Keratometry $= 42.00 @ 090; 43.00 @ 180$

Then: $\text{CRA} = \text{TRA} - \Delta K$

$= -2.00 \times 090 - (-1.00 \times 090)$

$= -1.00 \times 090$

EXAMPLE 2

Given: Spectacle Rx = $-2.00 - 1.50 \times 180$

Keratometry = 41.00 @ 180; 44.00 @ 090

Then: CRA = TRA − ΔK

$= -1.50 \times 180 - (-3.00 \times 180)$

$= +1.50 \times 180$ or transposed:

$= +1.50 - 1.50 \times 090$

$= -1.50 \times 090$

EXAMPLE 3

Given: Spectacle Rx = $+3.00 - 3.50 \times 180$

Keratometry = 40.00 @ 180; 43.00 @ 090

Then: CRA = TRA − ΔK

$= -3.50 \times 180 - (-3.00 \times 180)$

$= -0.50 \times 180$

EXAMPLE 4

Given: Spectacle Rx = $-8.00 - 2.50 \times 180$

Keratometry = 42.50 @ 180; 45.00 @ 090

$$\text{F90 (12 mm vertex distance)} = \frac{-10.50}{1 - 0.012\,(-10.50)} = -9.33 \text{ D}$$

$$\text{F180 (12 mm vertex distance)} = \frac{-8.00}{1 - 0.012\,(-8.00)} = -7.30 \text{ D}$$

Spectacle Rx (at corneal plane) = $-7.25 - 2.00 \times 180$

Then: CRA = TRA − ΔK

$= -2.00 \times 180 - (-2.50 \times 180)$

$= +0.50 \times 180$ or transposed to:

$= +0.50 - 0.50 \times 090$

$= -0.50 \times 090$

EXAMPLE 5

Given: Spectacle Rx = $+13.50 - 3.00 \times 010$

Keratometry = 41.00 @ 010; 44.00 @ 100

$$\text{F010 (12 mm vertex distance)} = \frac{+13.50}{1 - 0.012\,(+13.50)} = +16.11 \text{ D}$$

$$\text{F100 (12 mm vertex distance)} = \frac{+10.50}{1 - 0.012\,(+10.50)} = +12.01 \text{ D}$$

Spectacle Rx (at corneal plane) = $+16.00 - 4.00 \times 010$

Then: CRA = TRA − ΔK

$$= -4.00 \times 010 - (-3.00 \times 010)$$

$$= -1.00 \times 010$$

In Examples 4 and 5, the importance of vertexing the patient's refraction to the corneal plane is quite apparent. In both cases if vertex distance was ignored, the calculated residual astigmatism would equal zero.

If a GP spherical lens of standard thickness (to minimize or eliminate the effects of flexure) is selected for a diagnostic fitting, the predicted spherocylindrical overrefraction (OR) can be calculated by using the following guidelines[1]:

1. List the spectacle correction (Rx) and keratometric readings.
2. The effective power should be determined at the corneal plane (if indicated).
3. Determine the lacrimal lens power induced by the base curve radius (BCR) of the lens.
4. Add together the powers of the contact lens, lacrimal lens, and the difference between the keratometric readings of the principal corneal meridians.
5. With the following formula, subtract the value obtained in step 4 from the spectacle correction to obtain the overrefraction:

$$\text{Overrefraction (OR)} = \text{Spectacle Rx} - [\text{Contact Lens Power (CLP)} + \text{Lacrimal Lens Power (LLP)} + \Delta K]$$

The following example illustrates this principle:

EXAMPLE 6

1. Spectacle Rx	$= -2.00 - 2.50 \times 180$
Keratometry	= 43.00 @ 180; 45.00 @ 090
Diagnostic lens	= −3.00 D; 43.25 D base curve radius
2. At corneal plane, spectacle Rx	$= -2.00 - 2.25 \times 180$
3. LLP	= 43.25 − 43.00 = +0.25
4. CLP + LLP + ΔK	= LLP + ΔK = [−3.00 + (+)0.25] + (−)2.00 × 180
	$= -2.75 - 2.00 \times 180$
5. OR	= Spectacle Rx − (CLP + LLP + ΔK)
	$= -2.00 - 2.25 \times 180 - (-2.75 - 2.00 \times 180)$
	$= +0.75 - 0.25 \times 180$

Does the CRA correlate well with the residual astigmatism actually obtained after diagnostic lens application (i.e., actual residual astigmatism, or ARA)? There does appear to be some correlation, although often the ARA will be slightly less.[2–5] In one study of over 400 eyes fitted with spherical GP lenses, the mean CRA was found to be −0.51 D ×090, whereas the mean ARA was equal to −0.23 D × 090.[2] The difference between the CRA and ARA values could be caused by many factors, including inaccuracy of the keratometer for determining anterior corneal curvature (i.e., it evaluates only a few points on the paracentral cornea). In addition, examiner error in performing both refraction and keratometry could produce a difference between these two astigmatic values.

When a patient has refractive and keratometric cylinder axes that differ by >15 degrees, it can be assumed that the axes are unequal and the use of conventional crossed-cylinder equations are necessary to determine the CRA. Because of the time involved, unless the appropriate tables or a computer-assisted contact lens design program is available, the use of a GP, spherical diagnostic lens for overrefraction to determine the residual astigmatism is advisable.

Methods of Correcting Residual Astigmatism

A GP contact lens may cause a reduction in visual acuity that is unacceptable to a patient because of the amount of residual astigmatism. This depends on the amount of residual astigmatism, the patient's refractive error, and whether critical vision demands are common. Highly ametropic patients may be able to tolerate a higher amount of residual cylinder than low ametropes. Therefore, individual variance is determined by the amount of residual astigmatism necessary to contraindicate the use of a spherical GP lens; however, patients exhibiting >0.75 D often experience subjectively compromised vision. Methods of correcting residual astigmatism include spherical GP lenses, spherical soft lenses, soft toric lenses, and front surface toric GP lenses.

Spherical Gas-Permeable Lenses: Spherical GP lenses can be successfully fitted to patients exhibiting residual astigmatism if any one of the following conditions exists:

1. **ARA differs in amount from CRA.** For example, you may predict a CRA of -1.00×090, but your overrefraction results in a value of -0.50×090. Rechecking keratometry or the subjective refraction may determine where the error was made. However, the most important factor is to never allow the CRA to prevent spherical GP lens application because of the possibility of obtaining a lower ARA value.
2. **The lens can flex on the eye to reduce residual astigmatism.** In most cases, flexure or bending of a GP lens on the eye will increase the existent residual astigmatism. However, there is one case in which flexure will actually reduce or totally correct residual astigmatism. It has been found that when the corneal toricity is with-the-rule and the residual astigmatism is against-the-rule, a thin spherical GP lens will flex and reduce the amount of residual astigmatism.[6] This is illustrated in the following example:

EXAMPLE 7

Given: Spectacle Rx $= -2.00 - 1.00 \times 180$

Keratometry $= 41.00 @ 180; 43.00 @ 090$

Then: CRA = TRA − ΔK

$= -1.00 \times 180 - (-)2.00 \times 180$

$= +1.00 \times 180$ transposed to:

$= +1.00 - 1.00 \times 090$

A thin lens can flex between 0.25 to 0.50 D to correct some of this residual astigmatic error.[6,7] The use of a GP lens with high oxygen permeability (Dk) in a thin, large-diameter design fitted "steeper than K" (e.g., the Menicon Z thin design) should, in theory, correct even a greater amount of residual astigmatism.

3. **The demand on critical vision is low.**
4. **The patient's visual acuity is not decreased to an unacceptable level.**

Spherical Soft Lenses: There is one situation in which a spherical soft lens would definitely be indicated. If very little or no refractive astigmatism is present in the patient's spectacle correction, a spherical soft lens should provide acceptable visual acuity. This is demonstrated in Example 8.

EXAMPLE 8

Given: Spectacle Rx = −4.00 − 0.25 × 180

Keratometry = 43.00 @ 180; 44.50 @ 090

Then: CRA = −0.25 × 180 − (−)1.50 × 180

= +1.25 × 180 or transposed to:

= +1.25 − 1.25 × 090

The other advantage of spherical soft lens use is the avoidance of a more complicated and expensive lens design.

Soft Toric Lenses: The most common reason for the rapid decline in front surface toric GP lenses for correction of residual astigmatism is the optical quality, parameter availability, and disposability of soft toric lenses. With few exceptions, patients with ≥0.75 D of ARA can be fitted successfully into soft torics. The availability of large diagnostic sets incorporating numerous astigmatic corrections has also made this an easy option for fitting patients. The following examples illustrate representative applications for soft toric lenses in patients with a high amount of residual astigmatism:

EXAMPLE 9

Given: Spectacle Rx = −2.50 − 1.25 × 180

Keratometry = 43.00 DS

Then: CRA = TRA − ΔK

= −1.25 × 180 − 0

= −1.25 × 180

EXAMPLE 10

Given: Spectacle Rx = −2.50 − 1.25 × 180

Keratometry = 43.00 @ 180; 45.50 @ 090

Then: CRA = TRA − ΔK

= −1.25 × 180 − (−)2.50 × 180

= +1.25 × 180 or

= +1.25 − 1.25 × 090

In Examples 9 and 10, these patients exhibited no and high corneal astigmatism, respectively; however, they were both good candidates for soft toric lenses. Soft toric lenses are most successful when the refractive cylinder is between −0.75 D and −2.00 D and the cylinder axis is not oblique. The reasons for this are fourfold:

1. Most soft toric lenses are available in these parameters; higher-cylinder-power custom lenses are available at slightly more—to much greater—expense.
2. Most diagnostic sets and inventories are in these parameters.

3. In high refractive astigmatism, rotation of the lens with the blink may reduce visual acuity.
4. Oblique cylinder axes tend to result in greater lid effect on the lens edge; therefore, rotational instability is possible.

Front Surface Toric Gas-Permeable Lenses: Application of the patient's residual astigmatic correction onto the front of the GP lens surface was, until the introduction of soft toric lenses, the most common method of correcting this problem. It is still a recommended option in some cases, including patients who desire or benefit visually from a GP lens and those who have experienced soft lens-induced complications [i.e., edema, giant papillary conjunctivitis (GPC)]. Three stabilization methods have been used: (a) prism ballast, (b) prism ballast and truncation, and (c) periballast.

1. **Prism ballast.** Prism ballast can be incorporated into a GP lens to allow the patient's residual cylinder to be ground onto the front surface of the lens. The purpose of the prism is to stabilize the lens from possible rotational movement induced by the action of the lids. It is recommended when patients have lower lids at or below the lower limbus, when large palpebral apertures with loose lids are present, and whenever discomfort is experienced with truncated, prism-ballasted lens designs.[8]

The amount of prism to be incorporated into the lens design is the minimum amount that produces stabilization and is dependent on lens power. An amount equal to 0.75 to 1 Δ for moderate and high minus lenses and 1.25 to 1.5 Δ for low minus and plus lenses has been recommended.[9] A greater amount of prism is indicated with plus power lenses because of the thinner edge present in these designs.

Because of the greater center thickness (CT) of these lenses in comparison to spherical designs, a high-Dk lens material (>50) is recommended. A minimum overall diameter (OAD) of 8.8 mm is recommended, both to incorporate the prism effectively and help offset the possible effects of flare from a heavier, potentially inferiorly decentering lens design. To estimate the center thickness of a prism-ballasted lens, the following equation can be used[9]:

$$\text{Center thickness} \times 100 = \text{Prismatic power} \times \text{Overall diameter}$$

Therefore, if 1 Δ were used for stabilizing a 9.0-mm OAD, 0.09 mm would need to be added to a conventional spherical lens design of the same power (more plus meridian) to obtain an estimate of the CT in prism-ballasted form. If the conventional spherical CT for the lens power in the most plus meridian is 0.15 mm, in prism-ballasted form the CT would equal 0.15 + 0.09, or 0.24 mm.

If a diagnostic fitting set is present, a slightly "steeper than K" lens should be selected. As the center of gravity tends to be more anterior and the mass of these lenses tends to defy gravity somewhat, a plus tear film centrally should assist with centration. If the lens is riding inferiorly with little or no movement after the blink, a minus carrier should be indicated in the final order. A well-fitted lens will move slightly superiorly with the blink but with little or no rotation (i.e., a direct vertical movement).[10] Evaluating the amount of lens rotation with the blink is very important. This effect will vary as a result of such factors as the lid configuration, location, tightness, and forcefulness of the blink. As a result of the natural alignment or symmetry of the superior lid, there is a tendency for the lid to rotate nasally or excyclorotate. Therefore, the presence of tight lids or a forceful blink may contraindicate a front surface toric design. Assuming the base of the prism is dotted on the diagnostic lens, the amount of rotation can be evaluated in several ways, including the following:

a. **Trial frame.** The patient can also wear a trial frame in combination with a low-power cylinder trial lens having hash marks for judgement of rotation (Fig. 14.1). The marks on the spectacle trial lens can be aligned with both the prism base and the optical section beam, and the degree reading can be read directly from the trial frame.

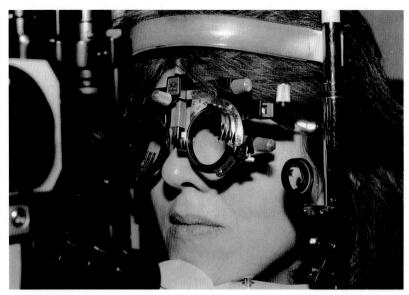

■ **FIGURE 14.1** Trial frame use with trial lens and hash marks to estimate toric lens rotation.

b. **Slit-lamp beam rotation.** Many of the slit lamps in use today allow the practitioner to rotate the optical section to align with the position of the prism base. The amount of rotation can be read directly from a scale on the slit lamp.

c. **"Guesstimate."** The most commonly used (and convenient) method is simply to estimate the amount of rotation with the blink. Because it is very easy to underestimate the amount of rotation, always think of the lens as a clock, with each hour equivalent to 30 degrees. If the prism base appears to be at approximately 6:30 (not 6 o'clock), the prism base has rotated 15 degrees. The importance of proper evaluation of rotational amount and stability is discussed further in the section of this chapter on soft toric lenses.

After the amount of rotation has been determined by one of the aforementioned methods, the contact lens powers must be adjusted accordingly. If, as you observe the lens, the right lens rotates 15 degrees nasally (to the observer's right) and the left lens rotates 15 degrees nasally (to the observer's left), then the LARS (left add, right subtract) principle is used (Fig. 14.2). In this case the axis of the final cylinder power of the right lens is decreased by 15 degrees, while the cylinder axis of the left lens is increased 15 degrees. On the average, prism-ballasted lenses tend to rotate 10 to 15 degrees nasally.

When a desirable lens-to-cornea fitting relationship has been achieved and an overrefraction performed through the ballasted sphere, the lenses can be ordered. If a diagnostic fitting set is not available (as is often the case), an overrefraction over the best-fitting spherical lenses will assist in determining the final lens powers. The calculations required to arrive at the final parameters are illustrated in the following example[1]:

EXAMPLE 11

	OD	OS
Spectacle Rx	$-1.50 - 1.00 \times 090$	$-2.50 - 1.25 \times 090$
Keratometry	43.25 DS	43.00 @ 090; 43.25 @ 180
Diagnostic lens	43.50 DS, -3.00 D	43.25 DS, -3.00 D
SLE	Good centration OU	
Overrefraction	$+1.25 - 1.50 \times 090$	$+0.25 - 1.00 \times 090$
Final power	$-1.75 - 1.50 \times 090$	$-2.75 - 1.00 \times 090$

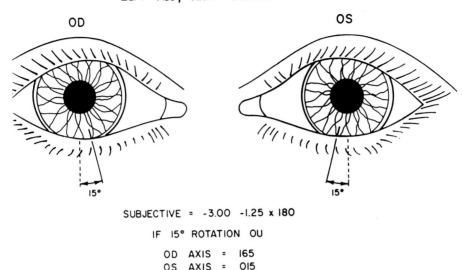

FIGURE 14.2 The LARS (left add, right subtract) principle.

The LLP can be obtained by subtracting the combined powers of the contact lens and the overrefraction from the spectacle correction.

The values obtained in the overrefractions above actually equal the predicted values. These can be obtained by performing the following calculations:

OD	OS

LLP = Spectacle Rx − (CLP + OR)

$$= [-1.50 - 1.00 \times 090] - \qquad [-2.50 - 1.25 \times 090]$$

$$[(-3.00) + (+)\, 1.25 - 1.50 \qquad -\, [(-3.00) + (+)0.25 - 1.00$$

$$\times\, 090] \qquad \times\, 090]$$

$$= [-1.50 - 1.00 \times 090] \qquad [-2.50 - 1.25 \times 090]$$

$$-\, [(-)1.75 - 1.50 \times 090] \qquad -\, [(-)2.75 - 1.00 \times 090]$$

$$= +0.25 + 0.50 \times 090 \qquad +0.25 - 0.25 + 090$$

The contact lens power can be derived simply by subtracting the LLP from the spectacle correction:

OD	OS

CLP = Spectacle Rx − LLP

$$= [-1.50 - 1.00 \times 090] \qquad [-2.50 - 1.25 \times 090]$$

$$-\, [+0.25 + 0.50 \times 090] \qquad -\, (+)0.25 - 0.25 \times 090$$

$$= -1.75 - 1.50 \times 090 \qquad -2.75 - 1.00 \times 090$$

As the cylinder will be ground on the front surface of the lens in plus cylinder form, the contact lens powers are transposed to:

OD

OS

$-3.25 + 1.50 \times 180$

$-3.75 + 1.00 \times 180$

As compensation for lens rotation is often desired, this could become:

OD

OS

$-3.25 + 1.50 \times 165$

$-3.75 + 1.00 \times 015$

The contact lens order could be written as follows:

Parameter	OD	OS
BCR	43.50 (7.76)	43.50 (7.76)
CLP	$-3.25 + 1.50 \times 165$	$-3.75 + 1.00 \times 015$
OAD	9.0	9.0
OZD	7.8	7.8
SCR/W (=BCR + 1 mm)	8.8/.3	8.8/.3
PCR/W (=SCR + 2 mm)	10.8/.3	10.8/.3
CT	0.26	0.25
Prism	1Δ, double dot base	1Δ, dot base
Material	Fluoroperm 60	Fluoroperm 60
Add. information	Minus carrier	Minus carrier

2. **Prism ballast and truncation.** In most cases in which a front toric GP lens is desirable, the lens of choice is a prism-ballasted truncated design. The addition of truncation assists in providing good rotational stability.

Most of the design and fitting information provided for prism ballast-only designs also pertains to lenses that incorporate prism ballast. The primary differences pertain to OAD, prism, and the shape of the inferior edge. Typically, vertical diameters are 8.7 to 9.2 mm, with horizontal diameters usually 0.4 to 0.5 mm larger.[8] Truncating a prism-ballasted lens reduces the ballast for minus lenses and increases it for plus lenses. Therefore, especially in high minus powers, the need for more prism ballast is imperative to maintain the truncation in contact with the lower lid; an amount equal to 1.25 to 1.5 Δ would be recommended, whereas a smaller amount is indicated for low minus and plus power lenses. Finally, the shape of the truncation is quite important. As the truncation should rest evenly against the lower lid, the edge should be flat to increase the distribution of lens pressure across as much of the lid as possible.[8] Anterior tapering of the lens edge may result in the truncation slipping under the lower lid; posterior edge tapering may result in subjective discomfort. Because of the typical nasal rotation of the base, ordering the truncation at approximately 15 degrees temporal to the base−apex line would be recommended. Referring back to Example 11, the order of a prism-ballasted truncated design might be similar to the following:

Parameter	OD	OS
Base curve radius	43.50 (7.76)	43.50 (7.76)
CLP	$-3.25 + 1.50 \times 165$	$-3.75 + 1.00 \times 015$

OAD	9.4/8.9	9.4/8.9
OZD	7.8 (decentered 0.5 mm) up	7.8 (same as OD)
SCR/W	8.8/0.3	8.8/0.3
PCR/W	10.8/0.3	10.8/0.3
CT	0.26	0.25
Prism	1.25 Δ	1.25 Δ
Material	Fluoroperm 60	Fluoroperm 60
Add. information	Double dot base	Dot base
	Truncation 15° temp OU	

The above examples assumed that diagnostic lenses were unavailable. Obviously, the success rate would be higher if diagnostic lenses were used. A recommended diagnostic set is provided in Table 14.1.

Prism-ballasted, front surface toric lens designs, both truncated and nontruncated, are associated with some problems that limit their use. These include the following[1]:

1. Vision is blurred.
2. Discomfort results from prism, truncation, or both.
3. Quality control is poor.
4. Inferior decentration causes flare and possibly corneal desiccation.
5. It is not possible to modify the front surface.
6. If unilateral, asthenopia can result from a vertical imbalance although low amounts of prism (i.e., $0.75 - 1 \Delta$) can usually be tolerated.
7. Edema can develop if a low-Dk GP lens material is used.

Verification of front surface toric lenses is straightforward. The back surface of the lens is placed against the lens stop of the lensometer and is rotated until the position of the target image indicates prism base down (axis = 90 degrees). If, for example, the left lens cylinder was ordered at axis 105, the base of the prism should be rotated nasally 15 degrees to obtain the power in that meridian. The lens is then rotated 90 degrees to obtain the power in the other

TABLE 14.1 CIRCULAR PRISM-BALLASTED TRIAL LENS SET (10 LENSES)				
BASE CURVE	OAD/OZD	CLP	SCR/W	PCR/W
1. 40.50 (8.33)	9.2/8.0	−3.00	9.30/0.3	11.30/0.3
2. 41.50 (8.13)	9.2/8.0	−3.00	9.10/0.3	11.10/0.3
3. 42.00 (8.04)	9.2/8.0	−3.00	9.00/0.3	11.00/0.3
4. 42.50 (7.94)	9.0/7.8	−3.00	8.90/0.3	10.90/0.3
5. 43.00 (7.85)	9.0/7.8	−3.00	8.90/0.3	10.90/0.3
6. 43.50 (7.76)	9.0/7.8	−3.00	8.80/0.3	10.80/0.3
7. 44.00 (7.67)	9.0/7.8	−3.00	8.70/0.3	10.70/0.3
8. 44.50 (7.58)	8.8/7.8	−3.00	8.60/0.3	10.60/0.3
9. 45.00 (7.50)	8.8/7.8	−3.00	8.50/0.3	10.50/0.3
10. 46.00 (7.34)	8.8/7.8	−3.00	8.30/0.3	10.30/0.3

CLP, contact lens power; OAD, overall diameter; OZD, optical zone diameter; PCR/W, peripheral curve radius/width; SCR/W, secondary curve radius/width.

meridian. The cylinder power of the lens is the same on the eye as in air when measured with the lensometer, as the cylinder is on the front surface only. If the lens was ordered with the power $-3.25 +1.25 \times 075$, this should be the power read with the lensometer.

3. **Periballast.** A periballasted lens design is cut in lenticular form with a high minus carrier. Two forms of this lens design are available. In one form, the final lens is cut with no flange at the top and with the entire 1.0 to 1.3 mm of flange left at the bottom to achieve the ballast. In the other form, the lens is manufactured such that a small amount of flange remains at the top to provide a minus carrier effect.

A periballast does reduce some of the prism ballast-induced problems. The advantages include better optical quality, a thinner design, and no vertical imbalance. However, it is rarely used because of the rotational instability and flange-induced discomfort.

High Astigmatism

The correction of high astigmatic error, defined as ≥ 2.50 D of corneal astigmatism, is quite different from correction of residual astigmatic error. In most cases, the selection of a carefully designed spherical or bitoric design will be successful with these patients. The latter design alternative is most often recommended, and these designs are easy to fit and evaluate. Other alternatives include aspheric designs, toric soft lenses, and back surface toric GP lenses.

Spherical Gas-Permeable Lenses

Although the benefits of a spherical design in high astigmatism include the use of an uncomplicated lens design and less expense, the selection of this alternative will, in most cases, eventually result in failure because of such problems as decentration-induced symptoms of visual flare, corneal desiccation resulting from excessive peripheral clearance, flexure-induced fluctuation in visual acuity, and lens rocking resulting in corneal staining.[10] In addition, although good centration is possible to achieve regardless of the amount of corneal astigmatism, these lenses will, as a result of poor corneal alignment, apply excessive pressure (i.e., bearing zones) against the cornea, possibly resulting in corneal distortion.[11] This condition is accelerated if poor centration is present.[12]

In many cases, it is not a bad idea to use a spherical lens as the initial diagnostic lens and evaluate vision, corneal alignment, and centration. A relatively low-Dk material (i.e., 25–50) should be selected to minimize flexure and facilitate manufacture. The BCR should be about one-third of the difference "steeper than K" to achieve a well-centered intrapalpebral lens-to-cornea fitting relationship. The CT in minus lens powers should be 0.02 to 0.04 mm thicker than with low astigmatic patients to minimize flexure. Overkeratometry should also be performed to rule out flexure. If toricity >0.50 D exists with overkeratometry, either a flatter BCR or a bitoric lens design should be considered.

Aspheric Designs

An aspheric design may provide better centration and a more uniform fluorescein pattern than a spherical lens design. In particular, designs with an elliptic back surface (i.e., the progressive and the so-called "biaspheric" designs) have been shown to exhibit good centration in patients having 2 to 3 D of corneal astigmatism (Fig. 14.3).[13] However, to minimize symptoms of visual flare, good centration is imperative with these designs.

Soft Toric

Improvements in quality control, enhanced quality of vision, and greater oxygen transmissibility currently make this modality an option to consider when a high astigmatic patient with no evidence of corneal distortion is strongly motivated toward soft lens wear.[14] In addition,

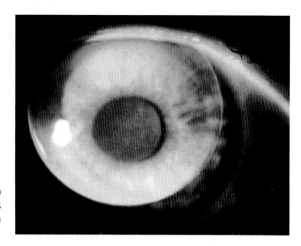

■ **FIGURE 14.3** An aspheric lens (Boston Envision) providing good centration and a less obvious "dumbbell-shaped" fluorescein pattern than present with a spherical design.

numerous companies manufacture custom soft toric lenses in practically any axis and power, and improvements in edge designs have resulted in better subjective comfort than was attained with previous-generation designs. Finally, computer-assisted lens design programs are available that are especially beneficial in cross-cylinder situations and currently are being used by both practitioners and manufacturers.[15] This type of program is capable of providing a recommended cylinder axis and power based on the patient's refractive data, the diagnostic lens parameters, and the amount of rotation on the eye.

Excellent quality control is imperative with these lenses, and they should also be stable on the eye; rotation of only a few degrees can significantly affect visual performance, especially with patients having more than 3 D of corneal astigmatism. If corneal distortion or irregular astigmatism is present, a much better visual result can be attained with the selection of a GP lens. Manufacturers' claims of success and accuracy may also be erroneous; therefore, it's important to consider toric soft lenses when the patient is motivated, astigmatism is regular, and the need for critical distance vision is not great.

Back Surface Toric

A back surface toric lens design has the advantage of providing greater alignment of the posterior lens surface to the cornea; therefore, better centration is present. In addition, problems such as flexure, lens rocking, and flare are minimized.

There are numerous philosophies on how to determine the base curve radii for any posterior surface (i.e., back surface or bitoric designs). The Mandell-Moore philosophy for determining the base curve radii is provided in Table 14.2.[16] To assist in achieving alignment between lens and cornea, toric peripheral curves may be beneficial.[17] To determine the specific peripheral curve radii to select, the following philosophy can be used:

> *Secondary curve radii (SCR)* = 1.0 mm flatter than the base curve radii [e.g., if the base curve radii are 41 D (8.23 mm) and 44 D (7.67 mm), the SCR would be 9.23/8.67 mm or rounded off to 9.2/8.7 mm].

> *Peripheral curve radii (PCR)* = 3.0 mm flatter than the BCRs; in the above case they would be equal to 11.2/10.7 mm.

If a spherical periphery is desired, simply add 1.0 mm to the average BCR to determine the SCR and add 3.0 mm to determine the PCR. In the above example, the average between 41 D and 44 D equals 42.50 D (7.94 mm); the SCR would equal (approximately) 8.9 mm and the PCR would equal 10.9 mm.

TABLE 14.2 MANDELL-MOORE FIT FACTOR

CORNEAL CYL	FIT FLAT MERIDIAN	FIT STEEP MERIDIAN
2.0 D	On K	0.50 D Flatter
2.5 D	0.25 D Flatter	0.50 D Flatter
3.0 D	0.25 D Flatter	0.75 D Flatter
3.5 D	0.25 D Flatter	0.75 D Flatter
4.0 D	0.25 D Flatter	0.75 D Flatter
5.0 D	0.25 D Flatter	0.75 D Flatter

From Mandell RB, Moore CF. A bitoric lens guide that really is simple. Contact Lens Spectrum 1988;3(11):83–85.

When determining the base curve radii, the tear layer power will result in a change in power. To determine these values, Sarver's formula can be used[18]:

$$Fs = Ff + Kf - Ks$$

where

Fs = the back vertex power of the contact lens in the steeper principal meridian (in air)
Ff = the back vertex power of the contact lens in the flatter principal meridian (in air)
Ks = the BCR of the contact lens in the steeper principal meridian
Kf = the BCR of the contact lens in the flatter principal meridian

All of this information can be incorporated into the following example:

EXAMPLE 12

Spectacle Rx: $+0.50 - 4.00 \times 180$

Keratometry: 40.50 @ 180; 44.50 @ 090

A spherical diagnostic lens with a BCR of 41.50 D was attempted. However, this lens resulted in inferior decentration and some flexure-induced uncorrected corneal astigmatism confirmed by toric readings by keratometry performed over the lenses. A back surface toric lens design, using the Mandell-Moore base curve philosophy, is then ordered. The parameters can be obtained from the following:

$$Kf = 40.50 + (-)0.25 = 40.25 \text{ D}$$

$$Ks = 44.50 - 0.75 = 43.75 \text{ D}$$

$$Ff = +0.50 + (0.25)(\text{LLP}) = +0.75 \text{ D}$$

$$Fs = +0.75 + (40.25 - 43.75) = -2.75 \text{ D}$$

The peripheral curves can be determined as follows:

$$\text{Average BCR} = \frac{40.25 + 43.75}{2} = 42.00 \text{ D } (8.04 \text{ mm})$$

$$SCR = 8.00 \text{ mm (rounded off from 8.04)} + 1.00 = 9.00 \text{ mm}$$

$$PCR = 8.00 + 3.00 = 11.00 \text{ mm}$$

Final order (empirical):

BCR	Power	SCR/W	PCR/W	OAD
40.25/43.75	+0.75	9.00/.3	11.00/.3	9.2
(8.38)(7.71)				

Unfortunately, the great majority of high astigmatic patients would not be able to achieve optimum visual acuity from a back surface toric design because of the problem of induced cylinder. A back surface toric GP contact lens in situ induces a cylinder in the optical system (contact lens-fluid lens) designed to correct the ametropia. The minus cylinder is the result of the difference between the refractive index of the contact lens (n = 1.44–1.49 in most cases; 1.49 will be used here) and the index of the tear lens (n = 1.336). The exact amount would be 0.456 times the back surface toricity. The minus cylinder axis will lie along the flatter principal meridian of the toric back surface of the contact lens. This induced cylinder rarely corrects and sometimes compounds the residual astigmatism.

The following contact lens conversion factors are important when determining the changes in power induced by a toric back surface contact lens.

1. From back surface lens toricity (measured with the radiuscope) to contact lens cylinder power in air (measured with the lensometer)—multiply by 1.452 (or approximately 1.5).
2. From back surface lens toricity (measured with the radiuscope) to the contact lens cylinder power measured in fluid (on the eye or induced)—multiply by 0.456 (or approximately one-half).
3. From contact lens cylinder power in air (measured with the lensometer) to the contact lens cylinder power in fluid (on the eye or induced)—multiply by 0.314 (or approximately one-third).
4. From the contact lens cylinder power in fluid (on the eye or induced) to the contact lens cylinder power in air (measured with the lensometer)—multiply by 3.19 (or approximately 3).

Essentially, this concept can be simplified to a 1:2:3 principle (Fig. 14.4). This would represent a fractional component by which if one component is known, the other two can be easily determined. If "2" equals the amount of base curve toricity verified with the radiuscope, "1" equals 1 divided by 2 or one-half the base curve toricity; "3" equals both three times the "1" value or 3/2 times the base curve toricity. If the base curve toricity equals 3 D, the induced cylinder predicted with lens wear is one-half this value or 1.5 D; the value verified with a lensometer is 4.5 D or 3/2 times the radiuscope value.

Referring back to Example 12, the amount of induced astigmatism would equal approximately 0.5 × ΔK (back surface or −3.50 × 180) = −1.75 × 180. A plus correcting cylinder of the same amount and axis is applied to the front surface; therefore, in this case, +1.75 D × 180 is the front surface cylinder power. This will result in a power of −3.50 × 180 while creating a spherical power effect (i.e., the lens can rotate on the eye without affecting vision); this will be discussed later in this section of the chapter.

The other factor to consider when verifying a back surface toric lens is that because the induced astigmatism is not corrected, when the cylinder power is verified with a lensometer, a value equal to approximately 1.5 times the back surface toricity (radiuscope cylinder) will be read. In the previous example, the amount of cylinder power recorded with a lensometer is −3.50 × 1.5 = −5.25 D × 180. This is a key factor when a back surface toric is differentiated from a bitoric lens because a bitoric design with the induced cylinder corrected on the front surface (unless a significant residual astigmatism is also being incorporated into the lens) will verify with a similar cylinder for both the radiuscope and the lensometer.

To summarize this discussion, it is apparent that to obtain both good centration and good visual acuity, a bitoric lens is indicated. There is one situation in which a back surface toric design would provide the preferable vision correction. This design is the lens of choice when

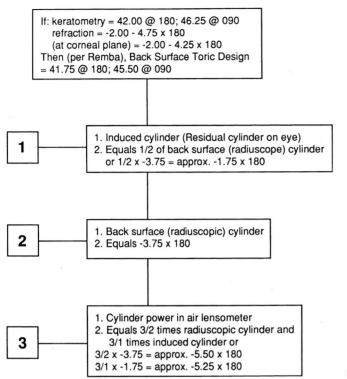

> If: keratometry = 42.00 @ 180; 46.25 @ 090
>   refraction = -2.00 - 4.75 x 180
>   (at corneal plane) = -2.00 - 4.25 x 180
> Then (per Remba), Back Surface Toric Design
> = 41.75 @ 180; 45.50 @ 090

1
1. Induced cylinder (Residual cylinder on eye)
2. Equals 1/2 of back surface (radiuscope) cylinder
   or 1/2 x -3.75 = approx. -1.75 x 180

2
1. Back surface (radiuscopic) cylinder
2. Equals -3.75 x 180

3
1. Cylinder power in air lensometer
2. Equals 3/2 times radiuscopic cylinder and
   3/1 times induced cylinder or
   3/2 x -3.75 = approx. -5.50 x 180
   3/1 x -1.75 = approx. -5.25 x 180

■ FIGURE 14.4 The 1:2:3 principle.

the corneal toricity is against-the-rule and the residual astigmatism is approximately 0.5 times the amount of back surface toricity of the lens (as measured with the radiuscope).

Bitoric Design

In most cases of high corneal astigmatism, a bitoric lens design should be used. The benefits of centration (Fig. 14.5) and, if the lenses are well designed and manufactured, satisfactory visual acuity are present with this option.

It was mentioned earlier that if the induced astigmatism that was created as a result of the toric anterior tear layer is corrected, a spherical power effect is created. In other words, if this front surface correction is ground onto the lens in the correct meridian relative to the principal meridian of the base curve, lens rotation will not alter the correction and the bitoric lens will provide a spherical effect when correcting only for the induced astigmatism.[19,20] This is

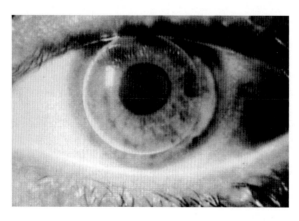

■ FIGURE 14.5 A well-centered bitoric lens on a highly astigmatic cornea.

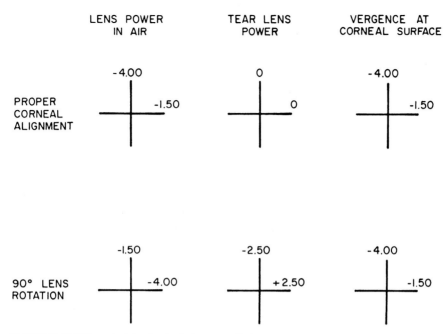

| LENS POWER IN AIR | TEAR LENS POWER | VERGENCE AT CORNEAL SURFACE |

FIGURE 14.6 The principle of spherical power effect.

shown in Figure 14.6 in which the extreme case of 90-degree rotation is provided. It is shown that the tear layer will compensate, and the front surface cylinder correction will still equal the new cylinder and axis of the induced cylinder.

Fitting Methods: A misperception of bitoric lenses is that they are very challenging to fit. However, this has not been substantiated by recent research.[21,22] In a survey of the Diplomates of the Cornea and Contact Lens Section of the American Academy of Optometry (AAO), approximately 90% responded that bitoric GP lenses varied from acceptable to very easy to fit.[22] These lenses are fitted either empirically or via a bitoric diagnostic set.

Empirical Methods: The lens powers and base curve radii of any back surface or bitoric lens design can be determined by several methods, including the previously demonstrated computational method.[10] Example 13 shows how these values can be determined for a bitoric design using both computational and optical cross methods:

EXAMPLE 13

   Keratometry: 42.50 @180; 45.50 @90

   Refraction (at corneal plane): $-6.00 - 3.00 \times 180$

1. *Computational method*
   (a) Calculate residual cylinder:

   Spectacle cylinder − corneal cylinder = $-3.00 \times 180 - (-)3.00 \times 180 = 0$

   (b) Select base curve radii via Mandell-Moore:

   $$Kf = 42.50 - (+)0.25 = 42.25 \text{ D or } 7.99 \text{ mm}$$

   $$Ks = 45.50 - (+)0.75 = 44.75 \text{ D or } 7.54 \text{ mm}$$

(c) Calculate back vertex powers:

$$Ff = -6.00 + (+)0.25 = -5.75 \text{ D}$$

$$Fs = Ff + (Kf - Ks) = -5.75 + (42.25 - 44.75) = -8.25 \text{ D}$$

Power of lens in air $= -5.75 - 2.50 \times 180$

2. *Optical cross method*

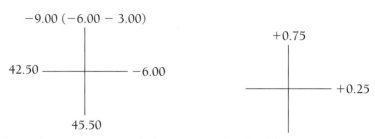

Spectacle power at corneal plane   Lacrimal lens power correction

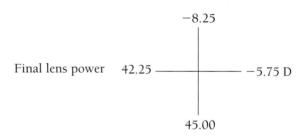

Final lens power

Bitoric lens correction: $-5.75/-8.25$ $42.25(7.99 \text{ mm})/44.75(7.46 \text{ mm})$

It is important for the laboratory to understand that these are the values that should be verified with the lensometer. Therefore, the powers should represent compensated values with the induced cylinder correction on the front surface. In this case, approximately 0.50×-2.50 (back surface cylinder) $= -1.25 \text{ D} \times 180$. $+1.25 \text{ D} \times 180$ will need to be added to the front surface to arrive at the final lens powers of $-5.75/-8.25$.

As the optical cross method illustrates, it is not necessary to use a formula to determine the final lens powers. Essentially, a bitoric design can be considered as two spherical designs when tear lens power calculations are performed. In this example, a BCR was selected that was 0.25 D "flatter than K" in the horizontal meridian. Using the SAM-FAP philosophy (i.e., steep add minus/flat add plus), the power in the meridian becomes 0.25 D more plus or -5.75 D. In the steep meridian, a BCR was selected that was 0.75 D "flatter than K" in the steep meridian; therefore, the final lens power becomes 0.75 D more plus or -8.25 D.

3. *Mandell-Moore Bitoric Lens Guide*

Another computational method for determining the bitoric lens specifications is the Mandell-Moore bitoric lens guide.[16] This is a simple reference guide in which the keratometric and refraction information is entered and the final values are derived using the recommended base curve radii. This is an excellent empirical method for determining powers and base curve radii in which it is not necessary to compute lacrimal lens effects. It has also been found to result in a comparable success rate when compared with diagnostic fitting of bitoric lenses.[23] An example of this method is provided in Figure 14.7. The form is downloadable from the GP Lens Institute website (www.gpli.info). There is also a calculator to perform the calculations on this website.

GP CLINICAL EDUCATION:
Mandell-Moore Bitoric Lens Guide
Click here for a blank guide, which you can then print for your office

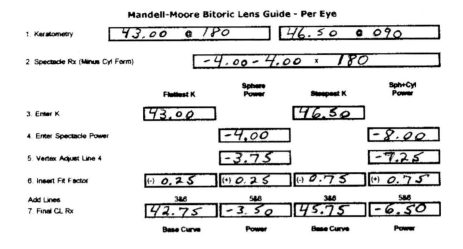

Mandell-Moore Bitoric Lens Guide - Per Eye

1. Keratometry   `43.00  @ 180`   `46.50  @ 090`

2. Spectacle Rx (Minus Cyl Form)   `-4.00 -4.00  x  180`

	Flattest K	Sphere Power	Steepest K	Sph+Cyl Power
3. Enter K	`43.00`		`46.50`	
4. Enter Spectacle Power		`-4.00`		`-8.00`
5. Vertex Adjust Line 4		`-3.75`		`-7.25`
6. Insert Fit Factor	`(-) 0.25`	`(+) 0.25`	`(-) 0.75`	`(+) 0.75`

Add Lines   3&6   5&6   3&6   5&6

7. Final CL Rx   `42.75`   `-3.50`   `45.75`   `-6.50`

Base Curve   Power   Base Curve   Power

Bitoric Lens Fit Factor

Corneal Cyl	Fit Flat Meridian	Fit Steep Meridian
2.0 Diopters	On K (0 D)	0.50D Flatter
2.5 Diopters	0.25D Flatter	0.50D Flatter
3.0 Diopters	0.25D Flatter	0.75D Flatter
3.5 Diopters	0.25D Flatter	0.75D Flatter
4.0 Diopters	0.25D Flatter	0.75D Flatter
5.0 Diopters	0.25D Flatter	0.75D Flatter

■ **FIGURE 14.7** Mandell-Moore bitoric lens guide.

Spherical Power Effect Bitoric Diagnostic Lenses: The use of bitoric diagnostic lenses is the preferable method of fitting these patients. Most Contact Lens Manufacturers Association (CLMA) member laboratories have bitoric diagnostic fitting sets available for loaner use as well as for purchase. Excellent success rates have been reported by fitting high astigmatic patients by using the Polycon II spherical power effect (SPE) bitoric diagnostic lenses (Ciba Vision Corp.).[24–26] In fact, in the aforementioned survey of AAO Diplomates, the Mandell-Moore Empirical Fitting Guide was the most commonly used empirical fitting method and the Polycon II SPE design was the most commonly used bitoric diagnostic fitting set.[21] This concept makes fitting bitoric designs as simple as fitting spherical lens designs, and many patients obtain visual acuity equal to or better than that achieved with their optimum spectacle correction.

Ten lens diagnostic sets are available with 2 D (recommended for <3 D of corneal astigmatism), 3 D (recommended for 3−5 D of corneal astigmatism), and 4 D (recommended for >5 D of corneal astigmatism) of back surface toricity. The 3 D diagnostic set is recommended for most bitoric fits. The base curve radii of the diagnostic lenses range from 40.50/43.50 to 45.00/48.00 in 0.50 D steps, all with powers of pl/−3.00 D. The induced cylinder correction is already incorporated into the lens.

The initial SPE diagnostic lens flat meridian BCR should be 0.12 D to 0.50 D flatter than the flat K reading. As the diagnostic lenses are designed in 0.50 D steps, there should only be one lens to meet this criterion. The determination of the final lens powers is a two-step procedure:

1. Perform a spherical refraction over the selected SPE diagnostic lens.
2. Add the overrefraction to the powers in the flat and steep meridians of the diagnostic lens.

Example 14 shows how the SPE concept is used in the diagnostic fitting process:

EXAMPLE 14

Spectacle Rx: $+2.00 - 3.00 \times 180$

Keratometry: 41.50 @ 180; 44.50 @ 090

Diagnostic lens parameters:

BCR = 41.00/44.00

Power: pl/-3.00

SLE: good centration; alignment fluorescein pattern

Overrefraction: $+2.50$ DS (visual acuity = 20/20)

Final order: BCR = 41.00 (8.23 mm)/44.00 (7.67 mm)

Power = $+2.50/-0.50$

Boston XO bitoric

In the above example, a higher-Dk lens material (>50) would be recommended because of the powers necessary. As there was no predicted residual astigmatism and assuming the visual acuity was acceptable with a spherical-only overrefraction, it can be concluded that it was negligible. In most cases, if there is <0.75 D of residual astigmatism, it is not necessary to incorporate it into the lens correcting power. However, if the patient's visual acuity is reduced significantly (typically, at minimum, one line worse than the optimum correction) with a spherical-only overrefraction but is optimally corrected with the residual cylinder present, a cylinder power effect (CPE) bitoric lens design is indicated. This design incorporates both the induced and the residual cylindrical error (as determined with a SPE bitoric diagnostic lens). The following steps summarize the CPE fitting process:

1. Select the recommended SPE diagnostic lens.
2. Perform a spherical overrefraction; if the visual acuity is reduced, perform a spherocylindrical overrefraction.
3. Use Silbert's rule[8] to determine the final lens powers: "If the axes are at or near the principal corneal meridians, add the appropriate power in the refraction to the air power of the corresponding meridian in the diagnostic lens, and order."

Examples 15 and 16 are representative examples of CPE bitoric fitting.

EXAMPLE 15

Keratometry: 41.50 @ 180; 44.50 @ 090

Spectacle Rx: $-0.75 - 4.00 \times 180$

Diagnostic SPE lens: 41.00/44.00

Power: pl/-3.00

Overrefraction (sphere): -0.25 DS 20/30 + 2

Overrefraction (sphere-cyl): $-0.25 - 1.00 \times 180$ 20/20

Add the overrefraction to the corresponding power in the diagnostic lens to obtain the final lens powers:

180 meridian: $-0.25 + \text{pl} = -0.25$ D

090 meridian: $(-0.25 + -1.00) + -3.00 = -4.25$ D

Final order: 41.00 (8.23 mm)/44.00 (7.67 mm) $-0.25/-4.25$

Fluoroperm 30 bitoric

EXAMPLE 16A

Keratometry: 41.50 @ 180; 44.50 @ 090

Spectacle Rx: $-0.75 - 2.00 \times 180$

Diagnostic SPE lens: 41.00/44.00

Power: pl/-3.00

Overrefraction (sphere): -0.25 DS 20/25 $- 2$

Overrefraction (sphere-cyl): $+0.75 - 1.00 \times 090$ 20/20

Add the overrefraction to the corresponding power in the diagnostic lens to obtain the final lens powers:

180 meridian: $-0.25 + $ pl $= -0.25$ D

090 meridian: $+0.75 + (-)3.00 = -2.25$ D

Final order: 41.00 (8.23 mm)/44.00 (7.67 mm) $-0.25/-2.25$

Fluoroperm 30 bitoric

As the Polycon II lens has such a low Dk value, a higher-Dk material, as shown in the two examples, should be ordered. In addition, it is important to mention that the incorporation of the residual astigmatic correction negates the benefit of an SPE lens. Therefore, rotation of a CPE bitoric lens could compromise vision. However, on high astigmatic corneas, bitoric lens designs typically orient properly on the eye and satisfactory vision is achieved.

To verify the base curve radii of a bitoric (or back surface toric) lens design, rotate the lens mount until one mire image comes into focus and record that value. Then turn the focusing knob until the image 90 degrees away comes into focus and record this value. Essentially, a bitoric lens will have the same radiuscopic appearance as a warped lens. Verifying the power is straightforward when the lensometer is used. For both SPE and CPE bitoric lenses, the air powers should equal what was ordered (i.e., with SPE lenses, the cylinder power amount should equal the toricity measured with the radiuscope). If a back surface toric lens was ordered, the air power cylinder should be approximately 1.5 times the radiuscopic cylinder.

Other Considerations: Other factors to consider when fitting bitoric GP lenses include (a) the CT, (b) peripheral curve design, (c) very high astigmatic corneas, and (d) irregular astigmatism.

1. Center thickness. Bitoric lenses are thin lens designs. The CT for a bitoric lens is equal to the CT of a spherical in the most plus bitoric lens power. For example, in Example 16A, if the recommended CT for a Fluoroperm 30 lens material in -0.25 D power is 0.19 mm, that would be the recommended CT for this bitoric lens design.
2. Peripheral curve design. Either spherical or toric peripheral curves can be ordered. The primary author's philosophy is when corneal toricity is <4 D, spherical peripheral curves should be used; if the corneal toricity is ≥4 D, toric peripheral curves should be used.[27] With <4 D of corneal toricity, the mean of the base curve radii should be used and 1 mm can be added for the SCR and an additional 2 mm can be added for the PCR. In Example 16A, the base curve radii are 41.00 (8.23 mm)/44.00 (7.67 mm). The mean value is 42.50 (7.94 mm). The peripheral curve radii would be (rounding the mean value to 7.9 mm) 8.9 mm and 10.9 mm. The final order would be the following:

EXAMPLE 16B

> BCR: 41 (8.23 mm)/44.00 (7.67 mm)
> Powers: −0.25/−2.25
> OAD/OZD: 9.4/8.2 mm
> CT: 0.19 mm
> SCR/W: 8.9/0.3 mm
> PCR/W: 10.9/0.3 mm
> Fluoroperm 30 bitoric

When the corneal toricity is ≥4D, toric secondary curve radii and peripheral curve radii can be applied. The secondary curve radii can be 1 mm flatter than the base curve radii. The peripheral curve radii can be 2 mm flatter than the secondary curve radii.

   3. Very high astigmatic corneas. It is not unusual to have a very highly astigmatic patient fitted with a bitoric diagnostic lens of much lesser toricity. The resulting fluorescein pattern is not alignment but actually somewhat astigmatic in appearance. When this is the case, the fit should proceed as in Examples 14 through 16. An overrefraction is performed and added to the diagnostic lens powers to achieve the lens powers. Next, the steeper base curve radius can be steepened to improve the fitting relationship and the power in that meridian increased in minus by the same amount. This is demonstrated in Example 17.

EXAMPLE 17

> Spectacle Rx: +2.00 − 5.50 × 180
>
> Keratometry: 41.00 @ 180; 46.50 @ 090
>
> Diagnostic lens parameters: BCR = 40.50/43.50
>
> Power: pl/−3.00
>
> SLE: good centration; mild bearing horizontally; excessive clearance vertically
>
> Overrefraction: +2.50 DS (equal to predicted; visual acuity = 20/20)
>
> Tentative order: 41.00 (8.23 mm) +2.50 D/44.00 (7.67 mm) −0.50 D
>
> Steepen vertical meridian 1.5 D to improve fitting relationship and add −1.50 D to power in that meridian
>
> Final order: 41.00 (8.23 mm) +2.50D/45.50 (7.42mm) −2.00D
>
> Toric peripheral curves: SCR = BCR + 1 mm; PCR = SCR + 2 mm
>
> SCR = 8.2/7.4 + 1 mm = 9.2/8.4 mm
>
> PCR = 9.2/8.4 + 2 mm = 11.2/10.4 mm

> Fluorex 700 bitoric

   4. Irregular astigmatism. There are some situations in which a bitoric lens would exhibit limited success. These are cases in which the keratometric axis differs significantly (usually 15 degrees or more) from the spectacle cylinder axis as a result of hypoxia, trauma, surgery, or other factors. In this situation, it may be preferable to use a spherical GP lens design. Bitoric lenses are most successful from both a fitting and a vision standpoint when the steep and flat meridians of the cornea are 90 degrees apart. The decision about whether to use a bitoric lens will depend on corneal topography. If the topography map exhibits a symmetric pattern and, in particular, the astigmatism is limbus to limbus (termed "global" astigmatism), a bitoric lens design should be successful.[28]

In summary, a recommended toric fitting guide is presented in Figure 14.8.

I. Residual Astigmatic Correction

Front Toric GP

1. Rarely indicated; used when soft lenses contraindicated
2. Example: keratometry = 42.00 @ 180; 43.25 @ 090
   refraction = -1.00 -2.75 x 180

Spherical GP

1. Can flex to reduce induced cylinder
2. Example: keratometry = 41 @ 180; 43 @ 090
   refraction = -2.00 -1.00 x 180

Spherical Soft

1. Indicated when refractive cylinder is low and corneal cylinder is moderate or high
2. Example: keratometry = 42.00 @; 43.50 @ 090
   refraction = -5.00 - 0.25 x 180

Soft Toric

1. Indicated when refractive astigmatism is between 1-2 diopters and significant residual astigmatism is present
2. Example: keratometry = 43.00 DS
   refraction = -3.00 -1.50 x 090

II. High Astigmatic Correction

Spherical GP

1. <3D corneal cylinder or when oblique astigmatism-especially in ATR cylinder
   Example: keratometry = 42.00 @ 145; 46.00 @ 055
   refraction = -2.50 - 4.50 x 162
2. Consider aspheric design with 2-3 diopters of corneal astigmatism-especially in ATR cylinder

Soft Toric

1. Any refractive astimatic patient with regular astigmatism and motivated for soft lens wear

Back Surface Toric

1. Indicated when corneal toricity is ATR and residual astigmatism = 0.5 x radiuscopic toricity; otherwise, BS torics are contraindicated
2. Example: keratometry = 42.25 @ 090; 45.00 @ 180
   refraction = -1.00 - 4.50 x 090
   back surface - 41.50 @ 090; 44.50 @ 180

Bi Toric

1. Indicated in all regular astimatic cases with ≥ 3D of corneal toricity
2. Example: keratometry = 41.00 @ 180; 45.00 @ 090
   refraction = -3.00 -4.75 x 180
   (at corneal plane) -3.00 - 4.00 x 180
   Two methods can be used:
   a. Empirical power: order BCR :40.75/44.25, powers -2.75/-6.25
   b. spherical power effect:
      select: 40.50/43.50 base curve radius pl/-3.00 powers
      predicted OR = -2.50 DS
   Final predicted lens design = 40.50/43.50   -2.50/-5.50

■ FIGURE 14.8 Gas-permeable toric fitting guide.

TABLE 14.3 BITORIC EDUCATIONAL RESOURCES AVAILABLE FROM THE GAS-PERMEABLE (GP) LENS INSTITUTE

1. Mandell-Moore Bitoric Lens Calculator and Guide
2. GP Lens Management Guide
3. GP Lens Grand Rounds Troubleshooting Guide
4. GP Online Symposia

It would be appropriate to mention that the most important problem with any toric lens design is hesitancy on the part of the practitioner to use it. Comments pertaining to the complexity of the design, the difficulty in fitting, expense (especially if numerous refittings occur), and the time involved are not uncommon. Even many practitioners who pride themselves on their ability to fit GP lenses rarely fit toric designs, often indicating that a spherical design will work just as well, if not better. Certainly, the selection of a laboratory that can fabricate a toric lens with good optical quality is paramount to success. Fortunately, the quality of bitoric lenses today is quite good and very consistent as a result of improvements in manufacturing technology. Numerous educational resources on bitoric design and fitting are available from the GP Lens Institute and are listed in Table 14.3.

■ SOFT (HYDROGEL AND SILICONE HYDROGEL) CONTACT LENS APPLICATIONS

It has been estimated that about 45% of a contact lens-seeking population have an astigmatic correction ≥0.75 D,[29] and 35% require ≥1.00 D.[30] If the criterion for significant astigmatism is taken at the 0.75 D level, then approximately 40% of the spectacle-wearing population are potential candidates for astigmatic-correcting soft lenses. Obviously, there is a considerable need for contact lenses that correct astigmatism, especially when a soft lens is the lens of choice. This need is currently being met in the United States as manufacturers continue to develop and improve toric lenses. This section of the chapter will present an overview and update of toric lens technology and its clinical application and will discuss the techniques necessary to fit these lenses successfully.

Patient Selection and Indications

Clinical success with toric soft lenses is based on the standard criteria of good physical and physiologic performance, along with other visual considerations, which include the following:

1. Good vision in all directions of gaze.
2. Stable vision, minimally affected by lid actions.
3. Sustained vision (i.e., minimal effects from dehydration or base curve change that may affect meridional orientation).

One of the most important benefits of soft toric lenses pertains to the −0.75 to −1.00 D astigmatic patient. Clinical studies have concluded that vision is significantly better with soft toric wear than with spherical soft lenses.[31,32] Careful patient selection and proper selection of lens type or brand maximize the probability of success. The following patient characteristics should be considered:

Patient History

First, patients must be good candidates for fitting with soft contact lenses. The usual contraindications for soft lens wear also apply to toric soft lens wear. Patients who have failed to adapt to GP lenses because of discomfort or edge awareness are often motivated by the comfort of soft lenses. Patients with astigmatism who wear GP lenses and demonstrate chronic 3- and 9-o'clock staining, poor bearing patterns, flare, excessive or insufficient lens movement, or poor wetting characteristics are often good candidates for soft lenses.[33] For first-time contact lens wearers, clinician and patient preference will determine if GP or soft lenses are selected. Both can correct all types of astigmatism effectively. Diagnostic evaluation of the lenses on the eyes is still the best method of selecting the appropriate lens type, and it also aids in designing the lens specifications.

Amount of Astigmatism

Uncorrected refractive astigmatism that is ≥ 0.75 D is usually unacceptable to patients with low spherical refractive errors. In these cases, the corrected vision is usually quite good, and patients are less tolerant of any compromise that might occur with the use of toric soft lenses. However, patients having corrections with higher spherical errors often tolerate an uncorrected cylinder better. It has been suggested that the performance of a spherical soft lens first should be tried and then assessed in cases in which the astigmatic correction is $<25\%$ of the spherical correction.[34] Spherical soft lenses in the high power range or those that are thicker or made of a stiffer material can produce a masking effect because of incomplete draping about the toric cornea, thereby neutralizing some corneal cylinder. Spherical equivalent lenses often will perform surprisingly well in these cases of marginal astigmatism. Lenses with aspheric surfaces have been said to improve visual acuity in some astigmatic patients, although no evidence exists demonstrating actual cylinder masking or correction.[35] Moderate astigmatism of 1.25 to 2.00 D is now easily managed with the stock toric soft lenses available today. High cylindrical corrections are more sensitive to axis rotation or mislocation and may require custom toric lenses; however, some frequent replacement toric designs are available in high cylinder powers. Currently, custom toric lenses are available in an unlimited range of cylinder powers, and their use should be considered a viable option in high astigmatism of any axis.[14,36,37]

The Axis of the Refractive Astigmatism

In the case of myopic astigmatism, uncorrected oblique and against-the-rule astigmatism cause more visual distress and asthenopia than does uncorrected with-the-rule astigmatism. For with-the-rule astigmatism, the optics are less critical and are therefore the easiest to manage with toric soft lenses. The axis of the correcting cylinder affects toric soft lens orientation and stability. The torquing effects of the blink cause more rotation in oblique cylinders because of the lid–lens interaction that occurs at the meridian of thickest edge (most minus powers). However, modern toric soft lenses with uniform edge thickness around the full circumference of the lens minimize this problem.[36,38,39]

Types of Astigmatism

Whenever the use of a toric lens is indicated, a quantitative comparison of the relative amount of corneal toricity and refractive astigmatism is essential. This simple calculation will predict any residual astigmatism and assist in the selection of the least complex and most appropriate GP or soft lens design. Certain general rules are helpful in lens selection.

If the calculated residual astigmatism is significant, a soft toric lens is preferred. It corrects the internal cylinder that would remain if a spherical GP lens were fitted and eliminates the need for a more complex prism ballast, front toric, or bitoric GP lens design. Internal astigmatism is found most commonly in conjunction with spherical corneas or moderately against-the-rule corneas and is usually in the range of -0.75 to -1.50 D at axes of 90 ± 15 degrees.

As a general rule, if the refractive astigmatism is less than the corneal toricity, a GP lens would be the least complex option. If the refractive astigmatism is greater than the corneal toricity, a soft toric is usually the lens of choice.

If the axes of the primary corneal meridians and the spectacle cylinder do not coincide, a GP lens is preferable.[39] The masking ability of a GP lens avoids the crossed-cylinder result that occurs with a toric soft lens because of its tendency to align with the primary corneal meridians and not with the refraction axis.

When the cylinder power in a toric soft lens is prescribed, only the total refractive cylinder needs to be considered. The relationship of the ocular lens surface and the cornea does not create a significant tear lens, as in the case of GP lenses. However, rotational and flexural effects of soft lenses may affect the final prescription and require lens power or axis compensations. Irregular astigmatism and keratoconus require GP lens correction for best vision, although toric soft lenses can be attempted when GP lenses cannot be tolerated.[40] In keratoconus, soft lenses should be considered as a last resort; despite unusual corneal curvatures in these cases, a median base curve often fits well because soft lenses are semiscleral with relatively large sagittal heights and therefore conform well to the usually normal peripheral corneal curvatures. With an accurate overrefraction, a satisfactory visual result can sometimes be achieved when custom toric lenses are used on certain keratoconic eyes.

Lid Configuration and Anatomy

Because the dynamics of lid action are one of the principal causes of lens mislocation and undesired rotation, eyelid anatomy and function are critical when toric lenses are fitted.[41] Lid anatomy, tension, aperture size, and lid closure dynamics, in addition to prescription and lens parameters, play a role in lens stabilization.[42,43] The ideal eye has a relatively wide aperture, normal lid tension, complete closure, a lower lid at the inferior limbus, and no raised conjunctival tissue. Lids that are unusually tight or eyes that have small palpebral apertures often produce excessive force on the lens and result in unpredictable orientation. When the lower lid is positioned higher than 2 mm above the limbus or is sharply angled from the horizontal plane, undesired axis mislocations often result. An incomplete blinking pattern adversely affects toric lenses because of localized dehydration and buildup of surface deposits at the inferior region. Reduced tear volume or an unstable tear film also may cause unwanted lens rotation as a result of dehydration of the lens during wear, with subsequent changes in lens adherence to the cornea.

Occupational Considerations

Toric soft lenses may be unacceptable for patients with intolerance to slight prescription changes or for people who have critical vision requirements at work. Patients with early presbyopia require special consideration because lens axis shifts in the downward gaze position can affect visual acuity and add stress to an already fatigued accommodative system. Use of toric soft lenses in presbyopic monovision can be successful, but several lenses may be required to optimize the correction. For patients needing only slight astigmatic corrections and for whom comfort is a factor, a toric soft lens may be the best option because the immediate comfort with these lenses is equal to that found with spherical soft lenses, and the attainable vision is often comparable as well. Several hydrogel toric multifocal designs are now available and have provided an additional contact lens option for these patients (Table 14.4).[37]

Lens Design and Stabilizing Techniques

The various methods of providing specific orientation to soft lenses include prism ballasting, truncation, dynamic stabilization with double-thin zones, periballasting, eccentric lenticulation, back toricity, and combinations of all of the above. No matter what method of stabilization is selected, orientation is achieved as a result of a thickness differential along the superior, central, and inferior portions of the lens. These techniques are described below.

TABLE 14.4 SOFT TORIC MULTIFOCAL LENSES

LENS	MANUFACTURER
Clearion Progressive Toric	Acuity One
Essential Soft Toric Multifocal	Blanchard Contact Lens
CO Soft 55 Custom Bifocal Toric	California Optics
Cibasoft Progressive Toric	Ciba Vision
Proclear Multifocal Toric	CooperVision
Triton Translating Toric Bifocal	Gelflex USA
Metrofocal Toric	Metro Optics
OCU-FLEX 53 Toric Multifocal	Ocu-Ease/Optech
OCU-Flex Plus Toric Multifocal	Ocu-Ease/Optech
High Definition Toric Aspheric	PolyVue Distribution
HDX Toric Progressive	PolyVue Distribution
C VUE 55 Toric Multifocal	Unilens Corporation
MVT Multifocal Toric	Unilens Corporation
UCL Multifocal Toric	United Contact Lens
UCL Sonic View Toric	United Contact Lens
Horizon 55 Bi-Con Toric	Westcon Contact Lens
Horizon Progressive Toric	Westcon Contact Lens

From Thompson TT. Tyler's quarterly soft contact lens parameter guide. 2007;25(1):9–53.

Prism Ballasting

Incorporating 0.75 to 2 D of base-down prism can stabilize a soft lens and allow it to resist rotational forces. The general principle behind prism ballasting is to balance the various forces acting on the lens to obtain stabilization, although other theories suggest that prism stabilizes by lowering the center of gravity on the lens.[44,45] Prism stability has been explained more accurately by the *watermelon seed principle*.[46] Essentially, if a moist wedge is squeezed, the resultant action is for the wedge to be expelled by the pressure in a direction away from the wedge apex. Thus, lid pressure squeezes the lens into the base-down direction.[47] The principle works in a similar way with both prism and nonprism toric lenses. The nonprism torics have thinner regions in the superior and inferior portions (double-thin zones) and a greater thickness in the center, thereby creating a biprism effect with bases joined along the horizontal plane at the center of the lens. Because of the insignificant role that gravity appears to play, in contrast to the lens–cornea adherence and the lid forces, toric soft lenses usually do not rotate on eyes while wearers are lying on their side, unlike some prism GP lenses.

Truncation

Prism ballasting is occasionally combined with truncation and is reasonably successful, particularly when utilized on lenses with thicker edges.[45] Truncated lenses result via removing an area of lens material 0.4 to 1.5 mm from the lower edge of the lens, with larger truncations used with larger OADs. Truncation is successful via assisting the inferior lens to position adjacent to the lower lid margin, which provides a shelf for stability. It is used more often with translating segmented bifocal GP lenses. Although truncation raises the center of gravity on a lens, the stability of orientation is not reduced because of the minor role of gravity.

Although truncated lenses have had some success, soft torics today are being designed as round, nontruncated lenses without loss of stable meridional orientation and with greater comfort as a result.[48]

Dynamic Stabilization

Thinning the upper and lower sections of a lens results in the thickest portion of the lens being in the center. The thin zones at the top and bottom are covered by the lids, and because of the *watermelon seed principle* described previously, the thicker center positions horizontally between the lids. These stabilization zones are beveled equally or are double slab off in form, and the lens is nonprismatic. This design is often referred to as "double slab off," "thin zone," or "reverse prism" and is one of the most commonly used methods of soft toric lens stabilization.[45] This thin zone design is most successful when the thickness differential of the horizontal and vertical profiles is greatest, as in higher myopic or against-the-rule cylinder corrections, because the wedge effect is maximized. Plus lenses in this design were less stable at first; however, design changes have incorporated a minus carrier before the thin zones are added, which allows the increased thickness differential to work in much the same way as it does for minus toric lenses. The thin zone design usually provides good comfort, good optics, sometimes unpredictable axis location, but reasonably good stability.[48] In cases in which fitting a toric lens on one eye might produce a vertical imbalance from a prism-ballasted toric lens, the double-thin zone design, which contains no prism, is especially beneficial. It is interesting to note that in practice, vertical imbalance is seldom a problem, even if one eye is fit with a toric prism lens incorporating up to 2.0 Δ base down. The effective prism of a contact lens on the eye is related to the position of the visual axis relative to its geometric center and to its refractive power.[49] Thus, the effective prism power of a prism contact lens varies along its vertical meridian. In addition, the effectiveness of the prism will depend on the refractive index of the surrounding media.

Accelerated Stabilization

This design utilizes four zones with a thicker profile placed at the midperiphery of the lens to minimize lens rotation. It is similar to dynamic stabilization in that the thinner portions of the lens rest under the open lids. The "active" portions of the lens with the accelerated thickness slope orient within the interpalpebral fissure to work with the lid dynamics to quickly reorient the lens when it becomes misaligned.[50,51]

Periballasting

The periballasted design differs from prism-ballasted lenses in that it has no prism in the optical portion of the lens, only in the periphery. The lens is fabricated by removing the superior portion of a high minus lenticular carrier, which reduces lid–lens edge interaction and produces a peripheral ballast in the inferior portion of the lens. Eliminating prism in the optical zone may reduce the CT, and improved optical quality is achieved.[52]

Eccentric Lenticulation

This is a front surface, off-center (eccentric), lenticular cut in the direction of the prism apex that is similar to periballast. The removal of excess material on the anterior surface provides several benefits, which include a reduced differential in edge thickness that increases both stability and comfort, a reduced mass of the lens so that it behaves similarly to a spherical soft lens, better limbal-scleral draping, and minimized compression on the scleral conjunctiva.

The eccentric lenticulation feature is especially important in front toric lens construction, in which edge thickness can vary significantly. The increased stability is particularly evident in oblique cylinder corrections, in which the lid margin closure first meets the thicker part of the lens at an oblique angle, often resulting in torsional mislocation.[53] The eccentric lenticulation creates superior and inferior thin portions and nearly equal thicknesses around the entire lens periphery, but the prism remains only in the central two-thirds of the lens. Many of the laboratories making toric soft contact lenses incorporate eccentric lenticulation into their lenses.

Back Toricity

Some clinicians using toric lenses have presumed that back cylinder construction may aid stability, especially on eyes with a corneal toricity >3.00 D.[34,54] No studies have been performed to isolate back toricity as a major stabilizing feature; however, it seems logical to expect that a wrapping effect similar to that observed with toric GP lenses is present and may enhance the stability of toric soft lens orientation. Many of the second-generation toric lenses and most custom toric soft lenses are made with back toricity and with the toric zone limited to the central optic area. Toric curves that are confined to the central optic zone reduce differential edge thickness, which minimizes lid blink-related torsional effects. Whether by design or by manufacturing preference, back surface toric construction functions very well in terms of predictable location and nonrotation, but only when combined with prism ballasting. There is no difference or advantage in front or back toric construction in terms of optical performance of soft toric lenses, as there is in GP toric lenses. As a general rule, corneas with low toricities are best fitted with front toric designs, and those with moderate and high toricities (≥1.50 D) are best fitted with back toric designs.

Fitting Principles and Problem Solving

Lens Selection

Toric contact lenses are available in a variety of replacement modalities including daily disposable, 2-week, 1-month, and 3-month replacement schedules. The increasing availability of frequent-replacement and disposable soft toric lenses has allowed practitioners to fit common lens parameters from inventory. Many manufacturers produce stock lenses in cylinder powers of −0.75 to −2.25 D with axes in 5- or 10-degree steps, often ranging from 0 to 180 degrees. Extended power ranges are also available in frequent-replacement modalities for higher cylinder corrections, often with 1-degree axis increments from 0 to 180 degrees.[45,55] Additionally, the advent of silicone hydrogel lens materials has allowed astigmatic patients the option of extended wear because of the increased oxygen transmissibility of the material. The availability of disposable lenses has also allowed patients to have spare lenses readily available, and deposit-related problems, such as giant papillary conjunctivitis, are minimized.[56,57] As materials and parameters of soft toric lenses continue to expand, the need for custom lenses on a conventional replacement basis is decreasing, although there will always be patients requiring corrections beyond these ranges.[45]

Axis Location and Orientation

The primary influence on lens orientation is the torsion forces of the lids during a blink. The temporal-to-nasal motion created by the upper lid during the blink process creates a tendency for nasal rotation upward (encyclorotation) of a contact lens, commonly observed with GP lenses. Other patient factors that have been found to influence lens orientation include the intercanthal angle, degree of myopia, and palpebral fissure size.[43] Lids with a higher outer canthus tend to create inferior-temporal rotation, whereas lids with a higher inner canthus tend to create inferior-nasal rotation.[42,43,58,59] Most toric lenses will stabilize within 5 and 10 degrees of the zero position and most will stabilize within 10 minutes of insertion. However, as different designs interact with the lids in unique ways, not all designs will orient in the same position on a given eye.[58,59] Several physical and physiologic variables noted below can make predicting orientation difficult, especially in the case of toric soft lenses.

Lens rotation and mislocation of axis are the major factors responsible for inadequate toric soft lens performance that results in reduced visual acuity.[60] The term *mislocation* simply means consistent lens rotation to some resting position other than the desired one. This generally occurs with tight-fitting lenses, tight lids, or inadequately ballasted lenses. The less common problem of blink-initiated rotation, or rocking, is usually caused by a loose fit or insufficient lens stabilization features or forces. The amount of visual disruption resulting from a nonstable lens depends on the power of the cylinder, the degree of rocking, and the speed of recovery as the lens regains its resting position following a blink or change of gaze. Selecting a steeper base curve radius, larger diameter, or additional prism often solves the problem of the unstable, or rocking, toric soft lens.

Diagnostic Lens Procedures

Clinical studies have found empirical fitting (i.e., without diagnostic lens application) to be quite successful.[61,62] This method of fitting has become increasingly popular with the emergence of frequent-replacement soft toric contact lenses and more consistent reproducibility of these lenses.[42] Nevertheless, diagnostic lens evaluation is strongly recommended when the use of toric soft lenses is being considered.[63] Differences in axis location between the best diagnostic lens and the initially ordered lens is a major reason for first-lens failure. Toric lens thickness profiles, power, and cylinder axis affect orientation. The following suggestions will help minimize any unpredictable orientation or mislocation of an ordered toric lens.

First, diagnostic lenses should be relatively close to the spherical and cylinder powers and axis (±20 degrees and ±1.00 D) of the manifest refraction of the eye to be fitted. Second, 10 to 15 minutes should be allowed for trial lens equilibration. Third, axis location on the eye should be accurately determined. Only a well-centered, freely moving lens that is accurately labeled can provide a basis for reliable axis correction on the next lens. As discussed in the section on front toric GP lenses, if the base-down position rotates to the left of the center line (clockwise), the amount of axis deviation to compensate for the mislocation in the ordered lens must be added to the spectacle axis. Conversely, if the rotation is to the right of the center line (counterclockwise), subtraction is needed (i.e., LARS).

The amount of axis mislocation should be estimated by using one of the aforementioned methods. It is beneficial that most slit lamps allow the examiner to rotate the beam to align with the axis identification mark(s) on the lens and be able to read the amount of rotation directly off of the slit lamp. If this is not available, it is not uncommon to use a gross estimate method, in which a clock dial is visualized on the lens, with each deviation of an hour (e.g., from 5 to 6, 6 to 7) being equivalent to a 30-degree arc. Obviously, this "guesstimate" method is limited and should not be applied to cylinder evaluations of ≥2.00 D, which are meridionally very sensitive.

The importance of an accurate spherocylindrical overrefraction when determining the powers to be ordered cannot be overemphasized.[64] When small amounts of lens rotation in high cylinder cases are being considered, spherocylindrical overrefraction data can be combined with the in-air lens powers in a crossed-cylinder calculation to determine the next (and corrected) lens specifications.[65,66] Some manufacturers offer desktop or personal digital assistant-based crossed-cylinder calculators. These programs typically apply a simple spherocylinder overrefraction formula for a precise determination of the corrected lens power and axis specifications. Online sources of crossed-cylinder calculator programs include http://www.ecp.acuvue.com, http://www.coopervision.com, http://www.eyedock.com, and http://www.procare.cibavision.com.[35] While spherocylindrical overrefraction is a useful tool, a clear overrefraction endpoint and accurately labeled toric contact lenses are important for success with this technique.[67]

Markings on soft toric lenses are used as reference points for assessing lens rotation and do not represent the cylinder axis of the lens. A useful guide is shown in Table 14.5 and Figure 14.9.

TABLE 14.5 SOFT TORIC IDENTIFICATION GUIDE

1. Durasoft Optifit (Ciba Vision)

2. Optima Toric (Bausch & Lomb)
   Soflens 66 Toric (Bausch & Lomb)
   CSI Toric (Ciba Vision)
   Hydrocurve 3 Toric (Ciba Vision)

3. Biocurve Toric (Biocurve)
   Biomedics Toric (CooperVision)
   Frequency 55 Toric (CooperVision)
   Hydrasoft Toric (CooperVision)
   Preference Toric (CooperVision)
   Proclear Toric XR (CooperVision)
   Vertex Toric (CooperVision)
   Preferred T (Preferred Vision Group)

4. Continental Toric (Continental Soft Lens)
   Ocuflex 53 Toric (Ocu-Ease/Optech)
   OCI Gold Toric (Optical Connection)
   C-Value 55 Custom Toric (Unilens)
   PR-46 (United Contact Lens)
   Tresoft Toric (United Contact Lens)
   UCL Toric (United Contact Lens)
   Horizon 55 Toric (Westcom Contact Lens)

5. Multi-Flex Custom (Eyecom)
   Kontur 55 (Kontur Kontact Lens)

6. CO Soft Toric (California Optics)
   Custom 55 Toric (California Optics)
   Synergy (Gelflex)

7. Clearion Custom Toric (Acuity One)
   Alden HP49 Toric (Alden Optical)
   Alden HP59 Toric (Alden Optical)
   Biocurve Advanced Aspheric Toric (Biocurve Soft)
   Cibasoft Progressive Toric (Ciba Vision)
   Torisoft (Ciba Vision)
   Proclear Multifocal Toric (CooperVision)
   Hydrokone Toric (Medlens)
   Reverse Geometry Toric (Medlens)
   XP Toric (Medlens)
   Definition AC Toric (Optical Connection)

8. Focus Toric (Ciba Vision)
   Air Optix for Astigmatism (Ciba Vision)
   Proclear Tailor Made Toric (CooperVision)

9. Proclear Multifocal Toric (CooperVision)
   SpecialEyes (SpecialEyes, LLC)
   Westhin Toric (Westcom Contact Lens)

10. Proclear Toric (CooperVision)

11. Freshlook Color Blends Toric (Ciba Vision)
    Freshlook Toric (Ciba Vision)

12. Extreme H2O Toric (Hydrogel Vision)

13. Acuvue Advance & Oasys for Astigmatism (Vistakon)
    Flexens Toric (Flexens)
    Metrosoft Toric (Metro Optics)
    Satureyes Toric (Metro Optics)

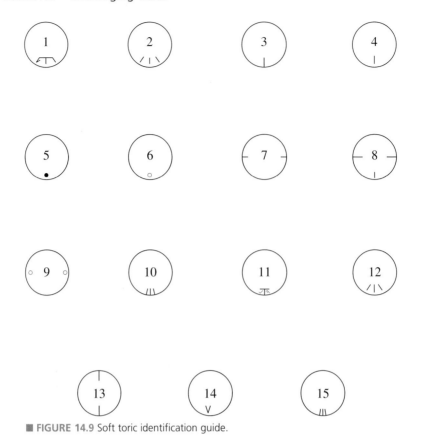

■ FIGURE 14.9 Soft toric identification guide.

Other Useful Suggestions for Evaluating Toric Lens Performance

Any mislocation caused by a tightly fitting lens should be determined. Steeply fitting lenses tend to lock at unpredictable and incorrect orientations. Lenses that move freely will respond properly to the orientation forces that stabilize them. In contrast, loosely fitting lenses often result in blink-initiated variable rotation by not allowing the lens-stabilizing forces to work.

Rotational velocity should be checked on the edge. This is the speed with which a poorly oriented toric lens will rotate in its effort to recover and to reorient.[48] After deliberate mislocation of about 45 degrees and then release, it should take no more than 15 seconds (with normal blinking) for the lens to return to its initial stable orientation. A tightly fitting lens will demonstrate stable lens orientation with a slow return to correct axis orientation. A loosely fitting lens will demonstrate unstable and inconsistent orientation.[45] A rapid return is desired and is particularly important for those patients who engage in demanding sports or occupations that require accurate vision.

Equilibration or a settling time of 20 minutes for most lens types should be adequate for reliable assessment of fit, with lower-water-content lenses requiring less time. If after equilibration a lens shows unpredictable rotation or a mislocation >30 degrees, a base curve change, a larger diameter, or a different type of toric lens should be considered. Small degrees of mislocation or rocking (0−5 degrees) are visually acceptable to most patients, especially in cylinder powers ≤2.00 D.[68]

Greater amounts of mislocation must be corrected using axis compensation. The result of cylinder mislocation is a spherocylinder overrefraction with the amount of the resultant cylinder equal to twice the power of the spherical component but of opposite sign.[29] Some clinicians have suggested undercorrecting the cylinder, as the patient is less sensitive to shifts of axis and the variable vision from crossed-cylinder effects.[69] Undercorrecting the cylinder by 20% is not uncommon with today's toric soft lenses and usually is successful. In addition, performing a spherocylindrical overrefraction is an important and accurate method of predicting success with soft toric fitting and gives the clinician an accurate means to evaluate whether poor visual acuity is caused by the fit of the lens or by poor optical quality.[68]

An interesting method of predicting soft toric success is the so-called "Becherer twist."[70] This is performed after the patient's best subjective refraction is in the phoropter. The cylinder knob is twisted, and when the patient observes a blurring or degrading of the sharpness of the image on the visual acuity chart, this value is recorded. If the twisting is >20 degrees in each direction, regardless of where the axis is located or the amount of cylinder, success will be achieved ≥90% of the time or greater with the first lens. If the twist is 15 degrees, then the success achieved will be about 90% with two lenses. If the twist is 10 degrees, then the success achieved will be 70% with three lenses necessary. If the twist is <5 degrees, any success will depend on how much decrease in contrast the patient is willing to accept.

Managing Poor Visual Response

Toric soft lenses, even when optimally fitted, may result in visual quality and acuity poorer than that attained with spectacles. This must be explained to the patient in advance, or expectations will be unrealistic. The lenses available today should correct the patient's sight to a consistent 20/20 acuity, and most unexpected visual responses can be managed. Common reasons for poor visual performance during the early fitting phase include axis mislocation, incorrect sphere or cylinder power, poor centration, flexure-related power effects, corneal curvature change, corneal edema, lens dehydration, and optically poor (defective) lenses (Fig. 14.10).

Several simple diagnostic tests may be used to isolate the factors causing the reduced vision. First, the correct axis location should be verified by relocating or dialing the contact lens base to either side of its stabilized position. The effect on vision should be noted as the lens is moved off axis and then allowed to return to its original position. If a slight off-axis movement reduces visual acuity significantly and equally on either side of the shift, then the axis is correctly positioned. If axis location is correct and consistent, a spherical overrefraction would be the next step to verify the spherical power, and finally the cylinder power can be verified with a hand-flip cylinder. If, on dialing, large axis shifts result in a minimal change in vision, poor optics or insufficient cylinder should be considered the cause of poor visual acuity, and the lens power and optical clarity should be checked with a lensometer.

Verification of suspect or poorly performing toric soft lenses by standard lensometry is advisable to identify the offending element in a toric soft lens failure. To do this, the lens is prepared by lightly "blot"-drying it with a lint-free cloth. The lens should then be geometrically centered over the lensometer stop, convex side up, with the prism base or lens marking positioned in the base-down (90 degrees) position. The use of a smaller aperture (3–4 mm) stop attachment to the vertically mounted lensometer is beneficial and eliminates peripheral aberrations, thus allowing more accurate power and axis measurements. These inexpensive plastic mounts are available for most lensometers. Measuring with the lens ocular surface down (back vertex) will determine the true axis, cylinder, and sphere. If the lens is placed convex side down on the aperture stop, the measured axis will be complementary or mirror reversed from the true axis (i.e., axis 80 degrees will be read as axis 100 degrees). A deflectometer has demonstrated much promise in accurate power determination for specialty lens practices.[71]

The use of the retinoscopic reflex will help assess the optical quality of a toric lens on the eye. A distorted retinoscopic reflex also can indicate an incorrect base curve relationship (usually too steep) or irregular wrapping of the back surface around the central cornea. Improperly draping lenses distort vision, which varies during the blink. This phenomenon may also be observed using overkeratometry, by noting the change in the shape and the clarity of the mires

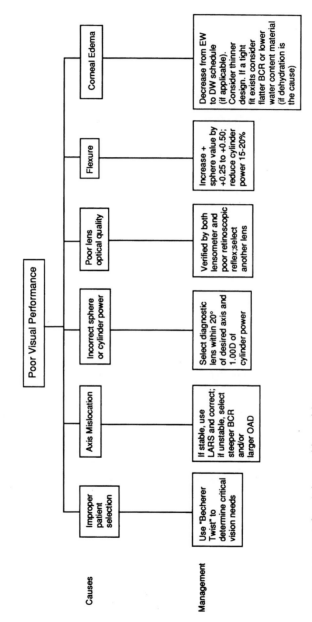

Causes

Poor Visual Performance

Improper patient selection | Axis Mislocation | Incorrect sphere or cylinder power | Poor lens optical quality | Flexure | Corneal Edema

Management

Use "Becherer Twist" to determine critical vision needs

If stable, use LARS and correct; if unstable, select steeper BCR and/or larger OAD

Select diagnostic lens within 20° of desired axis and 1.00D of cylinder power

Verified by both lensometer and poor retinoscopic reflex;select another lens

Increase + sphere value by +0.25 to +0.50; reduce cylinder power 15-20%

Decrease from EW to DW schedule (if applicable). Consider thinner design. If a tight fit exists consider flatter BCR or lower water content material (if dehydration is the cause)

■ FIGURE 14.10 Soft toric lens problem solving.

immediately following the blink. The best fit is the flattest lens that allows good centration and regular lens wrapping over the central cornea with no edge buckling.

In general, eyes with refractive astigmatism equal to the corneal toricity may be best corrected with a back toric design, and eyes that have refractive astigmatism with minimal or no corneal toricity may be best corrected with a front toric construction. However, the improved stability of toric soft lens designs blurs this distinction.[67] Soft lens flexure transfers toricity to either surface, from the back surface to the front surface, thus creating a bitoric form on the eye. Theoretically, a well-draping toric lens induces no significant unexpected optical power effects in situ. Power changes caused by flexure can result; these cannot be quantified in clinical practice. The general rules for power compensations (i.e., adding plus sphere and reducing cylinder power) have been learned and applied through clinical experience. The fitting guides of many manufacturers contain power compensation suggestions for their specific lens material, type, and thickness.

Induced Power Changes: The wrapping characteristics or flexure of a soft lens when placed on the eye can change its refractive power effect. Clinical observations suggest some general guidelines for empirical prescribing to compensate for flexure. Thinner toric lenses that are constructed with no prism and all toric hydrogel lenses in low power corrections (+2.00 to −3.00 D) need little, if any, power compensation. Thicker prism-ballasted designs should be adjusted by +0.25 to +0.50 D in spherical power. In higher corrections (i.e., ≥5.00 D), this power and adjustment should increase to +0.50 to +1.00 D. The spherical power compensation component should be considered relative to the amount of cylinder. It appears that higher cylinders (3.00 D) result in more flexure effects and require less cylinder power, and manufacturers recommend compensating for the spherical power with an additional +0.25 D for these higher cylinders.[72] The cylinder power correction of the ordered lens should be reduced whenever possible by 15% to 20% to allow for flexure effects and to reduce the possibility of variable vision caused by rotation or rocking. For example, for a spectacle prescription of −6.00 − 2.50 × 180 (13 mm) at the cornea, −5.50 − 2.12 × 180, the ordered lens powers might be −5.00 − 1.75 × 180 if no axis compensation is needed.

The improved accuracy and reproducibility of manufacturing have improved the reliability of labeled lens parameters, allowing greater confidence when the initial lens specification or lens reordering is based on a toric diagnostic fit or first-ordered lens and overrefraction. Most manufacturers provide liberal exchange policies and allow for often-needed fitting refinements without increased cost. An average of 1.4 to 1.6 toric lenses per eye needed to attain a successful result has been reported,[73] and this value appears to be decreasing. When using disposable soft toric lenses, typically a diagnostic lens is dispensed for 1 to 2 weeks' use to determine if the lens is the correct power and axis before ordering the lens multipacks.

Front versus Back Toricity: With the newer-generation, thinner toric lenses in the common cylinder powers of 0.75 to 2.50 D, there appear to be no advantages to either front or back surface toric construction. Toric soft lenses assume a bitoric configuration when draped over the toric cornea and, if properly prescribed, will result in a spherical power effect on the eye.[34] Soft lens toricity in situ is transferred from one surface to the other. From a manufacturing standpoint, a front toric design is less complex. Back toric fabrication requires more steps, but lenses can be made with higher cylinders more easily and probably more accurately. However, modern toric-generator lathes and molding techniques have simplified the manufacturing of back toric lenses.[67] Trends in lens fabrication technology are moving toward back toric designs.

There are special considerations, however, for a toric lens design on a nearly spherical cornea and in the case of high or oblique corneal toricity. It has been suggested that a back toric lens may provide better wrap and stability in highly toric corneas, and conversely, front toric construction may perform better on nearly spherical corneas with significant internal astigmatism.[74] It seems reasonable, then, to assume that spherical corneas may work best with front toric designs, and corneas with significant toricity (2.00 D) may be best fitted with back toric designs. If neither front nor back toric soft lenses yield acceptable quality of vision when all other criteria are met, then it is advisable to use a GP lens to achieve the best vision.

Physiologic Problems: A soft toric lens must fulfill the same physiologic criteria as a spherical soft lens. Because of the addition of cylinder and prism ballasting, the toric lens thickness is increased both centrally and regionally throughout most of the lens profile. While these lenses are thicker than spherical soft lenses, improvements in lens design have allowed for decreased overall thickness in most soft toric lenses.[45] The averaging of oxygen transmission throughout the entire lens determines the oxygen available to the cornea and the physiologic changes that may occur because of hypoxia.[75] An increased corneal swelling response induced by prism has been demonstrated in comparison to nonprism lenses.[76] The added thickness and increased mass of soft toric lenses suggest that they may impair normal corneal metabolism more often than spherical soft lenses.[77] Because of this, physiologic changes detected by the biomicroscope should be monitored. However, the availability of silicone hydrogel toric lenses has resulted in a reduction in physiologic problems associated with soft toric lenses. This material allows increased oxygen transmission throughout the entire lens and results in overall better eye health.[78]

Superficial punctate keratitis (SPK), if present with toric soft lenses, is usually observed in the inferior cornea. Edema, if present, also is observed more often at the lower hemisphere.[79] A probable cause of SPK, in addition to localized hypoxic edema, is localized dehydration of toric lenses.[80] With toric (nonrotating) lenses, dehydration is more common in the inferior region as evidenced by a tendency for surface deposits to form in this area.[79] This problem is more common in patients with partial blinking patterns. In addition, the flushing of tear debris may be impaired by nonrotating lenses, and this increases the likelihood of epithelial staining.

Conjunctival or scleral indentation from the pressure of lens edges is observed with larger lenses, bulky edges, tight fits, and base curve steepening caused by lens aging. If not resolved, this mechanical compression can lead to perilimbal congestion, limbal swelling, or an acute red-eye response.

Superior epithelial arcuate lesions (SEALs) are typically observed near the superior limbus and can result from mechanical pressure or rubbing of the lens at the superior peripheral cornea. While these lesions can occur with any type of soft lens, there is increased incidence with higher-Dk or silicone hydrogel materials.[81] A SEAL will typically resolve after discontinuing lens wear for a short period of time.

Corneal epithelial edema is a concern because of the increased thickness of toric lenses. This is especially true in lenses with a lower water content or thicker profiles. Studies have shown that corneal swelling of between 2.6% and 4.9% occurs after 3 hours of lens wear with some currently available toric soft lenses.[48] Although most patients wearing toric lenses on a daily-wear basis tolerate their lenses well when they follow a reasonable wearing schedule, for those with more sensitive or oxygen-demanding corneas, a higher-Dk silicone hydrogel soft toric lens or GP lens should be considered.

Neovascularization can be a response to a variety of factors, such as hypoxia, mechanical irritation, infections, allergies, or a toxin-mediated condition. The decreased oxygen supply that occurs with thicker toric lens designs increases the risk of neovascularization. Inferior corneal vascularization has been reported with extended-wear hydrogel toric lenses[82] and may be related to mechanical, as well as hypoxic causes. When corneal hypoxia secondary to soft toric contact lens wear is suspected, better oxygenation can be achieved with a silicone hydrogel material, a thinner lens design, or GP lenses.[35,45]

Higher-water-content hydrogel materials (55%) were once the best soft lens option available for patients who wear their lenses overnight and for patients whose corneas need increased oxygenation. With the introduction of extended-wear silicone hydrogel toric lenses, hydrogel lenses should be considered for a flexible-wear schedule at best. While the water content of silicone hydrogel lenses is lower than that of hydrogel lenses, the Dk value is higher.[78] This allows for much higher oxygenation and has resulted in improved patient tolerance and safety of extended-wear regimens.

■ SUMMARY

The ability to fit toric contact lenses successfully separates the expert from the novice contact lens clinician. The successful fitting of toric lenses requires clinical skills pertaining to contact lens evaluation and fit assessment; a familiarity with simple optical principles, product design, and availability; and eventually a feel for lens behavior on the eye. All these skills can be developed quickly by the clinician who resolves to practice full-scope contact lens care.

■ CLINICAL CASES

CASE 1

A patient enters your office with a strong desire to be refitted into GP contact lenses. His previous doctor fitted him with soft lenses 1 year ago, and he has experienced both blurred vision and frequent lens replacements because of lens surface deposits and fingernail tears.
    Your examination results in the following refractive data:

	OD	OS
Keratometry	42.25 @ 180; 44.25 @ 090	42.50 @ 180; 44.25 @ 090
Refraction	−2.00 − 0.75 × 180	−1.50 − 0.75 × 180
CRA	−1.25 × 090	−1.00 × 090

What lens material should this patient be fitted with?

SOLUTION: As the corneal astigmatism is with-the-rule and the residual astigmatism is against-the-rule, a high-Dk GP lens material should flex to reduce the residual astigmatism sufficiently. For example, the Menicon Z is a hyper-Dk material that is manufactured in a thin lens design. In addition, if it is fitted slightly "steeper than K" (i.e., 0.25 D), the flexure may be such that almost all the residual astigmatism will be compensated for by the flexing of the lens.

CASE 2

Your patient is being evaluated for possible contact lens wear. She has never worn contact lenses before and has no lens material preference. Your examination results in the following refractive data:

	OD	OS
Keratometry	44.00 @ 180; 44.25 @ 090	43.50 @ 180; 44.00 @ 090
Refraction	−3.25 − 1.25 × 180	−3.00 − 1.25 × 180
CRA	−1.00 × 180	−0.75 × 180

Assuming (based on all other examination findings) that she is a good contact lens candidate, into what lens material would you fit her?

SOLUTION: As the patient does not have a preference for lens material and the residual astigmatism may be of sufficient magnitude to compromise vision with GP lens wear, soft toric lenses are recommended. This patient has an excellent probability of success based on the refraction (i.e., low cylinder amount, regular astigmatism, and the availability of lens parameters).

CASE 3

Your patient has been a spherical GP lens wearer for 2 years after previously being a soft lens failure because of giant papillary conjunctivitis. Although he enjoys the wettability, ease of care, comfort, and durability of these lenses, he thinks his vision has never been "crisp." Your examination results in the following information:

	OD	OS
Keratometry	43.25 @ 010; 44.25 @ 100	43.75 @ 170; 44.25 @ 080
Refraction	+2.00 − 2.25 × 010	+1.25 − 1.75 × 170
CRA	−1.25 × 010	−1.25 × 170

Evaluation of current contact lenses:

	OD	OS
Visual acuity	20/25 − 2	20/25 − 1
Overrefraction	pl − 1.25 × 010	+0.25 − 1.00 × 170
	20/20 + 2	20/20 + 1
SLE	Good centration and lag	Good centration and lag
Lens parameters		
BCR	43.50 D (7.76 mm)	43.75 D (7.71 mm)
Power	+2.00	+1.00
OAD	9.4 mm	9.4 mm
CT	0.24 mm	0.22 mm
Edge	Minus lenticular	Minus lenticular

Into what material would you fit this patient?

SOLUTION: As a result of this patient's motivation to continue GP lens wear, a front surface toric lens design is recommended. If this is to be empirically designed, the following parameters can be ordered:

	OD	OS
BCR	43.50 D (7.76 mm)	43.75 D (7.71 mm)
Power	+2.00 − 1.25 × 175	+1.25 − 1.00 × 005
	or	or
	+0.75 + 1.25 × 085	+0.25 + 1.00 × 095

These values were determined by adding overrefraction of spherical lens to lens power and compensating 15 degrees for possible rotational effects.

OAD	9.4/9.0 mm	9.4/9.0 mm
CT	0.24 + 0.11 (1.25 × 9.0)	0.22 + 0.11
	= 0.35 mm	= 0.33 mm
Edge	Minus lenticular	Minus lenticular
Prism	1.25Δ	1.25Δ

A higher amount of prism is not indicated as truncation will actually increase ballast effect.

Lens   As a result of the CT, a minimum 50-Dk lens material is recommended.

CASE 4

This patient is a previous GP lens failure as a result of discomfort and is highly motivated for soft lenses. Your refraction reveals the following:

OD: −4.00 − 3.00 × 175   OS: −4.25 − 3.25 × 005

Assuming the ocular health is normal and all other tests indicate that contact lens wear is recommended, would you fit this patient into soft lenses?

SOLUTION: With the increase in optical quality accompanied by the availability of numerous, custom, soft toric lens designs, it would be worthwhile to attempt to fit this patient with soft lenses. If lens rotation is not excessive or unstable, soft toric lenses should be successful in this case. Likewise, if the patient is very motivated and does not have very critical vision demands, the probability of success is very high. However, if critical vision demands are accompanied by unstable lens rotation, a bitoric GP lens material should be recommended.

CASE 5

A patient who has recently moved to your town enters your office with a desire to have his current contact lenses evaluated and possibly refitted. He was fitted 6 months ago by an eye doctor who told him these lenses were "hard astigmatism contacts." Until today he had not worn the lenses for 2 months as a result of poor visual acuity. Your evaluation of these lenses reveals the following:

	OD	OS
Visual acuity	20/30 + 1	20/25 − 2
Overrefraction	pl − 1.50 × 180 20/20	pl − 1.25 × 180 20/20
SLE	Good centration/alignment	Good centration/alignment
	Fluorescein pattern	Fluorescein pattern
Lens parameters		
BCR	41.50 (8.13 mm)/44.50	42.00 (8.04 mm)/44.50
	(7.58 mm)	(7.58 mm)
Power	−1.50/−6.00	−2.00/−5.75

What type of lens design is this and how should you manage this patient?

SOLUTION: It is very apparent that these are back surface toric lens designs. This information matches the 1:2:3 principle exactly. The residual astigmatism equals one-half of the back surface toricity as verified with the radiuscope and equals one-third of the lensometry cylinder. This patient would benefit from application of a bitoric lens design. In this particular case, as the induced cylinder equals −1.50 × 180 OD and −1.25 × 180 OS, it would be compensated for by adding +1.50 × 180 OD and +1.25 × 180 OS to these respective lenses to create SPE bitoric lenses. The final powers (as determined in the absence of a bitoric diagnostic set and assuming the back surface toric lenses provided a good lens-to-cornea fitting relationship) would be obtained by simply adding the induced cylinder correction to the corresponding meridian of the back toric lens (i.e., the vertical meridian). The final lens powers would equal the following:

OD: −1.50/−4.50   OS: −2.00/−4.50

These values should be verified with the lensometer.

CASE 6A

A patient wants to wear contact lenses for the first time and exhibits no preference for lens material. Good motivation and normal ocular health are present. The refractive findings are the following:

	OD	OS
Keratometry	41.50 @ 180; 45.75 @ 090	41.00 @ 180; 44.50 @ 090
Refraction	−4.25 − 4.75 × 180	−3.50 − 4.00 × 180
Vertexed	−4.00 − 4.25 × 180	−3.50 − 3.50 × 180

What material/lens design would you fit this patient with?

SOLUTION: This appears to be an excellent candidate for a bitoric lens design, especially as the patient exhibits no preference for lens material. In addition, a back surface toric design should result in a significant amount of induced cylinder. If a bitoric diagnostic fitting set is not available, spherical lenses can be fit initially to evaluate both the patient's reaction to contact lens wear and the lens-to-cornea fitting relationship. An initial BCR approximately one-fourth the difference "steeper than K" can be selected (i.e., 42.50 D OD; 41.75 D OS). However, even if good centration is present, the fluorescein pattern will most likely exhibit areas of harsh bearing adjacent to regions of excessive clearance, which could ultimately result in excessive corneal curvature changes and possible distortion. Therefore, a bitoric lens design is recommended to provide an improved alignment relationship with the cornea. Two methods will be shown to arrive at the lens powers:

Method 1: Computational

BCR (Mandell-Moore):

OD	OS
41.25 (8.18 mm)/45.00 (7.50 mm)	40.75 (8.28 mm)/43.75 (7.71 mm)
$Ff = -4.00 + $ (tear lens correction)	$Ff = -3.50 + $ (tear lens correction)
$- 4.00 + (+)0.25$	$- 3.50 + (+)0.25$
$= -3.75$ D	$= -3.25$ D
$Fs = Ff + Kf - Ks$	$Fs = Ff + Kf - Ks$
$= -3.75 + (41.25 - 45.00)$	$= -3.25 + (40.75 - 43.75)$
$= -7.50$ D	$= -6.25$ D

Method 2: Consider as two spherical lens designs

BCR (Mandell-Moore):

OD	OS
41.25 (8.18 mm)/45.00 (7.50 mm)	40.75 (8.28 mm)/43.75 (7.71 mm)
Using "SAM-FAP," the powers become 0.25 D more plus in the horizontal meridian and 0.75 D more plus in the vertical meridian:	Using "SAM-FAP," the powers become 0.25 D more plus in the horizontal meridian and 0.75 D more plus in the vertical meridian:
$-4.00 + (+)0.25 = -3.75$ D	$-3.50 + (+)0.25 = -3.25$ D
$-8.25 + (+)0.75 = -7.50$ D	$-7.00 + (+)0.75 = -6.25$ D

Because no residual astigmatism is predicted with this design, addition of the induced cylinder correction on the front surface should result in an SPE bitoric design. The induced cylinder equals one-half of the back surface (radiuscope) toricity.

OD	OS
$IC = 0.5 \times -3.75 \times 180$	$IC = 0.5 \times -3.00 \times 180$
$= $ (approx.) -1.75 D $\times 180$	$= -1.50$ D $\times 180$
$+1.75$ D $\times 180$ should be added to front surface	$+1.50$ D $\times 180$ should be added to the front surface

Final Design

	OD	OS
BCR	41.25 (8.18 mm)/45.00 (7.50 mm)	40.75 (8.28 mm)/43.75 (7.71 mm)
Power	-3.75 D/-7.50 D	-3.25 D/-6.25 D
OAD	9.2 mm	9.2 mm
SCR	8.80 mm	9.00 mm
PCR	10.80 mm	11.00 mm
CT	0.14 mm	0.15 mm

Material Boston ES bitoric

CASE 6B

What would you predict the final bitoric lens design to be if an SPE bitoric diagnostic fitting set is used in the above case?

	OD	OS
Keratometry	41.50 @ 180; 45.75 @ 090	41.00 @ 180; 44.50 @ 090
Refraction (vertexed)	$-4.00 - 4.25 \times 180$	$-3.50 - 3.50 \times 180$

Select BCR 0.12 − 0.50 D flatter than flat K value:

	41.00 (8.23 mm)/44.00 (7.67 mm)	40.50 (8.33 mm)/43.50 (7.76 mm)
	pl/-3.00	pl/-3.00

Power (horizontal meridian)

	OD	OS
	$-4.00 + (+)0.50$ D	$-3.50 + (+)0.50$ D
	$= -3.50$ D	-3.00 D

SOLUTION: Because the diagnostic lens has a plano power in the horizontal meridian and residual astigmatism is not a factor in this case, the predicted overrefraction is spherical and equals the predicted lens power.

	OD	**OS**
Predicted OR	−3.50 DS	−3.00 DS

Final predicted lens powers = Diagnostic lens powers + OR

= pl + (−)3.50 = −3.50	= pl + (−)3.00 = −3.00
= −3.00 + (−)3.50 = −6.50	= −3.00 + (−)3.00 = −6.00

Final order (if good fitting relationship is obtained and lens powers equal predicted values):

BCR:	41.00 (8.23 mm)/44.00	40.50 (8.33 mm)/43.50
	(7.67 mm)	(7.76 mm)
Power	−3.50 D/−6.50 D	−3.00 D/−6.00 D
CT	0.14 mm	0.14 mm
SCR/W	42.50 (7.94mm) +1 mm	42.00 (8.04mm) + 1 mm
	= 8.9/0.3 mm	9.0/0.3 mm
PCR/W	SCR + 2 mm	SCR + 2 mm
	= 10.9/0.3 mm	= 11.0/0.3 mm
Material	Paragon HDS bitoric	

CASE 7

This patient enters your office with a situation identical to that of the patient in Case 6 except for refraction. Your findings reveal the following:

	OD	**OS**
Keratometry	41.50 @ 180; 45.75 @ 090	41.00 @ 180; 44.50 @ 090
Refraction	−4.25 − 5.75 × 180	−3.50 − 5.00 × 180
Refraction (vertexed)	−4.00 − 5.00 × 180	−3.50 − 4.25 × 180

With what lens material/design would you fit this patient?

SOLUTION: As with Case 6, you may want to fit a spherical GP lens design; however, if an SPE diagnostic fitting set is available, this would be the lens of choice in this case. To arrive at the predicted final lens parameters, the same diagnostic lenses as used in Case 6B should be used:

	OD	**OS**
BCR	41.00 (8.23 mm)/44.00 (7.67 mm)	40.50 (8.33 mm)/43.50 (7.76 mm)
	pl/−3.00	pl/−3.00

To arrive at the final predicted lens powers, perform the tear lens calculations:

Power (horiz. meridian) = −4.00 + (+)0.50 = −3.50 D (i.e., this meridian was 0.50 D flatter than flat K)	= −3.50 + (+)0.50 = −3.00 D (i.e., this meridian was 0.50 D flatter than flat K)
Power (vert. meridian) = −9.00 + (+)1.75 = −7.25 D (i.e., this meridian was 1.75 D flatter than steep K)	−7.75 + (+)1.00 = −6.75 D (i.e., this meridian was 0.50 D flatter than K)
or	or
−3.50 − 3.75 × 180	−3.00 − 3.75 × 180

Final predicted lens power = Diagnostic lens powers + OR; therefore, predicted OR = Final predicted lens power − Diagnostic lens powers

= (−3.50 − 3.75 × 180) −(pl − 3.00 × 180)	= (−3.00 − 3.75 × 180) − (pl − 3.00 × 180)
= −3.50 − 0.75 × 180	= −3.00 − 0.75 × 180

If these are the actual overrefractions found with these lenses, Silbert's rule can be used to determine the final lens powers:

Horizontal meridian: Add −3.50 D to pl = −3.50 D   Add −3.00 D to pl = −3.00 D

Vertical meridian: Add −4.25 D to   Add −3.75 D to −3.00 D
−3.00 D = −7.25 D   = −6.75 D

As can be observed, this is simply another method of obtaining the same values derived earlier.

Final order (if good fitting relationship exists and final powers equal predicted values):

	OD	OS
BCR	41.00 (8.23 mm)/44.00 (7.67 mm)	40.50 (8.33 mm)/43.50 (7.76 mm)
Power	−3.50/−7.25	−3.00/−6.75

Fluoroperm 30 bitoric

It should also be mentioned that 0.75 D residual astigmatism is borderline for determining whether a CPE design would be indicated. Obviously, this would be dictated by such factors as the patient's vision demands and the vision obtained with the best spherical overrefraction (not spherocylindrical) over an SPE bitoric diagnostic lens.

CASE 8

Your patient is deemed a viable candidate for bitoric GP lenses. The following refractive information has been obtained:

	OD	OS
Spectacle Rx:	−2.00 − 6.00 × 180	−1.50 − 5.00 × 180
(spectacle plane):	−2.00 − 5.25 × 180	−1.50 − 4.50 × 180
Keratometry:	42.00 @ 180; 47.25 @ 090	41.50 @ 180; 46.00 @ 090

With what bitoric lens design and material would you fit this patient?

SOLUTION: If, in fact, a 3 D SPE fitting set is the only option, the following lenses can be fitted and the vertical meridian compensated to achieve an improved fitting relationship. Likewise, toric peripheral curves would be recommended.

	OD	OS
Dx Lenses:	BCR = 41.50/44.50	41.00/44.00
	Power: pl/−3.00	pl/−3.00

SLE: Good centration; mild bearing horizontally; excessive clearance vertically OU

Overrefraction:	−1.50 DS (20/20)	−1.00 DS (20/20)
Tent. order:	41.50 (8.13 mm) − 1.50 D/	41.00 (8.23 mm) − 1.00 D/
	44.50 (7.58 mm) − 4.50 D	44.00 (7.67 mm) − 4.00 D

Steepen vertical meridian 1.5 D and add   Steepen vertical meridian by 1 D and add
−1.50 D to power in that meridian   −1 D to power in that meridian

Final order: 41.50 (8.13 mm) − 1.50 D/   41.00 (8.23 mm) − 1.00 D/
46.00 (7.34 mm) − 6.00 D   45.00 (7.50 mm) − 5.00 D

Toric peripheral curves: SCR = BCR + 1 mm; PCR = SCR + 2 mm

SCR = 8.1/7.3 + 1 mm = 9.1/8.3   8.2/7.5 + 1 mm = 9.2/8.5

PCR = 11.1/10.3 mm   11.2/10.5 mm

Material: Optimum Classic bitoric

CASE 9A

Your patient is a good candidate for soft toric lenses. The following refractive data has been obtained:

	OD	OS
Keratometry	42.25 @ 180; 43.50 @ 090	42.50 @ 180; 43.25 @ 090
Refraction	−2.50 − 1.25 × 180	−2.75 − 0.75 × 180

You apply the following soft toric diagnostic lenses:

BCR	8.6 mm	8.6 mm
Power	$-3.00 - 1.25 \times 180$	$-3.00 - 0.75 \times 180$

With slit-lamp evaluation, you estimate that the middle laser mark on the right lens has shifted 10 degrees to the right and 20 degrees to the left on the left eye.

What axis change would be indicated for the new diagnostic lenses? If a good, stable fit is achieved, what would be the predicted overrefraction and final lens powers?

SOLUTION: Using the LARS principle, you would subtract 10 degrees from the spectacle axis for the right lens axis and add 20 degrees for the left lens axis. The new diagnostic lenses would be:

$$\text{OD: } -3.00 - 1.25 \times 170 \qquad \text{OS: } -3.00 - 1.25 \times 020$$

If both a good fitting relationship and rotation stability exists with these lenses, the predicted overrefraction would simply equal the difference between the refraction and the diagnostic lens power:

$$\text{OD: } (-2.50 - 1.25) - (-3.00 - 1.25) = +0.50 \text{ DS}$$
$$\text{OS: } (-2.75 - 0.75) - (-3.00 - 1.25) = +0.25 \text{ DS}$$

Final predicted lens order:

OD: BCR = 8.6 mm   Power = $-2.50 - 1.25 \times 170$
OS: BCR = 8.6 mm   Power = $-2.75 - 0.75 \times 020$

CASE 9B

In the above case, what changes would you make if the right lens exhibited poor rotational stability—in other words, if it rotated excessively and periodically failed to return to its original position.

SOLUTION: The selection of a steeper BCR would be recommended (i.e., 8.3 mm, if available). Other possible options would be to select a lens with either a larger OAD or a greater amount of prism (if appropriate). As this problem is only present with one lens, it is quite probable that one of these options will result in a successful fit. However, if both lenses are exhibiting unstable rotation, these changes may not solve the problem. If this is the case, a different type of soft toric lens can be attempted (i.e., prism ballast if the previous lens was nonprism ballasted and vice versa). If this fails, a GP lens material is recommended.

CASE 10

You have recently fit a patient having the following refractive information with soft toric lenses:

	OD	OS
Refraction	$-2.50 - 2.75 \times 170$	$-2.00 - 2.25 \times 010$
Keratometry	42.50 @ 170; 45.50 @ 080	42.75 @ 010; 45.25 @ 100

Current lens parameters

BCR	8.6 mm	8.6 mm
Power	$-2.50 - 2.25 \times 160$	$-2.00 - 2.00 \times 020$
Design	Front toric	Front toric

At the dispensing visit, the patient complained of intermittent blurry vision, and SLE revealed poor rotational stability. Nevertheless, the patient was instructed to adapt to lens wear and return to the office in 1 week. At this visit, the same symptoms and clinical signs were present. How would you handle this situation?

SOLUTION: Because of the high amount of corneal astigmatism, it is possible that a back toric lens design might provide better stability. It is recommended that a back toric design be diagnostically fit to determine if better stability exists. If this design fails also, either a spherical or bitoric GP lens design can be used.

CASE 11

You have recently fit a patient with the following refractive information with soft toric lenses:

	OD	OS
Refraction	$-5.50 - 1.75 \times 180$	$-6.00 - 1.75 \times 180$
Keratometry	43.00 @ 180; 44.50 @ 090	42.50 @ 180; 44.00 @ 090

As appropriate diagnostic lenses were not available, the following lenses were ordered after empirical determination:

BCR	8.6 mm	8.6 mm
Power	$-5.25 - 2.00 \times 180$	$-5.75 - 2.00 \times 180$

At the 1-week follow-up evaluation, this patient complained of poor vision. What is the likely cause of this problem assuming good rotational stability is present?

SOLUTION: The solution should reside in the overrefraction. As this lens material was only available in cylinder powers of -1.25 D and -2.00 D, this practitioner ordered the -2.00 D power because this was closer to the -1.75 D refractive astigmatism value. In addition, the sphere was compensated for by reducing the minus by -0.25 D. However, the following two problems were created:

1. Vertex distance was ignored.
2. The effects of flexure were not considered.

Because of the effects of flexure, especially in high ametropic powers, the lens should be ordered in a slightly lower minus (greater plus) prescription and the cylinder correction should be less than the refractive astigmatism (i.e., -1.25 D).

CASE 12*

A 26-year-old patient presents wearing disposable spherical soft lenses, and is satisfied with the clarity of his vision. His lenses are worn on a daily-wear basis with occasional overnight wear.

Visual acuity with contact lenses:

OD	20/25−	Overrefraction: $+0.25 - 0.75 \times 180$ 20/20+
OS	20/25−	Overrefraction: $+0.25 - 0.75 \times 180$ 20/20+

Biomicroscopy with contact lenses:
OU Good centration and lens lag with the blink

Manifest refraction:

OD	$-3.00 - 0.75 \times 180$ 20/20+
OS	$-3.50 - 0.75 \times 180$ 20/20+

Keratometry:

OD	44.00 @ 180; 44.75 @ 090
OS	44.00 @ 180; 44.75 @ 090

SOLUTION: The uncorrected astigmatism would best be corrected by a soft toric lens. It was considered best to select a lens that would correct the refractive cylinder and could also be worn on a flexible-wear schedule.

He was fit with the following lenses:

OD	BCR: 8.6	Power: $-3.00 - 0.75 \times 180$ 20/20+
	Air Optix for Astigmatism (Ciba Vision)	
OS	BCR: 8.6	Power: $-3.50 - 0.75 \times 180$ 20/20+
	Air Optix for Astigmatism (Ciba Vision)	

---

* Cases 12 through 15 are modified from Bennett et al.[65]

Biomicroscopy with contact lens wear:
OU good centration and lens lag with the blink
These lenses were prescribed for daily wear with occasional overnight wear.

CASE 13*

A 23-year-old patient presented desiring contact lenses. She had been told by several previous doctors that she was a poor candidate for contact lenses. Several years earlier she had attempted GP lens wear and was unsuccessful.

Manifest refraction:

OD	+4.50 − 6.00 × 010 20/30+
OS	+3.75 − 5.50 × 180 20/25−

Keratometry:

OD	46.00 @ 010; 50.00 @ 100
OS	46.00 @ 180; 51.00 @ 090

SOLUTION: Custom soft toric lenses were designed using a company desktop or personal digital assistant-based crossed cylinder programmed calculator. The spectacle Rx conversion for vertex distance was entered and resulted in the following Custom Hydrasoft Toric EW (CooperVision) lenses:

OD	BCR 8.6 mm	OAD 15.0 mm	Rx +6.00 − 6.00 × 010
OS	BCR 8.6 mm	OAD 15.0 mm	Rx +4.75 − 5.50 × 180

These lenses were dispensed and re-evaluated at 1 week and then at 3 weeks. Although the patient was asymptomatic and was satisfied with her vision, at the 3-week follow-up evaluation, the right lens was torqued 6 degrees counterclockwise (i.e., the 6 o'clock mark shifted to the right) and the left lens was torqued about 5 degrees clockwise (i.e., the 6 o'clock mark was shifted to the left).

Visual acuity with contact lenses:

OD	20/50 (stable)	Overrefraction −0.50 − 0.50 × 127 20/25+
OS	20/30 (stable)	Overrefraction −0.25 − 0.75 × 043 20/25+

Biomicroscopy with contact lenses:

OU   Both lenses resulted in good centration and movement with the blink.

According to the LARS rule, the axis should be reordered at about 5 degrees for the right lens and 175 degrees for the left lens. However, a more accurate method would be to insert the overrefraction into a desktop or personal digital assistant-based crossed cylinder calculator, which is quite simple and quick. Using the cross-cylinder equations programmed into the calculator, the resultant powers were ordered. The following lenses were dispensed with the corresponding visual acuities:

OD	+5.00 − 5.50 × 007 20/25
OS	+4.25 − 5.50 × 003 20/25

CASE 14*

A 50-year-old gemologist wearing soft toric lenses for 16 years has become disillusioned with contact lens wear because of vision limitations. At work, she more often had to use a jeweler's loop to look at jewelry. Monovision was acceptable, although she was unwilling to compromise distance or near vision anymore. She required accurate distance, intermediate, and near vision for tasks at work and at home. A spectacle prescription was not an option for cosmetic reasons and because of the aberrations her present prescription provided. She was replacing her contact lenses every 18 months because of deposit buildup. This patient was on a daily-wear schedule using the Clear Care (Ciba Vision) disinfection regimen to clean and disinfect her lenses. She was not currently taking any medications. Her primary reason for requesting an eye examination was to investigate the possibility of improving her distance and near vision with soft toric daily-wear lenses.

Biomicroscopy:
Lid eversion revealed a slightly hyperemic appearance of the tarsal conjunctiva without papillae or follicles, a result of the present contact lens surface characteristics. When pressure was applied to the meibomian glands on the lid margin, normal contents were expressed. Lid appearance was slightly flaccid, typical for a 50-year-old woman. The inferior tear meniscus was adequate in height to support contact lens wear. Fluorescein staining revealed intact corneas without defects. Neither eye exhibited any signs of neovascularization or edema. Grade 1 bulbar conjunctival injection was present.

Manifest refraction:

OD	+1.75 − 2.50 × 100 20/20	Add +1.50 20/20 Dominant eye
OS	+1.75 − 2.00 × 70 20/20	Add +1.50 20/20

Keratometry:

OD	42.87 @ 180; 44.62 @ 090
OS	42.62 @ 180; 44.37 @ 090

Schirmer I without anesthetic:

OD	26 mm in 5 minutes
OS	24 mm in 5 minutes

Tear breakup time OD 10 seconds; OS 10 seconds

SOLUTION: The patient was determined to be a hyperopic astigmatic presbyope. She was not motivated to try GP lenses. An aspheric multifocal soft toric lens modality was an option that was available in her prescription. The commitment of office time and possible multiple lens orders were discussed to make the patient aware of the difficulties in achieving the visual requirement. The aspheric multifocal toric bifocal lens was fitted and ordered empirically because of the multiple visual demands at work and at home.

The contact lens specifications from CooperVision were as follows:

Proclear Multifocal Toric

Base curve: 8.8 mm (OD); 8.8 mm (OS)

Diameter: 14.4 mm (OD); 14.4 mm (OS)

Power: +1.75 − 2.00 × 100   Add +1.50 (OD) distance lens
       +1.75 − 2.00 × 70   Add +1.50 (OS) near lens

The patient was dispensed the soft toric multifocal contact lenses and educated about deposit build-up. Visual acuity and overrefraction exhibited the following:

OD	20/25− (distance and near) plano − 0.50 × 100
OS	20/20 (distance and near) − 0.25 − 0.25 × 70

Biomicroscopy with contact lenses:
The lenses centered well and revealed a 0.5-mm lag with the blink. The toric markings on both eyes were positioned at 3 and 9 o'clock and exhibited slight temporal rotation with the blink, although recovery was rapid. The lens surface appeared to be clean and wet evenly. A 1-week follow-up appointment was scheduled to discuss the acceptability of this lens design. The right lens was reordered to achieve better acuity.

CASE 15*

A 32-year-old man who is part owner of a very busy 24-hour restaurant was evaluated. His sleep habits were very erratic. He came into the office as a previously unsuccessful GP lens wearer because of intolerance; therefore, he was asking for soft contact lenses. He mentioned that eyeglasses were very troublesome, especially during warm weather. His primary reason for requesting an eye examination was to investigate the possibility of wearing soft extended-wear lenses.

Biomicroscopy:
Lid eversion revealed a normal satin appearance of the tarsal conjunctiva without papillae or follicles. Fluorescein staining revealed intact corneas without defects. Neither eye exhibited any signs of neovascularization or edema. Conjunctiva and sclera exhibited no inflammation or congestion. The tear meniscus was normal.

Retinoscopy:

	OD	$-3.00 - 1.50 \times 180$ 20/20 $- 2$
	OS	$-2.50 - 1.00 \times 180$ 20/20

Manifest refraction:

	OD	$-3.25 - 1.75 \times 165$ 20/20
	OS	$-2.50 - 1.25 \times 180$ 20/20

Keratometry:

	OD	40.00 @ 180; 41.75 @ 090
	OS	40.00 @ 180; 41.50 @ 090

Tear breakup time OD 12 seconds; OS 11 seconds

SOLUTION: He required a correction for his compound myopic astigmatism. Because of his visual demands, erratic work habits, and extended-wear criteria, monthly replacement PureVision Toric (Bausch & Lomb) contact lenses were prescribed. It was suggested that this patient be fitted with a monthly frequent-replacement toric extended-wear lens.

Lens specifications	OD	OS
Base curve	8.7	8.7
Diameter	14.0	14.0
Power	$-3.00 - 1.75 \times 180$	$-2.50 - 1.00 \times 180$

With dispensing, the following visual acuities were obtained:

	OD	OS
Visual acuity (distance)	20/20	20/20
Visual acuity (near)	J1	J1

The overrefraction was plano OU.

Biomicroscopy with contact lenses:
Good centration and lens movement with the blink were present OU. The toric markings at 6 o'clock on each lens showed slight nasal rotation with rapid recovery.

CLINICAL PROFICIENCY CHECKLIST

- CRA can be obtained by subtracting the patient's keratometric astigmatism from the refractive astigmatism. This value equals the predicted amount of astigmatism when a GP lens is placed on the eye.

- Because the ARA sometimes differs from the calculated, it is advisable to first use a spherical GP lens for diagnostic purposes.

- In certain cases, soft lenses are recommended when a high amount of residual astigmatism is present. If very little or no refractive cylinder is present, a spherical lens is often successful; if between -1.00 and -2.00 D of nonoblique refractive astigmatism is present, a toric soft lens is recommended.

- When a prism-ballasted, front surface toric design is used, use a high-Dk (>45) lens material, a minimum 8.8 mm overall diameter, slightly "steeper than K" BCR, and 0.75 to 1 Δ for moderate and high minus lenses and 1.25 to 1.50 Δ for low minus and plus power lenses (for prism-ballasted *and* truncated lenses, the prism amounts are reversed).

- A spherical lens design is rarely indicated in cases of high astigmatism (defined as ≥ 2.50 D) even if good centration is present. Poor alignment with the cornea can result in staining, corneal distortion, and flexure-related reduced visual acuity.

- Selecting the BCRs for a back surface or bitoric lens can be performed easily using an available philosophy such as Remba's. Determining the power in each meridian can be performed by calculating the tear lens power in each meridian (i.e., as if two spherical lenses were present).

(continued)

(Continued)

■ The primary problem with using a back surface-only GP toric lens is that this design will induce a cylinder amount equal to approximately one-half of the back surface toricity (as measured with a radiuscope); the lensometer (i.e., power in air) will measure a value equal to 3/2 times the radiuscope value and 3 times the induced amount, hence the term *1:2:3 principle*.

■ Correction of the induced cylinder requires adding the same amount of cylinder (but opposite in sign) to the front surface of the lens. If, for example, the induced cylinder equals -1.75×180 (i.e., the radiuscopic toricity was approximately -3.50×180), $+1.75 \times 180$ would need to be added to the front surface. With this plus cylinder addition, an SPE bitoric lens is created; this lens can rotate in any direction without having an effect on vision.

■ The use of a SPE bitoric diagnostic set is recommended. When the appropriate lens has been selected, a spherical overrefraction is performed and this value is then added to the diagnostic lens powers to derive the final powers. If less than optimum vision is obtained, a spherocylindrical overrefraction should be performed and the use of Silbert's rule is beneficial in deriving the final powers (i.e., add the over-refraction power to the power in the same meridian of the diagnostic lens).

■ Patients with astigmatism who are good contact lens candidates and are either first-time wearers motivated for soft lens wear or have failed with GP lenses be-cause of such factors as discomfort, chronic 3 and 9 o'clock staining, or a poor fit-ting relationship are good candidates for toric soft lenses.

■ Several methods of stabilizing toric soft lenses are used. Whereas truncation, prism ballast, and periballast have often been used in the past, dynamic stabilization (i.e., thinning the top and the bottom of the lens) and eccentric lenticulation (i.e., use of a front surface, off-center lenticular cut in the direction of the prism apex similar to periballast) are becoming popular.

■ When fitting a toric soft lens, it is important to use diagnostic lenses close to the patient's refractive sphere power, cylinder power, and axis values (i.e., ±1.00 D and ±20 degrees). If the lens rotates on the eye, the LARS principle (left add, right sub-tract) should be used. For example, if the lens moves 10 degrees to the right and the cylinder axis is 180 degrees, a lens with an axis equal to (180 − 10) or 170 de-grees should be ordered.

■ When in doubt, it is recommended to undercorrect the amount of cylinder power in a toric soft lens; this will often compensate for flexure effects while also making the patient less sensitive to axis shifts and the variable vision resulting from cross-cylinder effects.

■ One method of predicting toric soft success is, with the subjective refraction in the phoropter, having the patient twist the cylinder knob in both directions. If a blur-ring or degrading of the visual acuity chart occurs with <5 degrees of a twist, the chance for success is low.

■ Physiologic problems which can be induced by a toric soft lens include SPK, edema, scleral indentation, and neovascularization. For the more sensitive or oxygen-demanding cornea patients, a silicone hydrogel toric lens or GP lens should be considered.

REFERENCES

1. Bennett ES. Astigmatic correction. In: Bennett ES, Grohe RM, eds. Rigid Gas Permeable Contact Lenses. New York: Professional Press, 1986:345–380.
2. Sarver MD. A study of residual astigmatism. Am J Optom 1969;46(8):578–582.
3. Dellande WD. A comparison of predicted and measured residual astigmatism in corneal contact lens wearers. Am J Optom 1970;47(6):459–463.

4. Kratz JD, Walton WG. A modification on Javal's rule for the correction of astigmatism. Am J Optom 1949;26(7):295–306.
5. Carter JH. Residual astigmatism of the human eye. Optom Weekly 1963;54(27):1271–1272.
6. Harris MG, Chu CS. The effect of contact lens thickness and corneal toricity on flexure and residual astigmatism. Am J Optom 1972;49(4):304–307.
7. Harris MG. Contact lens flexure and residual astigmatism on toric corneas. J Am Optom Assoc 1970;41(3):247–248.
8. Silbert JA. Rigid lens correction of astigmatism. In: Bennett ES, Weissman BA, eds. Clinical Contact Lens Practice. Philadelphia: JB Lippincott, 1991;40:1–24.
9. Borish IM. Vision Correction with Contact Lenses. Clinical Refraction, 3rd ed. Chicago: Professional Press, 1970:971–1005.
10. Henry VA, Bennett ES. Contact lenses for the difficult-to-fit patient. Contact Lens Forum 1989;14(10):49–68.
11. Wilson SE, Lin DTC, Klyce SD, et al. Topographic changes in contact lens-induced corneal warpage. Ophthalmology 1990;97:734–744.
12. Wilson SE, Lin DTC, Klyce SD, et al. RGP decentration: a risk factor for corneal warpage. CLAO J 1990;16(3):177–183.
13. Seibel DB, Bennett ES, Henry VA, et al. Clinical evaluation of the Boston Equacurve. Contact Lens Forum 1988;13(5):39.
14. Snyder C. of "High-Cylinder" toric soft contact lenses. Int Contact Lens Clin 1997;24:160–164.
15. Budd J. Using your computer to design and evaluate lenses. Contact Lens Spectrum 1988;3(7):53–60.
16. Mandell RB, Moore CF. A bitoric lens guide that really is simple. Contact Lens Spectrum 1988;3(11):83–85.
17. Lowther GE. RGP bitoric lenses. Int Contact Lens Clin 1988;15(2):44.
18. Sarver MD, Mandell RB. Toric lenses. In: Mandell RB, ed. Contact Lens Practice, 4th ed. Springfield, IL: Charles C. Thomas, 1988:284–309.
19. Grosvenor TP. Optical principles of toric contact lenses. Optom Weekly 1976;67(2):37–39.
20. Bergenske PD. A recipe for SPE. Contact Lens Spectrum 2001;16(2):15.
21. Blackmore K, Bachand N, Bennett ES, et al. Gas permeable toric use and applications: survey of Section on Cornea and Contact Lens Diplomates of the American Academy of Optometry. Optometry 2006;77(1):17–22.
22. Kajita M, Ito S, Yamada A, et al. Diagnostic bitoric rigid gas permeable contact lenses. CLAO J 1999;25(3):163–166.
23. Pitts K, Pack L, Edmondson W, et al. Putting a bitoric RGP lens fitting guide to the test. Contact Lens Spectrum 2001;16(10):34–40.
24. Sarver MD, Kame RT, Williams CT. A bitoric rigid gas permeable contact lens with spherical power effect. J Am Optom Assoc 1985;56(3):184–189.
25. Kame RT, Hayashida JK. A simplified approach to bitoric gas permeable lens fitting. Int Contact Lens Clin 1988;15(2):53–58.
26. Weissman BA, Chun MW. The use of spherical power effect bitoric rigid contact lenses in hospital practice. J Am Optom Assoc 1987;58(8):626–630.
27. Bennett ES. Astigmatic correction. In: Bennett ES, Hom MM, eds. Manual of Gas Permeable Contact Lenses, 2nd ed. St. Louis: Elsevier, 2004:286–323.
28. McMahon TT, Szczotka-Flynn LB. Contact lens applications for ocular trauma, disease and surgery. In: Bennett ES, Weissman BA, eds. Clinical Contact Lens Practice. Philadelphia: Lippincott Williams & Wilkins, 2005:549–576.
29. Holden BA. The principles and practice of correcting astigmatism with soft contact lenses. Aust J Optom 1975;58:279.
30. Duke-Elder SW. Systems of Ophthalmology, vol. 5. London: H. Kimptom, 1970.
31. Dabkowski JA, Roach MP, Begley CG. Soft toric versus spherical contact lenses in myopes with low astigmatism. Int Contact Lens Clin 1992;19(11,12):252–255.
32. Kruse A, Lofstrom T. How much visual benefit does an astigmat achieve being corrected with a toric correction? Int Contact Lens Clin 1996;23(3,4):59–65.
33. Snyder C, Wiggins NP, Daum KM. Visual performance in the correction of astigmatism with contact lenses: spherical RGPs versus toric hydrogels. Int Contact Lens Clin 1994;21(7,8):127–131.
34. Remba MB. Clinical evaluation of toric hydrophilic contact lenses. II. J Am Optom Assoc 1981;52(3):220.
35. Bergenske PD. Prescribing soft toric contact lenses. Contact Lens Spectrum 2005;20(2):33–39.
36. Blaze P, Downs S. Fitting soft toric lenses in high astigmatics. J Am Optom Assoc 1984;55:12.
37. Thompson TT. Tyler's quarterly soft contact lens parameter guide. 2007;25(1):9–53.
38. Gasson A. Correction of astigmatism and hydroflex toric soft lenses. Contact Lens J 1979;8(2):3.
39. Dain SJ. Over-refraction and axis mislocation of toric lenses. Int Contact Lens Clin 1979;6(2):57.
40. Coast Vision, Inc. Irregular astigmatism correction with a toric soft lens [Newsletter]. March 1987.
41. Tomlinson A, Bibby MM. Lid interaction and toric soft lens axis location. Am J Optom Physiol Opt 1982;59(4):60.
42. Epstein AB, Remba MJ. Hydrogel toric contact lens correction. In: Bennett ES, Weissman BA, eds. Clinical Contact Lens Practice. Philadelphia: Lippincott Williams & Wilkins, 2005:515–529.

43. Young G, Hunt C, Covey M. Clinical evaluation of factors influencing toric soft contact lens fit. Optom Vis Sci 2002;79(1):11–19.
44. Ott W. Soft toric contact lenses. Optician 1978;4534:29.
45. Lindsay RG. Toric contact lens fitting. In: Phillips AJ, Speedwell L, eds. Contact Lenses. Edinburgh: Elsevier, 2007:255–270.
46. Knoll HA. The stability of the shape of the human cornea. Am J Optom Physiol Opt 1976;53(7):360.
47. Hanks A. The watermelon seed principle. Contact Lens Forum 1983;8(9):31.
48. Hanks AJ, Weisbarth RE, McNally JJ. Clinical performance comparisons of toric soft contact lens designs. Int Contact Lens Clin 1987;14(1):16.
49. Mandell RB. Contact lens optics. In: Mandell RB, ed. Contact Lens Practice, 4th ed. Springfield, IL: Charles C. Thomas, 1988:954–980.
50. Ficco CW. A model for fitting success. Contact Lens Spectrum 2006;21(7):s-2–s-4.
51. Edrington TB. Toric torque. Contact Lens Spectrum 2006;21(8):17.
52. Braff SM. A new corneal contact lens design for the correction of residual astigmatism. Optom Weekly 1970;61(1):24.
53. Holden BA. The principles and practice of correcting astigmatism with soft contact lenses. Aust J Optom 1975;58:279.
54. Strachan JPF. Further comments on the fitting of spherical hydrophilic lenses and the correction of astigmatism with toric lenses. Contacto 1971;20(5):22.
55. Gupta D. Upgrade your toric know-how. Optom Management 2003;38(9):63–67.
56. Choate W, Shaw R, West W, et al. A clinical evaluation of a custom toric lens for planned replacement. Contact Lens Spectrum 1997;12(9):2s–4s.
57. Cabrera JV, Rodriguez JB. Vision with disposable toric contact lenses and daily-wear toric contact lenses. Ophthal Physiol Opt 1998;18(1):66–74.
58. Voyles S, Henry VA, DeKinder JO, et al. Determining the most likely rotational direction of soft toric contact lenses. Poster presented at the Annual Meeting of the American Academy of Optometry, Denver, CO, December 2006.
59. Young G, Hickson-Curran S. Reassessing toric soft lens fitting. Contact Lens Spectrum 2005;20(1):42–45.
60. McMonnies C, Parker D. Predicting the rotational performance of toric soft lenses. Aust J Optom 1977:135.
61. Lieblein JS. To trial fit torics or not. Contact Lens Spectrum 1991;6(4):35–38.
62. Snyder AC, Bowling E. Diagnostic versus empirical fitting with the Eclipse toric soft contact lens. Contact Lens Spectrum 1990;5(12):29–36.
63. Hallak J. Standard soft toric lenses: a problem of orientation. Int Contact Lens Clin 1982;9(4):250.
64. Lindsay RD, Bruce AS, Brennan NA, et al. Determining axis misalignment and powers of toric soft lenses. Int Contact Lens Clin 1997;24(3):101–106.
65. Bennett ES, Davis RL. Toric grand rounds. In: Bennett ES, Weissman BA, eds. Clinical Contact Lens Practice. Philadelphia: Lippincott Williams & Wilkins, 2005:969–995.
66. Blaze P. Refining soft toric contact lens correction. Contact Lens Forum 1988;13(11):52.
67. Hom MM. Soft contact lenses for astigmatism. In: Hom MM, ed. Manual of Contact Lens Prescribing and Fitting with CD-Rom. Edinburgh: Butterworth Heinemann, 2000:219–230.
68. Myers RI, Jones DH, Meinell P. Using overrefraction for problem solving in soft toric fitting. Int Contact Lens Clin 1990;17(9,10):232–235.
69. Weissman BA. Theoretical optics of toric hydrogel contact lenses. Am J Optom Physiol Opt 1986;63(7):538.
70. Becherer PD. Soft torics: a viable modality. Contact Lens Update 1990;9(2):17–21.
71. Hough T. The Moire deflectometer: new technology to measure toric soft lenses. Contact Lens Spectrum 1996;11(9):37–42.
72. Coast Vision, Inc. Fitting Guide, 1989.
73. Kennedy JR. Clinical consideration of sub "K" findings. Contacto 1972;21(5):25.
74. Maltzman B, Rengel A. Soft toric lenses: an update. CLAO J 1985;11(4):335.
75. White P, Miller D. Corneal edema. Complications of Contact Lenses. Boston: Little, Brown, 1981.
76. Soni PS, Borish IM, Keech P. Ballasted contact lenses: topographical comparative changes in corneal thickness. Fifth National Research Symposium on Contact Lenses, Boston, August 1978.
77. Hallak J, Cohen H. Localized edema with soft toric contact lenses. J Am Optom Assoc 1985;56:12.
78. Hom M. Ten reasons to prescribe silicone hydrogel soft torics. Optom Management 2006;41(11):53–56.
79. Maltzman BA. Lipid protein precipitates in toric soft lenses. Contact Lens Forum 1988;13(1):74.
80. Clompus R. Custom correction for astigmats and soft torics. Rev Optom 1986;23(4):1986.
81. Bowling E, Shovlin JP, Russell GE, et al. The corneal atlas. Rev Optom 2007;144(1):19–20.
82. Westin E, Benjamin WJ. Inferior corneal neovascularization associated with extended wear of prism-ballasted toric soft lenses. Poster presented at the Annual Meeting of the American Academy of Optometry, Columbus, OH, December 1988.

CHAPTER 15

Bifocal Contact Lenses

Edward S. Bennett and Vinita Allee Henry

▇ INTRODUCTION

There is very little doubt that tremendous potential exists for expanding your contact lens practice in the ever-increasing presbyopic marketplace. It is rapidly growing and is currently the largest segment of the population as well as the largest relatively untapped segment of the contact lens market.[1–4] With 78 million baby boomers (i.e., those born in the United States between 1946 and 1964) now entering presbyopia, a large group of potential bifocal contact lens wearers will exist.[1] It is certainly evident that a contact lens that provides more natural vision will appeal to them, as would any product or service that claims to be all natural. The older cohort—those in the 45 to 54 age range—are in their peak earning period. They are willing to pay extra for features and benefits they perceive to be of value or that enhance the quality or services being provided.[1] Therefore, with the natural vision, binocularity, and cosmesis provided by bifocal contact lenses to a population in which vanity is important, the bifocal market has much potential in the coming decade.[1,5,6] Although this chapter will refer to this form of contact lens as "bifocals," most of these designs provide correction for more than two distances and would best be described as "multifocals." Other forms of presbyopic contact lens correction include single-vision distance-correcting contact lenses in combination with reading glasses, and monovision, in which one eye is optimally corrected for distance and the other eye is optimally corrected for near.

The primary question is: Will practitioners fit them? Although 18% of soft lenses in the United States are prescribed for presbyopia,[7] two-thirds are prescribed for monovision.[8] Worldwide, the values are much smaller, with 6% of presbyopes wearing soft lenses and only half of this group wearing bifocal or multifocal lenses.

Why is this percentage of contact lens-wearing presbyopes so low? Certainly, the reasons are multifold and include practitioner apprehension. Common comments from patients have indicated that when asked about bifocal contact lenses, it is not uncommon to hear such responses as: "I never knew bifocal contact lenses existed" or "I've heard of them but my previous doctor said they don't work." Actually, the latter is a true comment. Bifocal contact lenses are not successful—until they are diagnostically fit to the patient. This is confirmed by a study by Jones et al,[9] who divided subjects into "reactive" (i.e., contact lenses were not presented to them initially as an option) and "proactive" (i.e., contact lenses were actively discussed as a viable option). The results showed that, whereas 9 of 80 subjects were fit into contact lenses in the reactive group, 46 of 80 subjects, including 21 of 33 presbyopic patients, were fit into contact lenses in the proactive group.

Bifocal contact lens patients not only receive the binocular vision advantages and more natural vision, but they also can represent the most enthusiastic patients in the practice who can refer others and allow practitioners to build their contact lens practice. Patients being told either that there is no such option or that bifocal lenses are not successful or those automatically being fitted into monovision (one eye optimally corrected for distance, the other eye for near) are not being properly managed. Instead, these patients should be referred to a practitioner who is fitting bifocal contact lenses. There are numerous stories in the literature of how fitting presbyopic patients into bifocal contact lenses had a significant impact on their lives.[10,11]

Some explanations for the limited bifocal contact lens applications do have merit. Although translating gas-permeable (GP) bifocal designs can claim as good or better vision at distance and near versus progressive addition spectacle lenses (PALs), most contact lens bifocal/ multifocal designs do represent some compromise. Most designs have multiple vision corrections in front of the pupil at the same time, termed *simultaneous vision* designs. Although the compromise in vision may only be mild with some designs, it must be considered with patients having critical vision demands. In addition, the spectacle lens market is enjoying considerable success as a result of the enormous amount of publicity aimed at showing the glamour and beauty of today's fashion frames. Presbyopic spectacle sales also benefit practice income.

Nevertheless, presbyopic patients deserve the opportunity to be educated and, if interested, to be fitted with bifocal contact lenses. These specialty contact lenses are not for everyone, as will be discussed later in this chapter. However, consumer interest is increasing—and will continue to increase—as a result of several recent advancements with these designs including the following: (a) soft disposable multifocal and bifocal designs allow the ability of the presbyope to minimize lens deposit-related problems and to have replacement lenses readily available, while also allowing the practitioner the ability to trial a pair of lenses for a short time period (typically 1 week) and make any indicated changes; (b) silicone hydrogel materials in presbyopic designs have allowed a cohort of contact lens wearers who require high oxygen transmission to achieve this goal; (c) high add aspheric multifocal GP designs have allowed the more mature presbyope to see at all distances via an aspheric design; and (d) GP segmented, translating designs with intermediate vision capabilities allow the advanced presbyope with critical vision needs at all distances to meet these needs. In addition, members of this population are more active than their predecessors, making spectacle correction a less desirable option for visual freedom. As PALs often require numerous head movements to find the optimum position for computer use and other intermediate tasks, because of the varying corrective powers present during any eye movement, they can also represent compromise.[12–15] Also, as will be emphasized in this chapter as well, the fitting and problem solving of these designs are not nearly as complicated as one might perceive them to be. With the baby boomers becoming presbyopic, it makes good sense to present this option to all presbyopic patients in your office.

■ PATIENT SELECTION AND EVALUATION

Practice Promotion

The first important step toward achieving success with a potential bifocal contact lens patient is practice promotion of this contact lens option. Patient brochures can be displayed in the reception area as well as the examination rooms. This gives the patient every opportunity to review this material before the examination and introduce them to the possibility of wearing bifocal contact lenses. Obviously, practice newsletters and—an ever-increasingly popular modality—the practice website can be used to inform both current and potential future patients about bifocal contact lenses.

Comprehensive Preliminary Evaluation

Aging Changes

To determine if the patient is a good candidate, an understanding of normal changes occurring over time is important.[16,17] Aqueous tear production and stability of the tear film both decrease with age, making the patient more susceptible to dry eye, which can affect the wetting and comfort of contact lenses. In fact, it has been found that, whereas 28% of presbyopic patients reported dryness before contact lens wear, 68% reported dryness after 6 months of lens wear.[18] Older eyes are also more likely to have developed pingueculae and pterygia, which can further disrupt the tear film and decrease contact lens comfort. Loss of endothelial cells throughout the lifespan makes the cornea more susceptible to edema, and since most bifocal contact lenses are thicker by nature, materials must be chosen with oxygen transmission in mind. As a result of crystalline lens changes, reduction in light transmission, a decrease in retinal sensitivity, and reduced contrast sensitivity occur as well. Loss of eyelid tonicity occurs with age and can present problems with translating bifocals.

Tests to Perform

Fitting a patient who is not a good candidate for bifocal contact lenses will almost always result in failure, and with the high cost of chair time and patience, it is advisable to rule these patients out before any fitting begins. The preliminary evaluation tests to perform are listed in Table 15.1.

1. Case history. A comprehensive case history should be performed to determine the patient's goals, motivation (to be discussed), history of medications, history of surgery (notably cosmetic surgery), visual requirements, and occupational requirements. It is important to ask if the patient is currently taking any medications and record all medications being used. Numerous medications—including antihistamines, ibuprofen, estrogen, tricyclic antidepressants, anticholinergics, and the scopolamine patch—can reduce tear volume.[18] It's important to ask about previous surgeries. With cosmetic lid surgery becoming increasingly popular, this may affect GP bifocal and multifocal lens positioning by exerting excessive lifting with the blink.
2. Visual requirements. The patient's visual requirements need to be carefully evaluated. Open discussions between the doctor and the patient about life and work styles are mandatory if success is to be obtained. This will be further discussed in the forthcoming section on consultation.
3. Anatomic measurements. Performing anatomic measurements such as vertical fissure size, horizontal visible iris diameter, and pupil diameter will be beneficial. Pupil diameter determination should be obtained both in normal room illumination and with the lights

TABLE 15.1 PRELIMINARY EVALUATION TESTS FOR THE POTENTIAL PRESBYOPIC CONTACT LENS PATIENT

1. Case history
   - Medications
   - History of surgery
   - Visual requirements
   - Occupational environment
   - Goals

2. External findings
   - Vertical fissure size
   - Lid position and tonicity
   - Pupil size (normal room illumination; dim illumination)
   - Blink rate/quality

3. Tear volume and quality

4. Corneal integrity

5. Refraction: BVA at distance and near; add power

6. Keratometry/corneal topography

BVA, best corrected visual acuity.

dimmed. Patients wearing simultaneous vision designs will be impacted by the variance in pupil diameter with changes in illumination. In particular, patients with a large pupil diameter (>5 mm in normal room illumination), although relatively uncommon in the presbyopic population, would be contraindicated for a GP aspheric lens design because of the glare and ghosting of images that would occur during low illumination conditions.[15] In addition, patients with a "low" lower lid (i.e., over 1 mm inferior to lower limbus) will not be good candidates for GP translating bifocals because of poor or no alignment of lower lens to lid. Likewise, patients exhibiting poor (i.e., loose) lid tonicity/elasticity would be poor candidates for translating designs.

4. Tear film evaluation. The patient should blink completely and frequently (at minimum, every 5 seconds). The tear meniscus should be evaluated, and the customary tests for tear quality [tear breakup time (TBUT)] and quantity (i.e., Zone-Quick or Schirmer) should be performed. Patients exhibiting a TBUT of ≥ 10 seconds should experience successful all-day wear,[19] whereas those with less than this value should be advised that they will not typically achieve an all-day wearing period.[20] In particular, if the TBUT is between 6 and 9 seconds, patients should be informed that all-day wear may not be possible and extended wear is not recommended.[21] These individuals tend to optimize their wearing period via the use of either silicone hydrogel disposable lenses or GP lenses. They also benefit from regular cleaning of their lenses as well as frequent rewetting drop use. A TBUT of ≤ 5 seconds typically contraindicates contact lens wear, especially if the measurement is repeatable.[22]

5. Biomicroscopy. A careful biomicroscopic evaluation is important to rule out corneal dry spots or other causes of staining. Lid eversion will be important to ensure that significant papillary hypertrophy is not present.

6. Refraction. A refraction will help in determining motivation. The best candidates for bifocal contact lenses should have more than 1 D of hyperopia or more than 1.25 D of myopia.[23] Low hyperopic patients typically expect better vision through the contact lenses since spectacles were not necessary before presbyopia. Low myopic and emmetropic patients entering presbyopia are also difficult to please since they can typically see quite well at near without any correction. However, they should not be excluded if, in fact, they are motivated. These individuals may appreciate wearing one distance lens only (if exhibiting low myopia) or either one near lens or a soft bifocal lens on one eye if emmetropic. If the patient is amblyopic, unless an optimum translating bifocal fitting relationship can be achieved, a bifocal lens is often contraindicated because of possible further compromise in vision.

7. Corneal topography. Finally, corneal topography evaluation will assist in both determining whether the patient is a good candidate for bifocal lenses and what specific lens design would be indicated. Although corneal topography evaluation is not essential when fitting the presbyopic patient into contact lenses, it is beneficial in determining the size and location of the apex and the eccentricity of the cornea and, in some cases, assisting with the design parameters.[15] In particular, when GP lenses are the preferred option, a centrally positioned apex lends itself to an aspheric design, whereas an inferior positioned apex would be desirable for segmented, translating designs. Patients having keratoconus or other forms of irregular cornea are often poor candidates because of some compromise in distance acuity that may result with bifocal contact lenses.

The characteristics of good and poor candidates for bifocal contact lens wear are given in Table 15.2.

Patient Consultation

This is perhaps the most important factor when considering bifocal contact lens success. Good bifocal contact lens patients need to be sufficiently motivated to give their lenses appropriate

TABLE 15.2 GOOD AND POOR CANDIDATES FOR BIFOCAL CONTACT LENS WEAR

GOOD CANDIDATES	POOR CANDIDATES
• Motivated presbyopes (do not want to wear spectacles) • Vision demands are not very critical • Normal lid tonicity • Good ocular health; good tear quality (>10 sec TBUT) and volume	• Unmotivated • Critical vision demands • Poor tear quality (≤5 sec TBUT) and/or volume • Irregular cornea • Amblyopia

TBUT, tear breakup time.

care and should be made thoroughly aware of the level of visual quality to be expected well before the initial fitting. A comprehensive education program is extremely valuable, as it will help to develop the correct amount of optimism and realism concerning bifocal contact lens wear. A well-informed patient is your best patient.

What are the patient's expectations? Is poor cosmesis with spectacles present? If the patient spends most of the time performing critical near tasks, failure with bifocal contact lenses is probable. The questions about lifestyle/visual demand presented in Table 15.3 have been recommended for potential presbyopic bifocal contact lens wearers.[24]

TABLE 15.3 DETERMINING POTENTIAL BIFOCAL CONTACT LENS PATIENT SUCCESS

	GOOD CANDIDATE	QUESTIONABLE
1. Time spent in public eye?		
a. A lot	X	
b. Very little		X
2. Are spectacles undesirable when in the public eye?		
a. Yes	X	
b. No		X
3. How much time do you spend doing precise work like accounting?		
a. Very little	X	
b. A lot		X
4. How much time do you spend doing intense reading during the day?		
a. Very little	X	
b. A lot		X
5. Are spectacles bothersome in your sports and leisure activities?		
a. Yes	X	
b. No		X
6. Do you dislike spectacles?		
a. Yes	X	
b. No		X

From Friant RJ. When bifocal lenses are most likely to succeed. Contact Lens Spectrum 1986;1(6):14–23.

The process begins by always asking patients if they are interested in contact lenses. They may not be aware that you fit contact lenses, not to mention bifocal contact lenses. They may be assuming that bifocal spectacle wear is their only option. This simple invitation to try contact lenses may significantly change a patient's quality of life; nevertheless, it has been found that practitioners ask <20% of their spectacle-wearing patients if they would be interested in wearing contact lenses.[11] If patients show interest and appear to be qualified, they can be told about all of the patients who have experienced an enhanced quality of life through bifocal contact lenses, as they are free from spectacle lens wear. The availability of disposable bifocal lenses allows the practitioner the opportunity to prescribe them on a trial basis for those patients deemed good soft lens candidates.

It is important to determine what patients' goals from contact lens wear are and, specifically, to determine which distances are most important to them. How they spend their time during the day and what visual tasks are especially important and time consuming (i.e., computer use, driving, reading, etc.) should be asked about. The goal should be to satisfy their primary visual demands. Patients should not be guaranteed that spectacles will not be necessary if they are fitted into a presbyopic contact lens correction. Not only should they have a spectacle correction to use as a backup to contact lenses (perhaps for morning or evening wear or to have available if lens loss or an eye infection occurs), but also monovision wearers should be encouraged to wear overspectacles for critical distance tasks (especially driving), and some aspheric multifocal wearers appreciate additional plus power when reading fine print (especially in dim illumination) or perhaps some additional minus power when driving at night.

A positive, optimistic but realistic approach is best. It is particularly important to "underpromise and overdeliver" with presbyopic patients being fitted into contact lenses. They need to be aware of possible compromises, including the fact that they do not have the focusing ability of a teenager. Even with the best technology available, bifocal contact lenses will not meet all of their visual demands. They need to appreciate that bifocal contact lenses are different from spectacles. Patients should be told that they may not experience the same quality of vision as with spectacles as contact lenses are dynamic devices that sit directly on the eye, unlike spectacles, in which good near vision can be obtained via simply dropping the eyes to view through the bifocal segment. If patients appear to be quite satisfied with spectacle wear and/or are extremely concerned about any possible compromise in vision, they can be told that bifocal lenses may not be the best option for them. In that way their motivation can be assessed. Conversely, there are patients who will accept reasonable visual compromise to experience the benefits of contact lens wear. "20/Happy" is a phrase in common use today to describe patients who experience a slight decrement in acuity chart vision (often 20/25 to 20/30) but are extremely satisfied with their bifocal contact lenses.

Finally, it is important to review all of the contact lens corrective options with patients. Single-vision contact lenses, supplemented by reading glasses, can be mentioned first. Patients can be told that this option should provide them with their best vision at near and distance. They should also be informed that some patients do not like to put the spectacles on and take them off frequently (not to mention the wearing of spectacles in general). The second option to explain would be monovision. A surprising number of patients have already heard of this option, but it should be defined to patients nevertheless as an option in which one eye sees optimally at distance whereas the other eye sees well at near. The fact that the opposite eye will be somewhat blurred for any visual task and the need for supplemental vision correction (i.e., a second distance contact lens or "driving" glasses) for critical vision tasks should be explained. Finally, bifocal contact lenses can be presented. This option allows the patient the aforementioned benefits of visual freedom and binocularity. Although the higher cost should be mentioned (often one and one-half to two times the cost of conventional designs), as well as the possibility of a lens exchange or two to fine-tune the fit (although the patient rarely needs to discontinue lens wear during this period), patients can be told that if they are patient and motivated, there is a good likelihood for success.

■ SOFT BIFOCAL AND MULTIFOCAL LENSES

Soft contact lenses for presbyopia were introduced in the 1980s. The first lenses were expensive to manufacture and custom made; therefore, the cost to the patient was high. This, compounded with the inherent nature of soft lenses to deposit and tear, as well as the lack of success of the designs and product discontinuation, made this a less than desirable modality for practitioners and patients. Translating designs in GP lenses are beneficial for providing increased near vision; however, translating designs have not been very successful in soft contact lenses. Most soft contact lenses for use with presbyopia are a simultaneous vision design. This may result in compromised vision, as this design does not provide the same clarity as spectacles, but the patient may be satisfied with the vision. The simultaneous existence of a focused image and an out-of-focus image on the retina results in a reduction in retinal image quality.[6,25] Despite this, many patients experience satisfactory vision and success when wearing these lenses.

The introduction of disposable/frequent-replacement soft lenses and silicone hydrogel lenses has increased the popularity and success of soft bifocal and multifocal contact lenses. As the baby boomer population increases and their desire to remain lifelong contact lens wearers has increased, bifocal contact lens use is on the rise.[8,26] In addition to the disposable lenses and the increased oxygen transmission, material changes that aid dry-eye patients and the ease in fitting and dispensing trial lenses have been a large part of this upward trend in bifocal/multifocal use.

Patient Selection

Motivation is a key factor for these patients. Planting the seed in single-vision soft lens wearers before they require a presbyopic correction is beneficial to them remaining lifelong contact lens wearers. Although the process of fitting is easier than in the past, enthusiasm on the part of the practitioner and patient will affect patient motivation.[27]

Patient education is another key factor for success. This requires a thorough explanation for what is occurring in presbyopia and methods of correcting for it, including reading glasses over contact lenses, monovision, and bifocal contact lenses. The patient needs to know that these lenses are a little more complicated and may require some compromise, but with motivation and patience, success is obtainable. Thorough education makes patients feel a part of the fitting and makes the process more understandable. Their input is vital in arriving at a successful endpoint.

Normal age-related changes may affect the patient's ability to wear soft multifocals successfully. Ocular dryness may be an issue and may be managed by lens materials and solutions. More complicated age-related changes, like cataracts and macular degeneration, may result in unacceptable vision.

Good candidates for soft multifocals include successful single-vision soft lens wearers, dissatisfied monovision patients, those with low amounts of astigmatism (unless fitted in a toric multifocal), moderate myopes and hyperopes, and those with a healthy cornea and tears. The patient may have to accept some compromise, usually in one area, either distance, intermediate, or near (Table 15.4).

Lens Designs

Center-Near

Many of the soft multifocal lenses are aspheric with a center-near correction. Examples of disposable/frequent-replacement center-near multifocals are listed in Table 15.5. These center-near designs are discussed in this section.

The Soflens Multifocal and the PureVision Multifocal (Bausch & Lomb) are aspheric, center-near designs. The anterior surface is aspheric and the back surface is a spherical bicurve.

TABLE 15.4 SOFT MULTIFOCAL PATIENT SELECTION

- Motivation
- Successful soft lens patient
- Computer users
- Dissatisfied monovision wearer
- Healthy cornea, lids, and tear film
- Low astigmats (unless fitting a toric multifocal)
- Emmetropes and low myopes (hyperopes are less successful)

The Soflens Multifocal is available in two base curve radii (BCR) (8.5 and 8.8 mm) and is a 2-week replacement lens. The PureVision Multifocal is a silicone hydrogel lens, approved for daily, extended, or continuous wear (up to 30 days). It is available in one BCR (8.6 mm) and is a monthly replacement lens.

When fitting these lenses, the 8.5-mm BCR is used first on the Soflens Multifocal and the 8.6-mm BCR for the PureVision Multifocal. The lenses come with two add powers, low and high add. If the patient has a spectacle add ≤ +1.50 D, the low add is recommended to be used on both eyes. For an add power between +1.75 and +2.25 D, mixed adds are recommended, with the low add on the dominant eye and the high add on the nondominant eye. Adds ≥ +2.50 D are fit with the high add on both eyes.

C-Vue Multifocals and EMA Multifocals (Unilens Corp.) are both aspheric center-near designs with two adds, low and high, similar to the Bausch & Lomb lens designs. Quattro (Blanchard) is an aspheric center-near design that comes in two BCR (8.4 and 8.8 mm). It is available in an add power that corrects up to +2.50 D. When fitting this lens, the spherical power is based on the distant spherical equivalent power corrected for the required add (Table 15.6). If the patient has an add < +1.25 D, it is recommended that the dominant eye be fitted in a spherical distance lens and the nondominant eye be fitted with a lens of a power equal to the distance power (spherical equivalent, vertexed) with +1.25 added. For example, a patient with a −2.50 D OU and +1.00 Add right eye dominant would wear a spherical −2.50 D lens on the OD and a −1.25 D Quattro lens on the OS. BCR selection is 8.4 mm with a 14.2 mm diameter for keratometry readings ≥44.50 D, and 8.8 mm with a 14.5 mm diameter for keratometry readings ≤44.25 D.

Focus Progressive and Focus Dailies Progressive lenses (Ciba Vision) are aspheric, center-near designs with an add power that corrects up to +3.00 D. A formula is used to determine

TABLE 15.5 DISPOSABLE/FREQUENT-REPLACEMENT PRESBYOPIC SOFT CONTACT LENSES (CENTER-NEAR DESIGNS)

NAME	MANUFACTURER
Soflens Multifocal, PureVision Multifocal	Bausch & Lomb
Quattro	Blanchard
Focus Progressive, Focus Dailies Progressive	Ciba Vision
Proclear, Proclear XR, Frequency, and Proclear Toric Multifocal (N lenses)	CooperVision
C-Vue 55 and Toric Multifocal	Unilens
EMA Multifocal	Unilens

TABLE 15.6 QUATTRO POWER SELECTION (ADDED TO DISTANCE RX—SPHERICAL EQUIVALENT, VERTEXED)

ADD (YR OLD)	DOMINANT EYE RX	NONDOMINANT EYE RX
+1.25 (≤46)	1.00	1.25
+1.50 (47–48)	1.00	1.25
+1.75 (49–50)	1.25	1.50
+2.00 (51–52)	1.50	1.75
+2.25 (53–54)	1.75	2.00
+2.50 (≥55)	1.75	2.25

the distance prescription to select. The formula is based on adding half the patient's add power to their spherical equivalent, vertex-corrected distance prescription. For example, a patient with −3.00 D spectacle prescription and a +1.00 D add would require the following:

$$-3.00 + (0.50) = -2.50 \text{ D}$$

These lenses are labeled with only the distance prescription. This simplifies the fitting process, but limits the available choices for the patient. If the patient's distance vision is not acceptable, decreasing the amount of the plus power added to the distance prescription of, at minimum, the distance eye, may be beneficial.[28] The Focus Dailies Progressive is the only daily disposable multifocal lens, which can be advantageous for occasional wearers, frequent travelers, and those with allergies.

There are conventional replacement (6–12 months) center-near lenses available, which are fit similar to these lenses. Because of the number of conventional center-near lenses, they will not be discussed individually in this chapter.

Center-Distance

Currently available disposable/frequent-replacement center-distance lenses are listed in Table 15.7.

The Acuvue Bifocal (Vistakon) is a concentric bifocal with five alternating concentric rings and four add powers (+1.00, +1.50, +2.00, and +2.50 D). The central distance zone is 2 mm wide surrounded by a near zone, alternating distance and near for a total width of 8 mm (Fig. 15.1). The add power selection is based on the patient's age (Table 15.8).

This lens is less dependent on pupil size than aspheric designs because of the alternating zones within the pupil, which aid in providing an equal area of distance and near over a range

TABLE 15.7 DISPOSABLE/FREQUENT-REPLACEMENT PRESBYOPIC SOFT CONTACT LENSES (CENTER-DISTANCE DESIGNS)

NAME	MANUFACTURER
Biomedics EP	CooperVision
Proclear, Proclear XR, Frequency, and Proclear Toric Multifocal *(D lens)*	CooperVision
Acuvue Bifocal	Vistakon
UCL Multifocal	United Contact Lens

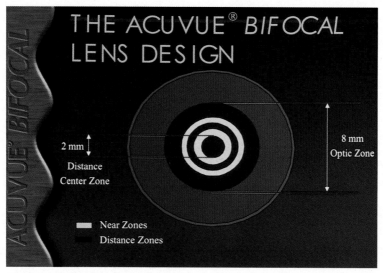

■ **FIGURE 15.1** The Acuvue Bifocal.

of pupil sizes.[29] One study found that the Acuvue Bifocal, when compared with progressive addition spectacles at varying illuminations, resulted in similar near performance.[30]

Biomedics EP (CooperVision) has a center spherical distance zone with a progressive aspheric zone that provides intermediate and near vision for emerging presbyopes (Fig. 15.2). The design is similar to the D lens of other CooperVision multifocals. This lens is easy to fit as there is only one BCR and the lens power is selected based on the patient's distance spectacle prescription. This lens can provide an effective add power of, at maximum, +1.50 D. No add power is recorded on the lens pack as it is the same for all lenses. This lens is made of omafilcon A (Proclear material); therefore, it is recommended for dry-eye patients. This is beneficial for those presbyopic patients that experience dryness.

Frequency 55 and Proclear Multifocals (CooperVision) have a unique design that allows creativity in fitting patients' visual needs. Both lenses are available in one base curve radius and four add powers (+1.00, +1.50, +2.00, and +2.50 D). A recent addition to this family of multifocals, the Proclear XR Multifocal, has expanded parameters for distance powers of ±20 D and add powers from +0.75 to +4.00 D in 0.50 D steps. This creates a wide range of multifocal lenses for almost every patient, regardless of their spectacle power. In the future, we can expect this design to be available in the Biofinity silicone hydrogel material.

These multifocals have a D lens, which is fitted on the dominant eye and has a center-distance spherical zone, surrounded by an aspheric progressive intermediate zone and then an outer spherical near zone. The N lens, fitted on the nondominant eye, has a center-near spherical zone, surrounded by the aspheric intermediate progressive zone and a distance spherical zone. This design is termed Balanced Progressive Technology (Fig. 15.3A,B). This lens design

TABLE 15.8 ACUVUE BIFOCAL RECOMMENDED ADD SELECTION

AGE (YR)	ADD (D)
40–46	+1.00
47–52	+1.50
53–59	+2.00
60+	+2.50

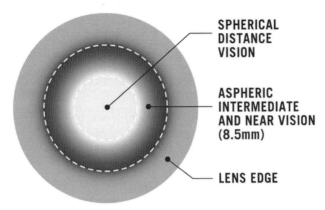

SPHERICAL
DISTANCE
VISION

ASPHERIC
INTERMEDIATE
AND NEAR VISION
(8.5mm)

LENS EDGE

■ FIGURE 15.2 Biomedics EP. (Courtesy of CooperVision.)

has been very successful. One study comparing the Soflens Multifocal with the Frequency Multifocal found that the Frequency lens had better near vision and superior stereopsis when compared by patients wearing the Soflens.[28,31]

When fitting this design, the initial power is based on the spherical equivalent of the current refraction, vertexed back to the cornea. The add should be equivalent to the add for spectacles unless it is between add powers; if this occurs, the lower add should be selected. As indicated

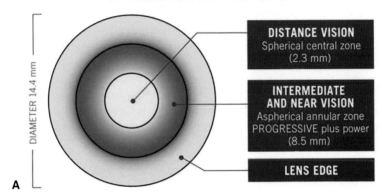

D LENS: DOMINANT EYE

DIAMETER 14.4 mm

DISTANCE VISION
Spherical central zone
(2.3 mm)

INTERMEDIATE
AND NEAR VISION
Aspherical annular zone
PROGRESSIVE plus power
(8.5 mm)

LENS EDGE

A

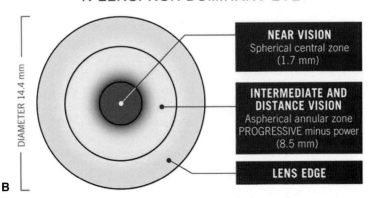

N LENS: NON-DOMINANT EYE

DIAMETER 14.4 mm

NEAR VISION
Spherical central zone
(1.7 mm)

INTERMEDIATE AND
DISTANCE VISION
Aspherical annular zone
PROGRESSIVE minus power
(8.5 mm)

LENS EDGE

B

■ FIGURE 15.3 **(A,B)** The Frequency 55 and Proclear Multifocals utilize a distance center ("D" in **A**) and near center ("N" in **B**). (Courtesy of CooperVision.)

previously, the D lens should be used on the dominant eye and the N lens on the nondominant eye. The manufacturer recommends that 20/20 vision be obtained binocularly at distance and near. Monocular visual acuities with the D lens should be 20/20 at distance and 20/40 or better at near. The reverse is true of the N lens, where distance visual acuity should be 20/40 or better and near visual acuity 20/20. If the visual acuity does not meet these criteria, then an overrefraction should be performed monocularly to improve the vision.[32] Conventional lens replacement materials, available in this center-distance design, include Satureyes Multifocal and Metrofocal (Metro Optics) and 4Vue and XTRA (Unilens Corp.).

Translating

The only soft lens currently available in a translating design is the Triton Translating Bifocal (Gelflex). Translation is more challenging with a soft lens bifocal than a GP bifocal, but can provide better vision than simultaneous designs. The thicker inferior edge may cause more lens awareness.[33] The Triton lens is available in sphere and toric conventional replacement lenses. It is a back surface design with biprism and truncation for stability and position.[34] The horizontal diameters are 14.5 and 15.0 mm with vertical diameters of 11.4 to 13.9 mm. The near seg is located 1 mm below the geometric center. Marker dots on the lens at the 3 and 9 o'clock positions mark the geometric center of the lens and aid the practitioner in adjusting the vertical size to affect the fit and seg position.[35] In the near future, we can expect more bifocal/multifocal designs and more silicone hydrogel multifocal lens materials.

Soft Toric Multifocals

Several manufacturers make soft toric multifocal lenses, which increases the range of refractive errors that can be corrected. Until there are more of this type of lens available in disposable/frequent-replacement modalities and silicone hydrogel materials, the lenses still will be limited in use. Two soft toric multifocals that are available in multipacks for frequent replacement are the Proclear Multifocal Toric (CooperVision), replaced monthly, and the C-Vue 55 Toric Multifocal (Unilens Corp.), replaced quarterly. Both designs are similar to their spherical counterpart. Both are available in a prescription of ±20 D and a large range of cylinder powers and full axis range. In addition, there are several conventional replacement soft toric multifocals, which include the Cibasoft Progressive Toric (Ciba Vision) and the Essential Soft Toric Multifocal (Blanchard).

Fitting

Preliminary Testing

The fitting process is important to the success of the bifocal contact lens fitting. Examination procedures that should be performed before lenses are placed on the eye include current refraction, add determination, keratometry readings, determination of dominant eye, pupil size, TBUT, and a discussion pertaining to the patient's visual needs. Initiating the process with a current refraction and add power aids in the selection of the initial diagnostic lenses. In cases where the lenses must be ordered empirically, errors in the refraction contribute to patient and practitioner frustration and increase chair time. Keratometry may not be crucial with every lens design, as many of the lenses are only available in one BCR; however, it is beneficial if the cornea is exceptionally steep or flat, or if the lenses are available in more than one BCR.

There are several methods of determining the dominant eye. One of the most common methods is to have patients view a 20/30 or 20/40 letter on the visual acuity chart with both eyes open. Patients are instructed to look through their hands, and upon closing their right eye, asked whether the letter is still visible. This is repeated with the left eye. The eye in which the letter disappears upon closure is the dominant eye. This can be confirmed by having the practitioner observe which eye the patient is using. Another common method is the use of a plus lens over each eye monocularly while viewing the visual acuity chart binocularly. This can be performed with the patient behind the phoropter or by simply placing a trial lens (+1.00 to +2.00 D) in front of each eye individually and asking the patient which eye has greater blur. The eye that observes greater blur is the dominant eye.[36] A final method is to hand patients a camera and ask them to hold the camera as they would if they were going to take a photograph. Typically they will look through the camera with their dominant eye. This method can be used to confirm the prior methods.

Pupil size may play a critical role in the resulting vision in simultaneous designs. A small pupil size may affect distance vision when wearing a center-near design or near vision for a center-distance design. A large pupil may lead to glare and poor image quality. A lens that is successful during the day may not be satisfactory at night. If pupil size appears to be affecting vision, try a different lens design.[28,37]

Successful soft contact lens wearers should be able to be refitted into a multifocal design that is a similar material or replacement modality as their current lenses. Those who have not worn contact lenses before or who have been unsuccessful may have similar challenges with the multifocal lenses. As with any contact lens patient, a healthy ocular surface and good tear quality aids in successful lens wear. As age-related changes may result in a dry eye, eliminating environmental issues, encouraging the patient to drink more water, and managing blepharitis or meibomian gland dysfunction can be beneficial. The use of either hydrogen peroxide solutions or multipurpose solutions especially formulated to increase wettability should be used. In addition, using a lens material, such as omafilcon or a silicone hydrogel, may add to patient comfort. Rewetting drops and blinking exercises should also be encouraged.[37]

Patients should be asked about their daily visual needs at work and for hobbies. Do they primarily have distance, near, or intermediate tasks? How much time do they spend performing these tasks? Someone who works all day on a computer has different needs than a truck driver or an accountant. Practitioners strive for 20/20 visual acuity at distance and near, but a computer user may not desire or require 20/20 visual acuity at near. Near point visual acuity charts that simulate everyday reading tasks (i.e., newsprint, phone book, map, music, menu, etc.) are helpful. If patients have a specific near task that they need to be able to see, they should be encouraged to bring it along to use for testing. Patients can evaluate their intermediate vision at a computer in the office if this is important to them. They should be encouraged to use good lighting and adjust their working distance to provide optimum clarity.[38] The benefit of disposable soft multifocals is the ability to send patients out into their everyday environment for a few days to try the lenses. Wearers who participate in sporting activities may desire one or two distance vision-only lenses for occasional wear.

Diagnostic Lenses

When selecting diagnostic lenses, the current refraction should be converted to the spherical equivalent for spherical lenses and vertexed back to the cornea for both spherical and toric lenses. Distance powers should represent the "least minus," "most plus" power accepted by the patient. Add powers should be selected as prescribed unless the add falls between add powers available; in that case the lower add power should be used. Typically, if there are two base curve radii available, the steeper base curve radius should be selected first, unless the manufacturer's fitting guide specifies differently. Fitting guides and manufacturer calculators can be helpful for selecting the initial diagnostic lenses and for troubleshooting. Table 15.9 contains information regarding online fitting guides and contact lens calculators.

The diagnostic lenses should be inserted and allowed to sit for 15 to 20 minutes before evaluating visual acuity at near and distance. During this period of time, patients should be cautioned not to judge their vision as the lenses are settling. Patients may want to take a walk around the office or outside the office to initially evaluate their lenses. If they choose to read during this period of time, they may become discouraged by their near vision and think the lenses will not be successful before allowing the lenses to settle.

TABLE 15.9 ONLINE CONTACT LENS FITTING GUIDES AND CALCULATORS

Bausch & Lomb: http://www.presbyopesinyourpractice.com/managing_fitting/fitting_assistant.php
Blanchard: http://www.blanchardlab.com/products/essential_soft/home.html
Ciba Vision: http://www.virtualconsultant.cibavision.com
CooperVision: http://www.coopervision.com
GelFlex: http://www.gelflex.com/gelcalc.html
Vistakon: http://www.ecp.acuvue.com

The fit of the lenses should be evaluated before checking the visual acuity. The lenses should fit like an acceptable soft spherical lens. The lenses should center, move with the blink, or have a positive push-up test. If the fit is not satisfactory and the BCR cannot be changed, then the lens should be removed and another design should be used.

Testing of the lenses should be done with normal illumination and with trial lenses or flippers (±0.25 and ±0.50D flippers). When overrefracting, 0.25 D steps can be significant to vision; therefore, the practitioner should be cautious about making large changes in power. Monocular overrefraction with the patient viewing binocularly is encouraged. Any overrefraction should be checked at distance and near so as not to compromise near vision to obtain good distance vision or poor distance to achieve good near vision. Vision should be checked binocularly at distance and near. If vision is reduced, monocular visual acuities and overrefraction should be checked to see if a change needs to be made. The patient should be encouraged to assess vision binocularly, not monocularly. Charts for testing near visual acuity should include paragraphs to be read, not individual letters, and should have examples of newsprint, music, maps, telephone books, and other everyday reading material.[38] Many of the manufacturers make near cards like this, but if not, the practitioner can keep a sample of different reading materials for multifocal fittings.

Modified Monovision

Some patients will benefit from creative combinations of lenses. This could include enhancing the distance vision or near vision in one eye depending on if it is the dominant or nondominant eye (this will be discussed in more detail in the next section), using unequal add powers, combining two different bifocal lens designs, or fitting a spherical or toric distance lens in the dominant eye and a multifocal lens in the nondominant eye. Occasionally, a patient may see well at distance with one type of lens design but be dissatisfied with near vision. Another design may yield good near vision but poor distance vision. In a case such as this, it is not out of the question to fit the dominant eye with the lens that provides good distance vision and the nondominant eye with the lens that provides good near vision. These two lenses would have to have similar replacement schedules (i.e., both 2-week or monthly replacement).

Although all of the aforementioned combinations may be a form of enhanced bifocal fitting, the use of a spherical lens in the dominant eye and a multifocal in the nondominant eye is an example of modified monovision. This is often successful for patients who require good distance vision and have few near visual tasks or those who need little to no correction for distance. The disposable/frequent-replacement multifocals make this an easier alternative as the patient can wear the same material and replacement schedule on both eyes, but have one lens that is a distance-only lens and one a multifocal (i.e., Proclear, Frequency, PureVision, Acuvue, Focus, etc.). As noted, typically the full distance prescription is provided in the contact lens to be placed on the dominant eye and the multifocal lens is placed on the nondominant eye. The multifocal lens should be adjusted so that distance and near visual acuity is good, priority being given to near vision.

Follow-Up Care/Problem Solving

If, upon fitting the initial diagnostic lenses, the patient has slightly reduced distance vision, monocular visual acuities should be checked to make sure that the distance correction is at least 20/40 or better in both eyes. If not, then an overrefraction should be performed over the lens that has reduced visual acuity. If both eyes have better than 20/40 distance visual acuity, then trial lenses or flippers should be used in an attempt to increase the power on the dominant eye by −0.25 D. If the overrefraction is > −0.50 D, reducing the add in the dominant eye may be the best alternative. Typically, the order for making alterations in the lens power for distance blur is:

1. To add −0.25 D steps to the dominant eye distance prescription.
2. To decrease the add power in the dominant eye.
3. To increase minus in the distance prescription of both lenses.

An example of this is:

OD lens −3.00 D, add +1.50 D dominant eye
OS lens −3.00 D, add +1.50 D

If this patient has poor distance vision, the first step would be to add −0.25 D to the OD lens, resulting in −3.25 D. If it requires > −0.50 D to improve the distance vision, then the add in the OD lens should be reduced to +1.00, rather than increasing the minus power.

When the patient is experiencing near vision blur, this is often solved by adding plus (+0.25 D) to the nondominant distance prescription. If the overrefraction at near is +0.50 D or greater, then the add in the nondominant eye should be increased. The order of making changes is:

1. Add +0.25 D to the nondominant eye distance prescription.
2. Increase the add in the nondominant eye.

An example of this is:

OD lens −3.00 D, add +1.50 D dominant eye
OS lens −3.00 D, add +1.50 D

If this patient has poor near vision, the first step would be to add +0.25 D to the left lens, resulting in −2.75 D. If it requires > +0.50 D to improve the near vision, then the add power in the left lens should be increased to +2.00 D, rather than increasing the plus power.

If there is blur at distance and near, the distance vision should be corrected first. If several lens changes have been made and the visual acuity is still not satisfactory, then another design should be used. When 20/20 vision is achieved or when vision is satisfactory, patients should be sent home with the lenses to try them in their natural environment. Patients should make a mental note of any visual concerns experienced with the lenses, so that at the follow-up visit (typically in 3–7 days) they can tell the practitioner what visual tasks are satisfactory and which ones are not satisfactory. Changes in the power, fit, or design can be made at this visit.

Care and handling of these lenses are no different than any other soft contact lens (see Chapter 12). If patients are new wearers, they may experience more difficulty handling the lens—notably inserting the lens—because of difficulty in seeing the lens at near and loss of manual dexterity. Care regimens that improve wettability or are preservative free may be helpful for patients with dry eye. A summary of fitting pearls can be found in Table 15.10.

▓ GAS-PERMEABLE LENS DESIGNS

Introduction

Traditionally, and also true today, GP multifocal and bifocal designs have enjoyed greater success than their soft lens counterparts. The optical quality achieved with a rigid lens, as well as

TABLE 15.10 FITTING PEARLS WITH SOFT MULTIFOCAL CONTACT LENSES

If there is more than one base curve radius, start with the steeper base curve radius.
Remind patients to have good light and adjust their working distance to the optimal distance.[38]
If the patient has slightly reduced distance and near vision, fix the distance vision before working with near vision.
Use normal room illumination.
Let lenses settle for 15–20 min before evaluating.
Assess vision binocularly.
Use handheld trial lenses or flippers to overrefract.
Overrefract in 0.25 D steps.
Overrefract monocularly with both eyes open and recheck any overrefraction at near and distance.
Use everyday reading material when evaluating patient's near vision.
Test vision at the distances required by the patient's visual needs (e.g., a computer user needs good intermediate vision and may accept reduced near vision).
Round add powers down.
It is acceptable to use unequal add powers.

the ability to achieve translation, is important in obtaining this success. These designs can be divided into aspheric multifocal and translating designs.

Types of Designs

Aspheric Multifocal

Aspheric lens designs have a gradual change in curvature along one of their surfaces (anterior or posterior) based on the geometry of conic sections. The eccentricity or rate of flattening of the lens surface is greater than with single-vision lens designs; therefore, an increase in plus power is generated toward the periphery of the lens. Although often available in a back surface aspheric, several front surface designs have been introduced. Aspheric multifocal GP lenses, unlike soft lens designs, often have very good optical quality and, like soft lenses, are relatively easy to fit. These are thin lens designs, fit steeper than K, in an effort to achieve optimum centration with very little (usually about 1 mm) movement with the blink. High success rates have been reported with these lenses, often >75%.[39–43]

Patient Selection: As aspheric designs utilize the simultaneous vision principle with near and distance power corrections in front of the pupil at the same time, the best candidates are early to moderate presbyopes. Some of the newer designs have been able to incorporate a higher add power into the lens via modification of the front surface; therefore, high add patients should not be excluded. GP aspheric multifocals are a good option for individuals with a high intermediate distance demand, including accountants, electricians, plumbers, and those with mechanical responsibilities.[44] Most important are individuals who devote much of their time to computer use. GP aspheric multifocals have been recommended for individuals spending, at minimum, one-third of their waking hours at a computer.[45] Early presbyopes who are current GP wearers also tend to prefer the ease of transition from a thin spherical design into a relatively thin aspheric design. It is important to select patients with a small-to-medium pupil size (i.e., <5 mm in room illumination), as glare and ghosting of images is possible at night with individuals having large pupil diameters because of the effect created by paracentral and mid-peripheral plus powers.[15] Patients with critical distance and/or near demands may obtain greater benefit from a translating design, although the vision achieved with the early presbyope

TABLE 15.11 GOOD CANDIDATES FOR GAS-PERMEABLE (GP) ASPHERIC MULTIFOCAL LENSES

- Early-to-moderate presbyopes
- Computer users
- Present single-vision GP wearers
- Small-to-medium pupil size
- Low and/or flaccid lower lid

having an optimum fit is often quite satisfactory. Part of this may be the result of a slight amount of shift, or translation, with downward gaze. Individuals who are still quite active athletically are good candidates for aspheric lenses because of their low risk of displacement. Individuals who are not good candidates for translating multifocals because of an inferior positioned and/or a flaccid lower lid are typically good aspheric candidates. Characteristics of good candidates for aspheric multifocal lenses are summarized in Table 15.11.

Lens Design/Fitting: Until recently, most aspheric designs were of such high eccentricity that the manufacturer recommended a base curve selection of as much as 3 D steeper than K. The VFL 3 lens from Conforma is an example of such a design. However, most lens designs in common use, whereas higher in eccentricity than single-vision lenses, are typically fit approximately 1 D steeper than K.

Low Eccentricity Back Surface Designs: There are a large and increasing number of lens designs that have a lower posterior rate of flattening and are fit in a more conventional manner (i.e., not as steep) than higher eccentricity designs. As with previously discussed lens designs, these lenses need to position centrally (or slightly superiorly) with limited lens movement with the blink. Approximately 1-mm lag is optimum with these designs. Although they are fit approximately 1 D steeper than K, the fluorescein pattern should exhibit an alignment or near-alignment pattern because of the back surface geometry (Fig. 15.4). There are numerous such designs on the market and the specific manufacturers with their designs can be located at http://www.gpli.info.

A representative example of a lower eccentricity posterior aspheric lens design is the ESSentials Multifocal from Blanchard. This design has three series of add powers, with the increase in add

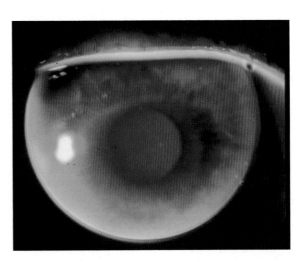

■ **FIGURE 15.4** A well-fitting aspheric gas-permeable multifocal lens.

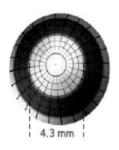

4.3 mm

■ FIGURE 15.5 The ESSential CSA lens design from Blanchard Contact Lens. The red region represents the area on the front surface in which additional add power is placed.

resulting from an effective decrease in the central distance power zone.[46] Series I is for the beginning presbyope, Series II is for the early to moderate presbyope, and Series III is for the moderate to high presbyope. However, it is not uncommon for advanced presbyopes, especially if they have small pupils, to require additional add power. The introduction of the Essential CSA design allows for more add power to be placed on a concentric ring surrounding the central distance zone—which is 4.0 to 4.6 mm in diameter—on the front surface of the lens (Fig. 15.5). If the patient, for example, is wearing the Series II design but requires an additional +0.75 D add power, this lens can be ordered with the identical parameters but specified with a +0.75 D CSA. This is one of several aspheric multifocal designs that can provide higher add powers. One multifocal lens design, the MVP Multifocal (ABBA Optical), is available in a 100 lens dispensing inventory.

High Eccentricity Back Surface Designs: Although not as popular as the lower eccentricity designs, very high eccentricity designs such as the VFL 3 Lens (Conforma) are available. This high eccentricity, posterior aspheric lens design is available in the Fluoroperm 30 and Boston ES lens materials. The "Super Add" lens design, incorporating a slightly higher add power, is available in the Paragon HDS material. It is typically fit several diopters steeper than K. In addition, its best application is in the early to moderate presbyopic patient; although a high add is obtained by fitting a steeper base curve radius, the "distance" zone is reduced and distance visual acuity can be compromised. Typically, good centration (which is essential) is obtained because of the steep base curve radius and the absence of prism ballast. A mild apical clearance fluorescein pattern will be observed (Fig. 15.6). The lens should not move more than 1.0 to 1.5 mm with the blink and, therefore, it often fails on flat corneas because of excessive lens lag with the blink.

Front Surface Aspheric Designs: Several laboratories have available front surface aspheric lens designs including the Naturalens Progressive (Advanced Vision Technologies) and the Renovation Multifocal (Art Optical). Although the amount of add generated with these designs can be limited, this is a viable option in cases in which the back surface design decenters and

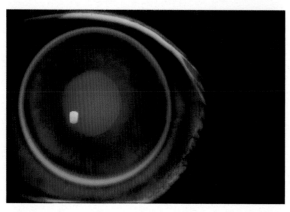

■ FIGURE 15.6 An optimum-fitting VFL 3 aspheric multifocal lens.

causes flattening and possibly distortion of the cornea. This is likely if the lens decenters superiorly and either adheres or moves very minimally. The front surface of the Renovation Multifocal has the additional benefit of being designed to reduce spherical aberration.

Problem Solving: Possible problems with these designs include decentration and blur at near because of insufficient near add power. If the lens moves excessively with the blink and decenters inferiorly, the base curve radius should be steepened, typically by 0.50 D.[22] Superior decentration, if excessive and resulting in undesirable corneal topography changes, should be solved by changing to a front surface aspheric design. A steeper base curve radius may be beneficial as well in this case. If lateral decentration is present, a larger diameter lens can be attempted, although if the decentration is because of a decentered corneal apex, the use of another lens design or material is recommended.

In some cases, patients experience blur at near because of insufficient add power being provided from these designs. As indicated previously, there are higher add designs available for the management of this problem. In addition, either via the use of unequal adds or a "modified bifocal approach" in which one lens is overplussed by a small amount (i.e., 0.25–0.50 D), this problem can be easily solved.

Summary: Aspheric multifocal fitting and problem solving is actually quite simple and straightforward. After proper patient selection, a good fitting relationship with minimal movement with the blink is required. It is recommended to have, at minimum, one of these designs, and the manufacturer can provide assistance with the management of patients wearing these designs.

Translating Bifocals

Translating or alternating vision bifocals are prism-ballasted, and sometimes truncated, lens designs that utilize the lower lid as a stop gap such that when patients drop their eyes inferiorly to read, the lens is pushed superiorly such that they are viewing through the inferior near portion of the lens. With this method, when properly fit, excellent vision can be obtained at distance and near. The segments represent many of the common types of spectacle segments including executive, crescent, and D-shaped. In addition, a few annular or concentric translating bifocal designs with a superiorly decentered distance zone are available as well. Some representative examples include executive (Tangent Streak, Firestone Optics, Kansas City, MO; Solitaire, Tru-Form, Euless, TX), crescent (Solutions, X-Cel, Duluth, GA; Metro-Seg, Metro Optics, Austin, TX), and concentric (Mandell Seamless, ABB-Concise, Coral Springs, FL). Translating GP bifocals have achieved a similar—if not higher—success rate than aspheric multifocals.[47,48]

Whereas these lenses may take more initial chair time to fit, they are not as difficult as a novice practitioner may perceive them to be. In fact, they often represent the bifocal lens of choice in many contact lens practices as a result of the excellent vision obtained.[49] Initial comfort is actually quite good as a result of the thin edge and limited movement with the blink desired with these lenses. In fact, because of the fact that both aspheric multifocal and segmented translating designs should move little with the blink, the initial comfort of these designs has been comparable to, if not slightly better than, spherical single-vision GP designs.[50] The fitting and problem-solving guidelines outlined in this chapter will be important for patient success.

Patient Selection: As mentioned previously, patients desiring excellent vision, or having critical vision demands, are good candidates for this form of bifocal lens. In addition, the ability to incorporate any add power makes this a good option for moderate to advanced presbyopes who have unsatisfactory vision at near with an aspheric lens design. Although there are an increasing number of segmented translating designs that provide intermediate vision, one limitation

TABLE 15.12 GOOD CANDIDATES FOR GAS-PERMEABLE TRANSLATING BIFOCAL LENSES

• All presbyopic add powers
• Critical vision demands
• Any pupil size
• Lower lid positioned near or above lower limbus
• Moderate-to-tight lid tension
• Inferior corneal apex

of translating bifocals is the inability to provide intermediate vision, limiting their use in patients needing vision at this distance (or requiring them to have overspectacles for either reading or intermediate work). When good centration and limited movement are not possible with an aspheric design or the patient has large pupils, a translating design will often be successful. These patients should, however, have a lower lid within 1 mm of the lower limbus. Conversely, if the palpebral fissure size is too small, the lens may position too superiorly and the segment may position in front of the pupil on straight-ahead gaze. Specifically, if the lower lid is positioned >1.5 mm above the lower limbus, it may be difficult to provide a sufficient seg height for acceptable near vision.[22] To allow translation to occur, lid tension should be moderate to tight. Characteristics of good candidates for GP translating bifocal lenses are summarized in Table 15.12.

Fitting: These lens materials are customarily available in a material with either high or hyper oxygen permeability (Dk) because of the thickness of the prism-ballasted design. Most laboratories have warranty programs that allow you to exchange lenses for a higher overall fee and this is recommended, especially for the novice fitter. Diagnostic fitting is extremely important for successful fitting of GP translating bifocals. Regardless of the lens design to be used, the manufacturer's fitting guide is typically not complicated and straightforward in regard to base curve selection and lens evaluation. As with aspheric multifocals, it is important to have in-office, at minimum, one diagnostic fitting set of these lenses. When in doubt about which set to use, contact your local Contact Lens Manufacturers Association (CLMA) member laboratory.

These lenses typically incorporate 1 to 3 Δ in an effort to position on or close to the lower lid. Likewise, they are fitted slightly flatter than K to increase the likelihood that the lenses will fall quickly to the lower lid and move not more than 1 mm with the blink. It is important to evaluate the position of the seg line to the pupil in normal room illumination with straight-ahead gaze. With few exceptions, the seg line should position at or near the lower pupil margin. If the patient is viewing even slightly superior or inferior, this will shift the position of the seg line to the pupil and could result in ordering an incorrect seg height. Patients with a slightly low lower lid (i.e., 0.5–1 mm below the limbus) would benefit from both a larger overall diameter and seg height, and vice versa for patients exhibiting a lower lid 1 to 1.5 mm above the limbus.

Translation should also be evaluated. While in the biomicroscope the patient should view inferiorly and, with the upper lid held back, the lens should push up or translate such that, at minimum, one-half of the pupil is covered by the seg as the practitioner views it in straight-ahead gaze. Alternatively, the ophthalmoscope can be used from an inferior position to simulate reading, in which case the seg should appear to be predominantly in front of the pupil. As with aspheric designs, the use of loose trial lenses or flipper bars is important when performing the overrefraction.

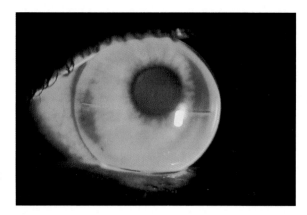

■ **FIGURE 15.7** An optimum-fitting Tangent Streak translating design gas-permeable bifocal lens.

Representative Examples

Prism Ballasted/Truncated (Tangent Streak): This is a prism-ballasted, often truncated, one-piece translating bifocal lens design. It is available in almost any lens material. It has an executive style seg line, which should be positioned at or slightly below the lower pupil margin (Fig. 15.7).

The 20-lens diagnostic set has base curve radii in 0.50 D steps for both +2.00 D and −2.00 D distance lens powers. Any seg is available; the seg power in the fitting set is +2.00 D. The overall diameter is 9.4 (horizontally)/9.0 mm (vertically) with a 4.2-mm seg height and 2 Δ base down. Any diameter, seg height, and prism can be ordered based on the diagnostic fitting relationship. For spherical corneas, a base curve radius 1 D flatter than K is recommended; for 0.50 D of corneal cylinder, a 0.50 D flatter than K base curve should be fit; for >1 D of corneal toricity, an "on K"to slightly steeper base curve radius can be selected.

Prism Ballasted Only (Solutions): This is a crescent design that utilizes diagnostic fitting set parameters as well as base curve fitting philosophies that are similar to the Tangent Streak lens (Fig. 15.8). The lens is available in low, medium, and high prism as well as five seg heights, in 0.5-mm increment differences. The benefit to the fitter is the ease of fitting because of the limited choices available, including the absence of prism.

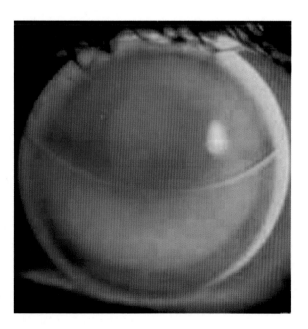

■ **FIGURE 15.8** An optimum position and fluorescein pattern for the Solutions Bifocal (X-Cel).

Concentric (Annular) Alternating Designs: These are also prism-ballasted designs with a central distance zone of approximately 4 mm in diameter, which is decentered slightly superior in an effort to be positioned directly in front of the pupil during distance gaze but in close proximity to the lower lid such that translation can occur with inferior gaze.[15,51] This is surrounded by a near concentric periphery. Increasing the central distance zone can result in improved distance vision but degraded near vision, and vice versa. These designs—like segmented designs—are often fit slightly flatter than K.

Segmented, Translating Designs with Intermediate Correction: There are several designs available including executive trifocal designs, such as the Tangent Streak Trifocal (Firestone Optics) and Llevations (Tru-Form); an aspheric intermediate zone, such as Presbylite (Lens Dynamics); and an aspheric back surface and segmented front surface, such as ESSential Solutions (X-Cel) and EZEyes Multifocal (ABBA Optical). Tru-Form Optics has a multitude of such designs and, in fact, has more types of segmented, translating designs than any other laboratory in the country. For patients who desire critical distance and/or near vision but spend much time every day at a computer, this type of design represents a preferable alternative to wearing a bifocal design accompanied by overspectacles for computer work.

Problem Solving: Problem solving translating lens designs can be divided into five categories: (a) excessive lens rotation with the blink, (b) lens positioned too superiorly, (c) poor lens translation, (d) poor distance vision, and (e) poor near vision.[52]

Excessive rotation with the blink is often the result of a base curve that is too steep. The apical clearance fitting relationship results in a lens that will attempt to position more centrally as opposed to fall inferiorly (Fig. 15.9). Therefore, the lens will be impacted more by the upper lid. Selecting a lens that is 0.50 D flatter in base curve radius should reduce or eliminate this problem. Another cause of excessive rotation is the presence of an upswept lower lid contour (Fig. 15.10).

When this is present, if the lenses can be truncated, the RALS (right add, left subtract) acronym can be used to determine the axis. For example, if both lenses rotate 15 degrees toward the nose because of the shape of the lower lid, the prism can be ordered at 105 degrees OD and 75 degrees OS.

When the lens is being lifted too superiorly with the blink such that the segment is in front of the pupil with distance gaze, increasing the prism ballast (again, by 0.50 Δ) should bring the lens down (Fig. 15.11). In addition, flattening the peripheral curve radius can be beneficial.

When the lens exhibits intermittent or no translation with the blink, the edge clearance of the lens should be increased (Fig. 15.12). This can be accomplished easily in-office by selecting a flatter base curve radius. Likewise, the peripheral curve could be made flatter and wider.

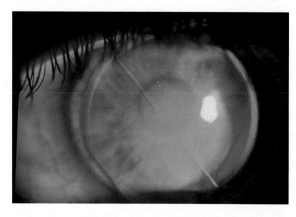

■ **FIGURE 15.9** Excessive rotation of a Tangent Streak bifocal lens fit 1 D steeper than K.

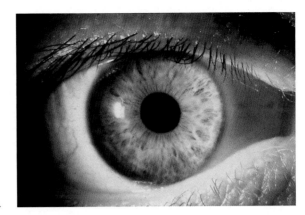

■ FIGURE 15.10 An upswept lower lid contour.

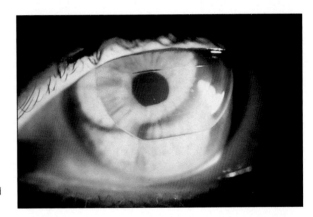

■ **FIGURE 15.11** A superiorly decentered translating bifocal.

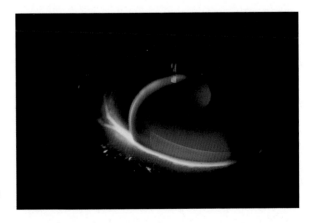

■ **FIGURE 15.12** Absence of translation in a segmented bifocal lens design.

TABLE 15.13 GAS-PERMEABLE TRANSLATING BIFOCAL PROBLEM SOLVING

PROBLEM	MANAGEMENT
Excessive rotation	1. Flatten BCR 0.50 D 2. Change prism axis
Lens positions too superiorly	1. Increase prism 0.50 Δ
Poor lens translation	1. Increase edge clearance (flatten BCR and/or PCR) 2. Increase prism and/or truncation
Blur at distance	1. Increase prism (if too high) 2. Increase OAD if too little pupil coverage 3. Lower seg height (if high)
Blur at near	1. Higher seg (if low) 2. Increase edge clearance (if poor translation) 3. Re-educate patient (if drops head, not eyes, to read) 4. Flatten BCR (if excessive rotation)

BCR, base curve radius; OAD, overall diameter; PCR, peripheral curve radius.

Another option would be to increase prism and/or truncation. If the lens continues to not translate, an aspheric design is indicated.

If poor distance vision is present, it is often the result of one of the following causes: (a) lens is too high/moves excessively (increase prism), (b) lens is not adequately covering the pupil with straight-ahead gaze (increase overall diameter), or (c) seg height is too high (reorder with smaller seg height). If poor near vision is present, it is often the result of one of the following causes: (a) seg height is too low (increase seg), (b) lens is not translating (increase edge clearance), (c) excessive rotation is present (flatten base curve radius), or (d) patient is dropping head—not eyes—when reading (re-educate patient).

GP translating bifocal problem solving is summarized in Table 15.13.

Gas-Permeable Multifocal and Bifocal Educational Resources

The most important educational resource to the practitioner who desires to fit GP presbyopic lens designs is the laboratory consultant. These individuals can provide useful information on lens designs, provide diagnostic fitting sets, and assist in the lens design, fitting, and troubleshooting process. In addition, many useful resources have been developed by the GP Lens Institute, the educational division of the CLMA. These include a comprehensive presbyopic tool kit entitled "Rx for Success," online fitting and problem-solving programs, and an online case grand rounds book. These programs are listed in Table 15.14.

TABLE 15.14 GAS-PERMEABLE (GP) LENS INSTITUTE GP PRESBYOPIC EDUCATIONAL RESOURCES

1. Rx for Success: Building Your Practice with GP Bifocals and Multifocals (CD-ROM and educational resources)
2. GP Multifocal Fitting and Troubleshooting lecture
3. GP Lens Grand Rounds Troubleshooting Guide
4. Correcting Presbyopia Tips (guide)
5. GP Lens Management Guide
6. Presenting GP Presbyopic Contact Lens Options card

■ OTHER FORMS OF PRESBYOPIC CONTACT LENS CORRECTION

Other contact lens options available for presbyopic patients include single-vision lenses in combination with reading glasses and monovision.

Single-Vision Contact Lenses/Reading Glasses

The use of single-vision lenses (soft or GP) in combination with reading glasses affords the benefits of ease of fit, optimum vision at distance and near, and limited expense. However, patients with varied near and distance tasks will complain of the inconvenience of frequently applying and removing their spectacles. In addition, many patients desire contact lenses to eliminate the need for spectacle wear. Nevertheless, it is important for this option to be presented to all potential presbyopic contact lens patients. Some patients will prefer to begin with this option; however, at a later date they may change to one of the other presbyopic contact lens options mentioned to them at the original fitting/consultation visit.

Monovision

Overview

Monovision was first reported as a form of presbyopic contact lens correction in the 1960s[53] and still represents the most popular form of contact lens correction for presbyopia.[54,55] The success rate for monovision is between 70% and 76%.[56,57] However, it is evident that for monovision to be successful, the brain must suppress blur from the defocused eye.[58] There has been much heightened consumer awareness about monovision because of a report of an aviation accident in which three passengers were injured in a plane in which the pilot was wearing a monovision correction.[59]

The advantages of monovision include[4,15,60] (a) ease of fitting, (b) uninterrupted vision out of each eye separately, (c) changing one lens only for present lens wearers, (d) less expense to patient and practitioner, and (e) avoidance of some of the problems present in multifocal contact lenses, including ghost images and fluctuating vision because of pupil size change.

Disadvantages/Problems

A major problem with monovision is a decrease in stereopsis. A decrease of anywhere from 37 to 150 seconds of arc has resulted when subjects have been refitted from monovision into multifocal contact lenses.[57,61,62] Several studies have demonstrated that stereoacuity loss increases with increasing monocular add powers.[63,64] Some monocular suppression of blur also occurs as the add increases.[65] Subjects with monovision correction have demonstrated contrast sensitivity loss and sometimes compromise on critical distance vision tasks.[66–68]. In addition, an increase in anisometropia of ≥0.50 D and as much as 1.25 D has been found in 29% of monovision wearers.[69]

Driving with monovision wear is also a concern and should, in fact, add to the problems presbyopes already experience with night driving.[70] As many as 80% of monovision patients have reported problems with night driving.[71] This would especially be true with glare.[72] It has also been found that monovision wearers have a very difficult time suppressing headlights while driving at night, with one-third of the subjects experiencing glare while night driving.[73] Interestingly, when evaluating habitual monovision wearers on several simulated driving tasks under daytime conditions, no difference was found in driving performance between monovision and their habitual distance correction.[74] Nevertheless, it has been advised for monovision patients to avoid driving or operating dangerous machinery during the first 2 to 3 weeks of adaptation.[75]

Patient Selection

The age and add powers of the patient are predictive of success, with lower-add-power patients (+1.25 to +2.00 D) being more successful than higher-add-power patients.[57,76] The visual needs as well as the lifestyle of the patient must be evaluated when considering monovision. If prolonged and critical distance vision is desirable, monovision is not a good option. Likewise, if depth perception is important to a given occupation (e.g., with construction workers), monovision would not be recommended.[77] Individuals in occupations like teaching, the performing arts, public speaking, and sales who desire the benefit of being able to constantly change viewing distances and still remain focused could benefit from monovision lens wear.

Because of an esophoric shift in eye posture, esophoria at distance and a reduction in nearpoint visual acuity and stereopsis have also been shown to indicate a poor prognosis for success with monovision.[75,78] A patient's personality has also been found to be important for monovision success.[79] A significant correlation between initial negative response and unsuccessful monovision wear has been found.[80] In addition, it has been found that introverted men tend to reject monovision most frequently, whereas the most successful patients were laid-back and optimistic.[81]

Lens Selection and Fitting Considerations

Both GP lenses, because of their resultant visual performance, oxygen permeability, and wettability, and silicone/hydrogel lens materials lend themselves well to monovision. As a result of the greater tendency for dryness and surface deposition, if soft lenses are deemed preferable, a disposable (daily to monthly) lens is essential for long-term success. If handling is challenging to the new monovision wearer, GP lenses would be a preferable alternative.

The eye to be selected for near depends on several factors. It has been found that in 95% of the cases it has been the nondominant eye.[57] The most popular method for establishing ocular dominance is to have patients extend both of their arms in front of them, forming an aperture with the fingers from both hands. Patients are then instructed to center a distance target in the opening of their hands. Whichever eye is found to be in alignment with the object when they are alternatively closed is the dominant eye. A "swinging plus" test, in which patients simply walk around the room holding a plus power trial lens equal to their required add over one eye, and repeating the procedure over the other eye, has been advocated.[82] This is also beneficial in simulating the impact monovision will potentially have on their quality of vision. The eye that the patients deem more comfortable with the overplus correction will be the eye corrected for nearpoint. The full distance and near powers are typically prescribed. It is possible that by overplussing the power of the distance lens and/or underplussing the power of the near lens, not only is the patient's vision compromised at one or both distances, but also the interocular suppression of blur may be suppressed, which is important for monovision to be successful.[4]

It is recommended to perform binocular vision testing to determine the effect of monovision on stereopsis. As indicated previously, it is important to strongly encourage—if not require—the patient to have overspectacles for use while driving and for any other critical distance vision tasks. Although full adaptation to monovision may take up to 2 to 3 weeks,[25] patients should be told that it may take as long as 4 to 6 weeks. If they experience difficulty in adapting (i.e., experience headaches, eye strain, blurred vision), switching the near- and distance-corrected eyes should be considered. If this is not successful, a bifocal or multifocal lens should be recommended. Important factors for successful monovision lens wear are provided in Table 15.15.

Problem Solving

Several problems induced by monovision and their clinical management have been reported[83]:

Asthenopia: If the patient reports frequent or prolonged asthenopic symptoms, the optics and power of the lenses should be verified and an overrefraction performed. Often poor optics,

TABLE 15.15 IMPORTANT FACTORS FOR MONOVISION FITTING AND PRESCRIBING

1. Monovision is most successful in early presbyopic patients, those who do not require long periods of critical distance vision, those who are optimistic in nature, and those who are realistic about the visual limitations.

2. Binocular vision testing should be performed to determine the effect of monovision on stereopsis.

3. The proper eye for near vision should be selected. This often is the nondominant eye and/or the eye in which vision is reduced relative to the other eye.

4. The indicated add power should be demonstrated to patients such that they can obtain a realistic impression of the resulting blur.

5. It is recommended to prescribe the full amount of correction and avoid the temptation of prescribing less plus power in the near-corrected eye and/or prescribing more plus power in the distance-corrected eye.

6. Patients should be strongly encouraged—if not required—to obtain a pair of driving spectacles (i.e., minus correction in the lens over the near-corrected eye) to wear for driving or any other critical distance tasks.

7. Although most individuals adapt within 2 wk, patients should be instructed that it could take up to 6 wk to fully adapt to monovision.

Modified from Bennett ES, Jurkus JM. Presbyopic correction. In: Bennett ES, Weissman BA, eds. Clinical Contact Lens Practice, 2nd ed. Philadelphia: Lippincott Williams & Wilkins, 2005:531–548.

inappropriate powers, or uncorrected cylinder are to blame. It is often necessary to fit a toric soft lens for a monovision wearer with astigmatism of 0.75 D.

Blur at Distance: If the patient's complaint is poor distance vision, it is first important to evaluate for optical problems. It may be necessary to completely correct the astigmatism in the distance eye or, in the case of a low add, the patient may not be suppressing at distance.

Blur at Intermediate Distances: Demand for intermediate vision may require the use of a modified monovision system that provides three optical corrections (often called trivision). Before attempting the more sophisticated fitting, it is important to determine if a slightly reduced add will allow a suitable compromise; by reducing the add by 0.50 D, the intermediate and near corrections may be sufficiently clear to allow useful, although not optimum, visual acuity.

If reducing the add is not sufficient, it is important to determine the zone of greatest demand, near or intermediate, and the time this zone is in use. For example, a patient who requires intermediate vision once each week when playing the church organ may be fitted with a third near lens with a reduced add.

If both the near and intermediate zones are used regularly and frequently (e.g., an executive who works on a computer and must read reports), the trivision system may prove worthwhile. In this case, a simultaneous bifocal lens is most often fit for the near eye. The distance zone of the bifocal lens provides intermediate power, with the add providing near vision.

Blur at Near: It is important to determine if the blur is constant or task specific. If the blur is constant, the add should be adjusted. You should then overrefract, adding plus to the near eye until clear vision is achieved. If clear vision is not achieved, the optics of the near lens should be evaluated. If the blur is task specific (e.g., most noticeable at work in near-intensive demands), a pair of overspectacles may be required.

Fatigue and Flare: A frequent complaint of monovision patients is eye strain or fatigue when performing an intensive amount of near work. Prescribing a pair of single vision glasses with plus over the distance eye and plano over the near will often alleviate the symptoms.

As for flare caused by a cosmetic fit, the cause of flare in monovision is too small of an optical zone for scotopic conditions. To verify the condition, it is important to examine the patient under both dim and normal room illumination. The pupil diameter should be measured under dim illumination, with 2 mm added to determine the minimum optical zone size.

Headaches: Some early presbyopes who have a reasonable amount of accommodation remaining only need a very low add and may be fighting excess plus power prescribed for near. They try to accommodate to clear their distance eye at near and, as a result, are overplussed on their near eye. If increasing the add to 1.25 D or 1.50 D does not alleviate the symptoms, the fitting should be deferred until a higher add is required. Hyperopic patients find being fitted with single-vision contact lenses optically provides them with an advantage, and monovision may not be necessary during the first year of lens wear.

Involuntary Eye Switching: Often patients will observe that, especially under visual stress, they momentarily switch eyes. An example of this is the executive fitted with the distance eye dominant who is reviewing annual budgets; as she concentrates on the budget, the dominant eye attempts to see the text. These are usually transient episodes of very short duration during adaptation. If eye switching continues after the first week of lens wear, the eyes are inappropriately fitted and the near eye should be refitted for distance, and vice versa.

Persistent Blur or Haze: If blurring and haze unrelated to the fit of the contact lens persist after 2 weeks of monovision wear, an adjustment is necessary. The practitioner must first ensure that the blur is not caused by edema as a result of a poorly fitting lens. If the lens is suspect, it should be adjusted before any other step is taken. If the fit of the lens is not the cause, the duration of the blur or haze should next be determined.

If the blur is constant, the optics of the lenses should be evaluated and an overrefraction should be performed. If the problem is optically induced, a new lens should correct the problem. If the blur is not related to the optics of the lens or refraction, the amount of add should be examined next.

In cases of low adds (<1.00 D), there may not be enough stimulus for the patient to learn to selectively suppress. In these cases increasing the amount of the add by 0.50 D has been successful in alleviating the symptom.

If the add is over 2.00 D, the patient may not be a suitable candidate for monovision. In some cases, reducing the add by 0.50 D has been successful, but most patients will not accept the near blur this creates. Often, the best solution is to abandon the monovision fitting for other bifocal corrections. If the add is between 1.00 and 2.00 D and blur persists, the lenses should be switched. Often, this symptom reflects an inappropriate eye being fitted for distance.

Slight or Intermittent Blur/Haze: This normal symptom of adaptation is encountered by most monovision patients at some time in their initial weeks of wear. It is generally found to be most common in circumstances requiring visual concentration under scotopic conditions (e.g., viewing television in a dim room). If the blur or haze is slight, intermittent, and transient, patients should be instructed that no correction is necessary. If possible, they should try to avoid these conditions in the first week of monovision wear. The practitioner should be alert for blur or haze caused by a poor contact lens fit and take action if necessary. If blurring or haze is persistent, an office visit is required.

Vague Complaints of Discomfort: Most nonspecific complaints can be alleviated by switching eyes: the dominant eye has not been fitted for the dominant task. This is more common in cases in which a clear eye dominance cannot be established during in-office testing. In the vast majority of cases, simply switching eye function between the eyes alleviates all symptoms, and the patient becomes successful. How to successfully evaluate this presbyopic contact lens option is summarized in Figure 15.13.

Comparison Studies

Spectacle Correction Versus Bifocal and Multifocal Contact Lens Designs

Recent studies have concluded that spectacle lens acuity (or best corrected spectacle acuity) has differed little between bifocal and multifocal contact lenses and spectacles. Fisher et al[12] found that distance and near acuity as well as stereoacuity and visuomotor task performance were somewhat better with the best spherocylindrical spectacle correction than with both an annular soft bifocal design and an aspheric soft multifocal design. However, Jimenez et al[30] found similar visual performance between progressive addition lenses and an annular soft bifocal under varying illumination conditions. Woods et al[84] found no statistical difference between the near and distance acuity of subjects wearing a GP aspheric design versus their spectacle acuities.

Monovision Versus Bifocal and Multifocal Contact Lens Designs

Recent studies with newer designs have resulted in different outcomes. Kirschen et al[61] found that not only was stereoacuity significantly better with the Acuvue Bifocal as compared to monovision, but also the soft bifocal resulted in a statistically significant decrease in the interocular difference in visual acuity at distance and near and improved binocularity. In several comparison studies in which patients had to make a forced choice between the two modalities, the bifocal/multifocal was preferred to monovision with preferences ranging from 68% (Acuvue Bifocal)[85] to 76% (SofLens Multifocal).[86] These results were similar to a study in which subjects wore GP lenses monovision for 6 weeks followed by 6 weeks in a GP aspheric multifocal (or vice versa).[87] At the conclusion of the study 75% preferred the multifocal design.

Monovision Correction Versus Soft Bifocal Lenses, Gas-Permeable Multifocal Lenses, and Spectacles

Recently, the visual performance of subjects wearing GP monovision lenses, soft bifocal lenses, GP aspheric multifocal lenses, and PALs was compared.[68] It was found that there was relative parity between the binocular high and low contrast acuity between PAL wearers and GP aspheric multifocal wearers followed by soft bifocal wearers and then monovision. The difference between monovision and the other three groups was most evident with high contrast acuity. In the contact lens groups, GP multifocal lens wearers had the highest binocular contrast sensitivity at all spatial frequencies, on parity with PAL wearers, except at the highest spatial frequency (18 cpd), in which PAL wearers performed superiorly.

■ SUMMARY

This chapter presented an overview of important fitting and problem-solving considerations, as bifocal contact lens designs progress well into the new millennium. It is hoped that this information will be of value in determining who is a good candidate and what lens material(s) would be most beneficial. It is not unreasonable to consider bifocal contact lenses for diagnostic fitting before monovision. Once experience is gained, a satisfactory (and sometimes excellent) success rate can result. It can be summarized by stating that two "certainties" exist with bifocal contact lenses:

1. It is the most exciting and potentially the biggest contact lens market.

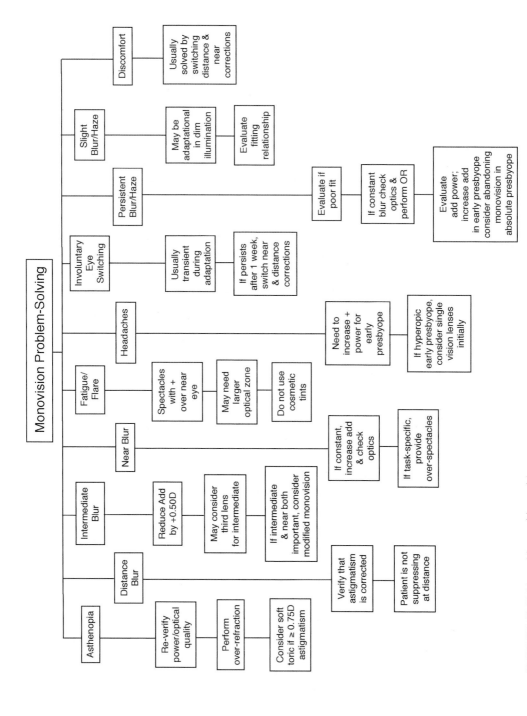

■ FIGURE 15.13 Monovision problem solving.

2. Many new and improved lens designs and materials will be added in the next few years, allowing practitioners the flexibility to use a presbyopic contact lens-fitting system approach for every interested and eligible patient.

■ CLINICAL CASES

CASE 1

A 56-year-old patient is undergoing an eye examination in your office. During the course of the examination, this patient "inquires" about contact lenses, showing mild interest. Her refractive findings are as follows:

$$OD +0.50 - 0.25 \times 180\ 20/20$$
$$OS +0.25 - 0.25 \times 180\ 20/20$$
$$Add +2.25\ D$$

Her TBUT is 4 seconds OU.

SOLUTION: Contact lens wear appears to be contraindicated for this patient. The ambivalent motivation, in combination with poor tear quality and small distance error, would most likely result in failure. After thorough education on fees, lens design and care, and ocular dryness, if the patient's motivation appears to be good, the patient might be fitted in a monovision lens for near or a bifocal lens on the nondominant eye only. A material like the Proclear or a silicone hydrogel material would be recommended because of her low TBUT.

CASE 2

A 46-year-old patient is strongly motivated for bifocal contact lenses. She is a first-time wearer who is especially interested in soft contact lenses. Her refraction is as follows:

$$OD -3.75 - 0.25 \times 180\ 20/20$$
$$OS -3.50 - 0.25 \times 180\ 20/20$$
$$Add +1.00\ D$$

Keratometry readings

$$OD\ 42.00/42.50\ @\ 090$$
$$OS\ 42.25/42.50\ @\ 090$$
Dominant eye: OD

The preliminary evaluation shows the presence of an inferiorly positioned lower lid (i.e., 1 mm below the limbus). All other findings indicate that she is a good bifocal contact lens candidate.

SOLUTION: This patient appears to be a good candidate for any of the available soft bifocal lens designs. All the options should be explained, and if she is still interested, one of these designs can be diagnostically fitted.
If the Acuvue Bifocal was selected, the trial lenses would be:

$$OD\ BCR\ 8.5\ mm,\ Rx\ -3.75,\ Add\ +1.00$$
$$OS\ BCR\ 8.5\ mm,\ Rx\ -3.50,\ Add\ +1.00$$

The patient sees 20/25 OU at distance and 20/20 OU at near. A -0.25 over the OD eye brings distance acuity to 20/20 OU and does not affect near vision. The patient is sent home to trial for 5 days the following:

$$OD\ BCR\ 8.5\ mm,\ Rx\ -4.00,\ Add\ +1.00$$
$$OS\ BCR\ 8.5\ mm,\ Rx\ -3.50,\ Add\ +1.00$$

CASE 3

A 53-year-old patient is strongly motivated for soft bifocal contact lens wear. She has worn spherical soft lenses before presbyopia developed. She then attempted monovision and failed because she did not like the loss of stereoacuity. She is currently wearing reading glasses over her distance vision soft lenses but desires to be spectacle free. Her refraction is as follows:

$$OD -3.00 - 0.25 \times 090 \ 20/20$$
$$OS -2.75 \ DS \ 20/20$$
$$Add +2.00 \ D$$

Keratometry readings:

$$OD \ 43.00/43.25 @ 090$$
$$OS \ 43.50/43.50 @ 090$$

Dominant eye: OD

Her TBUT is 10 seconds.

Her lower lid is positioned slightly above (0.5 mm) the limbus. All other findings indicate that she is a good bifocal contact lens candidate.

SOLUTION: This patient would be a good candidate for any soft bifocal lens design that can provide a +2.00 D add. If this patient is fit with the Proclear Multifocal, the following trial lenses would be selected:

$$OD \ BCR \ 8.7 \ mm, \ Rx -3.00 \ D, \ Add +2.00 \ D \ lens$$
$$OS \ BCR \ 8.7 \ mm, \ Rx -2.75 \ D, \ Add +2.00 \ N \ lens$$

With these lenses, her distance vision was 20/30 OU and her near vision 20/20 OU; monocular acuities should be checked. Monocular acuities were OD 20/30 at distance and 20/25 at near, and OS 20/30 at distance and 20/20 at near. A −0.25 D trial lens over the OD brings monocular distance acuity down to 20/20. The patient is sent home with the following lenses:

$$OD \ BCR \ 8.7 \ mm, \ Rx -3.25 \ D, \ Add +2.00 \ D \ lens$$
$$OS \ BCR \ 8.7 \ mm, \ Rx -2.75 \ D, \ Add +2.00 \ N \ lens$$

Distance and near acuities are 20/20 OU. The patient is to return for a 1-week follow-up visit.

CASE 4

Your 42-year-old patient is a long-term soft lens wearer. He has recently noticed that his near vision is not as good as it used to be. He is currently wearing Focus Dailies. His examination reveals:

$$OD -4.50 \ 20/20$$
$$OS -5.00 \ 20/20$$
$$Add +0.75 \ D$$

Keratometry readings:

$$OD \ 42.00/42.25 @ 090$$
$$OS \ 42.50/42.50 @ 090$$

Dominant eye: OS

His TBUT is 10 seconds.

SOLUTION: This patient is a good candidate for monovision or bifocal contact lens wear. With a low add, the patient may appreciate staying in his current lenses and just decreasing the power of the nondominant eye to −3.50 or −3.75 D to help at near. Another option would be to fit the nondominant eye with a Focus Dailies Progressive and leave the dominant eye in a spherical lens. The diagnostic lenses selected for this would be:

$$OD \ BCR \ 8.6 \ mm, \ Rx -3.75 \ or -4.00 \ D \ (-4.25 + 0.37) \ Focus \ Dailies \ Progressive$$
$$OS \ BCR \ 8.6 \ mm, \ Rx -4.75 \ D \ Focus \ Dailies \ Sphere$$

A third option is to fit the patient in the Biomedics EP lens. The diagnostic lens selected would be as follows:

$$OD \ BCR \ 8.7 \ mm, \ Rx -4.25 \ D$$
$$OS \ BCR \ 8.7 \ mm, \ Rx -4.75 \ D$$

The patient can be dispensed a trial pair of lenses and return for follow-up in 3 to 7 days.

CASE 5

A long-term soft toric patient, who has worn monovision for about 3 years, wants to try bifocal contact lenses. He replaces his current contact lenses on a monthly basis. His spectacle Rx is:

OD −2.50 − 1.25 × 180   VA 20/20
OS −2.00 − 1.75 × 180   VA 20/20
Add +1.50

Dominant eye: OD

Keratometry readings:

OD 43.00/44.00 @ 090
OS 43.00/44.25 @ 090

His TBUT is 9 seconds.

SOLUTION: This patient would be a good candidate for the Proclear Multifocal Toric lens. Diagnostic lenses can be ordered for the patient. For this patient, as no vertexing back to the cornea is necessary, contact lenses matching the spectacle prescription can be ordered and the identical add used. The OD lens should be a D lens and the OS an N lens. At the dispensing visit, acceptable vision is 20/20 at distance and near OU with 20/40 or better at near with the OD and 20/40 or better distance acuity with the OS. This lens is a monthly replacement lens and is good for less than ideal TBUTs. Ideally, the patient would have a TBUT ≥10 seconds for good tear quality. If the vision falls within the acceptable range at the dispensing, the patient should wear the lenses on a trial basis and return for follow-up within 3 to 7 days.

CASE 6

This 45-year-old patient is a current GP lens wearer who is beginning to be symptomatic at near. He enjoys playing squash and basketball. Your refraction shows the following:

OD: +4.00 − 1.00 × 180 20/20
OS: +4.50 − 1.25 × 005 20/20
Add +1.00 D

The pupil size is normal (4.5 mm), and the lower lid is positioned 1 mm below the limbus. All other findings indicate that this patient is a good bifocal contact lens candidate.

SOLUTION: All presbyopic contact lens options should be explained to this patient. If this patient is receptive to a bifocal design and is not particularly motivated for monovision, an aspheric design can be considered, especially since this patient is an early presbyope. The position of the lower lid and possibly the refractive error may contraindicate an alternating design. Likewise, he is very active and these lenses would be much less likely to dislodge than a translating design.

CASE 7

A 44-year-old patient had been a long-term spherical GP wearer and was recently refitted into a back surface aspheric GP lens design. The patient was pleased with both vision at all distances and comfort with these lenses. However, despite changes in both base curve radius and diameter, the lenses positioned superiorly and exhibited very little (if any) movement with the blink. Corneal topography revealed superior flattening (approximately 2.25 D change 2.5 mm superior from center and 3 D of steepening 3 mm inferior from center) immediately after lens removal. In addition, there was mild distortion evident superiorly OU.

SOLUTION: This is a good case for the use of a front surface aspheric GP design. The lens should position more centrally and the spherical back surface should minimize the topography changes that resulted with the back surface aspheric design.

CASE 8

A 50-year-old patient has been a 7-year wearer of the Essential Multifocal lens design (Blanchard). She has recently been experiencing blurred vision when performing critical near work, especially reading. Her refraction information is as follows:

Refraction:

OD: $-6.50 - 1.50 \times 172$ 20/20
OS: $-6.25 - 1.50 \times 006$ 20/20
Add +2.00 D

Keratometry:

OD: 43.00 @ 180; 44.25 @ 090
OS: 43.25 @ 180; 44.50 @ 090

Her anatomic measurements are the following:
Lower lid position: 1 mm below the limbus
Pupil size: 3.5 mm

She is wearing the following lenses in a "modified bifocal approach":

OD: Essentials Series II: BCR: 7.67 mm OAD: 9.5 mm Power: -7.00 D
OS: Essentials Series III: BCR: 7.63 mm OAD: 9.5 mm Power: -6.50 D
Visual acuity: 20/20 OD, OS, and OU at distance; 20/40 OD, 20/30 + 2 at near. A +1.00 D overrefraction over OD and +0.75 D over OS resulted in 20/20 at near.
Both lenses exhibited good centration and about 1 mm lag with the blink.

SOLUTION: Reorder the lenses in a Series II OU with the same lens parameters, but order with a +1.00 D CSA on the front surface OU. With the small pupil diameter, it is apparent that this patient required a higher add earlier than with most presbyopic patients. A 4.0-mm central distance zone is also recommended to optimize near vision via mild translation of the lens with downward gaze.

CASE 9

This 49-year-old patient is a former spherical GP lens wearer who discontinued contact lens wear 2 years ago after failing to achieve adequate vision at distance and near with monovision. Currently, he is wearing progressive addition spectacles, but as a result of his prescription, he is very motivated to return to contact lens wear. His refraction and keratometric measurements are as follows:

Refraction:

OD: $-5.00 - 1.00 \times 005$ 20/20
OS: $-4.50 - 1.50 \times 175$ 20/20
Add +1.75 D

Keratometry:

OD: 42.00 @ 180; 43.00 @ 090
OS: 42.50 @ 180; 44.00 @ 090

His anatomic measurements are the following:

Lower lid position: 0.5 mm above the limbus

Pupil size: 5.5 mm

All other findings indicate that this patient is a good bifocal contact lens candidate.

SOLUTION: Once all of the options have been explained to this patient, it is very likely he will be fitted with a translating design such as the Tangent Streak. Using the fitting guide, the following diagnostic lenses can be selected:

	OD	OS
BCR	8.08	7.94
OAD	9.4/9.0	9.4/9.0
Power	$-2.00/+2.00$ Add	$-2.00/+2.00$ Add

If the lens fits as predicted, the overrefraction is equal to the predicted value, and the seg position is at or near the lower pupil margin, the following lens design could be ordered:

	OD	OS
BCR	8.08	7.94
OAD	9.4/9.0 (11 − 2)	9.4/9.0 (11 − 2)
Power	−4.50/+1.75 D Add	−4.25/+1.75 D Add
	(the −4.50 results from vertexing the −5.00 D sphere to −4.75 and adding the +0.25 D tear lens power compensation)	(the −4.25 results from vertexing the −4.50 D sphere to −4.25)
Seg height	4.2 mm	4.2 mm
Prism	2.00 PD	2.00 PD

CASE 10

A Solitaire lens (Tru-Form Optics) diagnostically fitted to a motivated and qualified candidate both moves and rotates excessively after the blink on the right eye. The patient's refractive, keratometric, and lens design information is provided below:

Refraction: −2.00 − 0.75 × 170 20/20
              Add +2.00 D

Keratometry: 43.00 @ 180; 43.75 @ 090

Lens design:

              BCR: 7.85 mm (43.00 D)
              Power: −2.00/+2.00 D Add
              Prism: Standard

SOLUTION: A flatter base curve radius lens should be selected—for example, 42.50 D (remember: make the design change a *significant* one). If excessive rotation is still present, increasing the prism should be considered.

CASE 11

A 53-year-old wearer of the Solutions Bifocal (X-Cel) inquired if there was any way she could achieve better vision from her contact lenses when she is working at her computer. She spends several hours every day at her computer and for the past 2 years has been wearing a pair of +1.00 D reading glasses she bought at a pharmacy.

SOLUTION: With the increasing number of translating designs with an intermediate correction, this patient would benefit from any one of these designs. As she is already wearing the Solutions Bifocal, it would be recommended to refit her into the ESSential Solutions. The aspheric back surface will assist in providing an intermediate correction, while the segmented crescent front surface design will continue to provide her with both distance and near correction.

CASE 12

This early presbyope has been a 15-year soft lens wearer. She is very satisfied with soft lenses but is beginning to experience blur at near. Her refraction is as follows:

OD: −3.75 DS 20/20
OS: −3.50 DS 20/20
Add +1.00 D

All other findings indicate that she is a good contact lens candidate.

SOLUTION: Once again, all presbyopic contact lens options should be explained to this patient. If the patient chooses monovision over bifocal contact lenses, binocular function testing should be performed to evaluate the effect of monovision on stereopsis. In addition, the effect of this near add power should be demonstrated to the patient. If this is acceptable, the full add power should be prescribed for the indicated eye. If the patient is right eye dominant and all other indications tend to support this eye being fit for distance, a −2.50 D lens should be selected for the left eye. The patient should be told that a 4- to 6-week adaptation period may be necessary. A second distance lens or "driving" spectacles should also be encouraged. The use of a wettable lens material in a blue handling tint is recommended.

CASE 13

A monovision wearer has symptoms of fatigue when performing prolonged near work. These symptoms initiated after she changed to a job that required long periods of intense near work.

SOLUTION: Prescribing a pair of "overspectacles" is recommended. Plus is prescribed over the distance eye and plano over the near eye to relieve the visual fatigue caused by a monovision correction.

CLINICAL PROFICIENCY CHECKLIST

- Bifocal contact lenses are increasing in popularity, and new technology has resulted in better lens designs.
- Although monovision is an option for the presbyope interested in contact lens wear, the option of some type of bifocal contact lens should be discussed.
- The best candidates for bifocal contact lens correction include those who are very motivated, have good tear quality, and have >1 D of refractive error. Patients with poor tear quality, eye disease, amblyopia, or poor motivation should be ruled out.
- There are numerous simultaneous vision (i.e., the patient views through the distance and near zones at the same time) soft bifocal designs, including center-near and center-distance designs, either aspheric or concentric, and a translating design.
- The increased popularity of soft bifocal designs can be contributed to disposable/frequent-replacement lenses, silicone hydrogel materials, and toric multifocal lenses. Disposable/frequent-replacement lenses allow the practitioner to fit lenses from inventory and have the patient wear the lenses on a trial basis. In addition, deposit-related problems and torn lenses are less of an issue because of the regular replacement schedule and spare lenses.
- There are several available simultaneous vision GP bifocal lens designs, including aspheric and center-distance and center-near concentric designs. The primary benefit of the aspheric designs is good vision for early presbyopes and persons requiring good intermediate vision. The primary limitations include the need for good lens centration, achieving high add powers for advanced presbyopes, and reduced vision at distance if pupil size is large.
- Alternating vision bifocal designs include one-piece "no image jump" segmented designs, a fuse segmented design, and an alternating distance-center concentric design.
- The segmented, translating designs have a good probability of success, especially with advanced presbyopic patients. This is true because if the lenses are fitting and translating properly, the patient will be viewing through the distance zone when viewing at a distance and the near zone when viewing at near. Patients who have a low lower lid position (i.e., 1 mm or more below the lower limbus), very loose lower lid tension, or tight lids (creating excessive lens rotation) are not good candidates for these lenses.
- When fitting a segmented GP bifocal design, it is extremely important to take careful measurements of the patient's pupil size, corneal diameter, and distance from the lower lid to the center of the pupil.

(Continued)

- Monovision is the most commonly used method of presbyopic correction. With these patients, it is important to select a wettable contact lens material, perform binocular function testing to determine the effect of stereopsis, select the proper eye for near (often the nondominant eye, although it should be the eye with reduced vision or with higher myopia if anisometropia is present), and encourage either "driving" spectacles or a second distance contact lens.

- Another contact lens option for presbyopic patients is the use of reading glasses over a spherical (distance only) contact lens prescription. Although this option provides the benefits of ease of fit, optimum vision at distance and near, and limited expense, some patients will be unhappy with the frequent application and removal of spectacles, and others will not be interested in spectacle wear of any form.

ACKNOWLEDGMENTS

The authors would like to acknowledge information provided in the second edition by Drs. Jan Jurkus and Carol Schwartz.

REFERENCES

1. Schwartz CA. Portrait of a presbyope in 1999. Optom Today 1999;Suppl:5–7.
2. Meyler J, Veys J. A new pupil-intelligent design for presbyopic correction. Optician 1999;217:18–23.
3. Edwards K. Contact lens problem-solving: bifocal contact lenses. Optician 1999;218:26–32.
4. Bennett ES, Jurkus JM. Presbyopic correction. In: Bennett ES, Weissman BA, eds. Clinical Contact Lens Practice, 2nd ed. Philadelphia: Lippincott Williams & Wilkins, 2005:531–548.
5. Bennett ES. Bifocal and multifocal contact lenses. In: Phillips AJ, Speedwell L, eds. Contact Lens Practice, 5th ed. Oxford: Butterworth-Heinemann, 2006:311–331.
6. Pujol J, Gispets J, Arjona M. Optical performance in eyes wearing two multifocal contact lens designs. Ophthalmol Physiol Opt 2003;23:347–360.
7. Morgan PB, Woods CA, Knajian R, et al. International contact lens prescribing in 2007. Contact Lens Spectrum 2008;23(1):36–41.
8. Mack CJ. Contact lenses 2007. Contact Lens Spectrum 2008;23(1).
9. Jones L, Jones D, Langley C, et al. Reactive or proactive contact lens fitting – does it make a difference? J Br Contact Lens Assoc 1996;19(2):41–43.
10. Schwartz C, Bennett ES. How RGPs changed my life. Optom Management 1997;32(4):51–56.
11. Bennett ES. My second highest priority. Contact Lens Spectrum 1999;14(10).
12. Fisher K, Bauman E, Schwallie J. Evaluation of two new soft contact lenses for correction of presbyopia: the Focus Progressives Multifocal and the Acuvue Bifocal. Int Contact lens Clin 1999;26:92–103.
13. Martin DK, Dain SJ. Postural modifications of VDU operators wearing bifocal spectacles. Appl Ergonom 1988;19:293–300.
14. Afanador AJ, Aitsemaomo P, Gertzman DR. Eye and head contribution to gaze at near through multifocals: the useable field of view. Am J Optom Physiol Opt 1986;63:187–192.
15. Bennett ES. Contact lens correction of presbyopia. Clin Exp Optom 2008;91:265–278.
16. Jurkus JM, Nichols S. Contact lenses and the aging eye. Optom Today Suppl 1999;7(3):53–60.
17. Bennett ES, Weissman BA, Remba MR. Contact lenses and the older adult. In: Rosenbloom & Morgan's Vision and Aging. St. Louis: Elsevier, 2007:215–240.
18. du Toit, Situ P, Simpson T, et al. The effects of six months of contact lens wear on the tear film, ocular surfaces, and symptoms of presbyopes. Optom Vis Sci 2001;78:455–462.
19. Hansen DW. Current concepts of RGP multifocal contact lenses. Practical Optom 1992;3(2):70–78.
20. Andres S, Henriques A, Garcia ML, et al. Factors of the precorneal fluid break-up time (BUT) and tolerance of contact lenses. Int Contact Lens Clin 1987;4:81–120.
21. Bennett ES, Jurkus JM, Schwartz CA. Bifocal contact lenses. In: Bennett ES, Henry VA, eds. Clinical Manual of Contact Lenses, 2nd ed. Philadelphia: Lippincott Williams & Wilkins, 2000:410–449.
22. Bennett ES, Hansen D. Presbyopia: gas permeable bifocal fitting and problem-solving. In: Bennett ES, Hom MM, eds. Manual of Gas-Permeable Contact Lenses, 2nd ed. St. Louis: Elsevier Science, 2004:324–356.
23. Josephson J, Caffery B. Hydrogel bifocal lenses. In: Bennett ES, Weissman BA, eds. Clinical Contact Lens Practice. Philadelphia: JB Lippincott, 1991:43.1–43.12.
24. Friant RJ. When bifocal lenses are most likely to succeed. Contact Lens Spectrum 1986;1(6):14–23.

25. Gispets J, Arjona M, Pujol J. Image quality in wearers of a centre distance concentric design bifocal contact lens. Ophthalmic Physiol Opt 2002;22:221–223.
26. Kirby J. 2007 Annual contact lens update. Optom Management 2007;42(4):26–28.
27. Norman CW. Communicate and demonstrate soft multifocal benefits. Contact Lens Spectrum 2003;18(9):15.
28. Davis RL. Contact lens options for presbyopes. Optom Management 2004;39(4):37–43.
29. Bergenske PD. The presbyopic fitting process. Contact Lens Spectrum 2001;16(8):34.
30. Jimenez JR, Durban JJ, Anera RG. Maximum disparity with Acuvue bifocal contact lenses with changes in illumination. Optom Vis Sci 2002;79:170–174.
31. Rigel LE, Davis R, Schachet J, et al. A shift in presbyopic management. Contact Lens Spectrum 2005;20(2):42–47.
32. Henry VA. Soft multifocals – fitting and case presentations. Presented at the 47th Annual Meeting of the Heart of America Contact Lens and Primary Care Congress, Kansas City, MO, February 2008.
33. Gasson A, Morris J. Lenses for presbyopia. In: Gasset A, Morris J, eds. The Contact Lens Manual, 3rd ed. London: Butterworth-Heinemann, 2003:298–317.
34. Ezekial DF, Ezekial DJ. A soft bifocal lens that does not compromise vision. Contact Lens Spectrum 2002;17(6): 40–42.
35. http://www.gelflex.com/pdf/triton. Accessed February 28, 2008.
36. Quinn TG. The role of ocular dominance in presbyopic lens correction. Contact Lens Spectrum 2007;22(1):48.
37. Gromacki SJ. Preventing contact lens challenges for presbyopes. Contact Lens Spectrum 2004;19(8):S1–S8.
38. Richdale K. Presbyopic soft lens design options. Contact Lens Spectrum 2008;23(3).
39. Lieblein JS. Finding success with multifocal contact lenses. Contact Lens Spectrum 2000;14(3):50–51.
40. Byrnes SP, Cannella A. An in-office evaluation of a multifocal RGP lens design. Contact Lens Spectrum 1999;14(11):29–33.
41. Anderson G. A GP bifocal for active presbyopes. Optom Management 2003;38(6):74.
42. Smith VM, Koffler BH, Litteral G. Evaluation of the ZEBRA 2000 (Z10) Breger Vision bifocal contact lens. CLAO J 2000;26(4):214–220.
43. Bierman A. Beyond monovision. Optom Management 2003;38(4):70.
44. Hansen DW. RGP bifocals and computer users – the real world. Contact Lens Spectrum 1996;11(2):15.
45. Ames K. Fitting the presbyope with gas permeable contact lenses. Contact Lens Spectrum 2001;16(10):42–45.
46. Businger U, Byrnes S, Baker R. An RGP multifocal for moderate to high presbyopes. Contact Lens Spectrum 2000;15(10).
47. Kirman ST, Kirman GS. The Tangent Streak bifocal contact lens. Contact Lens Forum 1988;13(6):38–40.
48. Remba MJ. The Tangent Streak rigid gas permeable bifocal contact lens. J Am Optom Assoc 1988;59(3):212–216.
49. Bennett ES. The RGP bifocal patient: How to optimize success. Optom Today 1996;4(1):16–17.
50. Bennett ES. Researching GP multifocals. Contact Lens Spectrum. 2005;20(2).
51. Hansen DW. Multifocal contact lenses – the next generation. Contact Lens Spectrum 2002;17(11):42–48.
52. Bennett ES, Luk B. Rigid gas permeable bifocal contact lenses: an update. Optom Today 2001;15:34–36.
53. Fonda G. Trans Ophthalmol Soc Australia 1966;25:46–50.
54. Josephson JE, Caffery BE. Hydrogel bifocal lenses. In: Bennett ES, Weissman BA, eds. Clinical Contact Lens Practice. Philadelphia: JB Lippincott, 1990:43-1–43-20.
55. Harris MG, Kuntz S, Morris C, et al. Use of presbyopic contact lens corrections in optometric practices. Contact Lens Spectrum 2005;20(4):42–46.
56. Westin E, Wick B, Harrist RB. Factors influencing success of monovision contact lens fitting: survey of contact lens diplomates. Optometry 2000;71(12):757–763.
57. Jain S, Arora I, Azar DT. Success of monovision in presbyopes: review of the literature and potential applications to refractive surgery. Surv Ophthalmol 1996;40:491–499.
58. Collins MJ, Goode A. Interocular blur suppression and monovision. Acta Ophthalmol 1994;72(3):376–380.
59. Nakagawara VB, Veronneau SJH. Monovision contact lens use in the aviation environment: a report of a contact lens-related aircraft accident. Optometry 2000;71:390–395.
60. Gasson A, Morris J. Lenses for presbyopia. In: Gasset A, Morris J, eds. The Contact Lens Manual, 3rd ed. London: Butterworth-Heinemann, 2003:298–317.
61. Kirschen DG, Hung CC, Nakano TR. Comparison of suppression, stereoacuity and interocular differences in visual acuity in monovision, and Acuvue Bifocal contact lenses. Optom Vis Sci 1999;76:832–837.
62. Richdale K, Mitchell GL, Zadnik K. Comparison of multifocal and monovision soft contact lens corrections in patients with low-astigmatic presbyopia. Optom Vis Sci 2006;83(5):266–273.
63. Heath DA, Hines C, Schwartz F. Suppression behavior analyzed as a function of monovision addition power. Am J Optom Physiol Opt 1986;63:198–201.
64. Larsen WL, Lachance A. Stereoscopic acuity with induced refractive errors. Am J Optom Physiol Opt 1983;60:509–513.
65. Collins MJ, Goode A, Brown B. Distance visual acuity and monovision. Optom Vis Sci 1993;70:723–728.
66. Loshin DS, Loshin MS, Comer G. Binocular summation with monovision contact lens correction for presbyopia. Int Contact Lens Clin 1982;9:161–165.

67. Collins MJ, Brown B, Bowman KJ. Contrast sensitivity with contact lens correction for presbyopia. Ophthalmic Physiol Opt 1989;9:133–138.

68. Rajagopalan AS, Bennett ES, Lakshminarayanan V. Visual performance of subjects wearing presbyopic contact lenses. Optom Vis Sci 2006;83(8):611–615.

69. Wick B, Westin E. Change in refractive anisometropia in presbyopic adults wearing monovision contact lens correction. Optom Vis Sci 1999;76:33–39.

70. Wood JM. Aging, driving and vision. Clin Exp Optom 2002;85(4):214–220.

71. Josephson JE, Caffery BE. Monovision versus aspheric bifocal contact lenses: a crossover study. J Am Optom Assoc 1987;58:652–654.

72. Johannsdottir KR, Stelmach LB. Monovision: a review of the scientific literature. Optom Vis Sci 2001;78:646–651.

73. Hansen DW. It's time to minimize monovision. Contact Lens Spectrum 2001;16(1):15.

74. Wood JM, Wick K, Shuley V, et al. The effect of monovision contact lens wear on driving performance. Clin Exp Optom 1998;81(3):100–103.

75. Harris MG, Classe JG. Clinicolegal considerations of monovision. J Am Optom Assoc 1988;59:491–495.

76. Erickson P, McGill EC. Role of visual acuity, stereoacuity and ocular dominance in monovision patient success. Optom Vis Sci 1992;69:761–764.

77. Davis RL. Pinpoint success with GP multifocal lenses. Contact Lens Spectrum 2003;18(10):25–38.

78. McGill EC, Erickson P. Sighting dominance and monovision distance binocular fusional ranges. J Am Optom Assoc 1991;62(10):738–742.

79. MacAlister GO, Woods CA. Monovision versus RGP translating bifocals. J Br Contact Lens Assoc 1991;14:173–178.

80. du Toit R, Ferreira JT, Nel ZJ. Visual and nonvisual variables implicated in monovision wear. Optom Vis Sci 1998;75(2):119–125.

81. Erickson DB, Erickson P. Psychological factors and sex differences in acceptance of monovision. Percept Mot Skills 2000;91(3 Part 2):1113–1119.

82. Hom MM. Monovision and bifocals. In: Hom MM, ed. Manual of Contact Lens Fitting and Prescribing with CD-ROM, 2nd ed. Boston: Butterworth-Heinemann, 2000:327–354.

83. Schwartz CA, Jurkus JM. Trouble-shooting the monovision fit. Contact Lens Forum 1991;16(4):24–26.

84. Woods C, Ruston D, Hough T, et al. Clinical performance of an innovative back surface multifocal contact lens in correcting presbyopia. CLAO J 1999;25(3):176–181.

85. Situ P, du Toit R, Fonn D, et al. Successful monovision contact lens wearers refitted into bifocal contact lenses. Eye Contact Lens 2003;29(3):181–184.

86. Richdale K, Mitchell GL, Zadnik K. Comparison of multifocal and monovision soft contact lens corrections in patients with low-astigmatic presbyopia. Optom Vis Sci 2006;83(5):266–273.

87. Johnson J, Bennett ES, Henry VA, et al. MultiVision™ vs. monovision: a comparative study. Presented at the Annual Meeting of the Contact Lens Association of Ophthalmologists, Las Vegas, NV, February 2000.

CHAPTER 16

Extended Wear

Kathy Dumbleton and Lyndon Jones

■ INTRODUCTION

While the majority of patients choose to wear their lenses on a daily basis, removing them at the end of each day before going to sleep, this modality does not offer the convenience of permanent vision correction sought by many contact lens wearers. The opportunity for day and night lens wear has therefore been attractive to contact lens wearers since its very inception. This modality of contact lens wear is referred to as extended (up to 6 consecutive nights) or continuous (up to 30 consecutive nights) wear.[1] Overnight lens wear first became a reality some 30 years ago,[2–4] but its success has been extremely turbulent over this time.

Overnight contact lens wear has historically been associated with a high rate of complications[5–7] and, as a result, practitioners and patients alike have become concerned about the potential safety issues associated with extended wear. Hypoxic complications, resulting from poor oxygen supply to the cornea, were common.[8,9] Fortunately, with the advance of silicone hydrogel materials and high-oxygen-permeability rigid gas permeable (GP) materials, these complications are now relatively rare.[1,10–12] Unfortunately, the major concern with overnight lens wear, corneal infection, still remains.[13–17]

For overnight lens wear to be successful, contact lenses must not only be convenient, but they must also be safe and comfortable. While the risk of microbial keratitis remains the major source of anxiety associated with extended and continuous wear, comfort and dryness are also major limiting factors for patients desiring the convenience of this modality of lens wear.

■ HISTORY OF EXTENDED WEAR

Throughout the 1970s and early 1980s, manufacturers released a variety of materials that were intended for overnight wear. These early materials were often worn for up to a month at a time without being removed and achieved great commercial success, with John de Carle reporting success with over 2,000 patients in the early 1970s and other authors reporting similarly high levels of clinical success up to the mid-1980s.[18–22] As a result of such positive data, extended wear (EW) for cosmetic use for up to 30 days was approved by the Food and Drug Administration (FDA) in 1981, sparking an explosion in the number of patients being fitted with lenses for overnight wear. However, very soon afterward, reports of corneal ulceration with significant vision loss began appearing in journals,[23,24] and the safety of overnight wear was questioned in both peer-reviewed journals and the lay media. The Contact Lens Institute, in the United States, sponsored studies to investigate the relative risk and incidence of infectious keratitis. The results from these studies were published in 1989[5,6] and clearly demonstrated that overnight wear of lenses carried with it a significantly increased risk of corneal infection. As a result, the FDA immediately reduced the approved length of time for overnight wear without removal from 30 to 7 days.

In the mid-1980s, it was believed that the corneal infections observed with overnight wear were probably because of poor hygiene and compliance and that the principal factor driving such infection rates was because of patients reinserting poorly disinfected lenses. It was hypothesized that using lenses on a disposable or frequent replacement basis, in which the lenses were inserted once only and then discarded upon removal, would likely have an impact on the infection rates reported. Such a concept became a clinical reality with the introduction of disposable EW lenses to the United States in 1987. The first published large-scale study appeared to support such a concept,[25] but soon thereafter reports of infectious keratitis started to appear.[26] The final proof that disposability had no impact on the rate of ulceration with conventional hydrogel materials worn overnight came with the publication of a paper in 1999,[7] which showed that the rate of ulcerative keratitis was exactly that found 10 years previously in the United States,[6] before disposability was commonplace. This publication clearly showed that overnight wear with conventional soft lens materials should be discouraged because of the increased risk that such a modality had on the development of sight-threatening keratitis.

Despite this, patients still seek methods to liberate them of spectacles, with refractive surgery being extremely popular. Patients still sleep in lenses overnight even when told not to do so, with an estimated 40% of patients occasionally or frequently sleeping in their lenses.[27] Clearly, patients desire a lens that can be worn overnight and will do so whether their practitioner sanctions it or not. To determine the potential safety of materials to be worn overnight, at least from the perspective of hypoxia, requires a detailed knowledge of the oxygen requirements of the cornea.

■ CORNEAL OXYGEN REQUIREMENTS AND OXYGEN TRANSMISSIBILITY

The cornea is avascular and derives most of its oxygen supply from the atmosphere. Any contact lens acts as a potential barrier to oxygen transport, and the ability of a material to transport oxygen through the lens is a major factor in determining the clinical success of that material. The most widely cited figures for the minimum acceptable oxygen transmission (Dk/t) are 24×10^{-9} units for daily wear and 87×10^{-9} units for overnight or EW.[28] More recently, a level of 125×10^{-9} units has been reported as a requirement to prevent stromal anoxia during closed-eye conditions.[29] While these values are often quoted, it must be reiterated that these values are "averages," and patients exhibit widely different corneal oxygen requirements.[30,31]

In addition to understanding the corneal requirements for oxygen, an understanding of the factors relating to the lens that control oxygen transmission is also crucial. Oxygen delivery to the cornea through the lens depends on both the oxygen permeability (Dk) of the material and the thickness (t) of the lens in question. The Dk of conventional hydrogels is directly related to the amount of water that a polymer can hold, as the oxygen dissolves into the water phase of the material and diffuses through the lens from the anterior to the posterior lens surface. The Dk increases logarithmically with increasing water content of the material,[32] and can be determined from the water content using either the non–edge-corrected Fatt formula (Dk = $2.0 \times 10^{-11} e^{0.0411WC}$)[33] or the boundary- and edge-corrected Morgan and Efron formula (Dk = $1.67 \times 10^{-11} e^{0.0397WC}$),[34] in which WC is the quoted water content of the material concerned. The units of Dk are 10^{-11} (cm^2/sec)(mL O$_2$/mL $\times$ mm Hg) or "barrer." The term Dk/t describes the oxygen transmissibility of a lens and gives a quantitative indication of the amount of oxygen that a lens-wearing eye will receive through the lens and is a more clinically useful number than Dk, which gives no indication of the effect of lens thickness or lens design.[35] The units of Dk/t are 10^{-9} (cm/sec)(mL O$_2$/mL $\times$ mm Hg).

Once the Dk/t of the lens in question is known and it is appreciated that such a lens material and design would provide the cornea with suitable levels of oxygenation, then the issue becomes more related to the suitability of the patient to safely adapt to overnight wear.

■ PATIENT SELECTION FOR EXTENDED AND CONTINUOUS WEAR

Patient selection is crucial for success when prescribing contact lenses for any wearing modality, but is particularly important for EW and continuous wear (CW). Practitioners are fortunate to have a wide array of contact lens designs and materials available, such that almost every patient can be successfully fitted. However, care must still be taken to select only those patients suitable for overnight lens wear and then to prescribe the most appropriate lens type for their individual optical, physiologic, vocational, and environmental needs.

A thorough history is essential, not only to assess the patient's motivation and reasons for an overnight wearing modality, but also to evaluate his or her general and ocular health. Systemic disease, medications, allergies, dry eyes, and previous inflammation or infection may contraindicate how contact lenses are worn, and information about the patient's occupation, work environment, and leisure pursuits may also be crucial.

Suitable Candidates

While this appraisal is not intended to serve as an exhaustive list, there are several good reasons for considering an overnight wear modality. A group of obvious candidates for CW are patients with high refractive errors who are vulnerable as a result of their unaided visual performance. These patients benefit enormously from being able to see clearly at all times, particularly when waking during the night. Other prospective patients include those who have an active lifestyle or occupation in which spectacle wear is hazardous or impractical. These groups may include members of the emergency workforce, who often undertake shift work with unpredictable hours and schedules. CW may also be beneficial for parents of young children who demand functional vision within seconds of waking, day and night. There may also be situations where hygiene is a concern and patients are unable to disinfect or handle their contact lenses each day in a sanitary manner because of location. Examples include outdoor enthusiasts and military personnel.

An overnight wear modality may also be used for several therapeutic and bandage applications,[36–40] and in certain binocular conditions, where the likelihood of improving corrected visual acuity in the amblyopic eye is much greater with continuous visual correction. A group of potential candidates for EW or CW also worthy of mention is those individuals who are considering refractive surgery. These modalities of lens wear can be offered either in the short term, such that patients can experience 24-hour visual correction, or as a permanent alternative to irreversible surgical procedures. In addition, many current contact lens wearers admit to occasionally or regularly sleeping while wearing their lenses, and those individuals who report doing this should be proactively counseled on the options of EW and CW, when appropriate.

Unsuitable Candidates

Unfortunately, not all prospective EW and CW candidates are suitable, because of their lifestyle, general health, or ocular appearance. Patients who have a history of noncompliance with instructions for wearing time, replacement frequency, and lens care should probably be avoided, as the consequences of being noncompliant when wearing lenses overnight are potentially higher than in a daily wear mode, and these individuals have also been reported to be at greater risk of infection and inflammation.[41–43] Several studies have also reported a higher prevalence of infiltrative complications in smokers,[6,44,45] and while smoking is not strictly a contraindication to overnight wear, these patients should be counseled with respect to this factor. Another activity that has been reported to be associated with a higher risk of complications among lens wearers is swimming,[46,47] and for this reason EW and CW modalities should be avoided for regular swimmers. General health is also a consideration, and individuals with systemic conditions associated with increased inflammation or a slower healing response may be better suited to a daily wear modality.

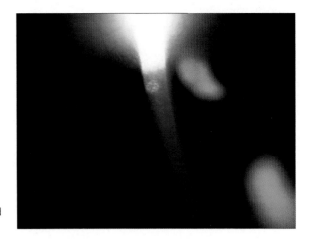

■ **FIGURE 16.1** Scar remaining from a resolved contact lens peripheral ulcer (CLPU).

There are also several ocular conditions that can preclude overnight wear with contact lenses. Patients with chronic blepharitis or meibomian gland dysfunction typically have a higher bacterial load (especially gram positive organisms) on the ocular adnexa,[48,49] increasing their risk for developing corneal infection or inflammation. Severely symptomatic dry eye patients should also be avoided, as their likelihood of successful wear is unlikely, and patients with chronic desiccation staining may also be better with a daily wear modality, as breaks in the epithelial barrier may lead to corneal infection.[50] The decision to fit patients with a history of inflammation will be dependent on the most likely cause of the infiltrates. Corneal scars should be regarded with great suspicion, particularly if they have the typical circular appearance indicative of a resolved contact lens peripheral ulcer (Fig. 16.1). Once there has been one corneal inflammatory response event, there is a much higher risk of the patient developing a further inflammatory event,[45,51–53] and overnight wear should either be avoided or the patient monitored extremely closely.

Once a decision has been made to fit lenses on an overnight basis, then the choice of contact lens material becomes the next important issue.

■ MATERIAL SELECTION FOR EXTENDED AND CONTINUOUS WEAR

Currently, practitioners have four major options for fitting patients who desire overnight wear:

Conventional Hydrogel Materials

As described above, oxygen diffuses through conventional hydrogel materials through the water phase. Unfortunately, this reliance on water to maximize Dk has been a severely limiting factor for the development of hydrogels for overnight wear, as water has a Dk value of only 80 barrer,[54] and thus the oxygen diffusion through the lens is limited. Using the Morgan and Efron formula,[34] it can be seen that the most basic of soft lens polymers, poly-HEMA, has a Dk of only 9 to 10 barrers. To increase the Dk of a conventional hydrogel contact lens material beyond that of poly-HEMA, it is necessary to incorporate monomers that will bind more water into the polymer.[35,55,56] These higher water content materials typically use HEMA or methyl methacrylate (MMA) as the "backbone" monomers, with more hydrophilic monomers such as N-vinyl pyrrolidone (NVP) or methacrylic acid (MA) increasing the water content to 60% to 70%, providing Dk values of close to 30 barrers.[35 55,56] Table 16.1 reports the Dk/t values for several commonly prescribed conventional hydrogel lenses, using the Morgan and Efron formula[34] to derive the Dk values from the published water contents and center thicknesses of

TABLE 16.1 COMMON CONVENTIONAL HYDROGEL CONTACT LENS MATERIALS

COMMERCIAL NAME	MANUFACTURER	WATER CONTENT	DK (EDGE AND BOUNDARY CORRECTED)	CT	DK/T
Frequency 38 (polymacon)	CooperVision	38.0	8	0.07	11
SofLens 38 (polymacon)	Bausch & Lomb	38.0	8	0.035	22
Preference Sphere (tetrafilcon A)	CooperVision	42.5	9	0.07	13
Biomedics 55 (ocufilcon D)	CooperVision	55.0	15	0.07	21
Focus 1–2 Week (vifilcon A)	CIBA Vision	55.0	15	0.06	25
Focus Monthly (vifilcon A)	CIBA Vision	55.0	15	0.10	15
1-Day Acuvue (etafilcon A)	Johnson & Johnson (Vistakon)	58.0	17	0.084	20
Acuvue 2 (etafilcon A)	Johnson & Johnson (Vistakon)	58.0	17	0.084	20
Proclear (omafilcon A)	CooperVision	62.0	20	0.065	30
Focus Dailies (nelfilcon A)	CIBA Vision	69.0	26	0.10	26
SofLens One Day (hilafilcon A)	Bausch & Lomb	70.0	27	0.17	16

CT, center thickness; Dk, oxygen permeability; Dk/t, oxygen transmission.

−3.00 D lenses. It must be remembered that these Dk/t values will be lower for positively powered lenses and high minus lenses because of the increased lens thickness inherent with such lens designs.

Inspection of Table 16.1 clearly shows that conventional hydrogel lens materials provide woefully inadequate oxygen transmissibilities for safe, edema-free overnight wear, given the required Dk/t values reported above for overnight wear. This awareness of the shortcomings of conventional hydrogel materials resulted in the development of novel materials that would provide increased amounts of oxygen to the corneal surface.

Silicone Elastomers

The first group of materials to provide significantly enhanced oxygen transmission was based on silicone rubber, and these "silicone elastomers" became clinically available in the early 1970s.[57,58] These lenses provided sufficient oxygen transport to the ocular surface for overnight wear, with Dk values >300 barrers,[59] and they were used for both therapeutic and pediatric applications for over 20 years.[60] However, despite their exceptional oxygen transmission and durability, several major limitations were associated with their use in clinical practice. Fluid is unable to flow through these materials, resulting in frequent lens binding to the ocular surface,[61] and the lens surfaces are extremely hydrophobic, resulting in marked lipid and mucous deposition.[62,63] A silicone elastomer lens is still available (Silsoft, Bausch & Lomb), but its clinical usage is very low because of its high cost, limited parameter availability. and poor surface wettability.

Rigid Gas-Permeable Materials

In the 1960s and early '70s, the only rigid lens material available was polymethyl methacrylate (PMMA). Despite their low cost and excellent biocompatibility, PMMA lenses gradually lost their popularity because of their lack of oxygen permeability, and in 1978 the first truly gas-permeable lens material (Boston 1) was introduced, which incorporated a silicon-containing monomer commonly called TRIS, which resulted in a marked increase in oxygen permeability.[64,65] Over the next decade polymer chemists started to increase the silicone content of rigid GP lenses in an attempt to increase oxygen permeability.[66] This strategy worked well, until a Dk value in the mid-1950s was reached, at which point the silicone content was so high that the surface acquired a small but significant electrostatic charge.[66,67] This negative charge attracted positively charged lysozymes from the patient's tear film and, after a few months of lens wear, tenacious protein deposits bound to the lens surface, preventing the surface from wetting properly and inducing inflammatory changes in some patients. In addition, such materials often displayed poor dimensional stability,[68] were relatively brittle,[69] easily scratched,[70] and occasionally exhibited lens "crazing" because of poor or variable polymerization procedures.[71–74]

In an attempt to reduce surface deposition but maintain gas permeability, manufacturers started to produce fluorosilicone acrylates in the late 1980s, in which fluorine was added to enhance wettability and oxygen permeability to levels above that previously available in silicone acrylates.[59,75] Studies have demonstrated that fluorosilicone acrylates deposit less protein than silicone acrylates[76] while maintaining high levels of oxygen transmission.

Silicone acrylate GP materials for overnight wear were initially fitted in the early 1980s and proved relatively successful.[77–79] However, some patients still showed hypoxic complications when lenses were worn for extended periods of time.[80] Improved manufacturing methods have now resulted in the development of several sophisticated GP lens materials that have Dk values of over 100 barrer (Table 16.2), which provides adequate oxygenation for overnight wear in the

TABLE 16.2 COMMON RIGID LENS MATERIALS

NAME	MATERIAL TYPE	MANUFACTURER-QUOTED DK	DK/T
Boston II	Silicone acrylate	12	8
Boston IV	Silicone acrylate	19	13
Boston 7	Fluorosilicone acrylate	49	33
Boston EO	Fluorosilicone acrylate	58	39
Boston Equalens	Fluorosilicone acrylate	47	31
Boston XO	Fluorosilicone acrylate	100	67
Boston Equalens II	Fluorosilicone acrylate	85	57
Fluoroperm 30	Fluorosilicone acrylate	30	20
Fluoroperm 60	Fluorosilicone acrylate	60	40
Fluoroperm 92	Fluorosilicone acrylate	92	61
Fluoroperm 151	Fluorosilicone acrylate	151	101
Menicon Z	Siloxanylstyrene-based fluoromethacrylate	163	125
Paragon HDS	Fluorosilicone acrylate	58	39
Paragon HDS 100	Fluorosilicone acrylate	100	67
Paraperm EW	Silicone acrylate	56	37

Dk, oxygen permeability; Dk/t, oxygen transmission at a "standardized" center thickness of 0.15 mm.

majority of patients.[81–83] Of these, the Menicon Z material is the only GP material that is FDA approved for up to 30 nights CW and has proven to be successful when worn in this way.[84–87]

Despite the fact that GP lenses have been successful from a physiologic perspective, issues relating to lens binding,[80,88,89] acquired ptosis,[90] and peripheral corneal staining[80,91] have limited their clinical usage.

Silicone Hydrogel Materials

Since the development of silicone acrylate GP and silicone elastomeric soft lens materials, the advantages of incorporating siloxane groups into contact lens materials, from an oxygen transmission perspective, have been well known. Since the late 1970s, manufacturers have tried to incorporate silicone into conventional HEMA-based hydrogel materials to develop high-Dk hydrogels. However, the chemistry required to successfully achieve this is very complex, and it was not until the late 1990s that this became commercially possible.

Eight silicone hydrogel lens materials are currently available, with their major features being summarized in Table 16.3. As described above, the incorporation of siloxane groups into hydrogel materials is complex, as silicone is inherently hydrophobic. A huge impediment to the development of silicone hydrogel lenses is related to the decreased surface wettability, increased lipid interaction, and accentuated lens binding previously seen in silicone elastomers. To make the surfaces of silicone hydrogel lens materials hydrophilic and more wettable, techniques incorporating plasma into the surface processing of the lens have been developed.[65,92–94] More recent techniques have involved incorporating hydrophilic monomers into the lens material that "migrate" to the surface of the lens and aid wettability.[95,96] The purpose of these surface modifications is to mask the hydrophobic silicone from the tear film, increasing the surface wettability of the materials and reducing lipid deposition. In addition to complications induced by poor surface wettability, the incorporation of siloxane moieties results in an increase in the modulus or "stiffness" of the lens materials, resulting in silicone hydrogel materials being significantly "stiffer" than their conventional hydrogel counterparts.

Space limitations prevent an extensive review of the technology behind these materials, and fuller reviews can be found elsewhere.[1,56,65,97] However, the differences that do exist are fairly closely related to the company that manufactures them, and thus a brief overview of the lenses will be provided by dividing them into the companies who currently have commercially available lenses.

Bausch & Lomb

Bausch and Lomb's PureVision material, balafilcon A, is a homogeneous combination of the silicone-containing monomer polydimethylsiloxane (a vinyl carbamate derivative of TRIS) copolymerized with the hydrophilic hydrogel monomer NVP.[92,98–100] PureVision lenses are surface treated in a reactive gas plasma chamber, which transforms the silicone components on the surface of the lenses into hydrophilic silicate compounds.[65,92,99,101] Glassy, discontinuous silicate "islands" result,[99,102] and the hydrophilicity of the transformed surface areas "bridges" over the underlying balafilcon A material. PureVision is one of only two lenses approved for up to 30 days of CW, and clinical trials have shown the lens to be effective when used in this way.[103–105] It is also one of only three silicone hydrogels approved for use as a therapeutic bandage lens, and several studies have demonstrated its value when used in this manner.[36,106,107]

CIBA Vision

CIBA Vision has four silicone hydrogel lenses. Focus Night & Day material, lotrafilcon A, employs a co-continuous biphasic or two channel molecular structure, in which two phases persist from the front to the back surface of the lens,[93] and their O₂OPTIX and AirOptix Aqua

TABLE 16.3 SILICONE HYDROGEL LENS MATERIALS

PROPRIETARY NAME	FOCUS NIGHT & DAY	AIROPTIX AQUA & O2OPTIX	PUREVISION	ACUVUE OASYS	ACUVUE ADVANCE	BIOFINITY	MENICON PREMIO
U.S.-adopted name	lotrafilcon A	lotrafilcon B	balafilcon A	senofilcon A	galyfilcon A	comfilcon A	asmofilcon A
Manufacturer	CIBA Vision	CIBA Vision	Bausch & Lomb	Johnson & Johnson	Johnson & Johnson	CooperVision	Menicon
Center thickness (@ −3.00 D) mm	0.08	0.08	0.09	0.07	0.07	0.08	0.08
Water content (%)	24	33	36	38	47	48	40
Oxygen permeability ($\times 10^{-11}$)	140	110	91	103	60	128	129
Oxygen transmissibility ($\times 10^{-9}$)	175	138	101	147	86	160	161
Surface treatment	25-nm plasma coating with high refractive index	25-nm plasma coating with high refractive index	Plasma oxidation process	No surface treatment. Internal wetting agent (PVP) throughout the matrix that also coats the surface	No surface treatment Internal wetting agent (PVP) throughout the matrix that also coats the surface	None	Plasma oxidation
FDA group	I	I	III	I	I	I	I
Principal monomers	DMA + TRIS + siloxane macromer	DMA + TRIS + siloxane macromer	NVP + TPVC + NCVE + PBVC	mPDMS + DMA + HEMA + siloxane macromer + TEGDMA + PVP	mPDMS + DMA + EGDMA + HEMA + siloxane macromer + PVP	FM0411M; HOB; IBM; M3U; NVP; TAIC; VMA	*1

*1, Principal monomers will be disclosed after USAN registration.

DMA, N,N-dimethylacrylamide; EGDMA, ethyleneglycol dimethacrylate; FM0411M, a-methacryloyloxyethyl iminocarboxyethyloxypropyl-poly(dimethylsiloxy)-butyldimethylsilane; HEMA, poly-2-hydroxyethyl methacrylate; HOB, 2-hydroxybutyl methacrylate; IBM, isobornyl methacrylate; MA, methacrylic acid; mPDMS, monofunctional polydimethylsiloxane; NVP, N-vinyl pyrrolidone; TEGDMA, tetraethyleneglycol dimethacrylate; TPVC, tris-(trimethylsiloxysilyl) propylvinyl carbamate; TRIS, trimethylsiloxy silane; M3U, α ω-bis(methacryloyloxyethyl iminocarboxy ethyloxypropyl)-poly(dimethylsiloxane)-poly(ω-methoxy-poly(ethyleneglycol)propyl methylsiloxane); NCVE, N-carboxyvinyl ester; PBVC, poly(dimethysiloxy)-di (silylbutanol)-bis(vinyl carbamate); PC, phosphorylcholine; PVP, polyvinyl pyrrolidone; TAIC, 1,3,5-triallyl-1,3,5-triazine-2,4,6($1H,3H,5H$)-trione; VMA, N-vinyl-N-methylacetamide.

lenses (lotrafilcon B) are based on very similar technology. These lenses are manufactured via a cast molding process, as are all the other silicone hydrogel lenses, with the exception of CIBA Vision's final offering, the O₂OPTIX Custom lens (sifilcon A), which is lathe-cut.[108] This lens is available in a wide variety of parameters[108] and is an ideal option for patients who require silicone hydrogels but are outside the conventional parameter range offered by the majority of frequent replacement lenses, thus needing a custom-made option.[109,110] The surfaces of all four lenses are permanently modified in a gas plasma chamber using a mixture of trimethylsilane oxygen and methane to create a permanent, ultrathin (25 nm), high refractive index, continuous hydrophilic surface.[93,99,102,111–113] Focus Night & Day is approved for up to 30 nights of CW and successful results have been reported with the lens used in this manner[52,105,114–119] and it is also approved for use as a therapeutic lens.[37–40,106,120,121] On a daily wear basis both lotrafilcon materials have proven to be clinically successful.[122–125]

CooperVision

CooperVision offers the Biofinity lens, which is manufactured from comfilcon A and reportedly has a higher oxygen permeability than would be predicted from its water content,[97,126] implying that the chemistry on which it is based is different from that employed in other silicone hydrogels. To date, little data have been published on the lens, but its performance appears comparable on overnight wear to other silicone hydrogels.[127,128]

Johnson & Johnson (Vistakon)

Johnson & Johnson's Acuvue Advance material, galyfilcon A, has the highest water content of all the silicone hydrogel materials (47%) and thus the lowest Dk and is only approved for daily wear. It has an ultraviolet (UV) blocker, with a reported class 1 UV protection, blocking >90% of UVA and >99% of UVB rays.[129–131] Acuvue OASYS lens (senofilcon A) also has class 1 UV-blocking capabilities.[131] The Acuvue Advance lens material was the first nonsurface-treated silicone hydrogel to become a commercial reality, closely followed by Acuvue OASYS. The senofilcon A material used to manufacture the Acuvue OASYS lens is based on similar chemistry to that of the galyfilcon A material in Acuvue Advance. Both materials incorporate a long chain high molecular weight internal wetting agent based on polyvinylpyrrolidone (PVP), which is designed to provide a hydrophilic layer at the surface of the material that "shields" the silicone at the material interface, thereby reducing the degree of hydrophobicity typically seen at the surface of siloxane hydrogels.[129,130] The Advance lens internal wetting agent is termed Hydraclear, and that used for the OASYS lens is HydraClear Plus, implying that more PVP is probably incorporated. The OASYS lens has been well received by the profession, clinically appears to deposit less than Acuvue Advance, and has been particularly successful in subjects with symptoms of contact lens-induced dryness.[132–134]

Menicon

The newest "kid on the block" is the PremiO lens from Menicon (asmofilcon A).[135] This lens is currently only available in a limited number of markets, and no data are yet available on its clinical performance. The lens uses a patented polymerization system to combine the siloxane and hydrophilic monomers (Menisilk) and uses a novel plasma surface treatment that, according to Menicon, combines the benefits of both plasma coating (as exemplified in the lotrafilcon A and lotrafilcon B materials from CIBA Vision)[94,102,136,137] and plasma oxidation (as seen in the surface treatment process used with the Bausch & Lomb balafilcon A material).[94,100,102] It is packaged in a unique heart-shaped blister and has an oxygen permeability that is higher than would be predicted from its water content.

■ CLINICAL PERFORMANCE OF SOFT CONTACT LENS MATERIALS WORN OVERNIGHT

Hypoxia and acidosis are perhaps the greatest challenges for any soft lens worn on an overnight basis. Acidosis results from hypercapnia (increase of carbon dioxide) and is often associated with hypoxia.[138,139] In addition, oxygen flow and the release of carbon dioxide waste products are impeded by the contact lens, and all these factors result in significant stresses on the cornea.

Of the four material options listed above, the majority of patients will wear either HEMA-based materials or silicone hydrogels. The potential complications associated with the overnight wear of these two materials are summarized in Table 16.4 and detailed below.

Potential Complications Associated with Conventional Hydrogel Materials

The major complications induced by overnight wear of HEMA-based materials are because of the fact that they provide insufficient oxygen to the cornea.

Striae and Folds

Hypoxia within the corneal stroma results in the accumulation of lactic acid and a subsequent influx of fluid from the anterior chamber, resulting in "edema" and a physical increase in corneal thickness.[140] This is an acute response to hypoxia and very often there are no symptoms associated with mild edema, but, in extreme cases, decreased vision, glare, halos, and photophobia can occur. With overnight wear of low-Dk conventional hydrogel lens materials, corneal swelling is typically in the order of 1% to 5% during the day, increasing to approximately 10% overnight.[141–144] Measurements of corneal thickness are made using a pachometer. Clinically, the presence of corneal swelling may be observed as the appearance of striae and folds, which occur as a direct result of corneal swelling.[145–148] Striae are vertical, grayish-white, wispy lines in the stroma seen with a parallelepiped and appear when edema exceeds 5%.[149] These folds appear as a physical "buckling" in the Descemet membrane, are seen as black, deep grooves with direct focal illumination, and are observed when edema of 10% or more occurs.[149] These acute responses are reversible on eye opening, but repeated overnight wear with conventional hydrogel lenses has been shown to result in many detrimental effects on corneal structure and function. The amount of oxygen required to eliminate edematous complications is a matter for some conjecture, with estimates suggesting that during overnight wear 87- to

TABLE 16.4 POTENTIAL COMPLICATIONS FOR HEMA-BASED AND SILICONE HYDROGEL MATERIALS WORN OVERNIGHT

HEMA-BASED HYDROGEL	SILICONE HYDROGEL	EITHER HYDROGEL
Stromal striae	Mucin balls	Contact lens acute red eye
Stromal folds	Superior epithelial arcuate lesions	Contact lens peripheral ulcer
Epithelial microcysts	Conjunctival flaps	Infiltrative keratitis
Endothelial polymegethism	Corneal erosions	Microbial keratitis
Limbal hyperemia	Papillary conjunctivitis	
Stromal neovascularization		
Reduced corneal sensitivity		
Reduced epithelial thickness		
Stromal thinning		

125-Dk/t units are necessary.[28,150–153] Conventional lenses clearly fall drastically short of these requirements (see Table 16.1), and edema can therefore be expected to occur for the vast majority of patients who wear these materials overnight. The same cannot be said for highly oxygen transmissible GP and silicone hydrogel lenses (Tables 16.2 and 16.3) and striae and folds would be expected to rarely, if ever, be observed in these patients.

Epithelial Microcysts

In addition to acute responses to hypoxia, the cornea also responds to chronic hypoxia. A common chronic response is the development of epithelial microcysts, which present as small (5–30 μm) inclusions or dots located in the epithelium.[154, 155] Low numbers of microcysts can occur without lens wear, but their prevalence increases when conventional hydrogel lenses are worn overnight,[156] and they are rarely observed in patients wearing silicone hydrogel lenses.[157,158] They are composed of necrotic cellular tissue or debris, which has a relatively high refractive index and results in the characteristic reversed illumination observed when viewed using marginal retroillumination.[156,159,160] Patients with microcysts are usually asymptomatic. Microcysts typically occur after approximately 2 months of chronic hypoxia and increase in number over the next 2 to 4 months, after which their numbers level off. Microcysts originate in the deeper layers of the epithelium and migrate anteriorly. If they reach the surface, they break through the epithelium, causing staining and occasionally a mild interference in vision. Treatment is discontinuation of lens wear or refitting with a contact lens of greater oxygen transmissibility. Recovery typically takes 4 to 6 weeks, and an initial increase in the numbers of microcysts usually occurs, as the cornea suddenly becomes reoxygenated.[161] The numbers of microcysts then gradually reduce over a 2- to 3-month period to the point where they are eliminated.[160]

Endothelial Polymegethism

The endothelium has also been shown to demonstrate changes in morphology because of chronic hypoxia. Polymegethism was first reported 25 years ago[162] and describes a change in size of the endothelial cells that occurs when low-Dk/t lenses are worn.[163–167] While this condition is initially asymptomatic, patients may eventually exhibit intolerance to contact lens wear.[168] Polymegethism does not occur in wearers of silicone hydrogel lens materials[157] or when hyperpermeable GP lenses are worn overnight.[169]

Limbal Hyperemia

Overnight lens wear with conventional hydrogel lenses frequently results in limbal hyperemia.[170] Increases in limbal redness are seen rapidly when conventional lens materials are worn, even on a daily wear basis, with detectable differences being seen within just a few hours of lens insertion.[151] Hypoxia has been shown to be a major contributing factor to limbal hyperemia, particularly in studies comparing the limbal response between silicone hydrogel lenses and conventional hydrogel lenses, where changes can be observed over both short- and long-term periods of time,[125,151,171,172] and extremely good evidence now exists to support the theory that limbal hyperemia is directly related to lens material oxygen transmissibility.[173] A rapid reduction in limbal redness can be observed when patients are refitted into silicone hydrogel lenses, even when they are worn on an overnight basis (Fig. 16.2A,B).

Neovascularization

In addition to limbal hyperemia associated with EW of conventional hydrogel lenses, chronic new vessel formation also frequently occurs. This "neovascularization" is defined as the formation and extension of capillaries into a previously avascular corneal area.[174] Studies have indicated that up to 65% of patients using conventional hydrogel lenses on an EW basis exhibit some level of neovascularization.[141] This is in comparison with no evidence of neovasculariza-

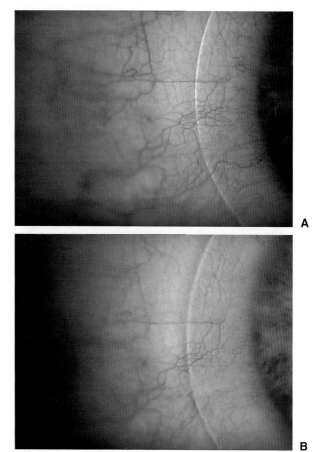

A

B

■ **FIGURE 16.2 (A)** Limbal hyperemia subsequent to conventional hydrogel lens wear on an extended wear basis. **(B)** Reduction in limbal hyperemia in the same eye as **A** when refitted with a silicone hydrogel lens for extended wear.

tion in patients using silicone hydrogel lens materials.[105,141,171] Patients who do exhibit neovascularization demonstrate regression of the vessel response following refitting with silicone hydrogels in as little as 1 month (Fig. 16.3A,B). The new vessels do not simply disappear, but "ghost vessels" remain,[175] and these ghost vessels can fill rapidly if adversely stimulated again.

Other Chronic Corneal Changes

Several other changes to the cornea frequently occur as a result of EW-induced hypoxia, but these may not be so apparent to the eye care practitioner. They include reduced corneal sensitivity,[176,177] reduced oxygen uptake by the epithelium,[164] decreased epithelial thickness,[164] and, perhaps of greatest concern, greater bacterial adherence.[178–181] In addition, although acute hypoxia is known to result in corneal swelling, chronic hypoxia can result in long-term stromal thinning.[164,182,183]

Myopic Shift

Chronic hypoxia is also the presumed cause of a myopic prescription shift, which can occur in some patients who wear conventional hydrogel lenses on an EW basis.[22,184,185] Similar to the reversal of other chronic responses to hypoxia, patients may show a hyperopic shift when refitted with silicone hydrogel lenses.[115,184,185] This can be clinically significant if a refitting occurs in a patient who is on the verge of presbyopia. Approximately 1 month after refitting, all patients should be carefully overrefracted, as the patient may be wearing a lens that is overminused or underplussed, possibly resulting in near vision problems.

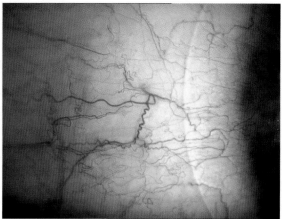

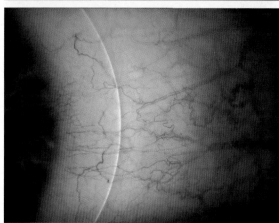

■ **FIGURE 16.3 (A)** Neovascularization subsequent to extended wear with a conventional low oxygen permeability lens. **(B)** Regression of neovascularization in the contralateral eye of the same patient as shown in **A** following refitting with a silicone hydrogel lens worn on an extended wear basis for 1 month.

Corneal Staining

A common complication observed with EW of conventional hydrogel lenses is corneal staining, also called superficial punctate staining (SPS) or superficial punctate keratitis (SPK). This can take on the appearance of small punctate spots to large, dense, confluent patches.[186] One of the possible causes of staining is hypoxia, and it is particularly important to monitor staining in EW and CW wearers because it represents a break in the epithelial barrier, which may act as a subsequent portal for the entry of bacteria.

The disadvantages of overnight wear with these HEMA-based materials relate to both the very low levels of oxygen provided by these lenses compared with silicone hydrogels[187,188] and the increased rates of complications reported when such lenses are worn overnight.[5–7] Given the long list of documented complications associated with the overnight wear of HEMA-based materials, it cannot any longer be considered clinically acceptable to support the use of these materials for overnight wear.

Potential Complications Associated with Silicone Hydrogel Materials

The principal advantage of silicone hydrogel lenses for overnight wear is their excellent ability to transmit oxygen,[65,150,188] which has resulted in the elimination of the hypoxic complications described earlier.[12,52,157] Despite these higher levels of oxygen available to the cornea when wearing silicone hydrogel lenses, mechanical, inflammatory, and infectious complications still occur. When silicone hydrogels were first introduced, limitations in parameter availability prevented every prospective patient from being able to realize their benefits for overnight wear, but with current ranges of powers, base curves, and lens designs, there are very few individuals who are now unable to be fitted with these lenses, if desired.

As discussed in the section on silicone hydrogel materials, the major disadvantages with these materials are their relatively hydrophobic surfaces and high modulus of elasticity. The first two silicone hydrogel lenses to be introduced (lotrafilcon A and balafilcon A) had very high modulus values compared with HEMA-based hydrogels, as they were primarily intended for overnight wear and thus oxygen transport was critical. This resulted in the lenses having high siloxane contents (providing very high Dk values), but correspondingly very high modulus values.[1,56,97] While this increased rigidity was beneficial for lens handling, it was certainly implicated in a variety of mechanical complications that were initially seen with these lenses, particularly when they were worn on a CW basis.[10,12,51,52,189] The silicone hydrogels that have more recently been introduced into the market tend to have lower modulus values[1,56,97] and mechanical complications with these lenses appear to be less common. Inflammatory and infectious complications remain a concern with overnight wear of silicone hydrogel lenses and appear to be more patient than material dependent. The following section will briefly review the complications that tend to occur with silicone hydrogel materials.

Mucin Balls

Post-tear lens debris often occurs with overnight lens wear, particularly with silicone hydrogel lenses. The most commonly reported debris is referred to as "mucin balls."[190–194] These are pearly, translucent, 20- to 100-μm spherical particles observed between the back surface of a contact lens and the cornea[10] (Fig. 16.4), which have been shown to consist of mucin and lipid.[194] They are believed to occur when relatively stiff lens materials "shear" the tear film and roll up small balls of mucin and lipid from the tear film. When the lenses are removed, transient depressions are left in the epithelium,[192,195] which pool with fluorescein.[10,190] In most cases, patients are asymptomatic and there is complete resolution within a few hours. Mucin balls have not been shown to be associated with any clinical complications, although a recent retrospective study has shown a three times greater risk of inflammation in daily wearers of silicone hydrogel lenses who have mucin balls compared with those who do not.[196]

Superior Epithelial Arcuate Lesions

Another mechanical complication that can occur with all hydrogel lenses, but that appears to be more common with silicone hydrogel lenses, is superior epithelial arcuate lesions (SEALs).[10,51,186,197–202] These typically present as an arcuate break in the epithelium approximately 1 mm from the limbus; however, in some silicone hydrogel wearers the lesion may be

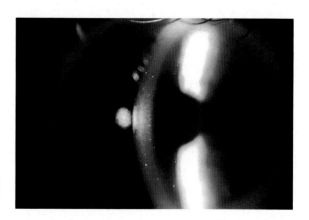

■ **FIGURE 16.4** Mucin balls observed between the back surface of a silicone hydrogel lens and the cornea.

closer to the central cornea.[198,201,203] The edges may be irregular, roughened, or thickened, particularly if the SEAL is associated with diffuse or focal infiltration. SEALs are frequently asymptomatic but may be associated with a mild foreign body sensation following lens removal.[10,52] SEALs can occur for several reasons, but are most likely the result of the stiff nature of silicone hydrogel materials and/or their inflexibility to conform to the limbus, causing increased mechanical pressure.[198,202] Management requires temporary discontinuation of lens wear for 1 to 2 days. Patients should be warned that their symptoms may increase initially, and ocular lubricants can be dispensed to relieve discomfort. In cases of reoccurrence, refitting with a different design or material may be indicated.[10,51] An example of a SEAL occurring in a silicone hydrogel lens wearer is described in Case 1 at the end of this chapter.

Bulbar Conjunctival Disruptions

Indentation and mild staining of the conjunctival tissue can occur with all soft lenses and is generally not too concerning if there is no subjective discomfort and associated adverse effects do not occur. A relatively new clinical finding affecting the bulbar conjunctiva associated with silicone hydrogel lenses, particularly when worn on an EW or CW basis, has been reported. It is referred to as *lens induced epithelial flaps* (LIFEs) or *conjunctival epithelial flaps* (CEFs).[204–207] These terms are used to describe areas of conjunctival epithelium that separate from the underlying tissue. They can be best appreciated with the use of fluorescein and a yellow barrier filter.[208] The "flaps" are usually observed up to 1 mm away from the lens edge superiorly and/or inferiorly and have a roughened or jagged appearance (Fig. 16.5). There does not appear to be any sign of associated inflammation in the area, and lens wearers are asymptomatic. While the condition appears benign, clinicians may choose to refit patients with alternative lens designs or materials if the presentation persists.

Corneal Abrasions and Erosions

Corneal abrasions and erosions can occur with all lens types. The etiology for these conditions is trauma from either a foreign body getting under the lens and abrading the superficial epithelial cells or the contact lens becoming "bound" to the epithelium and disturbing the cells when it regains mobility. This is more likely with overnight lens wear than daily lens wear,[51,189] and the severity of symptoms associated with these conditions varies considerably. The epithelium is disrupted (Fig. 16.6) and the affected area stains with fluorescein. In almost all cases simply removing the lens allows rapid resolution. Ocular lubricants may be used, but in most cases no medication is required. Severe cases may benefit from a prophylactic topical antibiotic, analgesics, or mydriatics.[189]

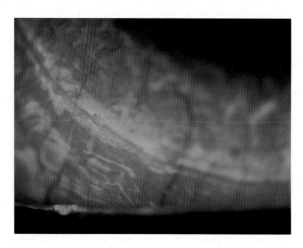

■ **FIGURE 16.5** Conjunctival disruption, as shown with fluorescein staining, subsequent to continuous wear with a silicone hydrogel lens ("epithelial flap").

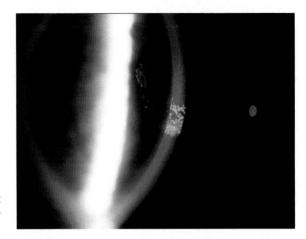

■ **FIGURE 16.6** Corneal erosion in a patient wearing silicone hydrogel lenses on a continuous-wear basis.

Contact Lens Papillary Conjunctivitis

Contact lens papillary conjunctivitis (CLPC) is believed to be both mechanical and immunologic in nature.[10,51,189,209–211] CLPC had become a relatively rare complication with conventional hydrogel EW since the introduction of frequent replacement lenses,[117,209,212–215] but the introduction of CW silicone hydrogels initially saw a resurgence of this condition.[10,189,216–219] A combination of the increased stiffness and edge designs of some of these lenses was implicated,[10,189] but newer designs and lower modulus silicone hydrogel materials appear to have diminished the prevalence once again. CLPC presents with changes to the palpebral conjunctiva, consisting of increased hyperemia and papillary excrescences. The papillae present either diffusely across the entire palpebral conjunctiva or may be in a localized area.[117,189,216,217] The symptoms associated with this condition in silicone hydrogel wearers are generally rapid in onset and include foreign body sensation or discomfort, itching, stringy or ropy mucous discharge, and in some cases lens mislocation, particularly during sleep.[10,189] Cases of CLPC that are mechanical in origin generally resolve very quickly, simply by ceasing lens wear and either wearing spectacles or daily disposable lenses for a period of approximately 2 weeks. A topical antihistamine/mast cell stabilizer may also be used to manage CLPC. Changes to wearing schedule, lens design, and material may then be required to prevent reoccurrence. An example of CLPC occurring in a silicone hydrogel lens wearer is described in Case 2 at the end of this chapter.

Potential Complications Associated with All Soft Materials

While the previous two sections have concentrated on the complications associated with conventional or silicone hydrogel lenses, it is important to emphasize that there are many complications that can occur with EW and CW of *all* soft lenses, and these are covered in the following section.

Contact Lens Acute Red Eye

Contact lens acute red eye (CLARE) is a unilateral, acute inflammatory condition that occurs with EW and CW in response to gram negative organisms (e.g., *Pseudomonas* spp.) colonizing the lens and releasing endotoxins.[220–224] A higher incidence of CLARE occurs in patients with upper respiratory infection, and these cases may be because of the presence of other gram negative organisms, including *Haemophilus influenzae*.[221] Patients with CLARE are typically woken in the early morning by a moderately painful (foreign body sensation) red eye, with associated epiphora and photophobia. Focal or diffuse subepithelial infiltrates are usually observed in the midperiphery of the cornea close to the limbus. The infiltrates rarely stain and rapidly resolve.[189] CLARE is self-limiting on removal of contact lenses. It is therefore generally managed with temporary discontinuation of lens wear and ocular lubricants during the acute stage.

Contact Lens Peripheral Ulcer

A contact lens peripheral ulcer (CLPU) is an inflammatory response that results in lesions often termed *sterile ulcers*.[225,226] The etiology of this condition is a hypersensitive reaction to the (usually gram positive) exotoxins released by pathogenic bacteria.[227,228] Signs include a single, small, circular, peripheral or midperipheral grayish-white lesion in the anterior stroma.[189,226] Symptoms include mild to moderate pain (foreign body sensation), mild lacrimation, and mild photophobia.[51,189,226] Following the acute presentation, the epithelium regenerates within a few days. Diffuse infiltration surrounding the lesion may develop. A very well-defined circular "scar" remains, gradually fading with time but still present several months after the event.[51,189,226] Differential diagnosis from microbial keratitis is extremely important.[51,229] An example of CLPU occurring in a silicone hydrogel lens wearer is described in Case 3 at the end of this chapter.

Infiltrative Keratitis

Infiltrative keratitis (IK) is a general term used to describe inflammatory events within the cornea. All cases of IK exhibit the presence of infiltrates within the cornea, which can be located anywhere but are usually peripherally situated in the limbal area, often with associated limbal hyperemia.[51,189,230] Many IK cases are because of the presence of gram positive exotoxins found on the lid margin.[223,230] Symptoms include mild to moderate irritation (often a foreign body discomfort), mild redness, lacrimation, photophobia, and occasionally mild discharge.[51,189,230] There is a large degree of variability in the severity of symptoms associated with IK, and in some cases there are no symptoms that are associated with the infiltrates. This condition is termed *asymptomatic infiltrative keratitis* (AIK) and its cause is unknown.[189] Temporary discontinuation of lens wear results in full resolution of signs and symptoms normally within a few days. In most cases no additional treatment is required; however, ocular lubricants may be dispensed to alleviate symptoms.[51]

Incidence of Inflammatory Complications

It is extremely difficult to accurately report the incidence rates for inflammatory conditions, as the percentages reported for corneal infiltrates vary significantly, depending on the study design and the criteria used for reporting infiltrates, which can vary widely.[231] A recent publication used a meta-analysis methodology to determine the incidence levels and relative risks for inflammatory complications with overnight wear in conventional and silicone hydrogel lens wearers.[232] This study concluded that there appears to be approximately twice the risk of developing inflammation in silicone hydrogel wearers compared with conventional lens wearers (14.4 and 7.7 per 100 eye-years, respectively) when the lenses are worn overnight. However, the majority of silicone hydrogel lenses were worn on a CW basis and conventional lenses were worn on an EW basis, and the number of nights of overnight wear may confound the overall results. What is clear is that there appears to be a patient predisposition for inflammatory events and approximately 10% to 25% of EW and CW patients in clinical trials have been reported to experience repeat episodes.[51,53,233] It may be advisable for those who do experience repeated events to switch to a flexible wear schedule, with only occasional overnight lens wear.

Microbial Keratitis

Microbial keratitis (MK) is the most serious complication associated with contact lens wear and was the greatest concern with EW of conventional hydrogel lenses. Fortunately, the prevalence of MK within the general population is extremely low, in part because of the exceptional defense mechanisms that protect the ocular surface.[234–236] The microorganisms most commonly associated with MK in contact lens wearers are the *Pseudomonas* spp. (principally *aeruginosa*),[237–239] but many different microorganisms have been cultured from cases of MK in contact lens patients.[240] The major risk factors for MK include overnight wear, poor compliance, epithelial trauma, smoking, and swimming in lenses.[231,241,242] The generally accepted figure for the annualized incidence of MK in conventional hydrogel daily wear patients is 4 per 10,000 wearers,[5,7,231] and EW has been reported to increase this risk by approximately five times.[5–7,231] Although it was initially hoped that the risks would be lower with CW of silicone hydrogels, study results now indicate that the risk level is similar to that found with conventional HEMA-based materials.[16,231,243]

Patients with MK usually experience severe pain, lacrimation, hyperemia, and photophobia.[51,189,229] Any area of the cornea may be affected, and the clinical appearance is usually of a single irregular infiltrative lesion with excavation of the epithelium, Bowman layer, and stroma. An anterior chamber reaction and lid edema are also common, and visual acuity may be reduced.[51,189,229] An example of MK occurring in a conventional hydrogel lens wearer is described in Case 4 at the end of this chapter.

MK is considered an ocular emergency, and treatment must be instigated immediately to achieve the best possible outcome.[242,244–247] Because most cases of MK in contact lens wearers are bacterial, treatment is with antibiotic agents unless other prognostic signs exist. Initial treatment is generally with fluoroquinolone monotherapy and supplemental cycloplegics and analgesics are given as required.[248–251] In severe cases, fortified antibiotics may also be prescribed.[252,253] Prognosis for most patients is good and most cases resolve without visual loss,[16] even though a scar remains, but this does depend on the causative organism. The recent cases of *Fusarium* keratitis[254–258] and *Acanthamoeba* keratitis[259–261] are typically much more severe and have frequently resulted in significant loss of best corrected vision, and in many cases, corneal transplantation is required.[257,262]

▪ PATIENT EDUCATION

Prescribing contact lenses for EW and CW represents some unique challenges, and certain adaptations to the contact lens fitting routine and management of patients using these lenses require discussion. In an increasingly litigious society, clinicians should exercise caution when fitting contact lenses that may result in an increased risk of complications. The most likely legal claim is one of negligence, and the most common causes of liability are inappropriate patient selection, providing inadequate instructions, prescribing improper wearing schedules, inadequate monitoring of ocular health, and incorrect management of contact lens-related complications. Appropriate patient education plays a key role in the success of overnight wearing modalities and reduces the likelihood of possible litigation.[263]

Informed Consent or Patient Agreement

It is highly recommended that practitioners develop documents that give clear information about the contact lenses to be worn, the overnight wearing modality (EW or CW), the risks and benefits for this modality, instructions on how to avoid complications, and what steps to take if a complication is suspected.[264–269] Several separate documents can be utilized or the information can be combined into one. An important element is either an informed consent or a patient–practitioner agreement, and examples of such documents have been previously described.[270]

Comfort and Adaptation

Properly fitted lenses are vital to provide optimum patient comfort and minimize the risk of mechanically induced adverse responses. Trial lens fitting should always be undertaken before the commencement of EW and CW and, if any problem with fit is observed or if significant discomfort is reported, an alternative design or product should be tried. Initial comfort during trial fitting greatly influences the patient's perception of contact lenses[271] and may have an effect on their ultimate success.

Lenses that decenter or do not provide complete corneal coverage should be avoided because they may result in corneal desiccation or limbal chafing. As discussed previously, the higher modulus of silicone hydrogel lenses renders them stiffer, and therefore the physical lens-to-cornea curvature relationship is more critical to successful fitting. A phenomenon that is consequently observed more often with silicone hydrogel lenses than conventional soft lenses is lens "fluting,"[272] which usually causes a foreign-body–like discomfort to the patient. Unfortunately, fluting does not reduce with increased wear and, if observed, an alternate base curve or design must be evaluated.

Adaptation to well-fitted lenses for overnight wear should be rapid. However, there is justification for recommending that patients who are new to contact lenses should adapt to daily wear for a period of at least 1 week, mainly to ensure that they are capable of wearing, handling, and looking after contact lenses before commencing EW or CW. When prescribing EW or CW for adapted wearers, these individuals should be instructed to commence overnight wear immediately. With highly permeable silicone hydrogel materials, a follow-up visit after the first night of lens wear is unnecessary, since the only reason for this visit would be to assess any possible acute hypoxic responses. It is more appropriate to see patients after approximately a week when they have had an opportunity to adapt to an overnight wearing modality. It is, however, very important to discuss how patients are likely to feel upon waking in their lenses. Changes in the tear film overnight may result in mild dryness and blurring of vision, which generally resolve with blinking but may also be alleviated with rewetting drops. Patients must also be instructed to contact their eye care practitioner if they experience any problems before their first follow-up visit is scheduled.

All wearers should be seen for an initial follow-up visit after the first week, to ensure that lenses are comfortable and they are able to tolerate overnight wear. Subsequent follow-up visits should occur after a further 2 to 3 weeks and then 3 months after commencing EW or CW. It is particularly important to assess patients who have been refitted into silicone hydrogel lenses from conventional hydrogel materials within the first weeks of wear, especially if they have been worn on an EW basis. Changes relating to recovery from chronic hypoxia may occur within the first month or so of lens wear, including a possible reversal of a previous myopic shift[184] and a transient appearance of microcysts.[158] Assessments of visual acuity and overrefraction and a careful slit-lamp biomicroscope examination are therefore recommended at each visit. Changes in lens parameters can be made before a supply of lenses is ordered for the patient. Subsequent follow-up visits should be scheduled at intervals of 3 to 6 months thereafter.

Wearing Schedule

The wearing schedule is determined by several factors. These include the current approvals of wearing time by the regulatory authorities (e.g., FDA, CE, etc.). Some lenses are only approved for up to 6 nights of overnight wear (EW) and others for up to 30 nights (CW). Even then, these approvals are the maximum recommended wearing schedule. The optimal number of consecutive nights should be considered for each patient on an individual basis, and it should be emphasized that patients can always remove their lenses after a shorter time period if they wish to. Flexibility in wearing schedule must be emphasized. If lenses are worn for shorter periods, they must be cleaned and disinfected with an appropriate care system before reinsertion. Regardless of wearing schedule, patients should be advised that they must NEVER continue to wear an uncomfortable lens or wear a lens when they have a painful or red eye.

Every 6 or 30 nights of overnight wear should be followed by 1 night with no lenses and lenses should either be discarded or, in the case of lenses approved for 6 nights, cleaned and disinfected and then reworn for a further 6-night period if this is indicated by the manufacturer. It is important that all patients replace their lenses according to the recommended schedule. Some practitioners suggest replacing monthly replacement lenses at the beginning or end of a month to improve compliance. Novel text messaging systems are also being used by some companies and practices to remind patients when they should be replacing their lenses.

Solutions and Rewetting Drops

Patients must be dispensed with a care regimen that they can use in the event of either a scheduled or unscheduled lens removal. Typically, multipurpose care regimens are prescribed because of their ease of use and relatively low cost, but care should be taken to ensure that there is compatibility between the lens material and the system. The use of a rub and rinse cycle is highly recommended, even with "no-rub" regimens, particularly for patients who are prone to lipid deposition.[273,274] An alcohol-based cleaner may also be helpful for some patients. Hydrogen peroxide systems can also be used if the practitioner prefers these systems. It is important to also provide rewetting drops to all EW and CW patients. These are very useful for the alleviation of eye dryness upon waking and during their normal wear. They can also be used at night if desired and should be recommended for patients exhibiting high numbers of mucin balls, since their regular use before sleep has been reported to decrease their frequency of observation.[190] Ideally, these drops should be of relatively low viscosity, to prevent blurring following their insertion. Rewetting drops with surface active agents have been shown to improve the clinical performance of silicone hydrogel contact lenses,[275] and patients experiencing lipid deposition may also find them helpful. Periodic lens removal with a rub and rinse with a care regimen containing a surfactant may also be helpful for some patients experiencing lipid build-up.[273]

Emergencies

Patients should be advised to remove their EW or CW lenses if they feel physically unwell, as they are often prone to adverse events during these times. Most importantly, they should be advised that they must NEVER sleep in an uncomfortable lens or when they have a painful or red eye and that they must check their eyes on waking each morning to ensure that they look "good," that they feel "good," and that they can see well, a three-point safety check they should perform every morning.[276] If they are at all concerned, they must remove the lenses and contact their practitioner. To facilitate this, they should be supplied with emergency contact details, which must include a 24-hour emergency contact number (via either a pager or practitioner home contact number). It may be possible for practitioners in a locality to arrange an on-call system, where practitioners rotate this duty.

Office staff play a vital role in the management of potential emergency situations for EW and CW patients. This is only possible with some degree of in-office training being undertaken, and such training is well worthwhile from both a clinical and a legal standpoint. It is particularly important that staff schedule patients with potential adverse responses quickly or arrange referral for an emergency appointment externally if necessary. Suitable in-office protocols should be developed and reviewed regularly.

Follow-Up Care

Contact lens follow-up is extremely important for EW and CW patients and is the best method of avoiding complications or identifying the cause of problems when they occur. It is important to emphasize the importance of follow-up visits to patients whether they are experiencing problems or not. They should be made aware of symptoms that may indicate a problem, but it is also crucial to explain that some complications may occur without any associated symptoms in the initial stages.

The visit should begin with a thorough history, preferably in the form of a patient discussion, and the use of "open" rather than "closed" questions is recommended. For example, the practitioner can ask, How would you describe your contact lens wear? or What seems to be the main problem with your contact lenses/eyes/vision?" Once the chief complaint is established, further questioning can follow. The measurement of visual acuity is extremely important, particularly if a complication is suspected or observed, and recording the best level of corrected acuity with and/or without the lenses in place is crucial both to establish whether any temporary or permanent loss of visual acuity has occurred and for the requirements of complete record keeping.

A thorough slit-lamp examination should be carried out at all follow-up visits. It is particularly important that lens surface characteristics and wettability be evaluated. After lens removal, the eyelids, lashes, margins, conjunctiva, and cornea should be examined using the appropriate illumination techniques. Lid eversion and fluorescein staining (with the use of an additional yellow barrier filter)[208] must be performed at all visits. The eye can be irrigated with saline before reinsertion of the lenses, and, as with all lens removals, patients should be advised to disinfect their lenses before wearing them again overnight. Evaluation of the anterior chamber for flare or cells may also be necessary for the differential diagnosis of certain complications.

Comprehensive record keeping is crucial for EW and CW patients. A record of all findings, verbal communication, and instructions must be clearly recorded in the patient's record.[266,267,277] The use of grading scales to rate the severity of ocular findings is strongly recommended.[269,278–280] Increasingly, photography and video recording are also being utilized as an accurate means of documenting findings.

■ SUMMARY

Overnight wear of contact lenses is certainly not for everyone, but does offer many advantages over daily wear for many patients. When discussing the opportunity for EW or CW with patients, it is important to provide a carefully balanced point of view. Patients appreciate learning about the potential disadvantages, as well as being informed of the positive aspects. Thorough follow-up examinations are crucial for patient success with overnight lens wear. While newer GP and silicone hydrogel materials appear to have solved hypoxia problems for the majority of patients choosing to wear lenses overnight, some patients will experience inflammation and mechanical complications, and practitioners must be equipped to handle these complications when they occur. Several strategies have been suggested to reduce a patient's risk of complications. The initiation of lid hygiene measures is also recommended for patients predisposed to inflammatory responses. Even though these new materials are an enormous improvement over older-generation materials, further modifications to lens designs and surface treatments are vital to the continuing success of overnight wear modalities.

■ CLINICAL CASES

CASE 1

AD is a 23-year-old Asian woman wearing Night & Day lenses (−3.00 D OU) on a CW basis with monthly replacement for 3 months. She came in for a routine follow-up visit with no symptoms. Visual acuities were 20/20 OD and OS. Slit-lamp examination revealed an arcuate lesion superiorly OS extending from 12 o'clock to 1 o'clock (Fig. 16.7). Following lens removal AD reported mild discomfort under her eyelid OS. The lesion stained with fluorescein (Fig. 16.8).

SOLUTION: A diagnosis of superior epithelial arcuate lesion was made. Ocular lubricants were dispensed q1h OS and contact lens wear was temporarily discontinued. AD was seen for follow-up the next day, at which time she was asymptomatic and the epithelium was intact in the affected area. She was refitted with O$_2$OPTIX lenses OU for EW with weekly removal without further complications. This case emphasizes the importance of reviewing all EW and CW patients at regular intervals, even when they do not report any problems.

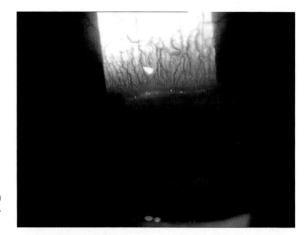

■ **FIGURE 16.7** Superior epithelial arcuate lesion (SEAL) subsequent to silicone hydrogel continuous wear.

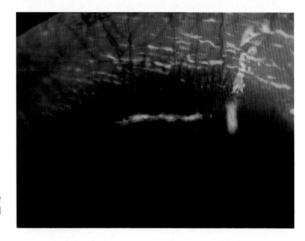

■ **FIGURE 16.8** The superior epithelial arcuate lesion (SEAL) seen in Figure 16.7 as observed with fluorescein staining.

CASE 2

JD is a 27-year-old Caucasian man wearing PureVision lenses (−4.00 D OU) on a CW basis for 1 month. He reported discomfort, mucus, and itchiness and suspected seasonal allergies. Visual acuities were 20/15 OD and OS. Slit-lamp examination of the cornea and bulbar conjunctiva showed no abnormalities. Lid eversion revealed hyperemia and an area of large papillae excrescences in the central area, adjacent to the lid margin OU (Fig. 16.9).

SOLUTION: A diagnosis of contact lens papillary conjunctivitis was made. JD was discontinued from PureVision CW and a supply of daily disposables was dispensed for sporting activities

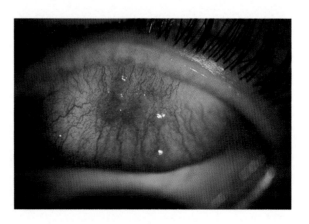

■ **FIGURE 16.9** Localized contact lens-associated papillary conjunctivitis (CLPC) subsequent to silicone hydrogel continuous wear.

only. At the follow-up visit 2 weeks later, the tarsal conjunctiva was smooth and no symptoms were reported. JD appreciated the convenience of daily disposable lenses and elected to remain in this modality.

CASE 3

JH is a 31-year-old Caucasian woman wearing PureVision lenses (OD −2.75 D, OS −3.50 D) on a CW basis for 3 years. She called to report pain, photophobia, and lacrimation OS, and a foreign body sensation that had started the previous day. She was instructed to immediately schedule an appointment. Visual acuities were 20/15 OD and OS. Slit-lamp examination revealed a small (0.3-mm) circular lesion in the paracentral cornea at 10 o'clock OS and sectoral bulbar and limbal hyperemia superior nasally (Fig. 16.10). The epithelium in this region stained with fluorescein (Fig. 16.11).

SOLUTION: A tentative diagnosis of contact lens peripheral ulcer was made. JH was directed to wear her spectacles and given ciprofloxacin drops qid prophylactically and ocular lubricants prn. Later that evening she reported a marked improvement in her symptoms and at a follow-up visit the next day she was asymptomatic and only showed mild epithelial disturbance in the area of the lesion. She continued the antibiotic therapy for a further 3 days and at the next follow-up visit the epithelium was intact and treatment was ceased. At the 1-week follow-up visit JH was anxious to resume lens wear and was recommended to commence with daily wear only. Six months later she had reverted to CW and experienced a second CLPU event. CW was discontinued and a daily/flexible wear recommended.

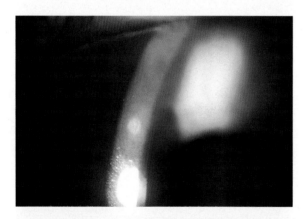

■ FIGURE 16.10 Contact lens peripheral ulcer (CLPU) subsequent to 30-night silicone hydrogel lens wear.

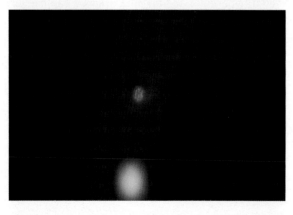

■ FIGURE 16.11 The contact lens peripheral ulcer (CLPU) seen in Figure 16.10 as observed with fluorescein staining.

CASE 4

SW is a 19-year-old Caucasian man wearing Acuvue 2 lenses (−2.50 D OU) on a daily wear basis with monthly replacement. He reported napping in his lenses the previous evening but removing them overnight and waking on the day of presentation with marked pain, photophobia, and redness in his right eye (Fig. 16.12). Visual acuities were 20/20 OD and 20/15 OS. Slit-lamp examination revealed a small irregular oval lesion in the midperiphery at 7 o'clock (Fig. 16.13). The epithelium stained with fluorescein and there was rapid stromal leakage. Anterior chamber examination showed grade 3 cells and flare.

SOLUTION: A diagnosis was made of probable microbial keratitis and the patient was treated with moxifloxacin HCL (0.5%). There was complete resolution of symptoms within 4 days and the epithelium was intact by day 5. A small scar remained, but the visual acuity returned to 20/15 OD. This case demonstrates that even daily wear patients do occasionally nap while wearing their lenses and can experience serious complications as a result. Careful counseling is crucial.

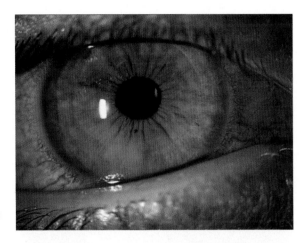

■ **FIGURE 16.12** Bulbar and limbal hyperemia associated with microbial keratitis.

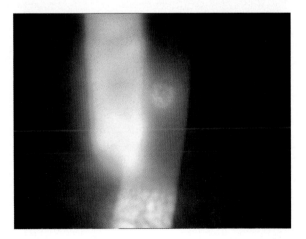

■ **FIGURE 16.13** Ulceration associated with microbial keratitis following napping in contact lenses.

CASE 5

MR is a 38-year-old Caucasian man wearing Night & Day lenses (OD −6.00 D, OS −6.50 D) on a CW basis for 2 years. MR is a volunteer firefighter, father of young children, and outdoor enthusiast.

SOLUTION: He initially started CW in a clinical trial and has subsequently continued in this modality with his own eye care practitioner. What he "loves" most about the lenses is that when he has to get up in the night for an emergency call or for one of his children, he immediately has functional vision without having to find spectacles or insert contact lenses. What he "hates" most about his lenses is that he has to take 1 night away from lens wear each month when he replaces his lenses and it is "Murphy's law" that this is always a night where he is called out!

CASE 6

SF is a 22-year-old Caucasian man who was successfully wearing FDA group IV Acuvue lenses on a daily-wear basis while using ReNu MultiPlus, but showed signs of limbal hyperemia. He was refitted into PureVision lenses and wished to wear them on a CW basis for up to 30 days. However, after 10 to 12 days the lenses continually appeared to be "greasy" and his comfort and vision was reduced.

SOLUTION: SF has mild meibomian gland dysfunction. He was advised to remove the lenses every 7 days, rub and rinse the lenses with his ReNu MultiPlus, soak the lenses overnight and insert them the next day for up to another 6 to 7 nights. In addition, he was given artificial lubricants and lid scrubs for his lid margin disease. This solved the problem and he now successfully wears the lenses on an EW basis with no complaints. This case is fairly typical of that which occurs with patients who have marginal tear film quality because of lid disease and wish to use their lenses on a CW basis. Acuvue lenses attract very little lipid deposition compared with silicone hydrogel lenses,[281,282] and switching a patient may result in symptoms because of deposition of the silicone hydrogel material. Reverting to a shorter period of wear without removal and using a rub and rinse process will help to control the lens deposition. It also demonstrates that not all patients who wish to wear their lenses for 30 nights can do so.

CASE 7

VM is a 54-year-old patient who presented having worn soft contact lenses for 30+ years. She wore her lenses for 7 days a week, 17 hours per day, with the last 5 to 6 hours being somewhat uncomfortable because of symptoms of dryness. On presentation she was wearing Acuvue 2 lenses in a monovision format (OD for near), with acuities of 20/40− and 0.8 M binocularly. Her spectacle prescription was OD −17.50−1.00 × 130 (20/40−) and OS −10.25−1.25 × 010 (20/40) with a +1.25 D reading add. Keratometry readings were OD 45.75 D × 46.50 D and OS 46.25 D × 47.25 D, and her horizontal visible iris diameter was 12 mm. Slit-lamp examination revealed extensive limbal hyperemia, obvious neovascularization, stromal striae, and endothelial polymegethism (OD > OS) because of chronic hypoxia.

SOLUTION: She was fitted with the O₂OPTIX Custom silicone hydrogel lens,[108,109] with 8.40:14.00 −14.50 D for the OD (near) and 8.40:14.00 −9.00 D for the OS (distance). On collection of the trial lenses she had best corrected distance acuities of OD 20/40 (with the distance overrefraction in place) and OS 20/30− and she managed 0.8 M binocularly.

At her 1-week follow-up visit her visual acuities were OD 20/30 and OS 20/20− and she managed 0.8 M with ease. There were no striae present and her limbal vessels appeared dramatically different, with an obvious reduction in both limbal hyperemia and neovascularization. Her wearing time was still 17 hours, but she reported a marked improvement in end-of-day dryness symptoms. The improvement in her ocular appearance continued over the next 3 weeks and at her 1-month visit all signs of chronic hypoxia (with the exception of endothelial polymegethism, which is not expected to recover substantially) were absent.

While not an example of a patient using his or her lens on an overnight basis, this case is typical of the kind of patient who will benefit greatly from the availability of custom-made silicone hydrogel lenses; their recent release will be of great benefit to patients and practitioners alike. The improved oxygen availability will also allow her to "nap" in her lenses without fear of hypoxic compromise.

CLINICAL PROFICIENCY CHECKLIST

■ EW and CW are not recommended for all contact lens patients, but these modalities can offer incredible convenience for many wearers.

■ Complications will occur with overnight wear as with daily wear, but the chances of them occurring can be reduced and, in the case of hypoxic complications, can be eliminated with current contact lens materials.

(Continued)

■ Only high Dk/t GP and silicone hydrogel materials should be prescribed for overnight wear unless no other alternatives exist.

■ Optimal lens fitting characteristics are vital for success with high Dk/t GP and silicone hydrogel materials.

■ Appropriate patient selection is crucial for overnight wear. Patients with a history of poor compliance and a prior history of complications should be avoided or meticulously counseled.

■ Certain changes can be expected when refitting low Dk/t wearers with high Dk/t materials for EW or CW. These include a transient microcyst response and rebound hyperopic prescription changes.

■ Mechanical complications can generally be reduced by changing lens designs or materials.

■ Inflammatory complications tend to be patient dependent. If they occur, pay close attention to the prospect of lid margin disease such as blepharitis or meibomian gland disease.

■ Differential diagnosis of inflammatory and infectious complications is crucial. If in doubt, the patient should be treated as if the case were infectious. If resolution is rapid, inflammation is the most likely etiology.

■ Inflammation can be prevented by suspending overnight wear during periods of ill health or stress.

■ Even if lenses are "approved" for wear for up to 6 or 30 consecutive nights, a flexible wearing schedule is recommended.

■ The risk of inflammation and infection can be reduced by avoiding swimming in contact lenses or at least cleaning and disinfecting the lenses before wearing them overnight after swimming and hot tub use.

■ Inflammation and infection can be reduced by careful and appropriate use of contact lens care products and following instructions for wearing schedules and lens replacement.

■ Thorough record keeping is essential.

■ All patients should be told that if they are "in doubt," they should "take their lens(es) out."

REFERENCES

1. Jones L, Dumbleton K. Soft lens extended wear and complications. In: Hom MM, Bruce A, eds. Manual of Contact Lens Prescribing and Fitting. Oxford: Butterworth-Heinemann, 2006:393–441.
2. Fatt I. Water flow conductivity and pore diameter in extended-wear gel lens materials. Am J Optom Physiol Opt 1978;55(1):43–47.
3. Kersley HJ. Contact lens in aphakia. Trans Ophthalmol Soc U K 1977;97(1):142–144.
4. Nesburn AB. Prolonged-wear contact lenses in aphakia. Ophthalmol 1978;85(1):73–79.
5. Poggio EC, Glynn RJ, Schein OD, et al. The incidence of ulcerative keratitis among users of daily-wear and extended-wear soft contact lenses. N Engl J Med 1989;321(12):779–783.
6. Schein OD, Glynn RJ, Poggio EC, et al. The relative risk of ulcerative keratitis among users of daily-wear and extended-wear soft contact lenses. A case-control study. Microbial Keratitis Study Group. N Engl J Med 1989;321(12):773–778.
7. Cheng KH, Leung SL, Hoekman HW, et al. Incidence of contact-lens-associated microbial keratitis and its related morbidity. Lancet 1999;354(9174):181–185.
8. Brennan NA, Coles ML. Extended wear in perspective. Optom Vis Sci 1997;74(8):609–623.
9. Donshik PC. Extended wear contact lenses. Ophthalmol Clin North Am 2003;16(3):305–309.
10. Dumbleton K. Noninflammatory silicone hydrogel contact lens complications. Eye Contact Lens 2003;29(1 Suppl):S186–189; discussion S190–191, S192–194.
11. Sweeney DF. Clinical signs of hypoxia with high-Dk soft lens extended wear: is the cornea convinced? Eye Contact Lens 2003;29(1 Suppl):S22–25.

12. Stapleton F, Stretton S, Papas E, et al. Silicone hydrogel contact lenses and the ocular surface. Ocul Surf 2006;4(1):24–43.

13. Lim L, Loughnan MS, Sullivan LJ. Microbial keratitis associated with extended wear of silicone hydrogel contact lenses. Br J Ophthalmol 2002;86(3):355–357.

14. Lee KY, Lim L. Pseudomonas keratitis associated with continuous wear silicone-hydrogel soft contact lens: a case report. Eye Contact Lens 2003;29(4):255–257.

15. Syam P, Hussain B, Hutchinson C. Mixed infection (Pseudomonas and coagulase negative staphylococci) microbial keratitis associated with extended wear silicone hydrogel contact lens. Br J Ophthalmol 2004;88(4):579.

16. Schein OD, McNally JJ, Katz J, et al. The incidence of microbial keratitis among wearers of a 30-day silicone hydrogel extended-wear contact lens. Ophthalmol 2005;112(12):2172–2179.

17. Landers JA, Crompton JL. Microbial keratitis associated with overnight wear of silicone hydrogel contact lenses. Med J Aust 2006;185(3):177–178.

18. Leibowitz HM, Laing RA, Sandstrom M. Continuous wear of hydrophilic contact lenses. Arch Ophthalmol 1973;89(4):306–310.

19. Ezekiel D. High water content hydrophilic contact lenses. Aust J Optom 1974;57:317–324.

20. Benson C. Continuous use of contact lenses. Trans Ophthalmol Soc N Z 1976;28:71–74.

21. Stark WJ, Martin NF. Extended-wear contact lenses for myopic correction. Arch Ophthalmol 1981;99(11):1963–1966.

22. Binder PS. Myopic extended wear with the Hydrocurve II soft contact lens. Ophthalmol 1983;90(6):623–626.

23. Hassman G, Sugar J. *Pseudomonas* corneal ulcer with extended-wear soft contact lenses for myopia. Arch Ophthalmol 1983;101:1549–1550.

24. Weissman BA, Mondino BJ, Pettit TH, et al. Corneal ulcers associated with extended-wear soft contact lenses. Am J Ophthalmol 1984;97(4):476–481.

25. Donshik P, Weinstock F, Wechsler S, et al. Disposable hydrogel contact lenses for extended wear. CLAO J 1988;14(4):191–194.

26. Killingsworth D, Stern G. *Pseudomonas* keratitis associated with the use of disposable soft contact lenses. Arch Ophthalmol 1989;107:795–796.

27. Jones L, Dumbleton K, Fonn D, et al. Comfort and compliance with frequent replacement soft contact lenses. Optom Vis Sci 2002;79(12s):259.

28. Holden BA, Mertz GW. Critical oxygen levels to avoid corneal edema for daily and extended wear contact lenses. Invest Ophthalmol Vis Sci 1984;25(10):1161–1167.

29. Harvitt DM, Bonanno JA. Re-evaluation of the oxygen diffusion model for predicting minimum contact lens Dk/t values needed to avoid corneal anoxia. Optom Vis Sci 1999;76(10):712–719.

30. Larke J, Parrish S, Wigham C. Apparent human corneal oxygen uptake rate. Am J Optom Physiol Opt 1981;58(10):803–805.

31. Efron N. Intersubject variability in corneal swelling response to anoxia. Acta Ophthalmol (Copenh) 1986;64(3):302–305.

32. Ng C, Tighe B. Polymers in contact lens applications VI. The 'dissolved' oxygen permeability of hydrogel and the design of materials for use in continuous wear lenses. Brit Polymer J 1976;8:118–123.

33. Fatt I, Chaston J. Measurement of oxygen transmissibility and permeability of hydrogel lenses and materials. Int Contact Lens Clin 1982;9(2):76–88.

34. Morgan PB, Efron N. The oxygen performance of contemporary hydrogel contact lenses. Contact Lens Anterior Eye 1998;21(1):3–6.

35. Jones L. Modern contact lens materials: a clinical performance update. Contact Lens Spectrum 2002;17(9):24–35.

36. Lim L, Tan DT, Chan WK. Therapeutic use of Bausch & Lomb PureVision contact lenses. CLAO J 2001;27(4):179–185.

37. Montero J, Sparholt J, Mely R, et al. Retrospective case series of therapeutic applications of lotrafilcon a silicone hydrogel soft contact lenses. Eye Contact Lens 2003;29(2):72–75.

38. Ambroziak AM, Szaflik JP, Szaflik J. Therapeutic use of a silicone hydrogel contact lens in selected clinical cases. Eye Contact Lens 2004;30(1):63–67.

39. Szaflik JP, Ambroziak AM, Szaflik J. Therapeutic use of a lotrafilcon A silicone hydrogel soft contact lens as a bandage after LASEK surgery. Eye Contact Lens 2004;30(1):59–62.

40. Ozkurt Y, Rodop O, Oral Y, et al. Therapeutic applications of lotrafilcon a silicone hydrogel soft contact lenses. Eye Contact Lens 2005;31(6):268–269.

41. Dart JK, Stapleton F, Minassian D. Contact lenses and other risk factors in microbial keratitis. Lancet 1991;338(8768):650–653.

42. Dart J. Predisposing factors in microbial keratitis: the significance of contact lens wear. Br J Ophthalmol 1988;72:926–930.

43. Cheung J, Slomovic AR. Microbial etiology and predisposing factors among patients hospitalized for corneal ulceration. Can J Ophthalmol 1995;30(5):251–255.

44. Cutter GR, Chalmers RL, Roseman M. The clinical presentation, prevalence, and risk factors of focal corneal infiltrates in soft contact lens wearers. CLAO J 1996;22(1):30–37.

45. McNally JJ, Chalmers RL, McKenney CD, et al. Risk factors for corneal infiltrative events with 30-night continuous wear of silicone hydrogel lenses. Eye Contact Lens 2003;29(1 Suppl):S153–156; discussion S166, S192–194.

46. Radford CF, Minassian DC, Dart JK. Acanthamoeba keratitis in England and Wales: incidence, outcome, and risk factors. Br J Ophthalmol 2002;86(5):536–542.

47. Stehr-Green JK, Bailey TM, Brandt FH, et al. Acanthamoeba keratitis in soft contact lens wearers. A case-control study. JAMA 1987;258(1):57–60.

48. Dougherty JM, McCulley JP. Comparative bacteriology of chronic blepharitis. Br J Ophthalmol 1984;68(8):524–528.

49. Groden LR, Murphy B, Rodnite J, et al. Lid flora in blepharitis. Cornea 1991;10(1):50–53.

50. Fleiszig SM. The Glenn A. Fry award lecture 2005. The pathogenesis of contact lens-related keratitis. Optom Vis Sci 2006;83(12):866–873.

51. Dumbleton K. Adverse events with silicone hydrogel continuous wear. Contact Lens Anterior Eye 2002;25:137–146.

52. Sweeney D, du Toit R, Keay L, et al. Clinical performance of silicone hydrogel lenses. In Sweeney D, ed. Silicone Hydrogels: Continuous Wear Contact Lenses. Oxford: Butterworth-Heinemann, 2004:164–216.

53. Sweeney DF, Stern J, Naduvalith T, et al. Inflammatory adverse event rates over 3 years with silicone hydrogel lenses. Invest Ophthalmol Vis Sci 2002;43(4 ARVO abstracts):40.

54. Fatt I. Now do we need 'effective permeability'? Contax 1986;July:6–23.

55. Tighe B. Soft lens materials. In: Efron N, ed. Contact Lens Practice. Oxford: Butterworth-Heinemann, 2002:71–84.

56. Tighe B. Contact lens materials. In: Phillips A, Speedwell L, eds. Contact Lenses. Edinburgh: Butterworth-Heinemann, 2006:59–78.

57. Zekman TN, Sarnat LA. Clinical evaluation of the silicone corneal contact lens. Am J Ophthalmol 1972;74(3):534–537.

58. Refojo MF. Contact lens materials. Int Ophthalmol Clin 1973;13(1):263–277.

59. Refojo MF. Mechanism of gas transport through contact lenses. J Am Optom Assoc 1979;50(3):285–287.

60. Gurland JE. Use of silicone lenses in infants and children. Ophthalmol 1979;86(9):1599–1604.

61. Rae ST, Huff JW. Studies on initiation of silicone elastomer lens adhesion in vitro: binding before the indentation ring. CLAO J 1991;17(3):181–186.

62. Huth S, Wagner H. Identification and removal of deposits on polydimethylsiloxane silicone elastomer lenses. Int Contact Lens Clin 1981;8(7/8):19–26.

63. Dahl AA, Brocks ER. The use of continuous-wear silicone contact lenses in the optical correction of aphakia. Am J Ophthalmol 1978;85(4):454–461.

64. Tighe B. Rigid lens materials. In: Efron N, ed. Contact Lens Practice. Oxford: Butterworth-Heinemann, 2002:153–162.

65. Tighe B. Silicone hydrogels: structure, properties and behaviour. In: Sweeney D, ed. Silicone Hydrogels: Continuous Wear Contact Lenses. Oxford: Butterworth-Heinemann, 2004:1–27.

66. Loveridge R. Dk 30, 60, 90 and 120 - can the cornea tell the difference? Optometry Today 1997;Feb 7:36.

67. Walker J. High Dk RGPs: the lens of first choice. Optician 1992;203(5337):18–25.

68. Schwartz C. Radical flattening and RGP lenses. Contact Lens Forum 1986;11(8):49–52.

69. Yokota M, Goshima T, Itoh S. The effect of polymer structure on durability of high Dk gas permeable materials. J Brit Contact Lens Assoc 1992;15(3):125–129.

70. Tranoudis I, Efron N. Scratch resistance of rigid contact lens materials. Ophthal Physiol Opt 1996;16(4):303–309.

71. Walker J. Handling high DK lenses. Optician 1989;197(5198):30–39.

72. Walker J. Cracking and crazing - a practitioner's viewpoint. Optician 1990;199(5245):19–21.

73. Lembach RG, McLaughlin R, Barr JT. Crazing in a rigid gas permeable contact lens. CLAO J 1988;14(1):38–41.

74. Arnestad J. Cracking of Persecon CE contact lenses. Contact Lens J 1989;17(3):86–87.

75. Bark M, Hanson D, Grant R. A guide to rigid gas-permeable contact lens materials. Optician 1994;207(5441):17–20.

76. Walker J. A clinical and laboratory comparison of the deposition characteristics of both silicone/acrylate and fluoro-silicone/acrylate lenses. J Brit Contact Lens Assoc 1988;11(Trans Ann Clin Conf):83–86.

77. Levy B. The use of a gas permeable hard lens for extended wear. Am J Optom Physiol Opt 1983;60(5):408–409.

78. Ichikawa H, Kozai A, MacKeen DL, et al. Corneal swelling responses with extended wear in naive and adapted subjects with Menicon RGP contact lenses. CLAO J 1989;15(3):192–194.

79. Koetting RA, Castellano CF, Nelson DW. A hard lens with extended wear possibilities. J Am Optom Assoc 1985;56(3):208–211.

80. Fonn D, Holden BA. Rigid gas-permeable vs. hydrogel contact lenses for extended wear. Am J Optom Physiol Opt 1988;65(7):536–544.

81. Ichijima H, Imayasu M, Tanaka H, et al. Effects of RGP lens extended wear on glucose-lactate metabolism and stromal swelling in the rabbit cornea. CLAO J 2000;26(1):30–36.

82. Ichijima H, Cavanagh HD. How rigid gas-permeable lenses supply more oxygen to the cornea than silicone hydrogels: a new model. Eye Contact Lens 2007;33(5):216–223.

83. Gardner HP, Fink BA, Mitchell LG, et al. The effects of high-Dk rigid contact lens center thickness, material permeability, and blinking on the oxygen uptake of the human cornea. Optom Vis Sci 2005;82(6):459–466.

84. Ladage PM, Yamamoto K, Ren DH, et al. Effects of rigid and soft contact lens daily wear on corneal epithelium, tear lactate dehydrogenase, and bacterial binding to exfoliated epithelial cells. Ophthalmol 2001;108(7):1279–1288.

85. Ren DH, Yamamoto K, Ladage PM, et al. Adaptive effects of 30-night wear of hyper-O_2 transmissible contact lenses on bacterial binding and corneal epithelium: a 1-year clinical trial. Ophthalmol 2002;109(1):27–39.

86. Gleason W, Albright RA. Menicon Z 30-day continuous wear lenses: a clinical comparison to Acuvue 7-day extended wear lenses. Eye Contact Lens 2003;29(1 Suppl): S149–1452; discussion S166, S192–194.

87. Maldonado-Codina C, Morgan PB, Efron N, et al. Comparative clinical performance of rigid versus soft hyper Dk contact lenses used for continuous wear. Optom Vis Sci 2005;82(6):536–548.

88. Swarbrick HA, Holden BA. Ocular characteristics associated with rigid gas-permeable lens adherence. Optom Vis Sci 1996;73(7):473–481.

89. Swarbrick HA, Holden BA. Effects of lens parameter variation on rigid gas-permeable lens adherence. Optom Vis Sci 1996;73(3):144–155.

90. Fonn D, Holden BA. Extended wear of hard gas permeable contact lenses can induce ptosis. CLAO J 1986;12(2):93–94.

91. Key JE, Mobley CL. Paraperm EW lens for extended wear. CLAO J 1989;15(2):134–137.

92. Grobe G, Kunzler J, Seelye D, et al. Silicone hydrogels for contact lens applications. Polymeric Materials Sci Eng 1999;80:108–109.

93. Nicolson PC, Vogt J. Soft contact lens polymers: an evolution. Biomaterials 2001;22(24):3273–3283.

94. Nicolson PC. Continuous wear contact lens surface chemistry and wearability. Eye Contact Lens 2003;29(1 Suppl):S30–32; discussion S57–59, S192–194.

95. Maiden A, Vanderlaan D, Turner D, et al. Hydrogel with internal wetting agent. 2002. US Patent #6,367,929.

96. McCabe K, Molock F, Hill G, et al. Biomedical devices containing internal wetting agents. 2006. US Patent #7052131.

97. Jones L, Subbaraman LN, Rogers R, et al. Surface treatment, wetting and modulus of silicone hydrogels. Optician 2006;232(6067):28–34.

98. Bambury R, Seelye D. Vinyl carbonate and vinyl carbamate contact lens materials. 1997. US Patent #5,610,252.

99. Lopez-Alemany A, Compan V, Refojo MF. Porous structure of Purevision versus Focus Night & Day and conventional hydrogel contact lenses. J Biomed Mater Res (Appl Biomat) 2002;63:319–325.

100. Kunzler J. Silicone-based hydrogels for contact lens applications. Contact Lens Spectrum 1999;14(8 supp):9–11.

101. Valint PL Jr, Grobe GL 3rd, Ammon DM Jr, et al. Plasma surface treatment of silicone hydrogel contact lenses. 2001. US Patent #6,193,369.

102. Gonzalez-Meijome JM, Lopez-Alemany A, Almeida JB, et al. Microscopic observation of unworn siloxane-hydrogel soft contact lenses by atomic force microscopy. J Biomed Mater Res B Appl Biomater 2006;76(2):412–418.

103. Nilsson SE. Seven-day extended wear and 30-day continuous wear of high oxygen transmissibility soft silicone hydrogel contact lenses: a randomized 1-year study of 504 patients. CLAO J 2001;27(3):125–136.

104. Brennan NA, Coles ML, Comstock TL, et al. A 1-year prospective clinical trial of balafilcon a (PureVision) silicone-hydrogel contact lenses used on a 30-day continuous wear schedule. Ophthalmol 2002;109(6):1172–1177.

105. Morgan PB, Efron N. Comparative clinical performance of two silicone hydrogel contact lenses for continuous wear. Clin Exp Optom 2002;85(3):183–192.

106. Foulks GN, Harvey T, Raj CV. Therapeutic contact lenses: the role of high-Dk lenses. Ophthalmol Clin North Am 2003;16(3):455–461.

107. Arora R, Jain S, Monga S, et al. Efficacy of continuous wear PureVision contact lenses for therapeutic use. Contact Lens Anterior Eye 2004;27(1):39–43.

108. Jones L, Dumbleton K, Woods J. Introducing a made-to-order silicone hydrogel lens. Contact Lens Spectrum 2007;22(2):23.

109. Jones L, Dumbleton K, Woods J. Fitting and evaluating a custom silicone hydrogel lens. Contact Lens Spectrum 2007;22(4):19.

110. Jones L, Dumbleton K, Woods J. Fitting a challenging case with a custom silicone hydrogel. Contact Lens Spectrum 2007;22(6):17.

111. Nicolson P, Baron R, Chabrecek P, et al. Extended wear ophthalmic lens. 1998. US Patent #5,760,100.

112. Weikart CM, Matsuzawa Y, Winterton L, et al. Evaluation of plasma polymer-coated contact lenses by electrochemical impedance spectroscopy. J Biomed Mater Res 2001;54(4):597–607.

113. Gonzalez-Meijome JM, Lopez-Alemany A, Almeida JB, et al. Microscopic observations of superficial ultrastructure of unworn siloxane-hydrogel contact lenses by cryo-scanning electron microscopy. J Biomed Mater Res B Appl Biomater 2006;76(2):419–423.

114. Montero Iruzubieta J, Nebot Ripoll JR, Chiva J, et al. Practical experience with a high Dk lotrafilcon A fluorosilicone hydrogel extended wear contact lens in Spain. CLAO J 2001;27(1):41–46.

115. McNally J, McKenney CD. A clinical look at a silicone hydrogel extended wear lens. Contact Lens Spectrum 2002;17(1):38–41.

116. Malet F, Pagot R, Peyre C, et al. Subjective experience with high-oxygen and low-oxygen permeable soft contact lenses in France. Eye Contact Lens 2003;29(1):55–59.

117. Stern J, Wong R, Naduvilath TJ, et al. Comparison of the performance of 6- or 30-night extended wear schedules with silicone hydrogel lenses over 3 years. Optom Vis Sci 2004;81(6):398–406.

118. Chalmers RL, Dillehay S, Long B, et al. Impact of previous extended and daily wear schedules on signs and symptoms with high Dk lotrafilcon A lenses. Optom Vis Sci 2005;82(6):549–554.

119. Bergenske P, Long B, Dillehay S, et al. Long-term clinical results: 3 years of up to 30-night continuous wear of lotrafilcon A silicone hydrogel and daily wear of low-Dk/t hydrogel lenses. Eye Contact Lens 2007;33(2):74–80.

120. Kanpolat A, Ucakhan OO. Therapeutic use of Focus Night & Day contact lenses. Cornea 2003;22(8):726–734.

121. Bendoriene J, Vogt U. Therapeutic use of silicone hydrogel contact lenses in children. Eye Contact Lens 2006;32(2):104–108.

122. Schafer J, Mitchell GL, Chalmers RL, et al. The stability of dryness symptoms after refitting with silicone hydrogel contact lenses over 3 years. Eye Contact Lens 2007;33(5):247–252.

123. Dillehay SM, Miller MB. Performance of lotrafilcon B silicone hydrogel contact lenses in experienced low-Dk/t daily lens wearers. Eye Contact Lens 2007;33(6 Pt 1):272–277.

124. Long B, McNally J. The clinical performance of a silicone hydrogel lens for daily wear in an Asian population. Eye Contact Lens 2006;32(2):65–71.

125. Dumbleton K, Keir N, Moezzi A, et al. Objective and subjective responses in patients refitted to daily-wear silicone hydrogel contact lenses. Optom Vis Sci 2006;83(10):758–768.

126. Jones L. Comfilcon A: a new silicone hydrogel material. Contact Lens Spectrum 2007;22(8):21.

127. Moezzi AM, Fonn D, Simpson TL. Overnight corneal swelling with silicone hydrogel contact lenses with high oxygen transmissibility. Eye Contact Lens 2006;32(6):277–280.

128. Brennan NA, Coles ML, Connor HR, et al. A 12-month prospective clinical trial of comfilcon A silicone-hydrogel contact lenses worn on a 30-day continuous wear basis. Cont Lens Anterior Eye 2007;30(2):108–118.

129. Steffen R, Schnider C. A next generation silicone hydrogel lens for daily wear. Part 1 - material properties. Optician 2004;227(5954):23–25.

130. Steffen R, McCabe K. Finding the comfort zone. Contact Lens Spectrum 2004;13(3):Supp 1–4.

131. Moore L, Ferreira JT. Ultraviolet (UV) transmittance characteristics of daily disposable and silicone hydrogel contact lenses. Contact Lens Anterior Eye 2006;29(3):115–122.

132. Sulley A. Practitioner and patient acceptance of a new silicone hydrogel contact lens. Optician 2005;230(6017):15–17.

133. Riley C, Young G, Chalmers R. Prevalence of ocular surface symptoms, signs, and uncomfortable hours of wear in contact lens wearers: the effect of refitting with daily-wear silicone hydrogel lenses (senofilcon A). Eye Contact Lens 2006;32(6):281–286.

134. Young G, Riley CM, Chalmers RL, et al. Hydrogel lens comfort in challenging environments and the effect of refitting with silicone hydrogel lenses. Optom Vis Sci 2007;84(4):302–308.

135. Jones L. A new silicone hydrogel lens comes to market. Contact Lens Spectrum 2007;22(10):23.

136. Weikart CM, Miyama M, Yasuda HK. Surface modification of conventional polymers by depositing plasma polymers of trimethylsilane and of trimethylsilane + O_2. II Dynamic wetting properties. J Colloid Interface Sci 1999;211(1):28–38.

137. Weikart CM, Miyama M, Yasuda HK. Surface modification of conventional polymers by depositing plasma polymers of trimethylsilane and of trimethylsilane + O_2. I Static wetting properties. J Colloid Interface Sci 1999;211(1):18–27.

138. Ang J, Efron N. Carbon dioxide permeability of contact lens materials. Int Cont Lens Clin 1989;16(2):48–57.

139. Ang JH, Efron N. Corneal hypoxia and hypercapnia during contact lens wear. Optom Vis Sci 1990;67(7):512–521.

140. Klyce S. Stromal lactate accumulation can account for corneal edema osmotically following epithelial hypoxia in the rabbit. J Physiol 1981;321:49–64.

141. Fonn D, MacDonald KE, Richter D, et al. The ocular response to extended wear of a high Dk silicone hydrogel contact lens. Clin Exp Optom 2002;85(3):176–182.

142. Holden BA, Mertz GW, McNally JJ. Corneal swelling response to contact lenses worn under extended wear conditions. Invest Ophthalmol Vis Sci 1983;24(2):218–226.

143. Fonn D, du Toit R, Simpson TL, et al. Sympathetic swelling response of the control eye to soft lenses in the other eye. Invest Ophthalmol Vis Sci 1999;40(13):3116–3121.

144. Fonn D, Sweeney D, Holden BA, et al. Corneal oxygen deficiency. Eye Contact Lens 2005;31(1):23–27.

145. Polse KA, Mandell RB. Etiology of corneal striae accompanying hydrogel lens wear. Invest Ophthalmol 1976;15(7):553–556.

146. Polse KA, Sarver MD, Harris MG. Corneal edema and vertical striae accompanying the wearing of hydrogel lenses. Am J Optom Physiol Opt 1975;52(3):185–191.

147. Kerns RL. A study of striae observed in the cornea from contact lens wear. Am J Optom Physiol Opt 1974;51(12):998–1004.

148. La Hood D. Daytime edema levels with plus powered low and high water content hydrogel contact lenses. Optom Vis Sci 1991;68(11):877–880.

149. Efron N. Stromal edema. In: Efron N, ed. Contact Lens Complications. London: Butterworth-Heinemann, 2004:133–140.

150. Alvord L, Court J, Davis T, et al. Oxygen permeability of a new type of high Dk soft contact lens material. Optom Vis Sci 1998;75(1):30–36.

151. Papas EB, Vajdic CM, Austen R, et al. High-oxygen-transmissibility soft contact lenses do not induce limbal hyperaemia. Curr Eye Res 1997;16(9):942–948.
152. Holden BA, Sweeney DF, Sanderson G. The minimum precorneal oxygen tension to avoid corneal edema. Invest Ophthalmol Vis Sci 1984;25(4):476–480.
153. Brennan NA. Corneal oxygenation during contact lens wear: comparison of diffusion and EOP-based flux models. Clin Exp Optom 2005;88(2):103–108.
154. Ruben M, Brown N, Lobascher D. Clinical manifestations secondary to soft contact lens wear. Br J Ophthalmol 1976;60:529–531.
155. Zantos S, Holden B. Ocular changes associated with continuous wear of contact lenses. Aust J Optom 1978;61:418–426.
156. Holden BA, Sweeney DF. The significance of the microcyst response: a review. Optom Vis Sci 1991;68(9):703–707.
157. Covey M, Sweeney DF, Terry R, et al. Hypoxic effects on the anterior eye of high-Dk soft contact lens wearers are negligible. Optom Vis Sci 2001;78(2):95–99.
158. Keay L, Sweeney DF, Jalbert I, et al. Microcyst response to high Dk/t silicone hydrogel contact lenses. Optom Vis Sci 2000;77(11):582–585.
159. Zantos S. Cystic formations in the corneal epithelium during extended wear of contact lenses. Int Contact Lens Clin 1983;10(3):128–146.
160. Efron N. Epithelial microcysts. In: Efron N, ed. Contact Lens Complications. London: Butterworth-Heinemann, 2004:116–121.
161. Keay L, Jalbert I, Sweeney DF, et al. Microcysts: clinical significance and differential diagnosis. Optometry 2001;72(7):452–460.
162. Schoessler J. Corneal endothelial polymegethism associated with extended wear. Int Cont Lens Clin 1983;10(3):148–155.
163. Efron N. Endothelial polymegethism. In: Efron N, ed. Contact Lens Complications. London: Butterworth-Heinemann, 2004:216–222.
164. Holden BA, Sweeney DF, Vannas A, et al. Effects of long-term extended contact lens wear on the human cornea. Invest Ophthalmol Vis Sci 1985;26(11):1489–1501.
165. Carlson KH, Bourne WM. Endothelial morphologic features and function after long-term extended wear of contact lenses. Arch Ophthalmol 1988;106(12):1677–1679.
166. Dutt RM, Stocker EG, Wolff CH, et al. A morphologic and fluorophotometric analysis of the corneal endothelium in long-term extended wear soft contact lens wearers. CLAO J 1989;15(2):121–123.
167. Polse KA, Brand RJ, Cohen SR, et al. Hypoxic effects on corneal morphology and function. Invest Ophthalmol Vis Sci 1990;31(8):1542–1554.
168. Sweeney D. Corneal exhaustion syndrome with long-term wear of contact lenses. Optom Vis Sci 1992;69(8):601–608.
169. Barr JT, Pall B, Szczotka LB, et al. Corneal endothelial morphology results in the Menicon Z 30-day continuous-wear contact lens clinical trial. Eye Contact Lens 2003;29(1):14–16.
170. Efron N. Limbal redness. In: Efron N, ed. Contact Lens Complications. London: Butterworth-Heinemann, 2004:88–93.
171. Dumbleton KA, Chalmers RL, Richter DB, et al. Vascular response to extended wear of hydrogel lenses with high and low oxygen permeability. Optom Vis Sci 2001;78(3):147–151.
172. du Toit R, Simpson TL, Fonn D, et al. Recovery from hyperemia after overnight wear of low and high transmissibility hydrogel lenses. Curr Eye Res 2001;22(1):68–73.
173. Papas E. On the relationship between soft contact lens oxygen transmissibility and induced limbal hyperaemia. Exp Eye Res 1998;67(2):125–131.
174. Efron N. Corneal vascularization. In: Efron N, ed. Contact Lens Complications. London: Butterworth-Heinemann, 2004:153–161.
175. McMonnies C. Contact lens induced corneal vascularisation. Int Contact Lens Clin 1983;10:12–21.
176. Millodot M, O'Leary DJ. Effect of oxygen deprivation on corneal sensitivity. Acta Ophthalmol (Copenh) 1980;58(3):434–439.
177. Millodot M. A review of research on the sensitivity of the cornea. Ophthal Physiol Opt 1984;4(4):305–318.
178. Fleiszig SM, Efron N, Pier GB. Extended contact lens wear enhances Pseudomonas aeruginosa adherence to human corneal epithelium. Invest Ophthalmol Vis Sci 1992;33(10):2908–2916.
179. Latkovic S, Nilsson SE. The effect of high and low Dk/L soft contact lenses on the glycocalyx layer of the corneal epithelium and on the membrane associated receptors for lectins. CLAO J 1997;23(3):185–191.
180. Ren H, Petroll W, Jester J, et al. Adherence of *Pseudomonas aeruginosa* to shed rabbit corneal epithelial cells after overnight wear of contact lenses. CLAO J 1997;23:63–68.
181. Ren DH, Petroll WM, Jester JV, et al. The relationship between contact lens oxygen permeability and binding of Pseudomonas aeruginosa to human corneal epithelial cells after overnight and extended wear. CLAO J 1999;25(2):80–100.
182. Holden B. The ocular response to contact lens wear. Optom Vis Sci 1989;66(11):717–733.

183. Liesegang TJ. Physiologic changes of the cornea with contact lens wear. CLAO J 2002;28(1):12–27.
184. Dumbleton KA, Chalmers RL, Richter DB, et al. Changes in myopic refractive error with nine months' extended wear of hydrogel lenses with high and low oxygen permeability. Optom Vis Sci 1999;76(12):845–849.
185. Jalbert I, Stretton S, Naduvilath T, et al. Changes in myopia with low-Dk hydrogel and high-Dk silicone hydrogel extended wear. Optom Vis Sci 2004;81(8):591–596.
186. Efron N. Corneal staining. In: Efron N, ed. Contact Lens Complications. London: Butterworth-Heinemann, 2004:108–115.
187. Bruce A. Local oxygen transmissibility of disposable contact lenses. Contact Lens Anterior Eye 2003;26(4):189–196.
188. Efron N, Morgan PB, Cameron ID, et al. Oxygen permeability and water content of silicone hydrogel contact lens materials. Optom Vis Sci 2007;84(4):328–337.
189. Sankaridurg P, Holden B, Jalbert I. Adverse events and infections: which ones and how many? In: Sweeney D, ed. Silicone Hydrogels: Continuous Wear Contact Lenses. Oxford: Butterworth-Heinemann, 2004:217–274.
190. Dumbleton K, Jones L, Chalmers R, et al. Clinical characterization of spherical post-lens debris associated with lotrafilcon high-Dk silicone lenses. CLAO J 2000;26(4):186–192.
191. Craig JP, Sherwin T, Grupcheva CN, et al. An evaluation of mucin balls associated with high-DK silicone-hydrogel contact lens wear. Adv Exp Med Biol 2002;506(Pt B):917–923.
192. Ladage PM, Petroll WM, Jester JV, et al. Spherical indentations of human and rabbit corneal epithelium following extended contact lens wear. CLAO J 2002;28(4):177–180.
193. Tan J, Keay L, Jalbert I, et al. Mucin balls with wear of conventional and silicone hydrogel contact lenses. Optom Vis Sci 2003;80(4):291–297.
194. Millar TJ, Papas EB, Ozkan J, et al. Clinical appearance and microscopic analysis of mucin balls associated with contact lens wear. Cornea 2003;22(8):740–745.
195. Jalbert I, Stapleton F, Papas E, et al. In vivo confocal microscopy of the human cornea. Br J Ophthalmol 2003;87(2):225–236.
196. Evans V, Carnt N, Naduvilath T, et al. Risk factors associated with corneal inflammation in soft contact lens daily wear. Contact Lens Anterior Eye 2007;30(5):302.
197. Hine N, Back A, Holden B. Aetiology of arcuate epithelial lesions induced by hydrogels. J Brit Contact Lens Assoc 1987;Trans Ann Clin Conf:48–50.
198. Holden BA, Stephenson A, Stretton S, et al. Superior epithelial arcuate lesions with soft contact lens wear. Optom Vis Sci 2001;78(1):9–12.
199. Jalbert I, Sweeney DF, Holden BA. Epithelial split associated with wear of a silicone hydrogel contact lens. CLAO J 2001;27(4):231–233.
200. Malinovsky V, Pole J, Pence N, et al. Epithelial splits of the superior cornea in hydrogel contact lens patients. Int Contact Lens Clin 1989;16(9&10):252–254.
201. O'Hare N, Stapleton F, Naduvilath T, et al. Interaction between the contact lens and the ocular surface in the etiology of superior epithelial arcuate lesions. Adv Exp Med Biol 2002;506(Pt B):973–980.
202. Young G, Mirejovsky D. A hypothesis for the aetiology of soft contact lens-induced superior arcuate keratopathy. Int Contact Lens Clin 1993;20(9/10):177–179.
203. O'Hare N, Naduvilath T, Sweeney D, et al. A clinical comparison of limbal and paralimbal superior epithelial arcuate lesions (SEALs) in high Dk EW. Invest Ophthalmol Vis Sci 2001;42(4):s595.
204. Lofstrom T, Kruse A. A conjunctival response to silicone hydrogel lens wear. Contact Lens Spectrum 2005;20(9):42–44.
205. Carnt N, Keir N. A conjunctival response to silicone hydrogel lens wear. http://www.siliconehydrogels.org/featured_review/may_06.asp 2006. 8/4/08 Last accessed.
206. Lin M. Conjunctival epithelial flaps: what are they and do we need to worry? http://www.siliconehydrogels.org/editorials/may_06.asp 2006. 8/4/08 Last accessed.
207. Santodomingo-Rubido J, Wolffsohn J, Gilmartin B. Conjunctival epithelial flaps with 18 months of silicone hydrogel contact lens wear. Eye Contact Lens 2008;34(1):35–38.
208. Cox I, Fonn D. Interference filters to eliminate the surface reflex and improve contrast during fluorescein photography. Int Contact Lens Clin 1991;18(9/10):178–181.
209. Katelaris CH. Giant papillary conjunctivitis—a review. Acta Ophthalmol Scand Suppl 1999;228:17–20.
210. Donshik PC. Contact lens chemistry and giant papillary conjunctivitis. Eye Contact Lens 2003;29(1 Suppl):S37–39; discussion S57–59, S192–194.
211. Stapleton F, Stretton S, Sankaridurg PR, et al. Hypersensitivity responses and contact lens wear. Cont Lens Anterior Eye 2003;26(2):57–69.
212. Nilsson SE. Ten years of disposable contact lenses—a review of benefits and risks. Cont Lens Anterior Eye 1997;20(4):119–128.
213. Porazinski AD, Donshik PC. Giant papillary conjunctivitis in frequent replacement contact lens wearers: a retrospective study. CLAO J 1999;25(3):142–147.
214. Marshall E, Begley C, Nguyen C. Frequency of complications among wearers of disposable and conventional soft contact lenses. Int Contact Lens Clin 1992;19(3/4):55–59.
215. Poggio EC, Abelson M. Complications and symptoms in disposable extended wear lenses compared with conventional soft daily wear and soft extended wear lenses. CLAO J 1993;19(1):31–39.

216. Skotnitsky C, Sankaridurg PR, Sweeney DF, et al. General and local contact lens induced papillary conjunctivitis (CLPC). Clin Exp Optom 2002;85(3):193–197.

217. Skotnitsky CC, Naduvilath TJ, Sweeney DF, et al. Two presentations of contact lens-induced papillary conjunctivitis (CLPC) in hydrogel lens wear: local and general. Optom Vis Sci 2006;83(1):27–36.

218. Donshik P, Long B, Dillehay SM, et al. Inflammatory and mechanical complications associated with 3 years of up to 30 nights of continuous wear of lotrafilcon A silicone hydrogel lenses. Eye Contact Lens 2007;33(4):191–195.

219. Santodomingo-Rubido J, Wolffsohn JS, Gilmartin B. Adverse events and discontinuations during 18 months of silicone hydrogel contact lens wear. Eye Contact Lens 2007;33(6 Pt 1):288–292.

220. Holden BA, La Hood D, Grant T, et al. Gram-negative bacteria can induce contact lens related acute red eye (CLARE) responses. CLAO J 1996;22(1):47–52.

221. Sankaridurg PR, Willcox MD, Sharma S, et al. Haemophilus influenzae adherent to contact lenses associated with production of acute ocular inflammation. J Clin Microbiol 1996;34(10):2426–2431.

222. Sankaridurg PR, Vuppala N, Sreedharan A, et al. Gram negative bacteria and contact lens induced acute red eye. Ind J Ophthalmol 1996;44(1):29–32.

223. Sankaridurg PR, Sharma S, Willcox M, et al. Bacterial colonization of disposable soft contact lenses is greater during corneal infiltrative events than during asymptomatic extended lens wear. J Clin Microbiol 2000;38(12):4420–4424.

224. Hume EB, Willcox MD. Adhesion and growth of Serratia marcescens on artificial closed eye tears soaked hydrogel contact lenses. Aust N Z J Ophthalmol 1997;25(Suppl 1):S39–541.

225. Grant T, Chong MS, Vajdic C, et al. Contact lens induced peripheral ulcers during hydrogel contact lens wear. CLAO J 1998;24(3):145–151.

226. Holden BA, Reddy MK, Sankaridurg PR, et al. Contact lens-induced peripheral ulcers with extended wear of disposable hydrogel lenses: histopathologic observations on the nature and type of corneal infiltrate. Cornea 1999;18(5):538–543.

227. Hume E, Wu P, Thakur A, et al. Contact lens induced peripheral ulcers (CLPU) are produced by an alpha-toxin deficient mutant of Staphylococcus aureus. Invest Ophthalmol Vis Sci 2001;42(4):s593.

228. Wu P, Stapleton F, Willcox MD. The causes of and cures for contact lens-induced peripheral ulcer. Eye Contact Lens 2003;29(1 Suppl):S63–66; discussion S83–84, S192–194.

229. Aasuri MK, Venkata N, Kumar VM. Differential diagnosis of microbial keratitis and contact lens-induced peripheral ulcer. Eye Contact Lens 2003;29(1 Suppl):S60–62; discussion S83–84, S192–194.

230. Willcox M, Sankaridurg P, Zhu H, et al. Inflammation and infection and the effects of the closed eye. In: Sweeney D, ed. Silicone Hydrogels: Continuous Wear Contact Lenses. Oxford: Butterworth-Heinemann, 2004:90–125.

231. Keay L, Stapleton F, Schein O. Epidemiology of contact lens-related inflammation and microbial keratitis: a 20-year perspective. Eye Contact Lens 2007;33(6 Pt 2):346–353, discussion 362–363.

232. Szczotka-Flynn L, Diaz M. Risk of corneal inflammatory events with silicone hydrogel and low dk hydrogel extended contact lens wear: a meta-analysis. Optom Vis Sci 2007;84(4):247–256.

233. Dumbleton K, Fonn D, Jones L, et al. Severity and management of contact lens related complications with continuous wear of high Dk silicone hydrogel lenses. Optom Vis Sci 2000;77(12s):216.

234. Smolin G. The defence mechanism of the outer eye. Trans Ophthalmol Soc U K 1985;104(Pt 4):363–366.

235. Knop E, Knop N. The role of eye-associated lymphoid tissue in corneal immune protection. J Anat 2005;206(3):271–285.

236. Meek B, Speijer D, de Jong PT, et al. The ocular humoral immune response in health and disease. Prog Retin Eye Res 2003;22(3):391–415.

237. Willcox MD. Which is more important to the initiation of contact lens related microbial keratitis, trauma to the ocular surface or bacterial pathogenic factors? Clin Exp Optom 2006;89(5):277–279.

238. Willcox MD. New strategies to prevent Pseudomonas keratitis. Eye Contact Lens 2007;33(6 Pt 2):401–403; discussion 410–411.

239. Willcox MD. Pseudomonas aeruginosa infection and inflammation during contact lens wear: a review. Optom Vis Sci 2007;84(4):273–278.

240. Willcox MD, Holden BA. Contact lens related corneal infections. Biosci Rep 2001;21(4):445–461.

241. Keay L, Edwards K, Naduvilath T, et al. Microbial keratitis predisposing factors and morbidity. Ophthalmol 2006;113(1):109–116.

242. Keay L, Edwards K, Naduvilath T, et al. Factors affecting the morbidity of contact lens-related microbial keratitis: a population study. Invest Ophthalmol Vis Sci 2006;47(10):4302–4308.

243. Keay L, Edwards K, Stapleton F. An early assessment of silicone hydrogel safety: pearls and pitfalls, and current status. Eye Contact Lens 2007;33(6 Pt 2):358–361.

244. Miedziak AI, Miller MR, Rapuano CJ, et al. Risk factors in microbial keratitis leading to penetrating keratoplasty. Ophthalmol 1999;106(6):1166–1170; discussion 1171.

245. Laspina F, Samudio M, Cibils D, et al. Epidemiological characteristics of microbiological results on patients with infectious corneal ulcers: a 13-year survey in Paraguay. Graefes Arch Clin Exp Ophthalmol 2004;242(3):204–209.

246. Butler TK, Males JJ, Robinson LP, et al. Six-year review of Acanthamoeba keratitis in New South Wales, Australia: 1997–2002. Clin Exp Ophthalmol 2005;33(1):41–46.

247. Titiyal JS, Negi S, Anand A, et al. Risk factors for perforation in microbial corneal ulcers in north India. Br J Ophthalmol 2006;90(6):686–689.
248. Smith A, Pennefather PM, Kaye SB, et al. Fluoroquinolones: place in ocular therapy. Drugs 2001;61(6):747–761.
249. Mather R, Karenchak LM, Romanowski EG, et al. Fourth generation fluoroquinolones: new weapons in the arsenal of ophthalmic antibiotics. Am J Ophthalmol 2002;133(4):463–466.
250. Pachigolla G, Blomquist P, Cavanagh HD. Microbial keratitis pathogens and antibiotic susceptibilities: a 5-year review of cases at an urban county hospital in north Texas. Eye Contact Lens 2007;33(1):45–49.
251. Parmar P, Salman A, Kalavathy CM, et al. Comparison of topical gatifloxacin 0.3% and ciprofloxacin 0.3% for the treatment of bacterial keratitis. Am J Ophthalmol 2006;141(2):282–286.
252. Rattanatam T, Heng WJ, Rapuano CJ, et al. Trends in contact lens-related corneal ulcers. Cornea 2001;20(3):290–294.
253. Leeming JP. Treatment of ocular infections with topical antibacterials. Clin Pharmacokinet 1999;37(5):351–360.
254. Yu DK, Ng AS, Lau WW, et al. Recent pattern of contact lens-related keratitis in Hong Kong. Eye Contact Lens 2007;33(6 Pt 1):284–287.
255. Saw SM, Ooi PL, Tan DT, et al. Risk factors for contact lens-related fusarium keratitis: a case-control study in Singapore. Arch Ophthalmol 2007;125(5):611–617.
256. Iyer SA, Tuli SS, Wagoner RC. Fungal keratitis: emerging trends and treatment outcomes. Eye Contact Lens 2006;32(6):267–271.
257. Chang DC, Grant GB, O'Donnell K, et al. Multistate outbreak of Fusarium keratitis associated with use of a contact lens solution. JAMA 2006;296(8):953–963.
258. Alfonso EC, Cantu-Dibildox J, Munir WM, et al. Insurgence of Fusarium keratitis associated with contact lens wear. Arch Ophthalmol 2006;124(7):941–947.
259. Thebpatiphat N, Hammersmith KM, Rocha FN, et al. Acanthamoeba keratitis: a parasite on the rise. Cornea 2007;26(6):701–706.
260. Joslin CE, Tu EY, Shoff ME, et al. The association of contact lens solution use and Acanthamoeba keratitis. Am J Ophthalmol 2007;144(2):169–180.
261. Foulks GN. Acanthamoeba keratitis and contact lens wear: static or increasing problem? Eye Contact Lens 2007;33(6 Pt 2):412–414; discussion 424–425.
262. Khor WB, Aung T, Saw SM, et al. An outbreak of Fusarium keratitis associated with contact lens wear in Singapore. JAMA 2006;295(24):2867–2873.
263. Foulks GN. Prolonging contact lens wear and making contact lens wear safer. Am J Ophthalmol 2006;141(2):369–373.
264. Classe JG. Liability for extended-wear contact lenses. Optom Clin 1991;1(3):51–62.
265. Harris MG, Dister RE. Informed consent for extended-wear patients. Optom Clin 1991;1(3):33–50.
266. Classe JG. Avoiding liability in contact lens practice. Optom Clin 1994;4(1):1–12.
267. Harris M. Informed consent for contact lens patients. J Brit Contact Lens Assoc 1994;17(4):119–134.
268. Classe JG. Informed consent and contact lens practice. J Am Optom Assoc 1996;67(3):132–134.
269. Brennan NA, Coles C, Jaworski A, et al. Proposed practice guidelines for continuous contact lens wear. Clin Exp Optom 2001;84(2):71–77.
270. Brennan NA, Coles C, Dahl A. Where do silicone hydrogels fit into everyday practice? In: Sweeney D, ed. Silicone Hydrogels: Continuous Wear Contact Lenses. Oxford: Butterworth-Heinemann, 2004:275–308.
271. Efron N, Brennan NA, Currie JM, et al. Determinants of the initial comfort of hydrogel contact lenses. Am J Optom Physiol Opt 1986;63(10):819–823.
272. Dumbleton KA, Chalmers RL, McNally J, et al. Effect of lens base curve on subjective comfort and assessment of fit with silicone hydrogel continuous wear contact lenses. Optom Vis Sci 2002;79(10):633–637.
273. Ghormley N, Jones L. Managing lipid deposition on silicone hydrogel lenses. Contact Lens Spectrum 2006;21(1):21.
274. Nichols JJ. Deposition rates and lens care influence on galyfilcon A silicone hydrogel lenses. Optom Vis Sci 2006;83(10):751–757.
275. Subbaraman LN, Bayer S, Glasier MA, et al. Rewetting drops containing surface active agents improve the clinical performance of silicone hydrogel contact lenses. Optom Vis Sci 2006;83(3):143–151.
276. Yamane S, Paragina S. Patient education. In: Bennett ES, Weissman BA, eds. Clinical Contact Lens Practice. Philadelphia: Lippincott, 1991:1–9.
277. Miller PJ. Liability issues in contact lens practice. J Am Optom Assoc 1986;57(3):227–229.
278. Efron N. Grading scales for contact lens complications. Ophthal Physiol Opt 1998;18(2):182–186.
279. Efron N, Morgan PB, Katsara SS. Validation of grading scales for contact lens complications. Ophthalmic Physiol Opt 2001;21(1):17–29.
280. IER. IER Grading Scales. In: Phillips A, Speedwell L, eds. Contact Lenses. Edinburgh: Butterworth-Heinemann, 2006:628–631.
281. Jones L, Senchyna M, Glasier MA, et al. Lysozyme and lipid deposition on silicone hydrogel contact lens materials. Eye Contact Lens 2003;29(1 Suppl):S75–S79.
282. Carney FP, Nash WL, Sentell KB. The adsorption of major tear film lipids in vitro to various silicone hydrogels over time. Invest Ophthalmol Vis Sci 2008;49(1):120–124.

CHAPTER **17**

Aphakia

Dennis Burger and Larry J. Davis

▓ INTRODUCTION

While the number of patients undergoing cataract surgery continues to increase, the number who remain aphakic following surgery has been declining rapidly since the mid-1980s. The quality of intraocular lenses (IOLs), the improved surgical techniques, and the safety of intraocular lenses have combined to be a driving force in reducing the number of aphakic patients. Although IOLs have resulted in greatly reducing the number of new aphakic patients, they have not eliminated aphakia for all patients requiring removal of the crystalline lens. The use of intraocular lenses is considered risky for some patients following trauma and complicated intraocular surgery and for relatively young patients, especially infants.

Perhaps no single population has experienced the benefits of contact lenses more than those who are aphakic. The thick spectacle lenses necessary for the aphakic eye (usually +12.00 D to +16.00 D) induce a magnification of at least 30%.[1] Restrictions of the peripheral visual field are also found while wearing spectacle lenses for the correction of aphakia. Prismatic effect is found to increase toward the edge of the lens, resulting in a ring scotoma. Although lenticular designs reduce the thickness and mass of these lenses, they may reduce the "optical" size of the lens, further restricting the visual field. Patients attempt to compensate for these effects by turning their head to scan the visual field. Contact lenses offer reduced magnification and better visual performance by eliminating visual field restrictions, and eliminate the use of the thick spectacle lenses, which are heavy, cosmetically unattractive, and optically inferior to contact lenses.[2,3]

▓ ADULT APHAKIC PATIENTS

Patient Selection

All contact lens wearers must perform routine lens care to maintain a lens with clear optical quality that is free from contamination. Once the decision is made to proceed with a contact lens correction, the patient, or in the case of extremely young or old patients, the guardian, should be advised of the required lens maintenance. Some factors to consider include specific visual requirements, best potential visual acuity, manual dexterity, willingness or ability to participate in lens care, and if indicated, social support system.

Ideally, the corneal astigmatism should be two diopters or less to maintain a well-fitting contact lens. In most cases (with the exception of infantile aphakia), this would mean fitting approximately 4 to 6 weeks following the primary surgical procedure. Against-the-rule corneal cylinder, which may occur from loose sutures or wound gape, can complicate the fitting of a contact lens. Therefore, while an attempt should be made to reduce the corneal cylinder as much as possible, having a moderate amount of with-the-rule cylinder is better than leaving the patient with even a small amount of against-the-rule corneal cylinder. Patients who have become aphakic as a result of blunt or penetrating trauma should be allowed sufficient time to reduce any intraocular inflammation. While a period of 4 to 6 weeks is also usually adequate in this group of patients, some may require a longer amount of time. This is usually of no consequence if the patient is beyond the critical period and without risk of refractive amblyopia and if good visual acuity is maintained in the paired eye. Correction of the pediatric aphakic patient should be performed as soon as possible. Most often this can be achieved within 5 days following the primary surgical procedure. This is especially true if small-incision techniques are used, which allow for a short healing period and reduced postoperative astigmatism.

Fitting Principles

Because of the large vertex powers and frequent unpredictability of lens dynamics while on the eye, diagnostic lens application is essential. During the prefitting evaluation, in addition to the usual evaluation of corneal curvature, refractive status, visual acuity, tear quality, and external disease, any results of undercorrecting the refractive cylinder should be evaluated. As the best corrected visual acuity in many of these patients is 20/40 or worse, residual cylinder may have no effect on their optimum visual acuity. Diagnostic fitting, using high-powered plus lenses, will improve the accuracy of the initial prescription by reducing any errors in compensating for vertex distance. It is also essential to evaluate lens movement and centration while performing a diagnostic fitting. When fitting gas permeable (GP) lenses, they will frequently be found to decenter and a careful fluorescein pattern evaluation is indicated. The use of a hydrogel lens requires careful evaluation of lens fit as well. Adequate lens movement is essential to reduce complications resulting from tight-fitting lenses.

Lens Materials

Gas Permeable Lenses

When to Use: Once the decision is made to proceed with contact lenses, practitioners are presented with an initial decision of whether to use a soft or GP contact lens design. Patients having no contact lens experience are usually fit with a rigid lens. This is especially true if the corneal curvatures are 43.00 D or flatter, with 2.00 D or less with-the-rule corneal cylinder, and if the upper lid is positioned at or below the superior limbus. Any amount of against-the-rule astigmatism can negatively influence centration of a rigid lens design. GP contact lenses offer several distinct advantages over their hydrogel counterparts (Fig. 17.1). Often, those patients most likely to reject GP contact lens wear are those having previous experience wearing a hydrogel contact lens. If, after proceeding with the fitting and evaluation of GP lenses, it is determined that an adequate fitting relationship or comfort cannot be achieved, refitting with a hydrogel lens design is usually well accepted by the patient. Patients who have experienced serious adverse reactions (e.g., tight lens syndrome, keratitis, severe giant papillary conjunctivitis) while using a hydrogel contact lens are more likely to successfully adapt to GP lenses than those wearing hydrogel lenses without apparent adverse effects. These patients must possess the motivation to accept the change in lid sensation, movement, and handling required for a GP lens design.

Lens Designs: Because of the high plus powers of aphakic lenses resulting in a large center thickness, those attempting to fit rigid lenses must be familiar with various design characteristics that may improve the fitting relationship and enhance patient comfort. In most cases, a minus lenticular type of design is indicated. This both reduces lens mass by decreasing center thickness and creates a more posteriorly positioned center of gravity, thus enhancing lens centration. Lenticulation also produces a thicker lens edge profile and creates greater lens-to-lid interaction. This enhances lens movement and improves centration of the optical zone diameter over the pupil. Because of intralaboratory variability in the manufacture of lenticular lens designs, it is advisable to specify a specific lenticular design for better consistency and performance. This is achieved, in part, by requesting a particular flange radius (lenticular curve)

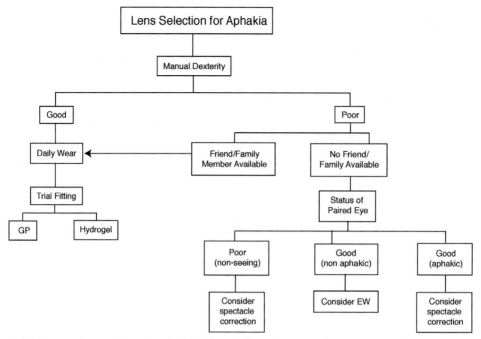

■ **FIGURE 17.1** Factors influencing the initial lens of choice for contact lens correction of aphakia.

and optic cap (front optical zone) to be used during lens manufacture (Fig. 17.2). While a flatter flange radius will usually assist in maintaining a superior lens-to-cornea fitting relationship, this may also result in increased lens awareness. An approximate, desired flange radius between 1.0 and 2.0 mm flatter than the base curve radius in millimeters is recommended.[4] For example, if a lens is ordered with a 45.00 D (7.50 mm) base curve radius, one would expect to order a flange radius of 8.5 to 9.5 mm. With few exceptions, the optic cap should be equal to the back optic zone diameter. A recommended diagnostic fitting set for lenticular lenses is found in Table 17.1.[5] Effective Power and Vertex Power optical considerations are provided in Appendix A and B respectively.

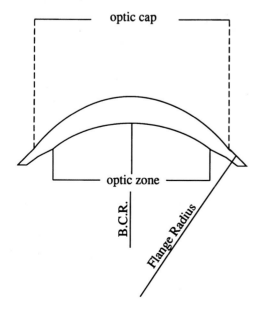

■ **FIGURE 17.2** Design of a minus carrier aphakic contact lens.

TABLE 17.1 SUGGESTED LENTICULAR APHAKIA TRIAL LENS SET (RECOMMENDED MATERIAL IS PMMA OR A LOW DK GAS PERMEABLE MATERIAL)

BASE CURVE	OAD	OZD	BACK VERTEX POWER	SCR/W	PCR/W	CT	FLANGE RADIUS
39.00	9.50	8.0	+13.00	BCR + 1.0 mm/.4	SCR + 1.5/.35	0.44	BCR + 1.50 mm
40.00	9.50	8.0	+13.00	BCR + 1.0 mm/.4	SCR + 1.5/.35	0.44	BCR + 1.50 mm
40.50	9.50	8.0	+13.00	BCR + 1.0 mm/.4	SCR + 1.5/.35	0.44	BCR + 1.50 mm
41.00	9.50	8.0	+13.00	BCR + 1.0 mm/.4	SCR + 1.5/.35	0.44	BCR + 1.50 mm
41.50	9.50	8.0	+13.00	BCR + 1.0 mm/.4	SCR + 1.5/.35	0.44	BCR + 1.50 mm
42.00	9.50	8.0	+13.00	BCR + 1.0 mm/.4	SCR + 1.5/.35	0.44	BCR + 1.50 mm
42.50	9.50	8.0	+13.00	BCR + 1.0 mm/.4	SCR + 1.5/.35	0.44	BCR + 1.50 mm
43.00	9.30	7.8	+13.00	BCR + 1.0 mm/.4	SCR + 1.5/.35	0.42	BCR + 1.50 mm
43.50	9.30	7.8	+13.00	BCR + 1.0 mm/.4	SCR + 1.5/.35	0.42	BCR + 1.50 mm
44.00	9.30	7.8	+13.00	BCR + 1.0 mm/.4	SCR + 1.5/.35	0.42	BCR + 1.50 mm
44.50	9.30	7.8	+13.00	BCR + 1.0 mm/.4	SCR + 1.5/.35	0.42	BCR + 1.50 mm
45.00	9.00	7.6	+13.00	BCR + 1.0 mm/.4	SCR + 1.5/.3	0.40	BCR + 1.50 mm
45.50	9.00	7.6	+13.00	BCR + 1.0 mm/.4	SCR + 1.5/.3	0.40	BCR + 1.50 mm
46.00	9.00	7.6	+13.00	BCR + 1.0 mm/.4	SCR + 1.5/.3	0.40	BCR + 1.50 mm
47.00	9.00	7.6	+13.00	BCR + 1.0 mm/.4	SCR + 1.5/.3	0.40	BCR + 1.50 mm
48.00	9.00	7.6	+13.00	BCR + 1.0 mm/.4	SCR + 1.5/.3	0.40	BCR + 1.50 mm

BCR, base curve radius; CT, center thickness; Dk, oxygen permeability; PCR/W, peripheral curve radius/width; PMMA, polymethylmethacrylate; OAD, overall diameter; OZD, optical zone diameter; SCR/W, secondary curve radius/width.

Reprinted with permission from Davis LJ, Bergin C, Bennett ES. Aphakia. In: Bennett ES, Weissman BA, eds. Clinical Contact Lens Practice. Philadelphia: Lippincott Williams & Wilkins, 2005:595–604.

Occasionally, patients having corneas >45.00 D may be fitted using a small-diameter, single-cut lens design. These lenses will require fitting at least 1 D steeper than K to improve lens centration. A recommended diagnostic fitting set for single-cut aphakic lenses is provided in Table 17.2.[5] Because of the large center thickness of these lenses, it is recommended to order aphakic designs in a lens material with medium to high oxygen permeability (Dk). These lenses demonstrate good stability even when materials having Dk values above 100 are used. Most lens designs are now available including spherical, front toric, bitoric, bifocal, and multifocal powers.

Hydrogel and Silicone Hydrogel Lenses

When to Use: Hydrogel and silicone hydrogel contact lenses offer potential advantages over their GP counterparts. Perhaps the most important advantage is immediate patient comfort. Second, a well-fitting contact lens is almost always obtainable. Therefore, one indication for using a hydrogel aphakic contact lens is when an inadequate fit occurs while using a GP lens design. In cases of low refractive astigmatism, hydrogel contact lenses usually perform quite well. If residual astigmatism reduces visual acuity, the appropriate cylindrical error can be incorporated into spectacles and worn over the contact lens. Finally, the ability to inventory most lens parameters provides immediate correction in cases of high refractive error without interruption of lens wear in the event of lens loss or damage. Patients who have become aphakic

TABLE 17.2 SUGGESTED SINGLE-CUT APHAKIA TRIAL LENS SET

BASE CURVE	OAD	OZD	(BACK VERTEX) POWER	SCR/W	PCR/W	CT
45.00	9.00	7.6	+13.00	BCR + 1.0 mm/.4	SCR + 1.5/.3	0.40
45.50	9.00	7.6	+13.00	BCR + 1.0 mm/.4	SCR + 1.5/.3	0.40
46.00	9.00	7.6	+13.00	BCR + 1.0 mm/.4	SCR + 1.5/.3	0.40
46.50	9.00	7.6	+13.00	BCR + 1.0 mm/.4	SCR + 1.5/.3	0.40
47.00	9.00	7.6	+13.00	BCR + 1.0 mm/.4	SCR + 1.5/.3	0.40
48.00	9.00	7.6	+13.00	BCR + 1.0 mm/.4	SCR + 1.5/.3	0.40

BCR, base curve radius; CT, center thickness; PCR/W, peripheral curve radius/width; OAD, overall diameter; OZD, optical zone diameter; SCR/W, secondary curve radius/width.

Reprinted with permission from Davis LJ, Bergin C, Bennett ES. Aphakia. In: Bennett ES, Weissman BA, eds. Clinical Contact Lens Practice. Philadelphia: Lippincott Williams & Wilkins, 2005:595–604.

secondary to trauma may also have iris defects resulting in large or ectopic pupils. These patients may benefit from a dark-tinted, hydrogel contact lens creating an artificial pupil and iris, which attenuates bright light. Hydrogel lens designs are more suitable for this application, as they more readily accept tint and encompass more of the corneal surface while providing better centration with decreased movement.

Lens Designs: Several hydrogel lens designs are available for aphakic contact lens fitting. As many aphakic patients are elderly and benefit from using an extended-wear contact lens material, various aphakic contact lenses have been designed for use on an extended-wear schedule. An attempt is made to increase oxygen transmission by reducing lens thickness using lenticulation, increasing the water content of the material, or both. It has been several years since any new hydrogel contact lens materials and/or designs have been investigated for use in aphakia on an extended-wear basis. Most recently, one silicone hydrogel lens (O$_2$OPTIX, O$_2$OPTIX Custom Ciba Vision) and numerous spherical, toric, and bifocal planned-replacement lenses in aphakic powers have been introduced. A list of these lens designs is provided in Table 17.3.[6]

Complications

The thick lens designs necessary for aphakia create a hypoxic environment for the cornea. It is thought that many contact lens-related complications such as corneal infiltrates, neovascularization, corneal edema, and the more serious complication of infectious corneal ulceration are caused in part by the relative hypoxia that occurs while wearing contact lenses. Contributing factors in the elderly population are reduced aqueous tear secretion, meibomian gland dysfunction, blepharitis, and possibly decreased activity of the immune system. Periodic evaluation of proper lens fit should be performed, at minimum, every 6 months. Occasionally, a hydrogel lens is found to fit tighter with age. Routine annual or semiannual lens replacement may be beneficial in reducing acute tight lens syndrome. It has been demonstrated that lens removal before sleep is an important factor reducing the frequency of serious lens-related complications. Therefore, it is advisable to discourage the use of extended wear for most aphakic patients.

Occasionally, patients are unable or reluctant to perform lens care. Many patients lack the necessary manual dexterity to insert and remove contact lenses. Others may have a psychological reluctance to be actively involved in the required lens manipulation and care. Routine removal and cleanings may then be performed by a friend or family member or as a last resort in the office.

TABLE 17.3 HYDROGEL AND SILICONE HYDROGEL PLANNED-REPLACEMENT LENSES IN APHAKIC POWERS

COMPANY	NAME	AVAILABILITY
I. SILICONE HYDROGEL		
Ciba Vision	O₂OPTIX Custom	Quarterly
II. HYDROGEL		
A. SPHERICAL		
Alden Optical	Alden HP49	4-pack
Alden Optical	Alden HP-59	4-pack
Metro Optics	Metrosoft II	4-pack
Metro Optics	Metrolite	4-pack
Metro Optics	Metrotint	4-pack
SpecialEyes	SpecialEyes 59 Sphere	4-pack
B. TORIC		
Alden Optical	Alden HP49 Toric	4-pack
Alden Optical	Alden HP59 Toric	4-pack
California Optics	CO Soft 55 Toric	4-pack
Gelflex	Synergy Quarterly	Quarterly
	Replacement Toric	
C. MULTIFOCAL AND MULTIFOCAL TORIC		
CooperVision	Proclear Multifocal XR	6-pack
CooperVision	Proclear Multifocal Toric	6-pack
Unilens	C Vue 55 Toric Multifocal	3-pack and 4-pack

From Thompson TT. Tyler's Quarterly 2007;24(4):5–10.

▩ PEDIATRIC APHAKIC PATIENTS

One of the most challenging and rewarding use of contact lenses is for the pediatric aphakic. Pediatric aphakia, although rare, is a condition that is made for the use of contact lenses. Cataracts can be either congenital or acquired and either monocular or binocular. Congenital cataracts are estimated to occur in approximately 1.4 to 2.3 per 10,000 births and can be unilateral or bilateral.[7–11] Although the incidence is rare, the visual implications are severe if the cataract is not removed early and the child is not properly treated (Fig. 17.3).

Treatment for congenital cataracts consists of early cataract extraction, contact lens correction, and amblyopia treatment before age 4 months to have reasonable expectation of good visual acuity in the affected eye.[12]

Treatment Options

Treatment options for the pediatric aphakics includes glasses, IOLs, and contact lenses. Glasses can be a viable option for the bilateral aphakic. Glasses allow both eyes to be corrected; however, there are significant limitations. Patients will experience reduced visual fields, magnification distortion (30% increase), and problems with achieving properly fitted frames, especially for infants (Fig. 17.4).

Unilateral aphakics have the additional problem of anisometropia and, as a result, cannot be effectively corrected in spectacles. The development of amblyopia is a major concern in unilateral

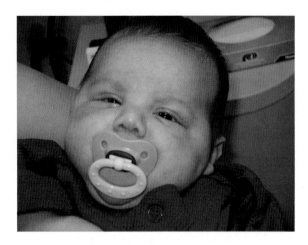

■ FIGURE 17.3 Two-week-old aphakic.

aphakics since it is unlikely that the patient is using both eyes. Bilateral aphakics are more successful as both eyes have similar refractive errors; the problem of anisometropia is eliminated.[13]

Intraocular lenses have been suggested for pediatric aphakics, but this is controversial.[14–19] Problems exist with this treatment modality in that the eye changes rapidly during the first 4 years of life because of axial length.[20] The average refractive error at the corneal plane for a 1-month-old infant is +31 D, while at age 4 it is +16 D.[21] Because of this change in refractive power, the IOL would either have to be changed multiple times or additional vision correction would be needed to properly correct the child's vision. Intraocular lenses would be best served in the aphakic population that is over the age of 4.

Currently, contact lenses are the best option for the pediatric aphakic. The power and fit of the lens can be easily changed as the eye grows.[17,18,22,23] The problem of anisometropia for the unilateral aphakic is significantly reduced to allow for binocular correction. There are multiple contact lens options for the pediatric patient. These options include soft lenses, rigid GP lenses, and silicone lenses.

Soft lenses are commonly used in the adult population or in the nonaphakic pediatric population. New materials, including silicone hydrogels, allow for long-term wear of lenses with minimal complications. Additionally, the disposable modality has allowed for ease of replacement for lost lenses with these patients. However, soft lenses are not extensively used in the pediatric population. The powers required for the pediatric aphakic are generally > +20 D. Many of these soft lenses need to be custom made (Table 17.4). Infants under the age of 1 year often

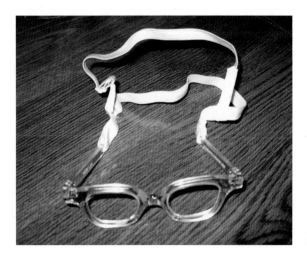

■ FIGURE 17.4 Headband frame.

TABLE 17.4 PEDIATRIC APHAKIC LENSES

LENS	MATERIAL	BASE CURVE	DIAMETER	POWER	DK	COST
California Optics Soft	Methafilcon 55%	8.4	13.5	pl–+30 D	18.8	$ 47
Alden Classic	38%	7.7–8.9		+10.25–+30 D	8.4	$ 50
Continental Pedi	Ocufilcon 55%	5.8–10.4	8.5–14.0	pl–+40 D	18.1	$ 40
Flexlens Pedi	Hioxfilcon B 45%	6.0–10.8	10.0–16.0	Any	13.2	$ 85
SuperNova	Hioxfilcon A 59%	5.0–22.0	6.0–18.0	Up to +50 D	21	$ 29
OcuEase Pedi	Ocufilcon B 53%	6.0–8.6	8.0–15.0	+10–+40 D	18.1	$ 75
Bausch & Lomb Silsoft	Elastofilcon A	7.5, 7.7, 7.9, 8.1	11.3, 11.3, 12.5, under +20	+11.50–+32 D	340	$126
Rigid Gas Permeable	Any	Any	Any	Any	Up to 163	Varies

Dk, oxygen permeability.

have lenses in the +25 to +32 D range. These lenses are extremely thick. Aphakic lenses in this power range are generally ≥1 mm thick. Additionally, the Dk of the soft lens material is low, in the range of 15 to 18.8. Therefore, these lenses are very thick with very low oxygen permeability. This creates a lens that has low oxygen transmissibility and can result in problems with acute red eye response. If soft aphakic lenses are used, they must be used as a daily wear option and should never be used in an extended-wear modality. Other problems associated with aphakic soft lenses are increased difficulty for insertion by the parents and some compromise in vision versus gas permeable lenses.

Gas permeable lenses are another option for the pediatric aphakic patient. Advantages of gas permeable lenses versus soft include that they are easier for the parents to handle, have higher oxygen transmissibility, offer better vision, can be obtained in any power, are the least costly contact lens alternative, and have good durability. There are several disadvantages: problems with comfort, the ease of displacement of the lens, the need for custom lenses, and the difficulty in fitting the lens. It is difficult to fit a rigid lens; keratometry readings may not be possible, diagnostic lenses have to be used, and the fitting on uncooperative children may need to be performed under general anesthesia in the operating room.

The last option is a flexible silicone elastomer, the Silsoft lens. Advantages of the Silsoft lens are that they have the highest oxygen permeability (Dk 340), they can be used as extended wear, they provide good comfort, there is availability of stock parameters, they stay in the eye better than a rigid lens, they are easier to handle for parents than soft lenses, and fluorescein can be used with the lens. Disadvantages are that they are the most expensive lens option, there is limited power availability (3 D steps), they attract lipid deposits and have to be replaced, and they can adhere to the eye and become excessively tight. Despite all these disadvantages, the Silsoft lens remains the workhorse lens for the pediatric aphakic. This lens has high oxygen transmissibility, good comfort, and the ability to stay in the eye, thus allowing it to be used as an extended wear lens with fewer complications than soft lenses. Silsoft lenses also have less irritation and, with the ability to be used in an extended wear modality, are more convenient for the parents than gas permeable lenses.

Anatomic Considerations

There are many differences between pediatric and adult eyes that the practitioner must be aware of: axial length, corneal diameter, corneal curvature, palpebral aperture, and pupil size.[21,24,25] All of these are important features to recognize when fitting a contact lens to a child.

The axial length is one of the key features, as it contributes so much to refractive error. In newborns, the axial length is typically 17 mm, whereas the adult eye's length is 24 mm. This short eye results in very high refractive errors. The typical aphakic power in an infant at 1 month is 31 D, but by the time the child is age 4, it has decreased to 17 D.[21] The average corneal diameter in infants is much smaller than adults. In infants, the average diameter is 9.8 mm, whereas in the adult eye it is between 11.5 and 12.5 mm.[21] The cornea also undergoes significant change during the first years of life. In premature infants, the average curvature is 49.50 D, in 1- to 2-month-old infants it is 47 D, and the 4-year-old it is 43 to 44 D.[21] The palpebral aperture in infants is also smaller and the tension of the lids tighter that the adult. This makes it a challenge to insert a contact lens onto the eye. The pupil diameter of the infant is also much smaller that the adult eye, with the average pupil size of an infant being 2 mm. With all these factors, the contact lens fit becomes critical. The contact lens has to fit these characteristics: relatively small in diameter to be inserted on the eye, steep in corneal curvature so the lens will stay centered, and high power because the refractive error is very high. Any contact lens that is used for the pediatric aphakic should also have exceptional oxygen permeability, as this lens may be used in an extended-wear modality.

Contact Lens Fitting

Determining Lens Parameters

Fitting a contact lens to an infant is one of the most challenging techniques that the contact lens practitioner must perform. Different age groups require different methods for successful contact lens fitting. Different strategies need to be employed for the infant, the toddler, and the young child. In general, it may not be possible to obtain corneal curvature measurements on children under the age of 4 to 5 years.[26,27] The practitioner will also not be able to obtain subjective responses. The use of an autorefractor may be limited to older children. Therefore, the practitioner needs to be skilled in performing retinoscopy. This will be the determining factor in deciding on the power of the contact lens. When determining an aphakic correction, it should be noted that the infant is going to have a very high refractive error and that the younger the child, the higher the refractive error.

Determining the initial power can be frustrating because of the lack of cooperation of the child. Retinoscopy can be performed several ways: using loose lenses, using retinoscopic lens bars, or using a single high plus lens. In using loose lenses, the practitioner places a lens in front of the child's eye and determines motion and then attempts a different lens depending on what was initially elicited. The problem is that the child often loses interest and the practitioner is constantly exchanging lenses. The use of a lens bar eliminates this, but typically the child will attempt to grab the bar. A simple way to determine the power is to take a high plus lens (e.g., +20 D) and move it away from the eye until neutralization is obtained (Fig. 17.5). If the distance is measured from where the lens is to the corneal plane, the power can be calculated for the lens using the following formula: $P_C = P_S/1 - dP_S$, where P_C is the power at the corneal plane and P_S is the power at the spectacle plane. This will yield an initial power for the contact lens. The practitioner should always keep in mind that the power of the eye will continue to change as the child gets older and it is not unusual for a newborn to have a lens with the power of +32 D while a 4-year-old may be only +17 D. In all cases, the first lens is a sophisticated diagnostic lens and retinoscopy needs to be performed over the lens to determine, with accuracy, the power needed for the patient.

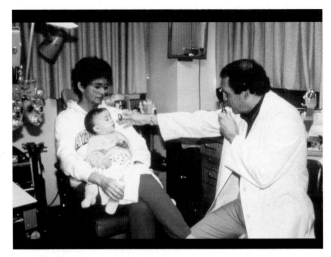

■ **FIGURE 17.5** Vertex lens technique.

Assessing the Lens-to-Cornea Fitting Relationship

All contact lenses should be assessed after they are in the eye. Determination of the power of the lens needs to be performed. Retinoscopy will yield how close the correction is. Typically, infants and toddlers are overplussed by 3 D. The reason for this is the fact that young infants and toddlers work in a near world, often holding things very close to their eyes. As the child ages, the correction changes until he or she is properly corrected for distance and uses reading overglasses, typically in the form of bifocals.

The fit of the lens needs to be evaluated. The primary author does not use soft lenses for pediatric aphakics who are under the age of 5. The use of gas permeable contact lenses and Silsoft lenses allows the practitioner to use fluorescein to determine the fitting relationship. Both types of lenses should center well and move easily. The fluorescein patterns should be minimal apical clearance. Rigid lenses will need to be fit a little larger than normal to help keep the lens centered. Whenever possible, the use of the slit lamp to access the lens-to-cornea fitting relationship is preferable. Even young children can be placed in the slit lamp for observation (Fig. 17.6).

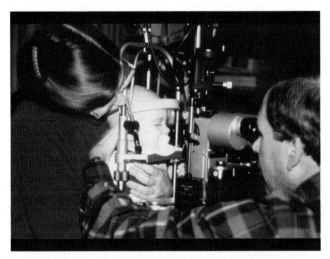

■ **FIGURE 17.6** Infant in slit lamp.

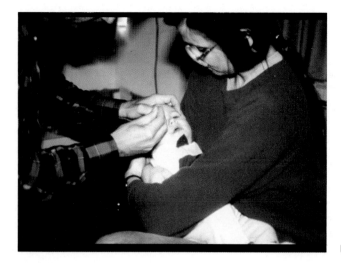

■ **FIGURE 17.7** Infant insertion.

Care should be taken to look for staining or lens binding. If these conditions are found, steps must be taken to eliminate them. The surface of the lens should also be evaluated. The Silsoft lens is a hydrophobic material that is coated to allow tears to cover the lens. A side effect of the coating is that it has an affinity for lipids and the lens will get deposited and have to be replaced.

Lens Handling and Care

Handling

Insertion for an Infant: Fitting a contact lens to an infant under the age of 1 year can be both frustrating and rewarding. The type of contact lens, the power, the overall diameter, and the base curve radius have to be selected. Once the lens has been selected, the lens must be inserted onto the eye. For the infant group, the most successful technique is to have the mother cradle the child against her breast and use her arms to secure the child so he or she cannot move (Fig. 17.7).

The lids are then separated and the lens is placed on the eye. Problems inserting the lens may exist if the child has very tight lids and the practitioner cannot get the lids sufficiently separated to get the lens in the eye. In situations like this, the use of a speculum to separate the lids will allow the practitioner to insert the lens on to the eye (Fig. 17.8).

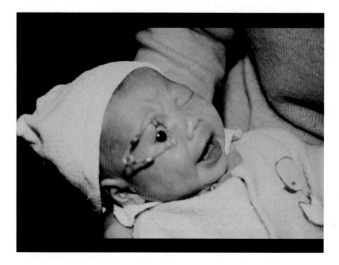

■ **FIGURE 17.8** Speculum on infant.

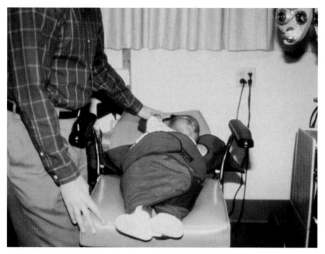

■ **FIGURE 17.9** Infant on papoose board.

Care should be taken not to express the contact lens when the speculum is removed. Although the technique with the speculum appears awkward and uncomfortable, it allows for fast insertion on an infant, who is challenging in applying a lens.

Insertion for a Toddler: Insertion for the toddler age group between 1½ to 4 years of age is the most difficult group in which to insert a lens. These children are very active and know what they want and what they don't want. The contact lens insertion is extremely difficult on an uncooperative child in this age group. They will turn their heads, squeeze their eyes shut, physically fight, and often generally resist. Many practitioners will use some form of restraint to aid in the insertion of the lens. The restraints will keep the child moderately immobile to allow lens insertion. Commercial restraints, such as the papoose board, have Velcro strips to hold the child still (Fig. 17.9).

The use of blankets or sheets will often be equally successful. When using a blanket, it is important to lay the child on the ground and then either roll the child in the blanket or wrap the blanket around the child, making sure that the arms and legs are securely within the blanket (Fig. 17.10). This then allows the practitioner to insert the lens on the eye with minimal movement of

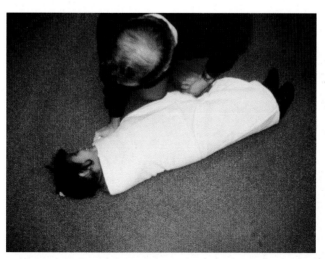

■ **FIGURE 17.10** Blanket technique.

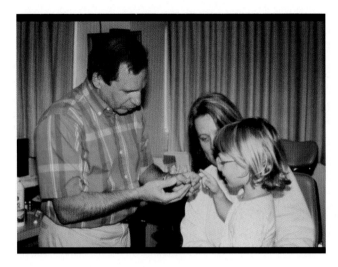

■ **FIGURE 17.11** Initial presentation of lens to child.

the child. Additionally, it frees the practitioner's hands to make lens insertion easier. In some of these cases, the practitioner may have to use the speculum as an aid to separate the lids to allow insertion. This technique is not as traumatic to the child as is a protracted lens insertion battle. Inserting the aphakic lens can be cumbersome. The lens is thick and heavy and will not stay on a finger. It is best to "pinch" the lens between two fingers to insert it. The lens should either be placed directly on center or, if not possible, the lens should be slid underneath the upper lid to allow the lens to adhere to the eye. These techniques should be used for all age groups. The practitioner should always remember that the goal is to place the contact lens on the eye because the child is aphakic and that this lens is therapeutically indicated.

Insertion for a Child: Children who are older (>5 years) are generally more cooperative; thus, determining the necessary contact lens is easier. Children of this age group can have keratometry performed, can use the autorefractor, and can tell you what they see and may be able to participate in a subjective refraction. This age group is the one that can be reasoned with. The technique that the first author uses is the following. A discussion of the contact lens is provided. A lens is then shown to the child (Fig. 17.11). The child can touch the lens and see how it feels (Fig. 17.12). The lens is then placed on different parts of the child such as the cheek, the nose, or the hand. At this point, the author then places a lens on his eye so the child can

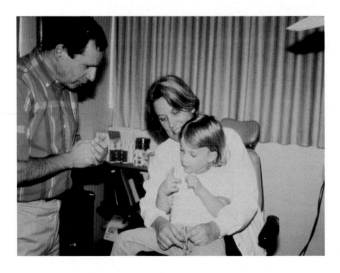

■ **FIGURE 17.12** Child handling lens.

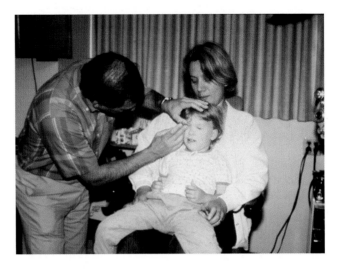

■ FIGURE 17.13 Insertion on child.

see that it is okay. The child then is allowed to handle the lens and the lens is placed on the child's eye (Fig. 17.13). The child is often rewarded for his or her effort after the lens is in place. Suitable rewards can be stickers, the surprise goody box, or, as we often use, some jelly beans.

Removal of the Lens: The technique for lens removal is the same for all age groups. The technique is the two-hand method using both lids to expel the lens (Fig. 17.14). To remove the lens, fingers from each hand should be placed at the lid margin of both the top and bottom lids. Pressure should be placed on the lids so the margin presses against the globe. The lids should then be pushed toward each other. Care should be taken not to evert the lids. When performed properly, the lens will be expressed from the eye. This technique will work for Silsoft, rigid, and even soft lenses. Soft lens solutions are used for Silsoft and soft lenses. Gas permeable solutions are used for GP lenses.

Care

Wearing Schedule: The wearing schedule for a pediatric aphakic will very depending on the age of the child and the contact lens modality used. If a soft aphakic lens is used, this lens must be removed on a daily basis. The low Dk and thick lens does not lend itself to an extended wear

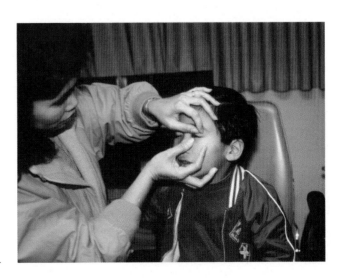

■ FIGURE 17.14 Two-hand removal.

modality. Rigid lenses have more flexibility. These lenses have higher oxygen permeability. This allows the child to sleep with a lens in place. The authors recommend removal of the rigid lens at night but leaving the lens in during daytime naps. The Silsoft lens, with its high permeability, is the most flexible. These lenses can be worn either as daily wear or as extended wear. The lens is durable enough to be removed every day if the practitioner chooses, or oxygen permeable enough that the lenses can stay in the eye for 1 week or more at a time. The practitioner will decide how long the lens should be used before removal. When the lens is removed, it is advised that the lens be cleaned and sterilized.

Follow-Up Appointments: Pediatric patients will be evaluated very frequently by the contact lens practitioner. The patient should be seen the day after dispensing to evaluate how the lens is being tolerated, especially if the lens is being worn in an extended wear modality. Follow-up visits should be scheduled at 1 week and again in 1 month. The child should then be evaluated every 2 to 3 months to monitor the fitting relationship of the lens and the resulting vision.

Potential Problems

With any type of contact lens there is a potential for problems. Pediatric patients are often more difficult to assess. In many cases they cannot verbalize the problem. The practitioner's first encounter of a problem may be a red eye. Parents should be made aware of signs of a normal and an abnormal response. Red eyes are the biggest concern. This can be secondary to erosion, an infection, or a tight lens. Parents should immediately have the child examined by a practitioner to determine the underlying cause. Once the cause is found, the practitioner should proceed with the proper treatment. Other less significant problems that will most likely be encountered include lens loss and lens degradation. Pediatric patients will lose lenses; this is always expected. A spare lens should always be available so the patient is not without a lens. Silsoft lenses will also degrade with use because of the film on the lens. Frequent removal and cleaning will help prevent this problem.

What Parents Need to Know

Successful contact lens wear for the pediatric aphakic patient is going to be directly related to the success achieved with the parents. Parents need to be informed of the child's condition, treatment, prognosis, and follow-up care. They need to be aware that they will be involved in all aspects of the child's lens care including insertion, removal, and cleaning. It is important that the parents are educated about the child's condition, are properly motivated, and have the ability and desire to make the contact lens work. They must be able to observe the eye for any potential complications secondary to lens use and need to recognize an adverse event. They need to be aware of the costs involved with the treatment. In the primary author's experience, the average pediatric aphakic uses six lenses per eye per year. Replacement of lenses can be because of loss, damage, or prescription change. Parents should also be aware that the contact lens is a long-term treatment and not a short-term management option. Parents need to be aware that not only will they have a contact lens to be responsible for, but, in all likelihood, the child will need treatment for amblyopia. They need to know that patching may be required to achieve the child's best possible vision. Once the parents are educated, it is important for them to comply. This will pertain to exhibiting proficiency with inserting, removing, cleaning, and recentering of the contact lens. Failure to perform these functions will cause failure of the patient to successfully wear the lens. Finally, it would be ideal to have a cooperative child but, in many cases, this will not be the result. Lenses have to be inserted and cared for by whatever means necessary and, especially if the child is not cooperative, perseverance is important. Although these patients are difficult to care for, the rewards can be extremely satisfying.

▧ SUMMARY

Aphakic patients are motivated by a strong desire to enhance their quality of vision. Despite this strong will to proceed with the indicated treatment of contact lenses, they often face disappointment from high expectations regarding convenience and best visual performance. This is especially true if the paired eye is phakic with excellent visual acuity or if the affected eye experiences glare. Reluctance to perform lens care or insertion/removal and persistent lens awareness may also result in dissatisfaction with contact lens wear. It is advisable to inform each potential contact lens candidate of the necessary lens care and handling before proceeding with fitting. This should be followed by fitting a lens that provides the best and most comfortable visual acuity and the best fit with the least lens awareness possible.

▧ ACKNOWLEDGEMENTS

The authors would like to thank Amy Langford, OD, for her contribution to this chapter.

▧ CLINICAL CASES

CASE 1

A 46-year-old man developed a cataract of the right eye following penetrating trauma. This has left him with aphakia and a small area of corneal scarring outside of the visual axis.

Manifest refraction:

OD: +12.50 − 0.75 × 145 20/25
OS: −4.00 − 0.75 × 180 20/20

Keratometry:

OD: 41.75 @ 150; 43.00 @ 60
OS: 41.00 @ 180; 42.00 @ 90

SOLUTION: Because of the relatively flat corneal curvatures and young age, this patient would be expected to perform well with a rigid contact lens. It is recommended to begin with a relatively large lens of about 9.50 mm in diameter with a base curve radius "on K." It would be expected that a lenticular edge design would be necessary to provide for adequate lens centration. The predicted lens design would be as follows:

Base curve radius (BCR)	41.75 D (8.08 mm)
Power +14.75 D (vertex distance = 12 mm)	
Diameter	9.50 mm
Optic zone	8.0 mm
Flange radius/optic cap	9.50 mm/8.0 mm
Peripheral curve radii/widths	9.0/0.4 mm, 12.0/0.35 mm

Another important consideration is the myopic refractive error of the paired eye. Aphakic contact lenses result in 3% to 5% image magnification. This, combined with the relative minification from the left spectacle lens, may result in aniseikonia-related asthenopia or diplopia (Appendix C). Therefore, overcorrecting the aphakic eye by 3 to 4 D will allow for a balanced spectacle prescription. Fitting both eyes with contact lenses would be an alternative method to reduce these magnification effects. If the keratometry readings were steeper (e.g., 45.00 @ 150; 46.00 @ 60), a smaller-diameter lens would be indicated. It is recommended to fit an initial lens that is approximately 0.50 D steeper than K using a 9.0-mm-diameter lens. A lenticular design will usually be indicated provided the upper eyelid is at or below the superior limbus. The predicted lens would therefore be as follows:

BCR	45.50 (7.42 mm)
Power +14.25 D (vertex distance = 12 mm)	
Diameter	9.0 mm

Optic zone	7.6 mm
Flange radius/optic cap	9.0 mm/7.6 mm
Peripheral curve radii/widths	8.5/0.4 mm, 11.0/0.3 mm

CASE 2

A 73-year-old aphakic patient has worn a hydrogel contact lens in her left eye with weekly removals for 5 years. She reports a 1-day history of discomfort in the eye with no discharge. The visual acuity in the affected eye is reduced to 20/50 but improves to 20/30 with a +2.00 D over-refraction. The best visual acuity 3 months previously was 20/30 using a plano overrefraction. Slit-lamp examination demonstrates a nonmoving hydrogel lens that is well centered. The conjunctiva is injected, and the cornea demonstrates stromal edema by the presence of several large striae. No corneal inflammatory cells are present. A diffuse, epithelial, punctate stain is apparent on instillation of fluorescein.

SOLUTION: These findings are consistent with acute tight lens syndrome. On dehydration, hydrogel lenses undergo parameter changes that result in a tighter fitting relationship. This, combined with corneal flattening from overnight corneal edema, may result in a lens adhering to the eye. Since aphakic hydrogel lenses with a medium to high water content can develop a large amount of dehydration, sufficient lens lag of at least 1.0 to 1.5 mm is indicated. Possible solutions would be to remove the lens more frequently, replace the lens more frequently (at minimum every 6 months), or loosen the fit by selecting a flatter base curve radius or smaller diameter. Another alternative would be to use a gas permeable lens design.

CASE 3

A 36-year-old man with a history of penetrating trauma is aphakic with a large iris defect in the affected eye. This results in a subjective complaint of glare. A corneal scar exists somewhat outside the visual axis. The best refraction of the right eye using a +14.00 D sphere provides a visual acuity of 20/40. There is no improvement with pinhole. The paired eye is emmetropic with a visual acuity of 20/20.

SOLUTION: In addition to correction of the aphakic refractive error, one must consider the large iris defect. Two options are available. First, the use of dark sunglasses while outdoors may improve the subjective comfort. If glare continues to be a problem while indoors, a tinted aphakic hydrogel lens with an artificial pupil would be indicated. The patient has excellent visual acuity with a spherical spectacle refraction. Therefore, a hydrogel lens design would also be expected to provide good visual acuity. It is recommended to begin with a hydrogel lens having a dark-tinted, opaque iris that also has a central clear pupil of about 3 mm. This design would allow for clear central visual acuity while reducing glare by simulating the natural iris.

CASE 4

A 65-year-old aphakic man wears a gas permeable lens for aphakia in the right eye. He reports lens intolerance for the past 3 to 4 days while wearing the lens. Upon examination, two to three areas of lens edge chipping are observed. Inspection of the lens demonstrates a very thin lens edge profile.

SOLUTION: The thin lens edge design has developed several chips that create lens awareness. A new lens must be ordered incorporating a thicker edge. This may be accomplished simply by increasing the lens center thickness. However, additional modifications may also be desirable since increasing lens center thickness may also produce a heavy lens that positions inferiorly. As this patient's lens had a very thin lens edge, it is likely that it did not have a lenticular design. Reordering a lenticular design would increase the lens edge thickness profile while reducing the lens center thickness. This is probably preferred in most cases as lens centration may also be improved.

CASE 5

A 73-year-old aphakic patient presents after 3 months of extended hydrogel contact lens wear. Her care regimen includes weekly lens removal, last removing the lenses 5 days previously. During the examination, her best visual acuity is 20/30 with an overrefraction of +1.50 D. A corresponding flattening of both corneal meridians is also found by keratometry after lens removal. Slit-lamp examination demonstrates two to three large Descemet folds in the central cornea. Consistent with previous examinations, the cornea also exhibits dot/fingerprint, epithelial basement membrane changes. The contact lens provides an excellent fitting relationship with approximately 1 to 2 mm of lens lag with the blink.

SOLUTION: This patient demonstrates corneal edema secondary to a high corneal oxygen demand. Despite a well-fitting contact lens, corneal hypoxia has resulted in corneal curvature and refractive power changes. If this patient continues with the present lens design and wearing schedule, more serious complications may result. Patients having vitreous prolapse touching the corneal endothelium may also demonstrate corneal edema with hydrogel lenses even when removed daily. The quality of vision may vary throughout the day because of fluctuating refractive error and corneal curvature changes. A reduction in wearing time is indicated. Alternatively, a silicone hydrogel contact lens material (e.g., O_2OPTIX, Ciba Vision) would provide much better oxygen transmission and, therefore, minimize the risk of serious lens-related complications. A hyper DK GP lens material is another option and should provide a more stable vision correction. She may also be considered for a secondary intraocular lens.

CASE 6

A 65-year-old aphakic patient wearing a hydrogel contact lens has experienced for the past 12 months recurrent episodes of giant papillary conjunctivitis, soiled lenses, and lens awareness. He is unable to care for the lens himself because of a tremor related to Parkinson disease. Lens maintenance includes weekly lens removal by his wife, followed by cleaning and disinfection overnight.

SOLUTION: This patient is found to have giant papillary conjunctivitis (GPC) along with poor tear layer and blepharitis. He is fortunate to have someone who can participate in lens care. However, weekly removals of a hydrogel lens have resulted in recurrent episodes of GPC. Therefore, more frequent lens removal is indicated. The patient also appears to have a tear layer that is incompatible with comfortable hydrogel lens wear.

The use of a GP lens may be advantageous in these cases. As the deposits are more easily removed with cleaning, lens soilage is reduced. These lenses can be worn overnight provided a good fit is obtainable and one of the new materials having a Dk of at least 70×10^{-11} is used. Another consideration is the patient's blepharitis and poor tear layer. Medical treatment in the form of hot packs and/or antibiotic/steroid drops is indicated for the lid disease. Tear supplements may be necessary to reduce lens deposits. GP contact lenses tend to become more comfortable following 1 or 2 days of overnight wear. If the patient is very motivated toward continuing soft lens wear, a planned replacement lens—preferably silicone hydrogel—would be recommended. Alternative therapy may include the use of a secondary intraocular lens.

CASE 7

An aphakic patient reports wearing a GP contact lens without complaints. The lens is observed to position inferiorly without movement on blinking. Heavy 3- and 9-o'clock staining is present along with distorted keratometer mires following lens removal.

SOLUTION: A low-riding aphakic rigid lens may result from a steep lens-to-cornea fitting relationship, a thin lens edge design, thick heavy lenses, or a loose upper eyelid. A recommended solution includes a lenticular design that will reduce the center thickness while increasing the edge thickness to maintain a superior lens fit. If the lens is already of lenticular design, flattening the flange radius and/or increasing the overall diameter may enhance the interaction between the lens and the upper eyelid, creating a higher lens fit (Fig. 17.15). In the event that

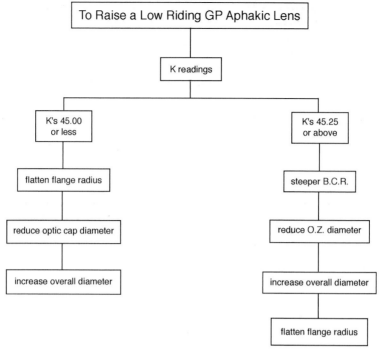

FIGURE 17.15 Raising a low-riding gas permeable aphakic lens.

a lens continues to drop with no improvement in corneal stain and distortion, hydrogel lenses should be considered. When indicated, the appropriate astigmatic correction is placed into a spectacle lens to be worn while wearing the soft lens.

CASE 8

A 9-year-old aphakic patient had cataract extraction because of lens subluxation secondary to Marfan syndrome. She presents for a contact lens follow-up. She wears her lenses daily wear and reports no problems. She is currently wearing the following:

OD BCR 8.3 mm   Dia. 13.8 mm Rx +15.00 D   Visual acuity (VA): 20/80
OS BCR 8.3 mm   Dia. 13.8 mm Rx +14.50 D   VA: 20/60 − 1

FlexLens, ReNu care system

Keratometry:

OD: 42.50 @ 090; 42.75 @ 180
OS: 40.00 @ 090; 42.75 @ 180

Horizontal visible iris diameter (HVID): 11.5 mm

Manifest refraction:

OD: +12.75 − 2.75 × 025   VA: 20/25
OS: +12.50 − 2.00 × 150   VA: 20/30

Slit-lamp examination revealed neovascularization, microcystic edema, and superficial punctate keratitis. The lenses were heavily deposited.

SOLUTION: Because of the anterior segment findings, the patient was refit into the O_2OPTIX Custom lens (Ciba Vision) to provide greater oxygen transmission. This lens was not yet available in a toric design, so spectacles were prescribed to be worn over the contact lenses to correct her astigmatism. The initial trial lenses ordered were:

OD BCR: 8.4 mm, overall diameter (OAD): 14.0 mm, Rx +15.00 D   Distance VA 20/50

Near VA 20/200

OS BCR: 8.4 mm, OAD: 14.0 mm, Rx +14.50 D   Distance VA 20/50

Near VA 20/70

Overrefraction:

OD: +1.25 − 2.25 × 15 Distance VA 20/25, near VA 20/50
OS: +0.50 − 2.00 × 165 Distance VA 20/30, near VA 20/50

A spherical overrefraction of +0.50 D OU gave the patient no blur at distance and 20/40 near vision. New trial lenses were ordered with the same parameters except the power, which was OD +15.50 D and OS +15.00 D. The patient was given a spectacle prescription to wear over the contact lenses at near or to correct the astigmatism as needed.

CASE 9

A 4-year-old patient has a history of congenital cataract in the left eye that was removed in the first year of life. She was initially fit with Silsoft contact lenses. At the age of 3, she became intolerant to the Silsoft lenses. Durasoft lenses were attempted, but the lenses decentered. She was successfully fit with Hydron Mini lenses (BCR 8.3 mm, OAD 13.0 mm, Rx +20.00 D). Four months after dispensing the Hydron Mini lens, the patient began to experience discomfort and the lens was decentering. The mother expressed interest in trying a different lens.

SOLUTION: O_2OPTIX Custom trial lenses are to be ordered. The patient's pertinent information is as follows:

Refraction:

OD: plano BCVA 20/20
OS: +15.00 BCVA 20/60

HVID: 10 mm

Keratometry values: unable to obtain because of the patient's age and cooperation. In young aphakic patients, keratometry readings cannot be taken with accuracy; therefore, it is best to perform a diagnostic fit. A trial fitting set of O_2OPTIX or Silsoft can be used as a basis for the base curve radius.

The following lens was ordered for her OS: O_2OPTIX Custom, BCR 8.0 mm, OAD: 13.2 mm, Rx: +20.00 D. (The power was chosen to make the patient artificially myopic to allow for clear vision at near because of lack of accommodation in the aphakic eye.)

At her follow-up visit, the results of testing were:

VA

OD: 20/20
OS: 20/100 with an overrefraction of ×4.00 + 1.00 × 180; visual acuity was still 20/100.

The lenses centered well. The patient was to continue patching for amblyopia. After 3 months of amblyopia treatment, her VA with contact lenses was OS 20/40. Her overrefraction was −0.50 + 2.00 × 135 for 20/30 acuity. A new lens was ordered with the same parameters, except the power was changed to +16.00 D. The lens centers well and provides a good fit.

CLINICAL PROFICIENCY CHECKLIST

- Diagnostic fitting using aphakic lenses is essential to provide for an accurate prescription and to evaluate fitting dynamics of these thick lens designs.
- Ideally, new wearers should be fit into a hyper Dk GP or silicone hydrogel lens material, provided a good fit can be achieved.
- Altering lens edge profile by using lenticular designs is essential to providing thin, well-fitting, GP aphakic contact lenses.

(continued)

(Continued)

- When indicated in unilateral aphakic patients, consider the refractive error of the paired eye to provide for a balanced spectacle prescription. Consider fitting both eyes with contact lenses, or if bifocal spectacles are to be worn, fit the aphakic eye and adjust the contact lens power to balance the spectacle prescription.
- Planned replacement of soft aphakic lenses reduces the effects of parameter changes and complications associated with soiled lenses.
- Hydrogel aphakic lenses having a water content of >45% require sufficient lens lag (1.5–2.0 mm) at the fitting visit to reduce complications resulting from tight lenses.
- Front vertex versus back vertex power specification may influence the accuracy of final lens power.
- Hydrogel aphakic lenses may produce significant corneal edema, especially in patients having a prolapsed vitreous making contact with the corneal endothelium. Methods of reducing edema include reduction in wearing time, the use of silicone hydrogel lenses, or using a hyper Dk GP contact lens material.
- Soft, large GP and silicone elastomer lenses are recommended for the pediatric aphakic patient, with the latter two options recommended for patients under the age of 5.
- The younger the child, the higher the refractive error; a newborn can have a refractive error of +32 D, which may be reduced to +17 D at age 4.
- A simple way to measure the power on a pediatric aphakic patient is to take a +20 D lens and move it away from the eye until stabilization has been achieved.
- For the pediatric infant, it is recommended to have the mother cradle the child for lens insertion; for the toddler, a papoose board can be used.

■ OPTICAL CONSIDERATIONS FOR APHAKIA

Appendix A: Effective Power

When moving a lens from the spectacle plane toward the cornea, the effective vergence of light rays is altered. Therefore, the same aphakic eye will require a different power in a spectacle lens placed 12 mm in front of the cornea than in a contact lens placed on the cornea. It is necessary to increase power in the positive direction when moving close to the cornea.

The following equation is used to determine the effective power:

$$Fe = \frac{F}{1 - dF}$$

where

Fe = effective power (diopters)
F = back vertex power of lens (diopters)
d = vertex distance, or distance lens is moved in meters; (+) if lens is moved toward cornea, (−) if lens is moved away from the cornea

For example, what would be the power of a lens placed on the cornea that would be equivalent to a +12.00 D lens placed at a distance of 12 mm in front of the cornea (vertex distance = 12 mm)?

$$Fe = \frac{+12}{1 - .012(12)} = +14.02 \text{ D}$$

Therefore, a contact lens having a power of +14.00 D would have an effective power equal to a +12.00 D lens placed in the spectacle plane.

Note: The magnitude of astigmatism increases at the corneal plane.

Appendix B: Vertex Power

The power of a spectacle and contact lens is measured from the surface along the visual axis. It is the dioptric power from this point that influences the plane of focus for light passing through these thick lenses. Since the lens shape is of meniscus form [front surface has (+) positive power, back surface has (−) negative power], the vertex power is different when measuring from a reference point on the front of the lens compared to one on the back of a lens. These values are dependent on the lens center thickness, according to the following equations:

$$\text{Front Vertex Power (Fv)} = \frac{F_2}{1 - t/n\, F_2} + F_1$$

$$\text{Back Vertex Power (Fv')} = \frac{F_1}{1 - t/n\, F_1} + F_2$$

where

   F_1 = power of front surface
   F_2 = power of back surface
   t = lens thickness (meters)
   n = power of back surface

For example, determine the front and back vertex powers of an aphakic contact lens that has the following parameters:

$$F_1(\text{air}) = +76.00 \; (r_1 = 6.32 \text{ mm})$$
$$F_2(\text{air}) = -64.00 \text{ D} \; (r_1 = 7.50 \text{ mm})$$
$$n(\text{air}) = 1.48$$
$$ct = .50 \text{ mm} (.0005 \text{ m})$$

$$Fv' = \frac{+76.00}{1 - \dfrac{.0005}{1.48}(+76.00)} + -64.00 = +14.00 \text{ D}$$

$$Fv = \frac{+76.00 + -64.00}{1 - \dfrac{.0005}{1.48}(-64.00)} = +13.35 \text{ D}$$

   In this example, there is a difference of 0.65 D between back vertex power and front vertex power. These differences increase in magnitude for lenses having higher vertex powers and increased center thickness.

Appendix C: Magnification

The spectacle-corrected aphakic eye is found to experience an image magnification of approximately 30%. These effects may be calculated from the following equations:

$$SM = \frac{1}{1 - t/n\, F_1} \times \frac{1}{1 - d Fv'}$$

where

 Fe = power of front surface
 Fv' = power of back surface
   t = lens thickness (meters)
   n = lens index of refraction
   d = distance from back of lens to eye's entrance pupil (meters)

Using our example of an eye that requires a spectacle lens with a power of $+12.00$ D and a contact lens having a power of $+14.00$ D gives the following result (vertex $= 12$ mm):

$$\text{Magnification: spectacle lens } \frac{1}{1 - \frac{.007}{1.49}(+15.00)} \times \frac{1}{1 - .015(12)}$$

$F_1 = +15.00$
$Fv' = +12.00$
$t = 7.0$ mm
$n = 1.49$ (plastic) $1.076 \times 1.219 = 1.31$
$d = 12 + 3 = 15$ mm   or 31% magnification

$$\text{Magnification: contact lens } \frac{1}{1 - \frac{.0005}{1.48}(+76.00)} \times \frac{1}{1 - .003(14)}$$

$F_1 = +76.00$
$Fv' = +14.00$
$t = .50$ mm
$n = 1.48$ $(1.026) \times 1.043 = 1.07$
$d = 3$ mm   or 7% magnification

The above example demonstrates that contact lenses decrease magnification to at least one-fourth of that produced using an aphakic spectacle lens. It can be shown that an IOL further reduces this magnification to one-half of that found with contact lenses.

REFERENCES

1. Boeder P. Spectacle correction of aphakia. Arch Ophthalmol 1962;68(6):870–874.
2. Davis JK, Torgersen DL. The properties of lenses used for the correction of aphakia. J Am Optom Assoc 1983;54(8):685–693.
3. Borish IM. Aphakia: perceptual and refractive problems of spectacle correction. J Am Optom Assoc 1983;54(8):701–711.
4. Nelson G, Mandell RB. The relationship between minus carrier design and performance. Int Contact Lens Clin 1975;2(2):75–81.
5. Davis LJ, Bergin C, Bennett ES. Aphakia. In: Bennett ES, Weissman BA, eds. Clinical Contact Lens Practice. Philadelphia: Lippincott Williams & Wilkins, 2005:595–604.
6. Thompson TT. Tyler's Quarterly 2007;24(4):5–10.
7. Abrahamsson M, Magnusson G, Sjostrom A, et al. The occurrence of congenital cataract in western Sweden. Acta Opthalmol Scand 1999;77(5):578–580.
8. San Giovanni JP, Chew EY, Reed GF, et al. Infantile cataract in the collaborative perinatal project: prevalence and risk factors. Arch Ophthalmol 2002;120:1559–1565.
9. Bhatti TR, Dott M, Yoon PW, et al. Descriptive epidemiology of infantile cataracts in metropolitan Atlanta, GA, 1968–1998. Arch Pediatr Adolesc Med 2003;157(4):341–347.
10. Wirthe MG, Russell-Eggitt IM, Graig JE, et al. Aetiology of congenital and paediatric cataract in an Australian population. Br J Ophthalmol 2002;86(7):782–786.
11. Rahi JS, Dezatraux C. Measuring and interpreting the incidence of congenital coular anomalies: lessons for a national study of congenital cataracts in the UK. Invest Oph Vis Sci 2001;42:1444–1448.
12. Beller R, Hoyt CS, Marg E, et al. Good visual function after neonatal surgery for congenital monocular cataracts. Am J Ophthalmol 1981;91:559–565.
13. Davis LJ. Complex refractive errors in pediatric patients: cause, management, and criteria for success. Optom Vis Sci 1998;75(7):493–499.
14. Anisworth JR, Cohen S, Levin AV, et al. Pediatric cataract management with variation in surgical technique and aphakic optical correction. Ophthalmol 1997;104:1096–1101.
15. Basti S, Ravishankar U, Gupta S. Results of a prospective evaluation of three methods of management of pediatric cataracts. Ophthalmol 1996;103:713–720.
16. Braverman DE. Pediatric contact lenses. J Am Optom Assoc 1998;69:452.
17. Ozbek Z, Durak I, Berk TA. Contact lenses in the correction of childhood aphakia. CLAO J 2002;28:28–30.

18. Chia A, Johnson K, Marrin F. Use of contact lenses to correct aphakia in children. Clin Exp Ophthalmol 2002; 30:252–255.
19. Buckley EG. Scleral fixated (sutured) posterior chamber intraocular lens implantation in children. J AAPOS 1999;3:289–294.
20. McClatchey SK, Parks MM. Myopic shift after cataract removal in childhood. J Pediatr Ophthalmol Strabismus 1997;34:88–95.
21. Moore BD. Changes in the aphakic refraction of children with unilateral congenital cataracts. J Pediatr Ophthalmol Strabismus 1989;26:290–295.
22. Ellis P. Extended wear contact lenses in pediatric ophthalmology. CLAO J 1983;9:317–321.
23. Cutler SI, Nelson LB, Calhoun JH. Extended wear contact lenses in pediatric aphakia. J Pediatr Ophthalmol Strabismus l985;22:86–91.
24. Chase WW, Fronk SJ, Micheals BA. A theoretical infant schematic eye. Presented at Annual Meeting of the American Academy of Optometry, St. Louis, 1984.
25. Enoch JM. The fitting of hydrophilic (soft) contact lenses to infants and young children. Mensuration data on aphakic eyes of children born with congenital cataracts. Contact Lens Med Bull 1972A:36–40.
26. Pratt-Johnson JA, Tillson G. Hard contact lenses in the management of congenital cataracts. J Pediatr Ophthalmol Strabismus 1985;22:94–96.
27. Saunders RA, Ellis FD. Empirical fitting of hard contact lenses in infants and young children. Ophthalmol 1981; 88:127–130.

CHAPTER 18

Keratoconus

Edward S. Bennett, Joseph T. Barr, and Loretta Szczotka-Flynn

Keratoconus is a progressive, asymmetric disease of the cornea that is characterized by steepening and distortion, apical thinning, and corneal ectasia.[1,2] The cause of keratoconus is unknown, although it is probably a genetic disease. The management of keratoconus is most often in the form of rigid gas permeable (GP) contact lenses; however, more severe cases require penetrating keratoplasty.

The Collaborative Longitudinal Evaluation of Keratoconus (CLEK) Observational Study was the largest multicenter, prospective, observational study designed to describe the course of keratoconus and the associations among its visual and physiologic manifestations. The CLEK study characterized the course of keratoconus and identified factors related to vision, progression, and corneal scarring in keratoconus. A total of 1,209 patients were enrolled between 1995 and 1996, at 15 participating clinics, and patients were re-examined annually for 8 years, through mid-2004. The results of the CLEK study will be referenced throughout this chapter.

■ CHARACTERISTICS

Keratoconus is bilateral in approximately 96% of the cases.[3] Typically, one eye is diagnosed earlier and progresses more than the fellow eye. It is often diagnosed in the early teens to early 20s.[4,5] There does not appear to be a significant difference in the incidence of keratoconus between left and right eyes nor between men and women.

Epidemiology

The prevalence of keratoconus is stated to be 1 per 2,000 persons. With 270 million Americans, this translates to 135,000 Americans with the diagnosis of keratoconus. However, the only estimate of the incidence and prevalence of keratoconus comes from a study conducted in Olmsted County in Minnesota, which identified 64 incident cases of keratoconus between 1935 and 1982 at Mayo Clinic.[6] Case ascertainment was based solely on medical record review with the diagnosis determined by the "examiner's description of characteristic irregular light reflexes observed during ophthalmoscopy or retinoscopy, or irregular mires detected at keratometry." Kennedy et al. estimated the overall average annual incidence rate at 2 per 100,000 population with a prevalence of 55 per 100,000. These estimates are most likely low given current diagnostic techniques such as corneal topography. Other groups have reported the prevalence as high as 86 per 100,000 in Denmark[7] and incidence as high as 25 per 100,000 in populations that have traditions of consanguineous marriages.[8] The higher incidence was suggestive of a genetic factor being significant in the etiology.

■ ETIOLOGY

The cause of keratoconus is unknown, although metabolic/chemical changes in the corneal tissue have been documented. However, the disease has been associated with atopy,[9–11] connective tissue disorders,[12–16] eye rubbing,[17,18] contact lens wear,[19–22] and inheritance.[23]

Histologic Changes

It is still unclear what causes the corneal changes that occur in keratoconus. A triad of classic histopathologic changes have been observed[1]:

1. Thinning of the corneal stroma
2. Breaks in the Bowman layer
3. Iron deposition in the basal layers of the corneal epithelium

Apparently, degeneration of the epithelial cells is followed by breaks in the Bowman layer. Specifically, fragmentation of the Bowman layer—possibly caused by degradative enzymes and reduced inhibitors in the epithelium—may represent an early change in keratoconus.[24,25] Abnormal enzymes in the corneal epithelium lead to excess collagenase and reduced protease inhibitors in the stroma, most likely resulting in keratocyte death.[26] This increased collagenase activation may slowly break down stromal collagen, resulting in stromal thinning.[27] Biochemical studies have shown the total amount of protein in the cornea to be decreased.[28] The pathology of collagen fibrils has shown abnormally low numbers of collagen lamellae.[29] It has been suggested that the lamellae are released from their interlamellar attachments or the Bowman layer and become free to slide, resulting in thinning without collagenolysis.[30]

Atopic Relationship

There appears to be a relationship between atopic conditions (i.e., eczema, hay fever, asthma) and keratoconus, as approximately 50% of keratoconic patients have some form of atopy.[1,3,31,32] As itching is a primary symptom in atopic conditions, it has also been found that most keratoconic patients are vigorous eye rubbers, although a cause-and-effect relationship has not been proven.[17,18,33]

Atopy and histologic changes are linked together via the "Cascade Hypothesis" from Kenney et al.[34–36] According to this theory, young patients have a propensity to produce high levels of reactive oxygen species (ROS, or free radicals) in the cornea. These free radicals are typically cleared by superoxide dismutase, ALDH3, and other enzymes that prevent accumulation of these potentially harmful substances. Some individuals are unable to produce protective healthy enzymes; therefore, free radicals accumulate, causing damage to the structural integrity of the cornea. This results in a cascade of events in which a compromised cornea weakens, thins, and becomes steeper in curvature. As exposure to ultraviolet B light generates free radicals, it is important for the appropriate eyewear protection to be used. Likewise, mechanical stress such as that caused by a poorly fitted contact lens or via eye rubbing can exaggerate ROS formation. If this is the case, these individuals need to avoid eye rubbing with the appropriate treatment of allergies and atopic conditions also advised. Antioxidative therapy, like those currently used in retinal treatments, could be a possible future option.[36]

Heredity

Several studies have suggested that keratoconus is genetic,[37,38] with reports from single families and twin studies also reported in earlier literature. Between 6% and 16% of patients with keratoconus have a history of familial disease.[32,39–41] Because the severity of the disease varies from asymptomatic forme fruste conditions to disabling scarring requiring corneal transplantation, the true incidence, prevalence, and familial aggregation is difficult to ascertain. Specifically, in asymptomatic conditions, keratoconus may only be detected using sophisticated instrumentation such as videokeratography. Some authors have shown that intermediate traits, as measured by videokeratography, are highly inheritable. Keratoconus has shown association with rare genetic syndromes, such as Woodhouse-Sakati syndrome[42] and Down syndrome,[43] further supporting the genetic hypothesis.

Contact Lenses

It has been suggested, in many reports, that rigid contact lenses may cause keratoconus because of such factors as mechanical pressure and hypoxia.[20,44–46] In one study, 27% of the keratoconic patients were contact lens wearers, all of whom were not diagnosed with keratoconus at the time of fitting.[46] It was found that these individuals were older at the time of diagnosis, had central (versus decentered) cones, and had a tendency toward flatter corneal curvatures. However, once again, it is difficult to establish a cause-and-effect relationship, as the incidence of keratoconus would be expected to be higher with contact lens wearers.[4] This is the age in which keratoconus typically is diagnosed, and these individuals may be corrected for their myopia before being diagnosed with keratoconus. A case report of one of the authors supports a hypoxic etiology. A long-term rigid lens wearer lost one of her gas permeable lenses and went back to wearing an older polymethylmethacrylate (PMMA) spare lens for 8 years. Keratoconus developed in the eye wearing the PMMA lens, whereas the eye wearing the gas permeable lens was unaffected.[47]

■ DIAGNOSIS

The earlier a patient can be diagnosed as having or possibly having keratoconus, the sooner the practitioner can institute the appropriate management and adequately educate the patient. For the condition to be diagnosed, the practitioner must be aware of the symptoms and clinical signs of keratoconus and encourage frequent follow-up care for monitoring progression.

Early Symptoms and Clinical Signs

The diagnosis begins with a thorough case history. The practitioner must ask the right questions and be a good listener, as the symptoms of incipient keratoconus are varied and frequently confused with psychogenic complaints. Quite often the patient has difficulty explaining the actual problem. Monocular diplopia or "ghost" images and blurring of images are common symptoms, but practitioners may fail to ask questions eliciting a description of image blur.[48] Vision may not actually be blurred but distorted; letters may be confused, and parts of letters may be missing or altered. Therefore, the practitioner should ask patients whether they are experiencing this distortion out of one eye only. In addition, if this condition had been previously undiagnosed, the patient may own several pairs of glasses, none of which is satisfactory. Finally, asthenopic complaints, polyopia, photophobia, and halos around lights may be reported.

A gradual decrease in visual acuity is often the first clinical sign of keratoconus. The vision of one eye will be affected before the other, and the blur will be present for both near and far distances. The patient may be able to see better by squinting or by holding printed material very close to the eyes. In addition, because of the conical distortion, an early clinical sign of keratoconus is a "scissors-like" motion observed during retinoscopy. In the early stages, manifest refraction will often result in satisfactory visual acuity; however, an increase in both myopia and regular or irregular astigmatism may be found. An absence of parallelism of keratometry mires and a localized region of corneal steepening is often observed with videokeratography (to be discussed).

Corneal Topography Change

Keratometry

Keratometry is beneficial in the diagnosis and monitoring of keratoconus. However, the limitations of keratometry, including the measurement of only a few paracentral points on the cornea, can make early diagnosis difficult, especially if the patient has a decentered apex of the cone.

What is often observed in early keratoconus is a lack of parallelism of the keratometric mires. The mires are somewhat distorted, and one may not completely overlap the other. The corneal astigmatism may increase and shift toward an oblique axis. A steepening of the corneal curvature may be observed. If the condition is incipient, the keratometry readings may be in the 43 to 48 D range. Once the condition advances beyond the curvature values of the keratometer, a +1.25 D ophthalmic lens can be mounted over the objective (patient end) to add approximately 8 D to the keratometer reading (Appendix 1).

Videokeratography

The use of videokeratography (VKG) has been an outstanding tool for the diagnosis and monitoring of patients with keratoconus. The location of the apex and the progression of the condition can be observed via evaluation of the color map. The localized area of steepening can easily be observed with a color map (Fig. 18.1).

Although definitive keratoconus cannot be diagnosed in the absence of several slit-lamp or retinoscopic findings, a keratoconus suspect can be determined quite easily via the appearance of the color map. These individuals can then be monitored to determine if further progression and diagnosis of the condition occurs. In addition, a compression of the mires will be present in the affected region via the reflection of the photokeratoscopic rings. Also, as the unaffected corneal region (typically superior) will not change, an inferior-superior dioptric asymmetry will be present.[1]

The impacted region or "cone" has traditionally been categorized as "nipple," oval (i.e., sagging), or globus.[49–51] The nipple cone is smaller and more centralized than the other two types. The oval cone is more inferior, whereas the globus cone is quite large in diameter. McMahon[52] reported on results from the CLEK study in which the impacted areas were divided into nipple (Fig. 18.2A), oval (Fig. 18.2B), globoid (Fig. 18.2C), and marginal (Fig. 18.1), with the latter group pertaining to a nonround or nonoval cone located in the periphery of the cornea (often inferior).

As shown in Table 18.1, most of the cones can be described as nipple or oval. It was also reported that 12.2% have an apex above horizontal with an average location at 262 degrees (inferior-temporal).[53]

Several VKG systems have developed applications for the screening and diagnosis of keratoconus.[48,54–57] This is particularly important, as the presence of keratoconus is a contraindication

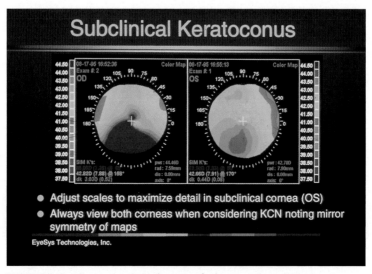

FIGURE 18.1 Representative color map of a keratoconic patient.

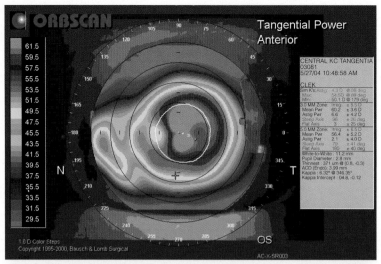

A

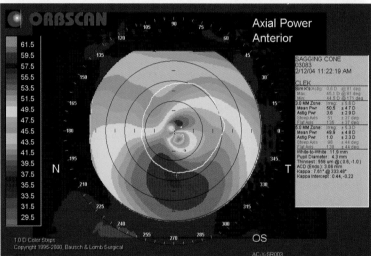

B

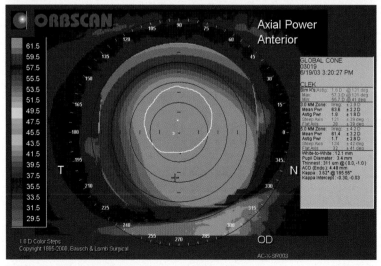

C

■ **FIGURE 18.2** A nipple cone is shown in **(A),** an oval or sagging cone in **(B),** and a globus or globoid cone in **(C).**

TABLE 18.1 CONE TYPES AND PREVALENCE

CONE TYPE	PREVALENCE
Nipple	28.7%
Oval	44.3%
Globoid	6.7%
Marginal	5.6%
Other	11.0%
PK	3.7%

From McMahon TT. Collaborative longitudinal evaluation of keratoconus update. Presented at the Annual Meeting of the American Academy of Optometry, Denver, CO, December 2006.

for refractive surgery and it has been found that as many as 5% to 7% of refractive surgery candidates have subclinical keratoconus.[58,59]

In research clinics, keratoconus has been defined using topographic indices only. VKG readings and differences in corneal shape have been used to diagnose keratoconus. Mandell et al.,[4,60] with the cone apex aligned with the optical system of a VKG, determined that a true apex power reading can be obtained and therefore compared to the normal range in the detection of keratoconus. It was concluded that if the cone apex power is 48 to 49 D, the patient should be considered a keratoconus suspect. For powers of 49 to 50 D, there is a very high likelihood of keratoconus, and for powers above 50 D, the diagnosis is almost certain. The modified Rabinowitz-McDonnell method[1,54,61] uses the following guidelines: if the central corneal power is >47.2 D or if the difference between the inferior and superior paracentral corneal regions (i.e., I-S value) is >1.4 D, then the cornea is considered keratoconus suspect. If the central corneal power is >48.7 D or the I-S value is >1.4 D, then the cornea is classified as keratoconus. Rabinowitz and Rasheed have also developed an index, the KISA%, to grade the presence or absence of keratoconus.[62] Although this index has the potential to define disease severity, the developers have only described its role in defining normals, keratoconus suspects, and those with the disease. The KISA index has been used to monitor changes in normal eyes of unilateral keratoconus patients[63] and genetic screening where KISA was used to distinguish keratoconus from normal individuals.[38]

The difficulty in using topographic-only methods to define keratoconus is that early forme fruste conditions—which may never progress—can be labeled as keratoconus with unnecessary worry imposed on the patient. Although topographic evidence of keratoconus should be a strong reason to avoid ablative refractive surgery, otherwise asymptomatic patients may not need any special therapeutic treatment other than monitoring. For that reason, a definitive diagnosis of keratoconus is usually made clinically by requiring either a slit-lamp sign of the disease (as discussed below), refractive and visual acuity changes suggestive of keratoconus, or distortion of the anterior cornea as measured by the red reflex.

Slit-Lamp Biomicroscopic Signs

Biomicroscopy is essential for the diagnosis of keratoconus. Only with the biomicroscope can the observer detect the subtle changes occurring within the cornea. The hallmark clinical signs of keratoconus, which are present in the majority of clinically confirmed cases, include Vogt striae, Fleischer ring, and scarring. Vogt striae are a series of vertical or oblique lines located in the posterior stroma or Descemet membrane (Fig. 18.3). They are most likely the result of the stretching of the corneal lamellae. They temporarily disappear when transient pressure is applied to the

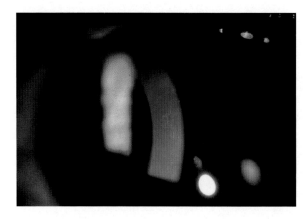

■ **FIGURE 18.3** Vogt striae.

globe through the upper lid.[64] The Fleischer ring can be observed in approximately 50% of all diagnosed cases of keratoconus.[65] It is a yellow-brown to olive-green discoloration appearing in a broken or interrupted ring encircling the base of the cone (Fig. 18.4). It appears to outline the base of the cone and represents hemosiderin deposits in the deep epithelium near the Bowman membrane. Irregular superficial scars can form at the apex of the cone as the condition progresses. They begin as discrete dots in the Bowman membrane; fibrillar connective tissue invades the space between the opacities, and they proceed to increase and become opaque[66,67] (Fig. 18.5).

Thinning of the cornea can be observed at the region of the cone via an optic section. Increased visibility of the nerve fibers can be observed at the corneo-scleral junction as a result of a change in their density. In severe cases, corneal hydrops can occur secondary to a rupture in the Descemet membrane, allowing aqueous humor from the anterior chamber to flow through the damaged endothelium, causing corneal edema and eventually scarring.

External findings include the Munson sign and Rizzuti phenomenon. In advanced cases, the shape of the lid will be altered because of the protrusion of the cone, and the Munson sign will be present. This can be confirmed by having the patient look down until the lower lid is at the equator of the cone. According to Rizzuti,[68] when illuminating the cornea with a penlight from the temporal side of the cornea, focused anterior to the iris, light is sharply focused on the temporal side of the nasal limbus.

Ophthalmoscopy

On ophthalmoscopy, a circular, oblong, or dumbbell-shaped shadow may appear that looks like a large indefinite cataract separating the central from the peripheral reflex.[48] On closer evaluation, this phenomenon is observed to be corneal in location. Fundus details are difficult to observe. A

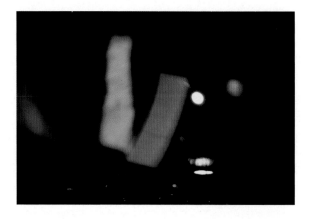

■ **FIGURE 18.4** Fleischer ring.

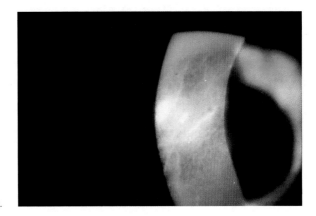

■ FIGURE 18.5 Corneal scarring.

technique called photodiagnosis has been useful in diagnosing and monitoring the size, shape, and location of advanced or severe cones. In this technique, the image of the cone is viewed against the red fundus reflex. With the dilated pupil, the examiner views the cornea through the direct ophthalmoscope at a distance of 2 feet. In advanced cases (>50 D), the cone can be easily observed against the red fundus reflex (Fig. 18.6). The image can also be recorded using a fundus camera with a high plus condensing lens.

The clinical signs of keratoconus are summarized in Table 18.2.

■ DIFFERENTIAL DIAGNOSIS

When diagnosing keratoconus, it is important to rule out other mimicking conditions such as corneal warpage syndrome, corneal molding from a high-riding GP lens, keratoglobus, and pellucid marginal degeneration.

Corneal Warpage Syndrome

Keratoconus and corneal warpage syndrome (CWS) can often be differentiated via a combination of the case history and a comprehensive clinical examination, including videokeratoscopy. Corneal warpage syndrome patients typically have a long-term history of contact lens wear. This condition occurs as a combination of corneal hypoxia and the mechanical effects induced by the contact lens. It has been most often reported with PMMA lens wear, although soft and GP lenses can induce CWS, the latter via a poor lens-to-cornea fitting relationship. Although corneal distortion and often a scissors-like retinoscopy reflex are present

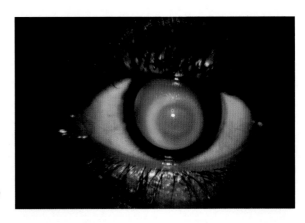

■ FIGURE 18.6 Photodiagnosis outlining the cone.

TABLE 18.2 KERATOCONUS CLINICAL SIGNS

External signs
   Munson sign
   Rizzuti phenomenon

Refractive signs
   Retinoscopic scissors reflex
   Increased myopia
   Increase in and irregularity of astigmatism

Keratometry signs
   Lack of mire parallelism
   Mire distortion
   Increase in and irregularity of astigmatism

Videokeratoscopy signs
   Compression of mires in affected region
   Color map shows increased power in isolated area of cone
   Inferior-superior dioptric asymmetry

Slit-lamp biomicroscopic signs
   Vogt striae
   Fleischer ring
   Scarring
   Increased visibility of nerve fibers
   Corneal thinning
   Hydrops

Ophthalmoscopy
   Cone can be observed against red fundus reflex in advanced cases

in both conditions, CWS patients typically manifest signs of corneal hypoxia while rarely exhibiting corneal steepening beyond 50 D.[69] In addition, the degree of mire irregularity or misalignment is typically less with CWS than in keratoconus. Videokeratoscopy will show a localized area of corneal steepening in keratoconus but not necessarily in CWS. Keratoconus can often be differentiated with a comprehensive biomicroscopy examination. Clinical signs such as corneal thinning, Fleischer ring, Vogt striae, and, in moderate to severe cases, corneal scarring are present in keratoconus and not associated with CWS, which is limited to changes in corneal contour.[70] The affected corneal region is limited in keratoconus, often of variable size, encompassing some of (but not limited to) the central and inferior regions. This can be verified via photodiagnosis. Keratoconus, unlike CWS, is a progressive condition, typically over a 5- to 10-year period, often resulting in a protruding conical region, easily observable via Munson sign in advanced stages. Corneal warpage syndrome, conversely, is remediated and often results in a healthy, regular cornea via discontinuation of contact lens wear and/or refitting into a lens material with higher oxygen permeability (Dk) exhibiting a well-centered lens-to-cornea fitting relationship. The differences in keratoconus and corneal warpage syndrome are summarized in Table 18.3.

High-Riding Gas Permeable Lens

A pseudokeratoconic corneal topography can result from wearing a highly positioned GP lens. This fitting relationship induces superior corneal flattening accompanied by inferior steepening, thus simulating a keratoconus color map. As with corneal warpage syndrome, none of the classical slit-lamp signs of keratoconus will be present. In addition, once the rigid lens is removed, the inferior cornea will flatten back toward baseline over the course of approximately 7 to 14 days.

TABLE 18.3 CORNEAL WARPAGE SYNDROME VERSUS KERATOCONUS: DIFFERENTIAL DIAGNOSIS

	CORNEAL WARPAGE SYNDROME	KERATOCONUS
1. Case history	• Long-term rigid lens wear: often PMMA or low Dk GP	• Not limited to rigid CL wear • Often atopic history
2. Slit-lamp evaluation	• Corneal hypoxia and possibly lens decentration	• Corneal thinning in affected region • Fleischer ring • Vogt striae • Scarring (in later stages)
3. Corneal topography	• Rarely steeper than 50 D • Mire irregularity often mild and improves with either discontinuation of CL wear or refitting into higher Dk material • VKG shows irregularity; not limited in location; if inferior steep region, need to rule out superior decentration	• Often steeper than 50 D at apex of cone • Continues to progress with increasing mire irregularity and steepening of affected region • Location of steepest area is often inferior

CL, contact lens; Dk, oxygen permeability; GP, gas permeable; PMMA, polymethylmethacrylate; VKG, videokeratography.

Pellucid Marginal Degeneration

As with keratoconus, pellucid marginal degeneration is a progressive disorder affecting both eyes. However, it is typically characterized by a peripheral band of thinning of the inferior cornea from 4 to 8 o'clock with a 1- to 2-mm unaffected area between the region of thinning and the limbus.[1] Slit-lamp evaluation should be beneficial in differentiating the regions of thinning between keratoconus and pellucid marginal degeneration. In addition, in pellucid marginal degeneration, the videokeratograph has a classical "butterfly" appearance demonstrating a large amount of against-the-rule astigmatism.[71] Many believe the two conditions are similar and perhaps share the same etiology and pathophysiology, yet different areas of the cornea are affected.

Keratoglobus

Keratoglobus is a condition in which the entire cornea thins, most notably near the limbus, as opposed to the localized thinning in keratoconus.[1,2] Although it is, like keratoconus, a bilateral condition, keratoglobus is typically present from birth and tends to be nonprogressive.

■ CLASSIFICATION AND PROGRESSION

There are various classification schemes for keratoconus, although no single classification scheme has been universally accepted. One comprehensive classification scheme is presented in Table 18.4, which includes visual symptoms, classical slit-lamp signs, and corneal curvature values as a method to distinguish among different degrees of severity. A recently introduced classification scheme (Table 18.5) utilizes slit-lamp findings, corneal topography map characteristics, and two easily determined topographic indices, average corneal power (ACP) and higher-order first corneal surface wavefront root-mean-square (RMS) error (HORMSE).[72]

Apical scarring is included to better delineate moderate to severe disease, since corneal scarring is associated with more advanced disease.[73] With the inclusion of higher-order RMS errors, normals from suspect cases are better delineated, as coma has been shown to be an excellent differentiator of suspected keratoconus and normal corneas.[74]

TABLE 18.4 KERATOCONUS CLASSIFICATION

STAGE 1
1. Fully correctable with spectacles
2. Slight increase in refractive astigmatism
3. Slight or no keratometric mire distortion
4. Normal keratometry readings
5. Mild area of steepening with videokeratoscopy
6. Mild scissors reflex with retinoscopy
7. Difficult to diagnose
STAGE 2
1. Definite corneal distortion and irregular astigmatism observed with keratometry and videokeratoscopy
2. Further increase in myopia and refractive astigmatism
3. Keratometer values exhibit 1–4 D of steepening
STAGE 3
1. Best corrected spectacle visual acuity is greatly decreased
2. Accurate keratometry readings are difficult to obtain because of mire distortion
3. Keratometry readings have steepened from 5–10 D
4. Increase in irregular astigmatism, commonly ranging from 2–8 D
5. Slit-lamp findings including corneal thinning, increased nerve fiber visibility, Vogt striae, Fleischer ring, and possibly scarring are often present
STAGE 4
1. Intensification of above signs, with the cornea steepening to >55 D
2. Scarring present at apex
3. Munson sign present

Patients first diagnosed with keratoconus want to know the prognosis for progression and loss of vision. Clinicians would like to be able to predict the rate of progression and to identify those patients who will advance to severe keratoconus. However, the rate of progression for a particular patient is impossible to predict. Some patients advance rapidly for 6 months to a year and then stop progressing, with no further change. Often, there are periods of several months with significant changes followed by months or years of no change; this may then be followed by another period of rapid change. However, it typically progresses over a time period of 3 to 8 years.[3] In the CLEK study, the slope of the change of flat K was approximately 0.20 D per year; over 7 years, this translated into an expected steepening of 1.44 D. Steepening of 3 D or more in either eye had an incidence of 23%.[75]

■ PATIENT CONSULTATION

As with almost all medical conditions, patients should be informed of the diagnosis (or possible diagnosis) as soon as possible. The progression of the disease can be described and, although most patients will not need a corneal transplant, the possibility of this option should be mentioned. These individuals are often very curious about their condition and desire more information. The internet is always a good source for information, but patients can also impose undue worry upon themselves if they retrieve faulty information or information not pertaining

TABLE 18.5 KERATOCONUS SEVERITY SCORE

Rules: The decision process flows down each grade. For grades 0–1, all of the parameters in a category must be met. For all grades the italicized features must be met. The worst of the remaining features is then assessed, with the "worst" of the features carrying the greater weight (as long as the italicized features are met).

0	Unaffected—normal topography *Definitely no scar (DNS)* *No slit-lamp signs for keratoconus* *Typical axial pattern* *ACP <47.75 D* *Higher-order RMS error <0.65*

1	Unaffected—atypical topography
	DNS
	No slit-lamp signs for keratoconus
	Atypical axial pattern
	    Irregular pattern
	    Asymmetric superior bowtie
	    Asymmetric inferior bowtie
	    Inferior or superior steepening no more than 3.00 D steeper than ACP
	ACP <48.00
	Higher-order RMS error <1.00

2	Suspect topography
	DNS or probably no scar (PNS)
	No slit-lamp signs for keratoconus
	Axial pattern with isolated area of steepening
	    Inferior steep pattern
	    Superior steep pattern
	    Central steep pattern
	ACP <49.00 D
	    or
	Higher-order RMS error >1.00, <1.50

3	Affected—mild disease *Axial pattern consistent with keratoconus* *May have positive slit-lamp signs* No corneal scarring consistent for keratoconus ACP <52.00 D or Higher-order RMS error 1.51–3.50

4	Affected—moderate disease
	Axial pattern consistent with keratoconus
	Must have positive slit-lamp signs
	ACP >52.01 D, <56.00 D
	    or
	Higher-order RMS error >3.51–5.75
	    or
	Corneal scarring grade up to 3.0 overall

5	Affected—severe disease
	Axial pattern consistent with keratoconus
	Must have positive slit-lamp signs
	ACP >56.01 D
	    or
	Higher-order RMS error >5.75
	    or
	Corneal scarring grade 3.5 or greater overall

ACP, average corneal power; RMS, root-mean-square.

to them or their specific disease state. One excellent source is the National Keratoconus Foundation site available online at http://www.nkcf.org. Keratoconus patients can contact a large number of sources of information here and find answers to commonly asked questions. Likewise, practitioners can utilize this information as well. Additionally, several cities have keratoconus support groups in an effort to allow patients the opportunity to share their experiences with others.

When monitoring these patients, it is important to empathize with the possible changes in their quality of life. Typical keratoconus has an onset early in life, often said to be at puberty.[76] The CLEK study reported a median age of 39 years at enrollment. Thus, keratoconus is a chronic disease with a long duration affecting people during their prime earning and childrearing years, which may relate to the reported adverse psychological effects reported by some authors.[77–80] In the CLEK study, visual acuity worse than 20/40 was associated with lower quality-of-life scores.[81] A steep keratometric reading >52 D was associated with lower scores on subscales representing Mental Health, Role Difficulty, Driving, Dependency, and Ocular Pain. Scores for keratoconus patients were between patients with category 3 and 4 age-related macular degeneration (AMD) except General Health, which was better than for AMD patients, and Ocular Pain, which was worse than for AMD patients.[81] This significantly impaired vision-related quality of life continues to decline over time.[82] Additionally, in those patients with worsening visual acuity and increasing corneal curvature, a significant 10-point decline over 7 years in National Eye Institute Visual Function Questionnaire (NEI-VFQ) scale scores is found.[82] Therefore, although keratoconus rarely results in blindness, its impact on patients is comparable to that of a person with advanced macular degeneration and, because it affects young adults, the magnitude of its public health impact is disproportionate to its reported prevalence and clinical severity.

Additionally, impact on the quality of life was confirmed by a study in which keratoconus patients were compared to normal controls and to age-matched patients with chronic, nonkeratoconic eye disease via use of a personality questionnaire.[41] Abnormal results were found on the same psychological scales (passive-aggressive, paranoid, hypomanic, disorganized thinking patterns, and substance abuse) in both the keratoconic and chronic eye disease patients.

▦ SPECTACLE MANAGEMENT

Spectacle correction is an uncommon form of correction in keratoconus. The CLEK study found that 16% of patients diagnosed with keratoconus wore spectacles as their primary form of distance correction.[32] As a result of the gradual progression of corneal irregularity, spectacles appear to have their best application early in the disease, before contact lens use. Spectacles do not impact the irregular nature of the corneal curvature. In addition, the refractive error can change quite rapidly and, as the condition progresses, anisometropia may exist because one eye is often more affected than the other eye.[65]

▦ CONTACT LENS MANAGEMENT

Rigid Lens Fitting

Keratoconus is best corrected with rigid gas permeable contact lenses. Even in the early stages of the disease when spectacle correction may still be an option, rigid contact lenses do the best job of correcting the irregular astigmatism and secondary aberrations that are induced from the irregular cornea. In the process of rigid lens fitting, the practitioner may be presented with a difficult fit as a result of an extremely decentered apex of the cone. This is particularly true in cases in which the apex is decentered several millimeters inferiorly, as the lens tends to position at the steepest region of the cornea.

In the CLEK study, 65% of patients were best corrected bilaterally with rigid lenses, and 8% unilaterally with a rigid lens.[32] This value is similar to the 75% of keratoconic patients wearing rigid lenses in the CLEK study[83] and is similar to other reports.[46,84]

A rigid contact lens will neutralize much of the distortion/optical aberrations of the anterior corneal surface, and the subsequent visual acuity can be increased several lines on the acuity chart.[85] However, even if visual acuity chart vision is "normal" with rigid contact lens correction, most likely there is some decrement in vision performance. Contrast threshold measurements have shown a vision loss at low spatial frequencies (0.25 c/deg) that is not improved by contact lens fitting.[86] Therefore, although rigid contact lenses can provide a significant improvement in visual acuity for keratoconic patients, there may still be residual loss of visual function.

Lens-to-Cornea Fitting Relationships

Three common rigid lens-to-cornea fitting relationships have been used in keratoconus. These include apical bearing, apical clearance, and three-point touch.

Apical Bearing: One previously practiced philosophy for fitting keratoconus has been to fit a large-diameter, flat base curve lens in an effort to supposedly slow down or halt progression of the condition. It was theorized to result in improved vision versus other fitting relationships. The resulting fluorescein pattern shows excessive central bearing accompanied by midperipheral and peripheral pooling (Fig. 18.7).

This method is now controversial and rarely used today, as it is believed that excessive pressure of the lens on a region of the cornea that is thin and fragile could encourage distortion and apical scarring.[87–89] It is possible that this fitting relationship could also encourage swirl staining, commonly observed over the apex of the cone in keratoconus. Korb et al.[87] compared corneal integrity with an apical bearing fitting relationship with a large-diameter, flat base curve radius lens versus an apical clearance fitting relationship achieved with a small-diameter, steep-fitting lens. Seven keratoconic patients exhibiting an absence of corneal scarring were fitted randomly such that one eye had the apical clearance design and the other eye had the apical bearing design. At the end of one year, four of the seven eyes in the apical bearing design exhibited scarring; none of the eyes with the apical clearance design had scarring.

Apical Clearance: In an attempt to contour the cornea with a small, steep lens design with total avoidance of bearing, some practitioners have recommended an apical clearance lens design.[87,88,90] This form of fitting relationship should result in minimum lens-induced apical corneal compromise. Essentially, this is accomplished with a small-diameter, steep base curve lens, which results in an apical clearance fluorescein pattern (Fig. 18.8).

In the CLEK study, the feasibility of this fitting philosophy was assessed using postfitting frequency of slit-lamp findings such as (a) moderate epithelial punctate staining, (b) moderate central corneal erosion, (c) corneal edema, (d) contact lens imprint, and (e) the development of central corneal scarring.[90] Investigators fitted 30 eyes with an apical clearance lens design

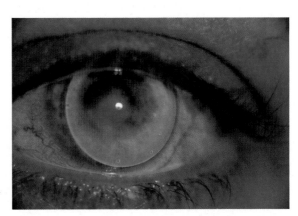

■ **FIGURE 18.7** An apical bearing fitting relationship in keratoconus.

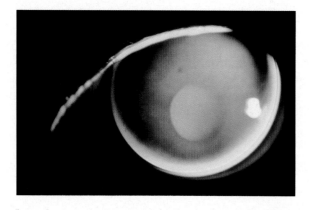

■ FIGURE 18.8 An apical clearance fitting relationship.

using the CLEK diagnostic fitting set (described below). All lenses had an 8.6-mm overall diameter with a 6.5-mm optical zone. An initial diagnostic lens was selected with a base curve radius equal to the steep keratometry value. After evaluation with fluorescein, lens changes would be made until the first definite apical clearance lens (FDACL), or the flattest lens that did not demonstrate central bearing, was obtained. Then all 30 eyes were assigned to wear steep-fitting lenses, defined as lenses with base curve radii 0.2 mm steeper than the FDACL lens, for a 12-month period. The results found that the average wearing time increased from a baseline of 10.5 hours per day to 13.7 hours per day at 12 months. In addition, there was not a decrement in visual acuity as compared to the baseline values. Only 1 eye out of 22 completing the study developed scarring. Nevertheless, if this philosophy is to be utilized, the fluorescein pattern should be monitored to ensure that peripheral seal-off and/or adherence of the lens to cornea do not occur.

Three-Point Touch: An especially popular lens-to-cornea fitting philosophy for fitting keratoconic patients is three-point touch. The goal, through diagnostic fitting, is to achieve mild or "feather" touch of the lens over the apex of the cone accompanied by, at minimum, two other areas of touch approximately 180 degrees from the apex at the corneal midperiphery.[48] This "feather touch" bearing of the apex and midperiphery creates a bulls-eye appearance upon fluorescein evaluation. Four zones are created: slight apical touch, paracentral clearance, midperipheral bearing, and peripheral clearance (Fig. 18.9). In this design, the weight of the lens is distributed across a healthy cornea and not focused on one specific area. It is theorized that mild apical bearing will provide some amount of regularity to the anterior corneal surface in that region and possibly improved visual acuity as compared to the apical clearance method. For this fitting relationship to be successful, it should have as little movement as possible that still allows some tear flow under the lens. In addition, it is important to monitor these patients to ensure apical bearing does not become excessive, possibly resulting in the aforementioned corneal complications occurring from apical bearing.

Author's Fitting Philosophy

One of authors (ESB) uses an approach that incorporates many of the principles used by other practitioners. The goal is to achieve a three-point touch fluorescein pattern with a spherical GP diagnostic lens and then design the lens to be consistent with the stage of the condition.

The Fitting Process: The use of a diagnostic fitting set is imperative when fitting a keratoconic patient with GP lenses. The first author's diagnostic fitting set is provided in Table 18.6.

If a GP fitting set is desired for keratoconic patients, it can be obtained from most Contact Lens Manufacturers Association (CLMA) member laboratories. Those providing rigid lens

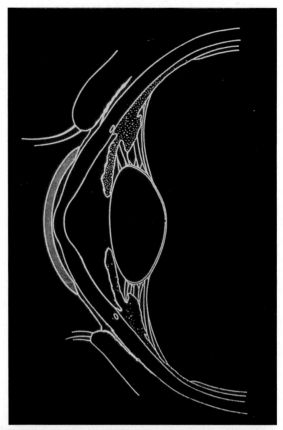

A

■ **FIGURE 18.9** Three-point touch: **(A)** A diagram showing mild apical touch and areas of mid-peripheral touch. **(B)** A three-point-touch fitting relationship.

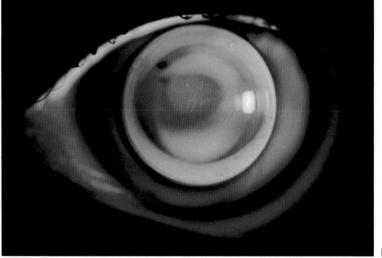

B

designs for keratoconus are listed in Table 18.7.[91] Many of these designs are also discussed later in this chapter.

When fitting a keratoconic patient, the application of a topical anesthetic is very beneficial. Keratoconic patients tend to be quite sensitive to initial lens application. Topical anesthetic application will minimize initial lens awareness and reduce chair time. The latter is particularly important, as several lenses may need to be attempted before obtaining an acceptable fitting relationship.[92]

TABLE 18.6 KERATOCONUS DIAGNOSTIC LENS FITTING SET (BENNETT)

LENS	OAD/OZD	BCR	SCR/W	ICR/W	PCR/W	POWER
1.	9.0/7.2	7.3	8.4/.3	10.2/.3	12.3/.3	−3.00 D
2.	9.0/7.2	7.2	8.3/.3	9.9/.3	12.2/.3	−3.00 D
3.	9.0/7.2	7.1	8.1/.3	9.7/.3	12.1/.3	−3.00 D
4.	8.8/7.0	7.0	8.0/.3	9.6/.3	12.0/.3	−4.00 D
5.	8.8/7.0	6.9	7.9/.3	9.5/.3	11.9/.3	−4.00 D
6.	8.8/7.0	6.8	7.8/.3	9.4/.3	11.8/.3	−5.00 D
7.	8.6/6.8	6.7	7.7/.3	9.3/.3	11.7/.3	−5.00 D
8.	8.6/6.8	6.6	7.6/.3	9.2/.3	11.6/.3	−6.00 D
9.	8.6/6.8	6.5	7.5/.3	9.1/.3	11.5/.3	−6.00 D
10.	8.4/6.6	6.4	7.3/.3	9.0/.3	11.4/.3	−7.00 D
11.	8.4/6.6	6.3	7.2/.3	8.8/.3	11.3/.3	−7.00 D
12.	8.4/6.6	6.2	7.1/.3	8.7/.3	11.2/.3	−8.00 D
13.	8.2/6.4	6.1	6.9/.3	8.5/.3	11.1/.3	−8.00 D
14.	8.2/6.4	6.0	6.8/.3	8.4/.3	11.0/.3	−9.00 D
15.	8.2/6.4	5.9	6.7/.3	8.3/.3	10.9/.3	−9.00 D

BCR, base curve radius; ICR/W, intermediate curve radius/width; OAD, overall diameter; OZD, optical zone diameter; PCR/W, peripheral curve radius/width; SCR/W, secondary curve radius/width.

The initial lens should have a base curve radius equal to the steep keratometry reading, as the CLEK study has found this to approximate, on the average, the FDACL.[93] The fluorescein pattern should not be viewed immediately after instillation, as a false pattern of apical clearance may exist when, in fact, after several blinks, bearing is present. Slit-lamp evaluation with both cobalt blue illumination and the use of a Wratten or Tiffen filter will dictate what change in base curve radius will be indicated. Often, a slight apical clearance fitting relationship will be present. The base curve can then be flattened in 0.50 to 1.00 D steps until apical bearing is first observed. At this time, a three-point touch or "bulls-eye" fitting relationship should be present. Careful evaluation of the peripheral fluorescein pattern is also important to ensure peripheral seal-off is absent. An alignment fluorescein pattern is not expected with this or other keratoconic designs; however, good centration is imperative. If the lens decenters inferiorly because of a corneal apex that is greatly displaced in that direction, either a larger diameter can be attempted in an effort to provide better centration or one of the other keratoconic designs discussed in this chapter may be necessary. A Burton lamp is also of great value for evaluating fluorescein patterns in keratoconus, as the greater field of view allows the practitioner the ability to more easily detect if a three-point touch relationship has been achieved.

Lens Design: Once three-point touch has been obtained, it is important to design the lens to be consistent with the changes in corneal topography. Generally, the optical zone diameter (OZD) should be decreased in size as the base curve radius steepens to maintain a well-centered lens. In this philosophy, the optical zone diameter is typically equal to the base curve radius in millimeters. For example, if the base curve radius is 7.00 mm, the optical zone diameter will, likewise, be 7.00 mm. Obviously, the OZD can vary depending on such factors as pupil size, fissure size, and lens position.

Multiple peripheral curves—typically three to four—are necessary to correspond with the rapidly flattening midperipheral and peripheral cornea. The peripheral curve should generally

TABLE 18.7 CONTACT LENS MANUFACTURER ASSOCIATION LABORATORIES WITH KERATOCONIC LENS DESIGNS

NAME	CONTACT INFORMATION
ABB-Concise	http://www.abboptical.com
ABBA Optical	http://www.abbaoptical.com
Acculens	http://www.acculens.com
Advanced Vision Technologies	http://www.naturalens.com
Art Optical	http://www.artoptical.com
Australian Contact Lenses	(email) eclaust@czemail.com.au
Beitler McKee Optical	http://www.beitlermckee.com
Blanchard Contact Lens	http://www.blanchardlab.com
CL Works Co.	http://www.clworks.com
Cardinal Contact Lens	(email) Cardinalcontact@aol.com
Carter Contact Lens	(email) carterlens@sbcglobal.net
Chessman's Contact Lens Lab	(email) chessman@ameritech.net
Conforma Contact Lens	http://www.conforma.com
Contex	http://oklens.com
Corneal Design Corporation	(email) DBellmd@aol.com
Corneal Contact Lens Corp. NZ	http://www.corneal-lens.co.nz
Custom Craft Service of Nevada	(email) cclenssv@lv.rmcl.net
Danker Laboratories	http://www.dankerlabs.com
Dist-o-con	(email) distocon@aol.com
Diversified Ophthalmics	http://www.divopt.com
E and E Optics USA	(email) eandeoptics@earthlink.net
Essilor USA—Contact Lens	http://www.essilorusa.com
Euclid Systems	http://www.euclidsys.com
Firestone Optics	http://www.firestoneoptics.com
Flexilens (India)	http://www.flexilens.com
Global Contact Lens	(email) globallens@bellsouth.com
Hawkins Contact Lens	(email) huskerba@networksplus.net
Herslof Contact Lens Service	800-558-7073
IVM Corporation	(email) ivmcontact@aol.com
Insight Contact Lens Labs	(email) insight01@msn.com
Int'l Contact Lens Labs	(email) dsicl@aol.com
Lancaster Contact Lens	(email) lcl@lancastercontactlens.com
Lens Dynamics	http://www.lensdynamics.com
Lens Mode	(email) lensmode@aol.com
Lensco	http://www.lensco.com
Luzerne Optical Labs	http://www.luzerneoptical.com
Medlens Innovations	http://www.innovationsinsight.com
Metro Optics—Arkansas	(email) blackburncharles@hotmail.com
Metro Optics of Austin	http://www.Metro-optics.com

(continued)

TABLE 18.7 CONTACT LENS MANUFACTURER ASSOCIATION LABORATORIES WITH KERATOCONIC LENS DESIGNS (Continued)

Mid-South Premier Ophthalmics	http://www.mspremier.com
New Era Custom Contacts	http://www.neweraopt.com
OPTIK K & R (Canada)	http://www.KandR.com
Oculus Limited (Singapore)	http://www.oculuslens.com
Opti Con	(email) opti-con@lpns.com
Paracon	(email) paraconinc@aol.com
Platt Contact Lens Service	(email) ncc1701lp@aol.com
Precision Optics	(email) precisionoptics1@aol.com
Progressive Vision Technologies	http://www.progressiveeyes.com
Rooney Optical	http://www.rooneyoptical.com
Safeway Contact Lens	(email) Safeway@cboss.com
Soderberg Contact Lens	http://www.soseyes.com
Sterling Contact Lenses	(email) sterlingcontacts@olypen.com
Tru-Form Optics	http://www.tfoptics.com
Ultralentes Ind. Optics (Brazil)	(email) ultralentes@ultralentes.com.br
Universal Contact Lens	(email) unidal@aol.com
Universal Contact Lenses of Florida	(email) ucl@bellsouth.net
Valley Contax	http://www.valleycontax.com
Visionary	http://www.visionarylens.com
Westlens	(email) WESTLENS@aol.com
Winchester Optical Company	(email) wocontacts@stny.rr.com

From Gas Permeable Lens Institute. Available online at http://www.gpli.info.

be flatter and wider than conventional designs to provide greater edge clearance and prevent peripheral seal-off and lens-to-cornea adherence.

As almost all lenses ordered will be in minus—if not high minus power—the center thickness should be 0.02 to 0.03 mm thicker than conventional designs to minimize flexure. Lenses with powers >-5.00 D should also be ordered with a plus lenticular or similar peripheral design to minimize edge thickness.

Lens Material: While lens design is the key factor in keratoconus, material selection is also important. Although very low Dk (i.e., <25) materials are still in use today because of their ability to correct corneal astigmatism while often providing excellent wettability, it is important to select a material that will not further compromise the cornea via hypoxia. With the fact that keratoconic lens designs are almost always of minus power and, therefore, thin in design, a fluoro-silicone/acrylate lens material with a minimum Dk value of 30 is often successful by providing satisfactory oxygen transmissibility while also providing sufficient rigidity to minimize the effects of flexure. Some believe higher Dk materials are warranted to protect the already compromised cornea, but then one must watch for flexure in thin lens designs. However, it also must be considered that keratoconic patients often will not (or cannot) wear spectacles; therefore, contact lens overwear is certainly possible. Extended wear is contraindicated in keratoconus because of the possibility of further compromising an already compromised cornea.

TABLE 18.8 KERATOCONUS PROBLEM SOLVING

PROBLEM	MANAGEMENT
1. Corneal abrasion/ severe swirl staining	D/C CL wear and allow abrasion to heal, then clean posterior surface or consider −0.50 D disposable as temporary piggyback; if BCR is too flat, refit with steeper BCR
2. Paracentral erosion	Most likely because of steep lens with sharp junction; blend PC junctions
3. Peripheral seal-off	Flatten/widen the peripheral curve
4. Adherence	Flatten/widen peripheral curve; also can flatten BCR and/or reduce OZD
5. Excessive inferior edge lift	Steepen BCR
6. Poor visual acuity	Select a flatter BCR
7. Flare	Change to a larger OZD lens
8. Poor centration	Larger OAD, steeper BCR, or use a piggyback design
9. Poor comfort	Ensure edges are thin; + lenticular use if indicated; consider piggyback design; R/O corneal abrasion

BCR, base curve radius; CL, contact lens; D/C, discontinue; OAD, overal diameter; OZD, optical zone diameter; PC, peripheral curve; R/O, rule out.

Problem Solving

The goal in fitting GP lenses is not necessarily to obtain a certain fluorescein pattern, but rather to allow adequate wearing time with acceptable comfort with best vision while minimizing tissue insult. Complications are often encountered, and a simple guide to problem solving is provided in Table 18.8.

As a result of the irregularity and fragility of the cornea, it is important that keratoconic patients are evaluated on a regular basis. Fortunately, these individuals are often receptive to follow-up care as a preventative measure to ensure the condition is successfully managed. When the condition is progressing, patients should be evaluated, at minimum, every 6 months. Once it has stabilized, annual, if not more frequent, examinations should be performed.

It is not uncommon for patients to experience corneal staining, especially at the more fragile apical region of the cone.[94] Unless this is coalesced, it can simply be monitored. If it coalesces to the point where the patient is symptomatic and an abrasion or severe swirl staining is present, lens wear must be discontinued until the staining has been resolved (Fig. 18.10). If necessary, a

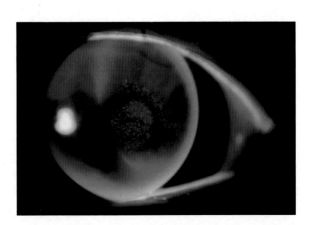

■ **FIGURE 18.10** Central corneal staining. (Courtesy of Craig Norman.)

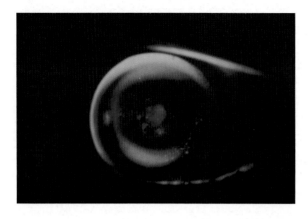

■ **FIGURE 18.11** Minimal edge clearance. (Courtesy of Dr. Larry Davis.)

soft lens can be used as a piggyback under the patient's GP lens during the healing process. The lens can then be cleaned and polished—especially the posterior surface—and an enzyme cleaner added to the care regimen if applicable. If the staining appears to be resulting from an excessively flat lens-to-cornea fitting relationship, a steeper base curve radius lens should be fitted. If a paracentral erosion is present from a steep-fitting lens, the midperiphery can be blended to reduce this problem. If the fitting relationship appears to be acceptable, it would be recommended to return the patient to the previous lens. It is not uncommon for keratoconic patients to overwear their lenses because of the poor vision often achieved with spectacles. If this is compounded by illness, allergies, or any other factor that may result in temporary dryness or hypoxia, significant staining may result.

Other problems may be a result of the lens-to-cornea fitting relationship. If peripheral seal-off is present (Fig. 18.11), the peripheral curve will need to be flatter and/or wider to increase edge clearance. If adherence is present, either flattening/widening the peripheral curve, selecting a flatter base curve radius, or decreasing the optical zone will typically result in lens movement with the blink. When excessive inferior edge lift is present (Fig. 18.12), the selection of a steeper base curve radius may reduce this problem. A better modern-day design change is to take advantage of new quadrant-specific peripheral curve steepening options available on the newest lathes from a few laboratories to solve this common problem. Representative designs include the steep-flat option from Lens Dynamics, the asymmetric corneal technology (ACT) from Blanchard, and the Quadra-Kone design from Tru-Form Optics. An example of the benefit of such a design is demonstrated in Figure 18.13A,B, which demonstrates an improved fitting relationship via refitting into a Quadra-Kone design, which has different peripheral eccentricities in each meridian.

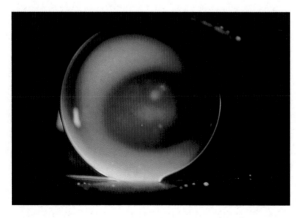

■ **FIGURE 18.12** Excessive edge clearance. (Courtesy of Craig Norman.)

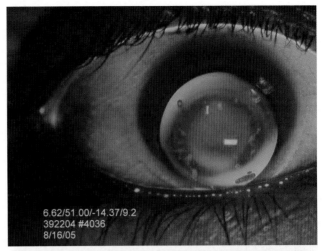

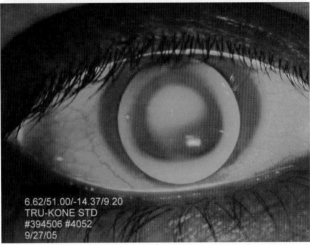

6.62/51.00/-14.37/9.2
392204 #4036
8/16/05

A

6.62/51.00/-14.37/9.20
TRU-KONE STD
#394506 #4052
9/27/05

B

■ **FIGURE 18.13 (A)** A decentered gas permeable lens on a keratoconic cornea with excessive edge lift in some peripheral regions and seal-off in others. **(B)** Same patient with a Quadra-Kone design resulting in a much more uniform peripheral pooling pattern.

Specific Corneal Gas Permeable Lens Designs and Fitting Methods

Many GP lens designs have been developed specifically for keratoconus. Typically, these consist of small-diameter, steep base curve radius lenses with either spherical or aspheric peripheral curves. These range from conventional designs such as the Soper Cone and McGuire lenses to more recently introduced designs such as the Rose K, ComfortKone, Dyna Z Cone, CLEK, amd I-Kone. The theory behind these designs will be discussed here; for detailed parameter presentation and selection, please refer to the manufacturer's fitting guides.

Small-Diameter Corneal Designs: These are intended to fit over the apex of the keratoconic cornea and, therefore, are steeper and smaller than conventional GP designs. For historical purposes, two classic designs will be outlined here, which were predominantly used in the 1980s: the Soper design and the McGuire design.

Soper Cone Design: The Soper Cone design is fit in an apical clearance manner in which support and bearing are directed off the apex of the cornea and onto the paracentral cornea.[95] This lens design is most effective for small cones, but is also successful for cones with their central apex displaced slightly inferior to the visual axis.[96]

The Soper Cone is a bicurve lens design. The two curves on the posterior surface consist of a steep central curve to vault the corneal apex and a flatter peripheral curve to align with the more normal peripheral cornea.[95] The secondary curve of the Soper lens is typically 7.5 mm or 45 D, which is one of the limitations of this design.[96] The constant base curve radius along with the large diameter of this lens results in an increased sagittal depth and, therefore, a steeper lens. A well-fitting Soper Cone lens will vault the central cornea and exhibit slight touch around the periphery.

A representative Soper Cone diagnostic fitting set, available from many CLMA member laboratories (see Table 18.7), is given in Table 18.9. The overall and optical zone diameters are selected dependent on the degree of keratoconus. In mild keratoconus, a 7.4/6.0-mm lens is used; in moderate keratoconus, an 8.5/7.0-mm lens is used; and in advanced keratoconus, a 9.5/8.0-mm lens is selected. If the initial lens shows excessive apical clearance and central air bubbles, increasingly flatter lenses with less sagittal depth should be used until a small central air bubble just appears. If the initial lens exhibits apical touch, an increasingly steeper base curve radius lens with greater sagittal depth may be applied until apical touch disappears or small bubbles appear.

McGuire Lens Design: Another classic and historical keratoconic lens design still available today from many laboratories is the McGuire lens. This is another apical clearance or alignment fitting relationship design. This lens design has a steep central curvature with four progressively flatter peripheral curve radii.[48,95] The peripheral curve radii are flatter than the base curve by 3 D, 9 D, 17 D, and 27 D. The three inner curves are 0.3 mm wide and the peripheral curve is 0.4 mm wide. It is available in three overall/optical zone diameters depending on whether the patient has a nipple cone (8.1/5.5 mm), oval cone (8.6/6.0 mm), or globus cone (9.1/6.5 mm) (Table 18.10). Fitting the McGuire lens is similar to the Soper lens. An advantage of the McGuire design is that it allows adequate edge clearance and movement in comparison to the Soper lens design.[62]

Other Corneal Lens Designs: Other, more contemporary corneal lens designs include the Rose K and Rose K2 lens (Blanchard Contact Lenses, Manchester, NH), Comfort Zone design (Abba Optical, Stone Mountain, GA), Dyna Z Cone design (Lens Dynamics, Golden, CO), CLEK design (Conforma, Norfolk, VA), and Ikone (Valley Contax, Springfield, OR). These designs are traditional multicurve designs; that is, the peripheral curve radii are spherical and continue to flatten from the base curve through to the final peripheral curve. These designs differ from the above two designs in that their peripheral curve systems are not immediately accessible to the

TABLE 18.9 SOPER KERATOCONUS DIAGNOSTIC LENS SET

BCR/SCR (D)	BCR/SCR (mm)	POWER (D)	OVERALL DIAMETER (mm)	OPTICAL ZONE DIAMETER (mm)	CENTER THICKNESS (mm)	SAGITTAL DEPTH (mm)
48.00/43.00	7.03/7.85	−4.50	7.50	6.0	0.10	.68
52.00/45.00	6.49/7.50	−8.50	7.50	6.0	0.10	.73
56.00/45.00	6.03/7.50	−12.50	7.50	6.0	0.10	.80
60.00/45.00	5.62/7.50	−16.50	7.50	6.0	0.10	.87
52.00/45.00	6.49/7.50	−8.50	8.50	7.0	0.10	1.00
56.00/45.00	6.03/7.50	−12.50	8.50	7.0	0.10	1.12
60.00/45.00	5.62/7.50	−16.50	8.50	7.0	0.10	1.22
52.00/45.00	5.62/7.50	−8.50	9.50	8.0	0.10	1.37
56.00/45.00	6.03/7.50	−12.50	9.50	8.0	0.10	1.52
60.00/45.00	5.62/7.50	−16.50	9.50	8.0	0.10	1.67

BCR, base curve radius; SCR, secondary curve radius.

TABLE 18.10 MCGUIRE CONE TRIAL SETS

BASE CURVE RADIUS (D/mm)	POWER (D)	OVERALL DIAMETER (mm)	OPTICAL ZONE (mm)	PERIPHERAL CURVE RADII/WIDTH (mm)
A. Nipple Cone				
50.00/6.75	−8.00	8.6	6.0	7.25/.3 8.28/.3 9.75/.3 11.75/.4
51.00/6.62	−9.00	8.6	6.0	7.10/.3 8.10/.3 9.60/.3 11.60/.4
52.00/6.49	−10.00	8.6	6.0	7.00/.3 8.00/.3 9.50/.3 11.50/.4
53.00/6.37	−11.00	8.6	6.0	6.85/.3 7.85/.3 9.35/.3 11.35/.4
54.00/6.24	−12.00	8.6	6.0	6.75/.3 7.75/.3 9.25/.3 11.25/.4
55.00/6.14	−13.00	8.6	6.0	6.65/.3 7.65/.3 9.15/.3 11.15/.4
B. Oval Cone				
50.00/6.75	−8.00	9.1	6.5	7.25/.3 8.28/.3 9.75/.3 11.75/.4
51.00/6.62	−8.00	9.1	6.5	7.10/.3 8.10/.3 9.60/.3 11.60/.4
52.00/6.49	−10.00	9.1	6.5	7.00/.3 8.00/.3 9.50/.3 11.50/.4
53.00/6.37	−10.00	9.1	6.5	6.85/.3 7.85/.3 9.35/.3 11.35/.4
54.00/6.24	−12.00	9.1	6.5	6.75/.3 7.75/.3 9.25/.3 11.25/.4
55.00/6.14	−12.00	9.1	6.5	6.65/.3 7.65/.3 9.15/.3 11.15/.4
56.00/6.03	−14.00	9.1	6.5	6.50/.3 7.50/.3 9.00/.3 11.00/.4
57.00/5.92	−14.00	9.1	6.5	6.40/.3 7.40/.3 8.90/.3 10.90/.4
58.00/5.82	−16.00	9.1	6.5	6.30/.3 7.30/.3 8.80/.3 10.80/.4
59.00/5.72	−16.00	9.1	6.5	6.20/.3 7.20/.3 8.70/.3 10.70/.4
60.00/5.63	−18.00	9.1	6.5	6.10/.3 7.10/.3 8.60/.3 10.60/.4
C. Globus Cone				
50.00/6.75	−8.00	9.6	7.0	7.25/.3 8.28/.3 9.75/.3 11.75/.4
51.00/6.62	−9.00	9.6	7.0	7.10/.3 8.10/.3 9.60/.3 11.60/.4
52.00/6.49	−10.00	9.6	7.0	7.00/.3 8.00/.3 9.50/.3 11.50/.4
53.00/6.37	−11.00	9.6	7.0	6.85/.3 7.85/.3 9.35/.3 11.35/.4
54.00/6.24	−12.00	9.6	7.0	6.75/.3 7.75/.3 9.25/.3 11.25/.4
55.00/6.14	−13.00	9.6	7.0	6.65/.3 7.65/.3 9.15/.3 11.15/.4

practitioner, and may be proprietary. Usually the designs are available with a peripheral geometry labeled as standard, flat, or steep. The best place to start in fitting these designs is to attempt the standard peripheral curve system in moderately advanced keratoconus, a steep peripheral system in advanced disease, and a flat peripheral system in moderate or early keratoconus.

Rose K and Rose K2 (Blanchard): Developed by a New Zealand optometrist, this very popular design utilizes a smaller than average optical zone diameter to minimize midperipheral lens impingement as well as pooling or bubbles at the base of the cone.[97] The optical zone ranges from 4.0 mm for a 5.10-mm base curve radius to a 6.5 mm for a 7.6-mm base curve radius. The peripheral lens design consists of a series of five to six computer-controlled spherical radii that clear the midperipheral and peripheral cornea. The curves are blended into a continuum for an aspheric-like periphery. The Rose K2 lens minimizes these aberrations by applying very small changes to the curves on both the front and back of the lens in an attempt to bring the light passing through the lens within the pupil zone to a single point.

As with all other designs, it is important to have their diagnostic fitting set when using this lens. It consists of 26 lenses with base curve radii ranging from 5.10 to 7.60 mm with a standard 8.7 mm overall diameter and a medium or standard edge lift. This diagnostic set is provided in Table 18.11. It is recommended to start with a base curve equal to the average of the two keratometer readings. A light, feather touch at the apex of the cone is desired. Although 8.7 mm is the standard diameter, any diameter is available, and smaller diameters of 8.1 to 8.3 mm tend to be more successful in advanced cases unless a globus cone or an inferior decentered apex exists.

CLEK Design: As part of the CLEK study, a rigid lens diagnostic fitting set was both designed and standardized.[98] This fitting set was developed and tested to simplify the fitting protocol for mild to moderate keratoconus patients. The diagnostic lens set and fitting method proposed allows the practitioner an easy-to-follow fitting protocol using an inexpensive diagnostic fitting set.

The parameters for the CLEK diagnostic lenses were standardized and are provided in Table 18.12.

TABLE 18.11   ROSE K DIAGNOSTIC FITTING SET[a]

BASE CURVE RADIUS (MM)	POWER (D)	OVERALL DIAMETER (mm)	PERIPHERAL CURVES	CENTER THICKNESS (mm)
5.10	−20.75	8.7	Std.	.10
5.20	−22.00	8.7	Std.	.11
5.30	−20.75	8.7	Std.	.12
5.40	−20.75	8.7	Std.	.10
5.50	−19.25	8.7	Std.	.11
5.60	−18.50	8.7	Std.	.11
5.70	−17.25	8.7	Std.	.12
5.80	−16.00	8.7	Std.	.13
5.90	−15.00	8.7	Std.	.10
6.00	−14.25	8.7	Std.	.13
6.10	−13.00	8.7	Std.	.14
6.20	−12.00	8.7	Std.	.14
6.30	−11.00	8.7	Std.	.14
6.40	−10.12	8.7	Std.	.14
6.50	−9.00	8.7	Std.	.15
6.60	−8.00	8.7	Std.	.16
6.70	−6.87	8.7	Std.	.17
6.80	−5.87	8.7	Std.	.18
6.90	−5.00	8.7	Std.	.19
7.00	−4.12	8.7	Std.	.19
7.10	−3.00	8.7	Std.	.20
7.20	−3.00	8.7	Std.	.19
7.30	−3.00	8.7	Std.	.20
7.40	−2.00	8.7	Std.	.20
7.50	−2.00	8.7	Std.	.19

[a]Optical zone diameter varies from 4.0–6.8 mm.

TABLE 18.12 COLLABORATIVE LONGITUDINAL EVALUATION OF KERATOCONUS DIAGNOSTIC SET

BASE CURVE RADIUS mm (D)	POWER (D)	OVERALL DIAMETER/ OPTICAL ZONE DIAMETER (mm)	SECONDARY CURVE RADIUS (mm)
8.00 (42.19)	−3.00	8.6/6.5	9.00
7.90 (42.72)	−3.00	8.6/6.5	9.00
7.80 (43.27)	−4.00	8.6/6.5	9.00
7.70 (43.83)	−4.00	8.6/6.5	9.00
7.60 (44.41)	−4.00	8.6/6.5	8.50
7.50 (45.00)	−4.00	8.6/6.5	8.50
7.40 (45.61)	−6.00	8.6/6.5	8.50
7.30 (46.23)	−5.00	8.6/6.5	8.50
7.20 (46.87)	−5.00	8.6/6.5	8.50
7.10 (47.54)	−7.00	8.6/6.5	8.50
7.00 (48.21)	−6.00	8.6/6.5	8.50
6.90 (48.91)	−6.00	8.6/6.5	8.50
6.80 (49.63)	−8.00	8.6/6.5	8.50
6.70 (50.37)	−7.00	8.6/6.5	8.50
6.60 (51.14)	−6.00	8.6/6.5	8.50
6.50 (51.92)	−8.00	8.6/6.5	8.50
6.40 (52.73)	−8.00	8.6/6.5	8.50
6.30 (53.37)	−7.00	8.6/6.5	8.50
6.20 (54.44)	−9.00	8.6/6.5	8.50
6.10 (55.33)	−8.00	8.6/6.5	8.50
6.00 (56.25)	−7.00	8.6/6.5	8.50
5.90 (57.20)	−9.00	8.6/6.5	8.50
5.80 (58.19)	−8.00	8.6/6.5	8.50
5.70 (59.21)	−7.00	8.6/6.5	8.50
5.60 (60.27)	−9.00	8.6/6.5	8.50
5.50 (61.36)	−8.00	8.6/6.5	8.50
5.40 (62.50)	−8.00	8.6/6.5	8.50
5.30 (63.68)	−8.00	8.6/6.5	8.50
5.20 (64.90)	−8.00	8.6/6.5	8.50
5.10 (66.18)	−8.00	8.6/6.5	8.50
5.00 (67.50)	−10.00	8.6/6.5	8.50

All diagnostic lenses are polymethylmethacrylate with a third curve radius of 11.00 mm and a third curve width of 0.2 mm. The lenses are lightly blended, and the center thickness is 0.13 mm.

From Edrington TB, Szczotka LB, Barr JT, et al. Rigid contact lens fitting relationships in keratoconus. Optom Vis Sci 1999;76:692–699.

The overall diameter was established at 8.6 mm and the optical zone diameter was set at 6.5 mm. The secondary curve radius was either 8.5 or 9.0 mm and the peripheral curve radius was 11.00 mm. The contact lens power gradually increased in minus as the base curve became steeper. The diagnostic lenses were fabricated in PMMA material because of its durability, dimensional stability, and low cost. As mentioned previously, a lens fit equal to the steeper keratometry value would represent a good starting point. Based on the fluorescein pattern, the lens would be changed until first definite apical clearance has been achieved.

Ikone: The IKone (Valley Contax), developed by Dr. Rob Breece, has a back surface designed to minimize pressure points, while the front surface asphericity reduces aberration-induced problems. As with many of the current designs, the optimum fitting relationship is one that exhibits either mild apical touch or slight clearance.

Multizone Lens Designs: There have been attempts to design multizone lenses for keratoconus in which the cone is advanced and located, at minimum, 1 mm away from the line of sight.[4] Such designs have included the Duozone and the Menicon Decentered OZ (Con-Cise, San Leandro, CA).

Aspheric Lenses

Back surface aspheric lenses have often been used in the fitting of the keratoconic cornea. Many of the designs are progressive asphics, which gradually flatten from the center of the lens to the periphery to provide better alignment with a highly prolate ectatic cornea. In normals, the central cornea has a mean eccentricity (e) of 0.45, with most corneas falling between 0 and 1.0. Aspheric GP lenses designed for nonkeratoconic eyes are usually not sufficient except for a mildly keratoconic cornea. However, aspheric back surface lenses designed to correct presbyopia have eccentricities of approximately 1.0, and these fit well on some keratoconic patients. In aspheric contact lenses, the degree of asphericity or eccentricity increases as the rate of flattening increases.[96] E-values of 0.4 to 0.6 are ellipsoidal in shape and fit a mild or nipple cone most effectively, while e-values of >1.0 are paraboloidal and hyperboloidal shaped and fit more advanced or oval-shaped cones.[99]

Examples of aspheric lenses useful for the keratoconic eye include the Abba Kone design from Abba Optical (Stone Mountain, GA), Apex Aspheric Cone design (X-Cel Contacts, Duluth, GA), and Conforma-K design (Conforma Laboratories, Norfolk, VA). These aspheric designs are available in flat, standard, and steep peripheral geometries for use in patients with moderate, moderately advanced, and advanced keratoconus, respectively. Historically, aspheric lenses not specifically intended for keratoconus that have been successful include VFLII and Ellip-See-Con (Conforma, Norfolk, VA).

Finally, there are spherical center/aspheric peripheral designs specifically intended for keratoconus. One such lens is the Comfortkone (Metro Optics, Austin, TX). The Comfortkone lens is designed with a spherical 4.0-mm optical zone diameter that fits the peak of the cone. This lens design incorporates a triaspheric curve in the periphery to maximize overall corneal lens alignment. The aspheric periphery flattens into the aspheric "A" curve. This "A" value is the fitting curve of the lens and depicts the rate of change from the central base curve to the peripheral fitting portion of the lens.[100] The greater the "A" value, the greater the change from the base curve to the peripheral fitting curve.

Intralimbal Rigid Gas Permeable Lenses

The advent of high oxygen transmissible rigid gas permeable lens polymers has allowed us to fit with much larger-diameter designs without the concern of hypoxic complications. In this chapter, large overall diameter lenses, or intralimbal lenses (because they can fit from limbus to limbus), will be referred to those lenses 10.5 to 12.8 mm in diameter. Examples include

Dyna-Intralimbal design (Lens Dynamics), GBL lens (Concise Laboratories), Rose K2 IC (Blanchard), and PMD lens (ABB-Concise).

The beauty of an intralimbal lens is that it tends to center better than smaller GP lenses as a result of greater pressure distribution over the midperipheral and peripheral cornea. Generally, these lenses have a large optical zone, which makes the lens forgiving if it decenters in terms of visual function. This is especially important with patients who have globus or decentered cones. These designs can be fitted by following with three-point touch or with minimal apical clearance. However, because of the deep sagittal depth often quickly achieved because of the large chord diameter and steeper base curves, bubbles can easily become trapped in the area surrounding the base of the cone. If this happens, one has to decrease the sagittal depth by either decreasing the optical zone size or flattening the base curve. Additionally, because of the large optical zone size, the required base curve will likely be flatter than expected to achieve clearance over the conical cornea.

Bitoric Lens Applications

Although keratoconic corneas typically have a high level of toricity, which, in theory, would benefit from a toric lens, toric back surface lenses have little application in keratoconus. In a back or bitoric lens, the toric curvatures and corresponding power corrections are 90 degrees apart. This is often not the case in the irregular astigmatism presented in keratoconus, especially in moderate and advanced cases. If the apex of the cone is decentered, a successful fit is difficult to achieve as well.[4] The corneal toricity error from the central cornea to the apex varies from 0 to 3 D when the apex is decentered by 1 mm and from 0 to about 6 D when the cone is decentered by 2 mm.

If the cone apex is well centered and if keratoconus is not advanced, the fitting of a bitoric is possible and has been found to be successful.[4,101,102] However, if the condition continues to progress, other designs will most likely be indicated.

Semi-Scleral Lens Designs

As is true for the intralimbal designs, semi-scleral designs have become available because of the highly oxygen permeable materials allowing us to fit very large lenses without compromise to corneal oxygenation. Semi-scleral lenses are usually, at minimum, 13.8 mm in diameter, and can be manufactured up to about 18.5 mm. They are differentiated from scleral (haptic) lenses, which range in size from 21 to 28 mm in diameter. Semi-scleral lenses are manufactured in one of a few GP materials that are available in the required material button size. Common materials include Boston XO, Tyro 97, or Equalens II. Examples include the Semi-Scleral design (Abba Optical), So$_2$Clear lens (Dakota Sciences), Jupiter lens (Medlens), and msd design (Blanchard).

Perhaps counterintuitive, large semi-scleral lenses are very comfortable when fitted well as a result of the large diameters, which minimize lens movement and lid interactions. If possible, an apical clearance fitting relationship is desirable; however, in advanced keratoconus, this may not be possible and apical bearing will have to be acceptable. If this is the case, the classic three-point-touch fit may not be achieved as the large diameter lens will likely vault over the rest of the cornea and limbus and rest on the peripheral limbus and sclera. In the central bearing type of fit, the apex of the cone usually tolerates the flat fit well (compared to small diameter corneal lenses) because these lenses usually do not move sufficiently for the apex of the cone to become irritated. In addition, as the sclera bears the weight of the lens surface, it is unnecessary to achieve a close alignment between cornea and lens, as compared to smaller designs.[103] This has been found to result in good visual acuity in irregular cornea patients because of the larger and flatter optical zone diameter.

Some patients may find the excess bulk of the lens to be irritating, and the physical size of the lens can discourage patients. Removal of these lenses can also be a problem because of the suction created by the lens–sclera interface. In cases of lens intolerance or discomfort with traditional lenses, however, semi-scleral GP lenses are a viable option to postpone or prevent surgical intervention.

Scleral (Haptic) Lenses

Scleral lenses made in PMMA materials were historically the first type of contact lenses created. These large lenses are approximately 21 to 28 mm in diameter and the goal in fitting this type of lens is to vault the keratoconic cornea. The major disadvantages of scleral lenses are the time, skill, and expense required to fit them. Only a few centers in the United States are proficient in fitting these lenses. Historically, these lenses were made by creating a negative mold of the patient's eye with dental molding. From this, a PMMA positive mold was created. The laboratory then lathed the optical zone, back curvatures, and refractive power.

Modern scleral contact lenses are made of high Dk GP materials, which are not thermoplastic, and, therefore, they cannot be molded in the manner of PMMA as described above. Preformed GP scleral lenses are available and can be fitted from an existing fitting set such as the one from Gelflex Laboratories (Donald Ezekial, Perth, Australia) or Innovative Sclerals, Ltd. (Kenneth Pullum, Hertford, UK). In the United States, Dr. Perry Rosenthal, who founded the Boston Foundation for Sight (Boston, MA), has established a small network of scleral lens fitters in a few centers nationwide. Nevertheless, fitting true scleral lenses on keratoconic patients is, therefore, reserved for the most advanced patients and/or in those where surgery is contraindicated.

Soft Lens Fitting

As with bitoric GP lens designs, spherical and toric soft lenses have little application in keratoconus. Corneal irregularity in keratoconus is best neutralized, and the vision optimum, with a GP lens design. Soft lenses have their best application in the mild forms of this condition before the onset of significant irregular astigmatism.[104] Several designs are commercially available. A popular design is the Hydrokone from Medlens. This design is also available in toric powers and practically every conceivable parameter is available (Table 18.13). However, soft lenses still have their primary application in piggyback designs. If a keratoconic patient is experiencing difficulty adapting to rigid lenses, it would be preferable to attempt a piggyback design first.

Piggyback Lenses

These designs either consist of a rigid lens fit over top of a soft lens or some form of integration of a rigid lens into a soft lens carrier. It is often a viable option in individuals who cannot tolerate a rigid lens or if a good lens-to-cornea fitting relationship cannot be obtained. The underlying

TABLE 18.13 THE HYDROKONE DIAGNOSTIC SET (MEDLENS)

BCR/FITTING	POWER	DIAMETER
8.5/8.9 mm	+2.00 D	14.8 mm
8.1/8.9 mm	Plano	14.8 mm
7.7/8.9 mm	−2.00 D	14.8 mm
7.3/8.9 mm	−4.00 D	14.8 mm
6.9/8.9 mm	−6.00 D	14.8 mm
6.5/8.9 mm	−8.00 D	14.8 mm
6.1/8.9 mm	−10.00 D	14.8 mm
5.7/8.9 mm	−12.00 D	14.8 mm

BCR, base curve radius.

(or adjacent) soft lens improves tolerance while the GP provides optimum vision. The soft lens also offers some amount of protection to the cornea. Two forms of piggyback-type designs will be discussed: (a) traditional piggyback designs and (b) the countersunk rigid lens–soft lens carrier.

Traditional Piggyback Designs: With this combination design, a highly oxygen transmissible soft lens is fitted initially so that both good movement and centration are achieved. A disposable lens, preferably a silicone hydrogel, is recommended. The use of a manufacturer who makes custom soft lenses in steeper base curve radii may be necessary if stock disposable lenses result in edge standoff. The O$_2$OPTIX Custom lens (Ciba Vision) is recommended in these cases.

Once the soft lens has been fit, keratometry is performed over the anterior surface of the soft lens. A high or hyper-permeable GP lens should be fit with both minimal edge and center thickness to promote good centration and decreased lid sensation[48,105] (Fig. 18.14). This is quite important as the rigid lens is now farther away from the cornea as a result of the presence of the soft lens. There are several accepted concepts in the selection of a soft lens power. Some practitioners prefer to fit with negligible power (+ or −0.50 D) and then fit the rigid lens in the same manner as would have been fit without the soft lens in place. This method is especially useful if the patient uses piggyback lenses intermittently for comfort or if the soft lens is expected to be discontinued as the patient's adaptation to the rigid lens improves. Alternatively, some practitioners prefer to fit with a plus lens design. This effectively moves the apex of the fitting surface to a centered position. If this method is used, the rigid lens is typically fitted 0.5 to 1.0 D flatter than the steep keratometry value. The lenses should move independently. That is, the rigid lens and the soft lens should not adhere nor move as one unit. Therefore, the rigid lens should not be fitted too steep to encourage lens adherence. The fluorescein patterns of GP lenses can be evaluated on top of silicone hydrogel lenses, because these soft lenses will not readily imbibe the fluorescein molecules. Fluorescein of high molecular weight is required for this purpose when conventional hydrogel lenses are worn.

A care system approved for both GP and soft lenses should be used on both systems for ease (e.g., Clear Care, Ciba Vision). However, if needed for wettability, the rigid lens can be cleaned with a compatible rigid lens cleaner and stored in an approved rigid lens storage solution. Most importantly, the rigid lens should be rinsed with soft lens solution (never water) before inserting over the soft lens. Patients should be instructed to insert the soft lenses first, but the rigid lenses are removed first.

Countersunk Rigid Lens–Soft Lens Carrier: The Flexlens piggyback system (X-Cel Contacts/Walman Optical) was first introduced in the 1970s.[106] It consists of a hydrogel lens with a cut-out section in the center for a rigid lens to fit. It is available in a 45% water content hefilcon A or 55% water content methafilcon A. The overall diameter of the soft lens is 14.5 mm

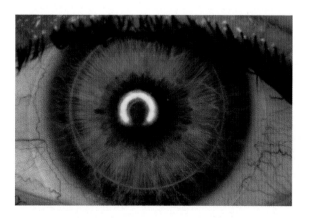

■ FIGURE 18.14 A piggyback lens.

FLEXLENS PIGGYBACK LENS

Front View

Sectional View

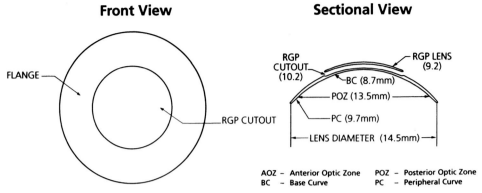

AOZ – Anterior Optic Zone   POZ – Posterior Optic Zone
BC – Base Curve   PC – Peripheral Curve

■ **FIGURE 18.15** The Flexlens (X-Cel Contacts/Walman Optical).

with a typical cut-out diameter of 10.2 mm. A standard thin GP lens design that is 1.0 mm smaller (9.2 mm) is placed within the recessed cut-out[107] (Fig. 18.15). The main purpose of the Flexlens piggyback is to assist in the centration of the rigid lens. The biggest drawbacks of this lens include the low Dk hydrophilic material and nondisposability of the product.

Hybrid Lenses

Hybrid lenses incorporate a rigid lens center and a soft periphery. One lens system provides certain benefits over piggyback options such as ease of care, less handling, and perhaps improved comfort, as there is no sensation of the rigid lens edge. There are two available hybrid lenses: the SoftPerm (Ciba Vision, Duluth, GA) and the SynergEyes Lens (SynergEyes, Inc., Carlsbad, CA). The SoftPerm lens utilizes an 8 mm diameter styrene-based rigid lens center with a Dk of 25. The periphery of this 14.3-mm overall diameter lens is a 20% water content soft lens. It is also available in steep base curve radii for the keratoconus patient, beginning with 6.5 mm. The introduction of a peripheral curve into the rigid lens section of the design has assisted in providing lens movement with the blink. Nevertheless, problems with this design include adherence, corneal hypoxia because of the relatively low Dk of both materials, and tearing of the lens at the rigid–soft lens junction.[108,109]

The SynergEyes lens was long awaited by many practitioners as a way to solve the hypoxic complications of the low Dk SoftPerm lens. This lens incorporates a central 8.2-mm rigid lens center made of Paragon HDS 100 and a 14.5-mm nonionic 27% water hydrophilic skirt. There are four types of lenses available, including designs for typical ametropias (SynergEyes A), ker-

TABLE 18.14 SYNERGEYES KC LENS PARAMETERS

I. Made to order	
Diameter:	14.5 mm
Base curve:	5.7–7.1 in 0.2-mm steps
Sphere power:	+4.00 to −16.00 D in 0.50 D steps
Skirt curve radius:	Steep, median, and flat
II. Custom	
Diameter:	14.5 mm
Base curve:	5.7–7.1 in 0.2-mm steps
Sphere power:	+4.50 to +20.00 D in 0.50 D steps
	−16.50 to −20.00 D in 0.50 D steps
Skirt curve radius:	Steep, median, and flat

TABLE 18.15 KERATOCONUS CONTACT LENS SELECTION

I. TYPE OF CONE	RECOMMENDED DESIGNS
Nipple	Small OAD/OZD
Oval	Small design or intralimbal (if large oval)
Globus	Intralimbal or mini-scleral (secondarily a piggyback or hybrid design
Marginal	Same as globus
II. PROGRESSION	RECOMMENDED DESIGNS
Mild	Conventional GP, small K cone design or specialty soft lens
Moderate	Small K cone, intralimbal (mini-scleral if intralimbal decenters)
Severe	Intralimbal, mini-scleral, piggyback, or hybrid (unless nipple cone)

GP, gas permeable; OAD, overall diameter; OZD, optical zone diameter.

atoconus (SynergEyes KC), multifocals (SynergEyes M), and oblate postsurgical cases (SynergEyes PS). This lens is promoted to be fit with apical clearance to allow for a fluid tear layer beneath the rigid portion to avoid adherence and corneal compromise. Multiple skirt radii are available to assist in lens centration and movement. The SynergEyes KC trial set parameters are provided in Table 18.14.

A recommended lens selection guide based on type of cone and progression of the condition is provided in Table 18.15.

■ ALTERNATIVE METHODS OF MANAGEMENT

Surgery

Keratoconus represents the most common corneal thinning disorder. As a group, it comprises the second most common indication for corneal transplantation in the United States, totaling nearly 16% of all cases in 2006: in 2006, keratoconus accounted for 15.9% of the 33,962 keratoplasties performed in the United States.[110] Anywhere from 10% to 22% of patients diagnosed with keratoconus will require a corneal transplant.[3,4,6,73,111–113] When surgery is indicated, a full-thickness penetrating keratoplasty (PKP) is the primary procedure performed. In the CLEK study, 9.8% of patients at baseline had a PKP in one eye, and, during the course of the 8-year study, 12% of those patients who started the study free of PKP in either eye proceeded to a PKP in one or both eyes.[114]

The primary indications for the need for a penetrating keratoplasty primarily pertain to cases in which a stable contact lens fit was not possible to achieve—or tolerated—and/or extensive axial corneal scarring was present, which resulted in unacceptable visual acuity and possibly extreme corneal thinning.[6] Corneal transplantation is highly successful with as high as 96% resulting in clear grafts.[70,115,116] This appears to be related to the integrity of the peripheral cornea in keratoconus. Risk factors for the eventual need for a penetrating keratoplasty appear to be (a) onset at a young age (<20 years of age), (b) >55 D keratometry readings, (c) best corrected visual acuity <20/40, and (d) apical scarring.[3,117] Studies have confirmed, however, that penetrating keratoplasty can be delayed or avoided by the application of contact lenses in the large majority of cases.[113,118,119] It is imperative that every attempt be made to achieve a successful contact lens fit before considering a surgical option.

After PKP, the patient is subject to moderate risk of graft rejection or other complications (e.g., infection, high postoperative astigmatism, wound dehiscence after blunt trauma). Other available procedures such as deep anterior lamellar keratoplasty (DALK) and intrastromal ring segments (INTACSs) have reduced some of the complications of PKP such as endothelial rejection, but they are not as popular and their long-term success is not known. In the DALK procedure, the posterior cornea and endothelial layer remain, which eliminates the risk of endothelial rejection; however, it is more difficult to perform and the graft is still subject to rejection in other layers. The INTACS procedure utilizes PMMA ring segments implanted in the midperiphery of the cornea, which serve to flatten the central ectatic area. This procedure was initially utilized for the correction of low to moderate amounts of myopia but is now primarily used for keratoconus. However, it is limited to the successful treatment of early cases of the disease and patients still have to use contact lenses postoperatively to achieve their best visual potential.

Riboflavin Cross-Linking

Spoerl et al.[120–122] have demonstrated some success with reducing keratoconus via increasing corneal rigidity. In this procedure, the surgeon removes corneal epithelium over a 9 mm diameter and adds riboflavin 0.1% to the stroma to ensure absorption. Following this procedure, the cornea is exposed to 30 minutes of ultraviolet A radiation, which increases the thickness of the collagen fibrils and results in a more rigid anterior half of the cornea.[36] In one study of 22 keratoconic eyes, the progression was halted in all treated eyes and, in 16 eyes, regression of the maximal keratometry readings by 2.01 D and of the refractive error by 1.14 D was found.[122]

▥ CODING AND REIMBURSEMENT

A common challenge among practitioners who are fitting, refitting, and problem solving keratoconus patients is the matter of appropriate coding for reimbursement to occur. As keratoconic patients often experience a significant improvement in vision with contact lenses versus spectacles, it is important to emphasize the medical need to third-party plans. The National Keratoconus Foundation has several useful resources including an insurance reimbursement form available to send to third-party plans, a brochure on medically necessary contact lens prescribing, and an article on "How to Code" from Dr. Carla Mack.

▥ SUMMARY

Keratoconus is a condition that warrants proper management accompanied by careful monitoring. In most cases, the fitting of contact lenses will delay and often preclude surgical intervention. The most successful option has been the fitting of rigid gas permeable contact lenses. However, other options including spectacles and soft lenses (in early cases) and piggyback or hybrid or semi-scleral designs (in advanced cases) should be used when indicated.

■ CLINICAL CASES

CASE 1

A 16-year-old patient, who is new to your office, presents with symptoms of a slight decrease in vision and a mild ghosting of images. She indicates a desire to simply have her spectacles updated. Your examination reveals the following:

Manifest refraction:

OD: −3.75 − 1.75 × 162   20/25
OS: −2.00 − 0.75 × 006   20/20

Keratometry:

OD: 44.12 @ 165; 46.00 @ 075 (slight mire distortion)
OS: 43.25 @ 180; 44.25 @ 090 (good mire quality)

Retinoscopy: scissors reflex present OD

Slit-lamp biomicroscopy: Vogt striae present OD

Videokeratoscopy: localized region of steepening (steepest area equaled 49.00 D) 1 to 2 mm below corneal center

SOLUTION: This patient has keratoconus based on the presence of Vogt striae, a scissors reflex with retinoscopy, and the 49 D region inferocentrally. In addition, the presence of mild irregular astigmatism in one eye only confirms the pattern of keratoconus, in which one eye progresses before the other eye.

CASE 2

A patient enters your office with symptoms of blurred vision through his spectacle correction. He has been a 20-year rigid lens wearer (10 years PMMA followed by 10 years in a 12 Dk lens material). Your examination reveals the following:

Manifest refraction:

OD: −4.75 − 1.25 × 022   20/25−
OS: −5.00 − 2.25 × 162   20/30

Keratometry

OD: 42.12 @ 025; 44.00 @ 118 (slight mire distortion)
OS: 42.25 @ 160; 44.75 @ 071 (slight mire distortion)

Slit-lamp biomicroscopy:

With lenses: superior decentration OU
Without lenses: mild central corneal edema OU

Videokeratoscopy: superior flattening accompanied by inferior steepening with mild distortion OU

SOLUTION: This appears to be corneal warpage syndrome. There is an absence of classical slit-lamp signs (i.e., Vogt striae, Fleischer ring, scarring), and the patient appears to have complications relating to contact lens-induced hypoxia. It is also likely that the superior fitting relationship is inducing a pseudokeratoconic color map because of superior molding accompanied by inferior steepening. This can be verified by having the patient remove his lenses and rechecking corneal topography a few hours (or days) later. The superior region should steepen, accompanied by inferior flattening.

CASE 3

An 18-year-old patient had been diagnosed with keratoconus 3 years ago. He has been wearing a spectacle correction but his vision has reached a point where he has decided that contact lenses may be a viable option for him. Your examination reveals the following:

Manifest refraction:

OD: −4.75 − 2.50 × 159   20/30−
OS: −4.00 − 1.25 × 010   20/25 + 1

Keratometry (simulated):

OD: 47.12 @ 155; 50.00 @ 039 (mire distortion); apex (paracentral; slightly inferior-temporal)
OS: 45.25 @ 012; 46.75 @ 105 (mire distortion); apex: same as OD
Pupil size: 4 mm (normal room illumination) OU

SOLUTION: This patient would appear to be a good candidate for GP lenses. One method of fitting the patient would be to select a diagnostic lens with a base curve radius (BCR) equal to the steep keratometry value. For example, in the right eye in this case that would equal 6.75 mm. Topical anesthetic can be used before lens application. If the fluorescein pattern shows apical clearance, a flatter lens can be used. If apical touch is obtained with a base curve radius equal to 6.89 mm and the power determined by adding the spherical overrefraction to the diagnostic lens power, the following lens can be ordered:

BCR: 6.89 mm
Secondary curve radius/width (SCR/W): 8.00/.3 mm
Intermediate curve radius/width (ICR/W): 9.60/.3 mm
Peripheral curve radius/width (PCR/W): 12.00/.3 mm
Overall diameter (OAD)/OZD: 8.8/7.0 mm
Power: −6.50 D
Paragon HDS

CASE 4

A patient was diagnosed with keratoconus 6 years ago and has been wearing rigid GP lenses for the past 4 years. He has observed an increase in lens awareness as well as fluctuating vision over the past 12 months. Your examination reveals the following:

Keratometry:

OD: 46.12 @ 015; 48.00 @ 108 (slight mire distortion)
OS: 50.25 @ 152; 54.75 @ 071 (moderate mire distortion)

Slit-lamp biomicroscopy:

With lenses: inferior decentration with 3 mm of lag with the blink OU
Videokeratoscopy: an inferiorly displaced cone (approximately 2–2.5 mm) is shown OU

SOLUTION: This would be a good candidate for one of the keratoconus lens designs recommended for an inferiorly displaced cone. An intralimbal design would be recommended initially. If this design exhibits excessive inferior edge lift, the inferior edge can be "tucked in" via ordering the change recommended by the manufacturer (i.e., "steep-flat," "ACT," "Quadra-Kone," etc.). If this is not successful, a hybrid (i.e., SynergEyes), piggyback, or semi-scleral design can be used.

CASE 5

An advanced keratoconus patient reports to your office with symptoms of gradual left lens awareness for the past 6 months. Your examination reveals the following:

Slit-lamp biomicroscopy:

With lenses: lens adherence is present OS; the fluorescein pattern shows mild apical
  clearance and peripheral seal-off
Without lenses: central staining is accompanied by an outer compression ring

Lens design: OS: BCR: 7.00 mm; SCR: 8.00/.4 mm; PCR: 10.00/.3 mm; OAD/OZD: 9.2/7.8 mm

SOLUTION: The first step in this case would be to apply a flatter peripheral bevel (i.e., 12.00 mm). An additional option that could be helpful would be to decrease the optical zone diameter (e.g., from 7.8 to 7.2 or even 7.0 mm). Polishing the back surface of the lens will remove any trapped debris that tends to accumulate and assist in adhering the lens to the cornea.

CASE 6

An advanced keratoconus patient reports to your office with symptoms of intolerance with her GP lenses. Over the past 3 years she has worn a variety of lens designs, all unsatisfactory from a comfort standpoint. She is very motivated to continue contact lens wear as a result of the vision benefits. Your examination reveals the following:

Slit-lamp biomicroscopy:

With lenses: lenses are decentering inferiorly
Without lenses: mild central staining is present

SOLUTION: This patient would be a good candidate for a piggyback or hybrid (i.e., SynergEyes) lens design. In any case in which comfort and/or lens centration is an ongoing problem, a piggyback or modified piggyback lens system can be used. One of the benefits of the piggyback system is that one can quickly determine whether it will be successful or not (i.e., do both the GP and soft lens fit properly?). The selection of a silicone hydrogel lens material (if a moderate to severe case is present, the O₂OPTIX Custom is recommended) in combination with a hyper-permeable GP material is very important. The use of disposable lenses provides the capability of trying a piggyback design on a trial basis. For example, if the patient is already wearing a high or hyper-permeable Dk GP material, a disposable silicone hydrogel lens can be worn with the conventional GP lens for a short period of time to see if the patient is more satisfied and comfortable with this lens combination.

CASE 7

An advanced keratoconus patient reports to your office with symptoms of intolerance with her GP lenses. She has been wearing GP lenses on an intermittent basis for 5 years but has experienced lens awareness, dryness, and several episodes of corneal abrasion. She had never been very motivated for contact lens wear but had been told it was necessary because of her condition. Piggyback lenses have been attempted without success because of inability of the rigid lens to properly position on the soft lens blanket. Your examination reveals the following:

Visual acuity (with GP lenses):

OD: 20/30 − 2   Overrefraction (best sphere): −0.75 DS 20/30
OS: 20/25 − 2   Overrefraction (best sphere): −0.50 DS 20/25

Slit-lamp biomicroscopy:

With lenses: lenses are decentering inferiorly
Without lenses: moderate apical scar formation is present (OD > OS). With optical section it is apparent that her corneal is thinner in the affected region. Mild central staining is present. Moderate peripheral corneal desiccation is present. Tear breakup time is 8 seconds OU.

Keratometry: very distorted OU

OD: (approximately) 53.12 @ 036; 56.50 @ 118
OS: (approximately) 56.00 @ 151; 60.25 @ 068
(+1.25 D ophthalmic lens used to extend range of keratometer OU)

SOLUTION: This would be an excellent candidate for a semi-scleral lens or a hybrid design. If she is not motivated toward these options, a corneal transplant consultation would be recommended as she has an advanced case of keratoconus, suspect motivation, apical scarring and thinning, and borderline tear quality. At minimum, the potential for this surgical procedure should be discussed if it has not been discussed previously.

CLINICAL PROFICIENCY CHECKLIST

- Keratoconus is a progressive, asymmetric disease of the cornea that is characterized by steepening and distortion, apical thinning, and corneal ectasia.
- It is likely to be genetic in origin and often has an association with atopic conditions.
- Early symptoms include gradual blurring, ghost image formation, and distortion of vision.
- Early clinical signs include a scissors reflex with retinoscopy, an increase in irregular astigmatism, lack of parallelism with keratometry mires, and a localized area of steepening as shown with videokeratoscopy.
- Videokeratoscopy is important in the diagnosis and monitoring of keratoconus. The modified Rabinowitz-McDonnell criteria indicate that if the central corneal power is >47.2 D or if the difference between the inferior and superior paracentral regions is >1.4 D, keratoconus should be suspected. If the central corneal power is >48.7 D and the I-S value is >1.4 D, keratoconus can be diagnosed.
- Classic clinical signs of keratoconus as diagnosed with the slit-lamp biomicroscope are Vogt striae, the Fleischer ring, and apical scarring.

(continued)

(Continued)

- Keratoconus can be differentiated from corneal warpage syndrome in that it is progressive, it may not be related to contact lens wear, it often progresses to >50 D, the aforementioned slit-lamp signs, and a localized affected region is identified via videokeratoscopy.

- One fitting philosophy utilizes a three-point touch relationship in which a diagnostic lens equal to the steep K reading is selected and, based on the fluorescein pattern, changes are made to result in minimum apical touch.

- The optical zone diameter should decrease as the condition progresses. It is not uncommon for the optical zone diameter to approximate the base curve radius in millimeters unless a globus cone or a decentered apex is present.

- The use of a topical anesthetic during the diagnostic fitting process will be beneficial with keratoconic patients.

- A wide, flat peripheral curve radius will reduce the risk of peripheral seal-off and adherence.

- A fluoro-silicone/acrylate lens material with a minimum Dk of 30 is recommended.

- A large-diameter (intralimbal) design is recommended when a small lens does not exhibit good centration. This design is recommended in cases of an inferior decentered apex or a large (globus) cone. A semi-scleral lens design can also be beneficial in these cases as well as moderate to severe keratoconus cases in which centration cannot be achieved with other, smaller designs.

- When comfort and/or centration are problematic, a piggyback or hybrid lens can be used.

- Corneal transplantation is highly successful in moderate to severe keratoconus cases in which a stable contact lens fit was not possible (or tolerated) and/or extensive apical corneal scarring was present.

REFERENCES

1. Rabinowitz YS. Keratoconus. Surv Ophthalmol 1998;42:297–319.
2. Krachmer JH, Feder RS, Belin MW. Keratoconus and related non-inflammatory corneal thinning disorders. Surv Ophthalmol 1984;28:293–322.
3. Tuft SJ, Moodaley LC, Gregory WM, et al. Prognostic factors for the progression of keratoconus. Ophthalmol 1994;101(3):439–446.
4. Mandell RB. Contemporary management of keratoconus. Int Contact Lens Clin 1997;24:(3,4):43–58.
5. Jimenez JL, Jurado JC, Rodriquez FJ, et al. Keratoconus: age of onset and natural history. Optom Vis Sci 1997;74(3):149–151.
6. Kennedy RH, Bourne WM, Dyer JA. A 48 year clinical and epidemiologic study of keratoconus. Am J Ophthalmol 1986;101:267–273.
7. Nielsen K, Hjortal J, Aagaard Nohr E, et al. Incidence and prevalence of keratoconus in Denmark. Acta Ophthalmol Scand. 2007;85:890–892.
8. Georgiou T, Funnell CL, Cassels-Brown A, et al. Influence of ethnic origin on the incidence of keratoconus and associated atopic disease in Asians and white patients. Eye 2004;18:379–383.
9. Bawazeer AM, Hodge WG, Lorimer B. Atopy and keratoconus: a multivariate analysis. Br J Ophthalmol 2000;84(8):834–366.
10. Galin MA, Berger R. Atopy and keratoconus. Am J Ophthalmol 1958;45(6):904–906.
11. Harrison RJ, Klouda PT, Easty DL, et al. Association between keratoconus and atopy. Br J Ophthalmol 1989;73(10):816–822.
12. Al-Hussain H, Zeisberger SM, Huber PR, et al. Brittle cornea syndrome and its delineation from the kyphoscoliotic type of Ehlers-Danlos syndrome (EDS VI): report on 23 patients and review of the literature. Am J Med Genet A 2004;124(1):28–34.
13. Capaccini A, Lampis R, Brogi M. [Incidence of mesenchymosic manifestations in keratoconus.] Ann Ottalmol Clin Ocul 1963;89(Suppl):1118–1122.
14. Gasset AR, Hinson WA, Frias JL. Keratoconus and atopic diseases. Ann Ophthalmol 1978;10(8):991–994.

15. Goodman RM, Gazit E, Katznelson MB, et al. Four new heritable disorders of connective tissue. Birth Defects Orig Artic Ser 1975;11(6):39–51.

16. Greenfield G, Stein R, Romano A, et al. Blue sclerae and keratoconus: key features of a distinct heritable disorder of connective tissue. Clin Genet 1973;4(1):8–16.

17. McMonnies CW. Abnormal rubbing and keratectasia. Eye Contact Lens 2007;33(6 Pt 1):265–271.

18. McMonnies CW, Boneham GC. Keratoconus, allergy, itch, eye-rubbing and hand-dominance. Clin Exp Optom 2003;86(6):376–384.

19. Macsai MS, Varley GA, Krachmer JH. Development of keratoconus after contact lens wear. Patient characteristics. Arch Ophthalmol 1990;108(4):534–538.

20. Gasset AR, Houde WL, Garcia-Bengochea M. Hard contact lens wear as an environmental risk in keratoconus. Am J Ophthalmol 1978;85(3):339–341.

21. Phillips CI. Contact lenses and corneal deformation: cause, correlate or co-incidence? Acta Ophthalmol (Copenh) 1990;68(6):661–668.

22. Sommer A. Keratoconus in contact lens wear. Am J Ophthalmol 1978;86(3):442–444.

23. Edwards M, McGhee CN, Dean S. The genetics of keratoconus. Clin Exp Ophthalmol 2001;29(6):345–351.

24. Tuori AJ, Virtanen I, Aine E, et al. The immunohistochemical composition of corneal basement membrane in keratoconus. Curr Eye Res 1997;16(8):792–801.

25. Sawaguchi S, Fukuchi T, Abe H, et al. Three-dimensional scanning electron microscopic study of keratoconus corneas. Arch Ophthalmol 1998;116(1):62–68.

26. Zhou L, Sugar J, Yue BYJT. Normal lysosomal enzyme staining in skin tissues of patients with keratoconus. Cornea 1996;15:409–413.

27. Rehany U, Lahav M, Shoshan S. Collagenolytic activity in keratoconus. Ann Ophthalmol 1982;14:751.

28. Critchfield JW, Calandra AJ, Nesburn AB, et al. Keratoconus: I. Biochemical studies. Exp Eye Res 1988;46:953–963.

29. Pouliquen Y, Graf B, de KY, et al. Morphological study of keratoconus. Arch Ophtalmol Rev Gen Ophtalmol 1970;30:497–532.

30. Polack FM. Contributions of electron microscopy to the study of corneal pathology. Surv Ophthalmol 1976;20:375–414.

31. Kemp EG, Lewis CJ. Immunoglobin pattern in keratoconus with particular reference to total and specific IgE levels. Br J Ophthalmol 1982;66(11):717–720.

32. Zadnik K, Barr JT, Edrington TB, et al. Baseline findings in the Collaborative Longitudinal Evaluation of Keratoconus (CLEK) study. Invest Ophthalmol Vis Sci 1998;39(13):2537–2546.

33. Ridley F. Eye rubbing and contact lenses. Br J Ophthalmol 1961:631.

34. Kenney MC, Brown DJ, Rajeev B. The elusive causes of keratoconus: a working hypothesis. CLAO J 2000;26(1):10–13.

35. Kenney MC, Brown DJ. The cascade hypothesis of keratoconus. Contact Lens Anterior Eye 2003;26:139–146.

36. van der Worp E. Keratoconus: what do we know? Contact Lens Spectrum 2007;22(10).

37. Owens H, Gamble G. A profile of keratoconus in New Zealand. Cornea 2003;22(2):122–125.

38. Wang Y, Rabinowitz YS, Rotter JI, et al. Genetic epidemiological study of keratoconus: evidence for major gene determination. Am J Med Genet 2000;93(5):403–409.

39. Assiri AA, Yousuf BI, Quantock AJ, et al. Incidence and severity of keratoconus in Asir province, Saudi Arabia. Br J Ophthalmol 2005;89(11):1403–1406.

40. Lee LR, Readshaw G, Hirst LW. Keratoconus: the clinical experience of a Brisbane ophthalmologist. Ophthalmic Epidemiol 1996;3(3):119–125.

41. Rabinowitz YS, Garbus J, McDonnell PJ. Computer-assisted corneal topography in family members of patients with keratoconus. Arch Ophthalmol 1990;108(3):365–371.

42. Al-Swailem SA, Al-Assiri AA, Al-Torbak AA. Woodhouse Sakati syndrome associated with bilateral keratoconus. Br J Ophthalmol 2006;90(1):116–117.

43. Shapiro MB, France TD. The ocular features of Down's syndrome. Am J Ophthalmol 1985;99(6):659–663.

44. Steahly LP. Keratoconus following contact lens wear. Ann Ophthalmol 1978;10:1177–1179.

45. Hartstein J. Keratoconus that developed in patients wearing corneal contact lenses. Arch Ophthalmol 1968;80:345–396.

46. Macsai MS, Varley GA, Krachmer JH. Development of keratoconus after contact lens wear. Arch Ophthalmol 1990;108:435–538.

47. Szczotka L. PMMA lens wear: a probable cause of keratoconus. Contact Lens Spectrum. November 1999. http://www.clspectrum.com/article. aspx?article=11727. Accessed December 27, 2007.

48. Bennett ES. Keratoconus. In: Bennett ES, Grohe RM, eds. Rigid Gas-Permeable Contact Lenses. New York: Professional Press, 1986:297–344.

49. Caroline PJ, Doughman DJ, McGuire JR. A new contact lens design for keratoconus: a continuing report. Contact Lens J 1978;12(1):17–20.

50. Perry HD, Buxton JN, Fine BS. Round and oval cones in keratoconus. Am Acad Ophthalmol 1980;87(9):905–909.

51. Fiol-Silva Z, Siviglia D. Keratoconus: fitting and managing. Ophthalmol Clin North Am 1989;2(2):291–297.

52. McMahon TT. Topography guided fitting of contact lenses in keratoconus. Presented at the Global Keratoconus Congress, Las Vegas, NV, January 2008.
53. McMahon TT. Collaborative longitudinal evaluation of keratoconus update. Presented at the Annual Meeting of the American Academy of Optometry, Denver, CO, December 2006.
54. Probst LE. Case 13: LASIK with forme fruste keratoconus. In: Machat JL, Slade SG, Probst LE, eds. The Art of Lasik. Thorofare, NJ: SLACK Inc., 1999:504–505.
55. Caroline PJ, Andre MP. Help for screening abnormal corneal topographies. Contact Lens Spectrum 1998; 13(12):56.
56. Klyce SD. Corneal topography in refractive keratectomy. In: Thompson FB, McDonnell PJ, eds. Color Atlas/Text of Excimer Laser Surgery: The Cornea. New York: Igaku-Shoin Medical Publishers, 1993:19–36.
57. Wilson SE, Klyce SD, Husseini ZM. Standardized color-coded maps for corneal topography. Ophthalmol 1993;100: 1723–1727.
58. Wilson SD, Klyce SD. Screening for cornea topographic abnormalities before refractive surgery. Ophthalmol 1994;101:147–152.
59. Nesburn AB, Bahri S, Berlin M, et al. Computer-assisted corneal topography (CACT) to detect mild keratoconus in candidates for photorefractive keratectomy. Invest Ophthalmol Vis Sci 1995;33/4(suppl):995.
60. Mandell RB, Chiang CS, Yee L. Asymmetric corneal toricity and pseudokeratoconus in videokeratography. J Am Optom Assoc 1996;67(9):540–547.
61. Rabinowitz YS, McDonnell PJ. Computer-assisted corneal topography in keratoconus. Refract Corneal Surg 1989;5:400.
62. Rabinowitz YS, Rasheed K. KISA% index: a quantitative videokeratography algorithm embodying minimal topographic criteria for diagnosing keratoconus. J Cat Refract Surg 1999;25:1327–1135.
63. Li X, Rabinowitz YS, Rasheed K, et al. Longitudinal study of the normal eyes in unilateral keratoconus patients. Ophthalmol 2004;111:440–446.
64. Davis LJ, Barr JT, VanOtteren D. Transient rigid lens induced striae in keratoconus. Optom Vis Sci 1993;70(3): 216–219.
65. Zadnik Z, Burger DS. Keratoconus. In: Bennett ES, Weissman BA, eds. Clinical Contact Lens Practice. Philadelphia: JB Lippincott, 1995:45-1–45-11.
66. Reinke AR. Keratoconus: a review of research and current fitting techniques. Part 1. Int Contact Lens Clin 1975;2(3):66–80.
67. Barr JT, Schectman KB, Fink BA, et al. Corneal scarring in the Collaborative Longitudinal Evaluation of Keratoconus (CLEK) Study: baseline prevalence and repeatability of detection. Cornea 1999;18(1):34–45.
68. Rizzuti AB. Diagnostic illumination test for keratoconus. Am J Ophthalmol 1970;70:141.
69. Shovlin JP, DePaolis MD, Kame RT. Contact lens-induced corneal warpage syndrome. Contact Lens Forum 1986;11(8):32–36.
70. Davis LJ. Keratoconus: current understanding of diagnosis and management. Clin Eye Vis Care 1997;9:13–22.
71. Maguire LJ, Klyce SD, McDonald ME, et al. Corneal topography of pellucid marginal degeneration. Ophthalmol 1987;94:519–524.
72. McMahon TT, Szczotka-Flynn L, Barr JT, et al. A new method for grading the severity of keratoconus: the Keratoconus Severity Score (KSS). Cornea 2006;25(7):794–800.
73. Zadnik K, Barr JT, Gordon MO, et al. Biomicroscopic signs and disease severity in keratoconus. Collaborative Longitudinal Evaluation of Keratoconus (CLEK) Study Group. Cornea 1996;15:139–146.
74. Gobbe M, Guillon M. Corneal wavefront aberration measurements to detect keratoconus patients. Contact Lens Anterior Eye 2005;28:57–66.
75. McMahon TT, Edrington TB, Szczotka-Flynn L, et al. Longitudinal changes in corneal curvature in keratoconus. Cornea 2006;25(3):296–305.
76. Feder RS, Kshettry P. Noninflammatory ectatic disorders. In: Krachmer JH, Mannis MJ, Holland EJ, eds. Cornea, 2nd ed. St. Louis: Mosby, 2005:955.
77. Cooke CA, Cooper C, Dowds E, et al. Keratoconus, myopia, and personality. Cornea 2003;22:239–242.
78. Giedd KK, Mannis MJ, Mitchell GL, et al. Personality in keratoconus in a sample of patients derived from the internet. Cornea 2005;24:301–307.
79. Mannis MJ, Morrison TL, Zadnik K, et al. Personality trends in keratoconus. An analysis. Arch Ophthalmol 1987;105:798–800.
80. Vitale S. CLEK study reports on the quality of life. Am J Ophthalmol 2004;138:637–638.
81. Kymes SM, Walline JJ, Zadnik K, et al. Quality of life in keratoconus. Am J Ophthalmol 2004;138:527–535.
82. Kymes S, Walline J, Zadnik K, et al. Changes in the quality of life of people with keratoconus. Am J Ophthalmol 2008;145:611–617.
83. Zadnik K, Gordon MO, Barr JT, et al, the CLEK Study Group. Biomicroscopic signs and disease severity in keratoconus. Cornea 1996;15:139–146.
84. Lass JH, Lembach RG, Park SB, et al. Clinical management of keratoconus: a multicenter analysis. Ophthalmol 1990;97:433–455.
85. Griffiths M, Zahner K, Collins M, et al. Masking of irregular corneal topography with contact lenses. CLAO J 1998;2492:76–81.

86. Carney LG. Contact lens correction of visual loss in keratoconus. Acta Ophthalmol 1982;60(5):795–802.

87. Korb DR, Finnemore VM, Herman JP. Apical changes and scarring in keratoconus as related to contact lens fitting techniques. J Am Optom Assoc 1982;53:199–205.

88. Soper JW, Jarrett HA. Results of a systemic approach to fitting keratoconus and corneal transplants. Contact Lens Med Bull 1972;5:50.

89. Ruben M. Treatment of keratoconus. Aust J Optom 1979;62(4):152–157.

90. Gundel RE, Libassi DP, Zadnik K, et al. Feasibility of fitting contact lenses with apical clearance in keratoconus. Optom Vis Sci 1996;73(12):729–732.

91. Gas Permeable Lens Institute. Available online at http://www.gpli.info. Accessed July 15, 2008.

92. Bennett ES. A common sense approach to fitting keratoconus with RGP lenses. Optom Today 1997;5(3):25–27.

93. Edrington TB, Szczotka LB, Begley CG, et al. Repeatability of two corneal curvature assessments in keratoconus: keratometry and the first definite apical clearance lens. Presented at the Annual Meeting of the American Academy of Optometry, San Antonio, TX, December 1997.

94. Weissman B, Chun MW, Barnhart LA. Corneal abrasion associated with contact lens correction of keratoconus- A retrospective study. Optom Vis Sci 1994;71(11):677–681.

95. Mannis MJ, Zadnik K. Contact lens fitting in keratoconus. CLAO J 1989;15:282–289.

96. Burger D. Contact lens alternatives for keratoconus: an overview. Contact Lens Spectrum 1993;8:49–55.

97. Caroline PJ, Norman C, Andre M. The latest lens design for keratoconus. Contact Lens Spectrum 1997; 12(8):36–41.

98. Edrington TB, Szczotka LB, Barr JT, et al. Rigid contact lens fitting relationships in keratoconus. Optom Vis Sci 1999;76:692–699.

99. Henry VA. Irregular cornea. In: Bennett ES, Henry VA, eds. Clinical Manual of Contact Lenses. Philadelphia: JB Lippincott, 1995:438–453.

100. Connelly S, Broe D. Comfort for the keratoconus patient: a comparison of lens designs. Contact Lens Spectrum 1999;14(5):42–44.

101. Miller B. Systematic application of toric contact lenses for high astigmatism – aspheric and asymmetric decentered lenses for advanced keratoconus. Contactologia (German) 1994;16(1):13–18.

102. Neumann S. Improving the fit and visual acuity by using bitoric keratoconic lenses. Presented at the Global Keratoconus Congress, Las Vegas, NV, January 2007.

103. Pullum KW, Buckley RJ. A study of 530 patients referred for rigid gas permeable scleral contact lens assessment. Cornea 1997;16(6):612–622.

104. Zadnik K. Meet the challenge of fitting the irregular cornea. Rev Optom 1994;131(4):77–83.

105. Young K, Eghbali F, Weissman BA. Clinical experience with piggyback contact lens systems on keratoconic eyes. J Am Optom Assoc 1995;66(9):539–543.

106. Caroline PJ, Doughman DJ. A new piggyback lens design for correction of irregular astigmatism: a preliminary report. Contact Lens J 1979;13:39–42.

107. Caroline PJ, Andre M. Custom soft contact lenses. Contact Lens Spectrum 1998;13(4).

108. Maguen E, Caroline PJ, Rosmer IR, et al. The use of the SoftPerm lens for the correction of irregular astigmatism. CLAO J 1992;18(3):173–176.

109. Maguen E, Martinez M, Rosner I, et al. The use of Saturn II lenses in keratoconus. CLAO J 1991;17(1):41–43.

110. Eye Banking Statistical Report. Washington, DC: America EBAo, 2006.

111. Eggink FAGJ, Pinckers AJLG, Van Puyenbroek EP, et al. Keratoconus, a retrospective study. Contact Lens J 1988;16:204.

112. Sayegh FN, Ehlers N, Farah I. Evaluation of penetrating keratoplasty in keratoconus. Nine years follow-up. Acta Ophthalmol 1988;66:400.

113. Smiddy WE, Hamburg TR, Kracher GP, et al. Keratoconus: contact lens or keratoplasty? Ophthalmol 1988;95:487.

114. Gordon MO, Steger-May K, Szczotka-Flynn L, et al. Baseline factors predictive of incident penetrating keratoplasty in keratoconus. Am J Ophthalmol 2006;142(6):923–930.

115. Boruchoff SA, Jensen AD, Dohlman CH. Comparison of suturing techniques in keratoplasty for keratoconus. Ann Ophthalmol 1975;7:433–436.

116. Martin WRJ, Smith EL. Some points in the surgical technique of keratoplasty. Am J Ophthalmol 1963;55: 1199–1208.

117. Crews MJ, Driebe WT, Stern GA. The clinical management of keratoconus: a 6 year retrospective study. CLAO J 1994;20(3):194–197.

118. Kastl PR. A 20-year retrospective study of the use of contact lenses in keratoconus. CLAO J 1987;13:102.

119. Belin MW, Fowler WG, Chambers WA. Keratoconus: evaluation of recent trends in the surgical and nonsurgical correction of keratoconus. Ophthalmol 1988;95:335.

120. Spoerl E. Biomechanical effect of combined riboflavin-ultraviolet A (UVA) treatment for keratoconus. Paper presented at the Global Keratoconus Congress, Las Vegas, NV, January 2007.

121. Spoerl E, Huhle M, Seiler T. Induction of cross-links in corneal tissue. Exp Eye Res 1998;66:97–103.

122. Wollensak G, Spoerl E, Seiler T. Riboflavin/ultraviolet-A-induced collagen crosslinking for the treatment of keratoconus. Am J Ophthalmol 2003;135(5):620–627.

CHAPTER 19

Postsurgical Contact Lens Fitting

Michael DePaolis, Joseph Shovlin, Julie Ott DeKinder, and Christine Sindt

One of the most challenging and rewarding aspects of contact lens practice involves the postsurgical fit. In each case, the clinician is faced with a complex ocular surface, one in which both structure and function have been altered. As the patient's contact lens needs are more therapeutic than cosmetic, and as there are few definitive prescribing guidelines, clinicians must be cautious, creative, and conservative. Although the fitting process can be an arduous one, patient gratification is often well worth it.

In this chapter, we will address the most common reasons for postoperative contact lens fitting, including penetrating keratoplasty (PK), radial keratotomy (RK), photorefractive keratectomy (PRK), laser-assisted in situ keratomileusis (LASIK), laser epithelial keratomileusis (LASEK), intrastromal ring segments (Intacs), and ocular trauma. For each application, we will discuss the rationale for perioperative and postoperative contact lens use. We will also review the topographic and physiologic challenges and the recommended fitting philosophies given these limitations. Finally, additional surgical options, should the patient prove to be contact lens intolerant, will be briefly discussed.

■ PENETRATING KERATOPLASTY

Full-thickness PK remains the surgical procedure of choice for many corneal conditions. In 2006, 33,962 PKs were performed in the United States, which was an increase from the 31,952 preformed the previous year.[1] PKs are performed regularly for a variety of reasons, including keratoconus, Fuch corneal dystrophy, pseudophakic bullous keratopathy, and herpes simplex stromal leukoma. A 20-year retrospective study determined that the most common indication for PK was aphakic/pseudophakic bullous keratopathy, followed by keratoconus and corneal scars.[2] Through the development of improved tissue typing and harvesting, microsurgical techniques, and postsurgical immunomodulating therapeutics, PK has become a very safe and efficacious procedure. Unfortunately, as we are introducing a different donor cornea to the recipient bed, component ametropia often results, which can be quite varied from the fellow eye, with resultant anisometropia. Furthermore, as graft–host junction wound healing occurs in a radially variable fashion, irregular astigmatism often prevails. Given these scenarios, an otherwise successful surgical endeavor can be obscured by a poor outcome with traditional spectacle correction.

Contact Lens Rationale

Over time, several methods have been tried to treat postkeratoplasty irregular astigmatism. These include wedge resections, relaxing incisions,[3] customized laser ablation,[4] laser in situ keratomileusis,[5] and photorefractive keratectomy.[6] In consideration of the latter three surgical procedures, LASIK has become the surgical method of choice, but it, like the other two, is still plagued with unintentional complications such as undercorrection or overcorrection, haze, and possible rejection of the graft,[7] leaving contact lenses as the most logical solution. A retrospective chart review of patients who had LASIK following PK showed 3-month follow-up results of 20/60 or better in all eyes; however, only one eye was reported to have achieved 20/20 vision. The success rate was significant in myopic eyes, but not in hyperopic eyes.[8] Corneal contact lenses in general, and rigid gas permeable (GP) lenses in particular, are well recognized for their ability to compensate for anisometropia and irregular astigmatism. In the case of unilateral PK, the patient may prefer an ipsilateral contact lens in which the prescription is balanced with the contralateral spectacle-wearing eye. In the case of bilateral PK, particularly when significant astigmatism is involved, the patient may prefer a bilateral contact lens correction. In addition to their role in long-term ametropia management, contact lenses are often used after PK for bandage purposes. In certain PK procedures, the graft is slow to reepithelialize, often requiring more than the traditional 1-week period of time. For these individuals, a bandage contact lens often provides protection to the sliding epithelium. The most prudent approach involves a hydrophilic bandage lens worn on an extended wear basis until epithelial closure occurs. As this is often a critical time from a graft rejection and infectious keratitis perspective, patients must receive concomitant topical antibiotic and steroid therapeusis. Additionally, the patient must be closely monitored on a 24- to 48-hour basis. Another reason for a hydrophilic bandage lens during the perioperative period involves the use of interrupted sutures in which the knots are not buried. Many surgeons attempt to modulate postsurgical astigmatism through the use of a continuous suture in conjunction with 6 to 12 interrupted sutures. While the continuous suture may remain in place for 12 months or longer, interrupted sutures are often removed as early as 8 weeks after surgery. Until their removal, however, the interrupted sutures can cause a significant foreign body sensation as well as papillary conjunctivitis. In these cases, a hydrophilic bandage lens can significantly reduce suture awareness and progression of papillary conjunctivitis. The bandage lens is often left in place for up to a week at a time, and ultimately discontinued when the interrupted sutures are removed. In both of these applications, disposable lenses have demonstrated good clinical efficacy.[9] Disposable lenses offer significant benefits over more time-honored conventional hydrophilic bandage lenses. Moreover, disposable silicone hydrogel lenses offer the greatest benefits. Silicone hydrogel disposable lenses lend greater oxygen transmissibility than disposable hydrophilic lenses and have become the modality of choice in PK patients. The primary advantage of a disposable bandage lens is that of preventing the immunogenic, toxic, and mechanical sequelae of a spoiled contact lens. As the perioperative PK eye is often inflamed and requires numerous topical agents, bandage lens spoilage is quite common. When using a disposable bandage lens, the patient has the opportunity of discarding the lens on a weekly basis. Another advantage of disposable bandage lenses involves ease of replacement. During the perioperative phase, PK patients can inadvertently dislodge the bandage lens with their eye drops or while sleeping, and frequent replacement of a conventional lens can be quite cost prohibitive relative to a disposable lens. Silicone hydrogel disposable contact lenses have obvious advantages over hydrophilic disposable lenses as extended wear bandages. Hydrophilic disposable contact lenses, when worn as extended wear bandages, must be monitored for relative corneal hypoxia because of their relative low oxygen permeability (Dk) value. Limiting corneal hypoxia is especially important during the perioperative phase when contact lens-related edema can either mimic or exacerbate graft rejection. Disposable lenses have essentially rendered conventional lenses obsolete; the one exception may be when extreme curvature changes are necessary or when a very large lens (15–20 mm) is necessary (i.e., for healing an associated leaking bleb). Custom hydrogel and, more recently, custom silicone hydrogel lenses offer good comfort, reproducibility, and quality for the management of challenging irregular cornea patients.

Special Considerations

As is true of any surgically altered cornea, the PK patient presents with a variety of special considerations and relative contraindications to contact lens wear. These alterations can affect both structure and function. Structural changes most often involve topographic alterations, whereas functional changes pertain to adverse physiologic sequelae.

The topographic alterations associated with PK can be profound. First and foremost is the fact that a donor cornea, often of significantly different curvature, is placed in the recipient bed. The actual apposition between host and recipient often alters the cornea's natural asphericity. The overall resulting curvature is further influenced by surgical technique and wound healing. Most PK surgeons attempt to trephinate a recipient bed, which is slightly smaller than the donor button. In doing so, the surgeon is able to ensure good wound coaptation (i.e., alignment and adhesion of the wound), maintain adequate anterior chamber depth, avoid peripheral anterior synechiae, and reduce the risk of postoperative glaucoma. However, if the recipient bed is too small or the donor button too large, a "proud" or very steep topography results. In the opposite scenario, one in which the donor button is too small for the recipient bed, the patient may encounter poor wound coaptation, a shallow chamber with peripheral synechiae, and increased risk of glaucoma. As a result of the donor cornea being drawn across the recipient bed, the topography is often "plateaued" or oblate. Either an excessively steep or flat cornea can be further complicated by graft "tilt." It is extremely important to qualitatively assess topographic morphology as this often influences the initial lens design selection.

In addition to the topographic morphologic changes associated with penetrating keratoplasty, the contact lens clinician must also manage a significant amount of astigmatism. It is not uncommon for the post-PK patient to manifest 5 D or more of astigmatism.[10] Although varying suturing technique and removal strategies can assist in reducing the probability of increased amounts of astigmatism, the surgeon is still at the mercy of individual wound healing. Furthermore, the astigmatism is often complicated by an irregular presentation. In fact, it is prudent to view the post-PK steep corneal meridian as two hemi-meridians that are not always orthogonal to the flat meridian.

The physiologic alterations associated with PK are numerous. Although many improvements have been made in tissue harvesting, transportation, and transplantation, the endothelium is still prone to cell loss. Given the fact that a viable endothelium is necessary to avoid graft rejection and expiration, it is especially important that the contact lens does not exacerbate polymegethism. Although the donor epithelium is entirely replaced by recipient epithelium within the first month, it is imperative that this tissue is protected throughout the graft's life. Poorly fit contact lenses that result in chronic epithelial edema, superficial punctate keratitis, or corneal abrasion can ultimately precipitate epithelial graft rejection.[11] Microcystic edema may be present, however, which is entirely independent of contact lens wear. Contraindications to fitting contact lenses include epithelial defects, inflammation, corneal edema, and loose sutures.[7] Additionally, many PK patients manifest some degree of corneal neovascularization that may be because of the preexisting corneal condition or a result of a volatile postoperative course. Regardless of its cause, corneal neovascularization must be held in check when prescribing contact lenses. A poorly fit contact lens can result in inflammation and progression of corneal neovascularization. Another aspect of PK surgery is the total hypoesthesia that ensues. Although some reinnervation occurs after PK, it rarely does so completely. As a result, the PK patient experiences decreased corneal sensitivity and an iatrogenic keratitis sicca.[12] Of course, contact lenses can aggravate the already dry eye, which, in turn, can limit contact lens wear.

Contact Lens Options

In light of the aforementioned alterations in corneal structure and function, it is understandable why contact lens fitting can be such a challenge. Contact lenses can be prescribed for visual restoration as early as 3 months post-PK on clear grafts.[13] The course of suture removal is highly dependent on the individual surgeon, but the presence of sutures should not be a contraindication to contact lens fitting. While a suture may complicate corneal topography, a contact lens fit can be highly successful, without increased risk of complications.

Gas Permeable Contact Lenses

GP lenses are the most frequently prescribed contact lenses after PK, largely because of their ability to mask significant irregular astigmatism as well as to provide for an excellent physiologic response. However, given the often unusual post-PK topography, achieving an adequate fit can be difficult (Fig. 19.1).

Lens Materials: The excellent oxygen transmission, good surface characteristics, and flexure resistance of most fluoro-silicone/acrylate (F-S/A) lens materials make this category a reasonable choice for post-PK fitting. An ultrathin, hyper Dk material is a reasonable option when considering maximum oxygen transmissibility; however, the highly flexible nature of this material still places it as a second choice behind lower Dk F-S/A materials.

Overall Diameter: The concept of a small diameter (7.0–8.0 mm) GP fit within the graft–host junction has been abandoned in recent years as poor comfort, inconsistent positioning, and easy displacement often prevails. Today's post-PK GP lenses are often 9.5 to 12.0 mm in diameter. In addition, several mini-scleral and semi-scleral designs have been introduced with diameters often in the 13.5- to 19-mm range. This larger diameter philosophy provides for better centration and stability, even in those patients manifesting unusual topographies or graft tilt. Of course, larger diameters often require nontraditional optical zone and peripheral curve relationships.

Optical Zone Diameter: GP optical zone diameters should be as large as possible to facilitate centration and minimize glare, but not so large as to result in harsh bearing, minimal movement, or lens adherence. In those situations, in which a large diameter (>10.5 mm) is necessary for lens centration and stability, a disproportionately small (<8.5 mm) optical zone diameter may be necessary to mitigate against a steep sagitta with attending tear stagnation.

Base Curve Radius: A reasonable starting point for post-PK GP fitting is to select a base curve radius that straddles the keratometric measurements.[14] Fluorescein evaluation is employed to refine the base curve radius to achieve a divided support fit. In recent years, corneal topography has been recommended as an alternate means for base curve radius selection. In this approach, the contact lens clinician selects the base curve radius based on the average dioptric

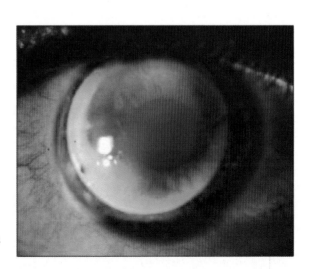

■ **FIGURE 19.1** Well-fitting gas permeable lens after penetrating keratoplasty.

value at approximately 3 mm from the topography map's center.[15] When using this approach, it is prudent to select the dioptric value from sagittal maps. While spherical base curve radius GP lenses are still used in post-PK fitting, back surface low aspheric lenses represent the majority of designs in use today in those patients with atypical topographies. The back surface aspheric geometry provides for a smoother transition from lens center to edge, resulting in a more even fluorescein pattern. On rare occasions, a bitoric GP design is indicated. This design is usually reserved for those patients with significant amounts of regular astigmatism where the astigmatism is on the host as well as the graft, and for whom spherical or aspheric designs prove inadequate. Of course, the caveat for prescribing a bitoric is that the astigmatism must be regular and symmetric. If corneal topography reveals major meridians that are not orthogonal, a back surface toric is contraindicated. Likewise, a bitoric lens will not remain stable if the periphery of the lens does not land on a toric peripheral cornea. Therefore, in these cases, a nontoric base curve with a toric periphery should be considered.

Peripheral Curve Systems: There is no consistent relationship between lens base curve radius and peripheral curves in post-PK fitting. In most patients, peripheral curve radii and widths are secondary to overall diameter, optical zone diameter, and base curve radius in facilitating lens centration and movement. Occasionally, a very large diameter lens may result in peripheral lens binding, in which case a series of flatter and wider peripheral curves is warranted. Conversely, in a proud graft or plateau-type graft, a traditional peripheral curve system might result in excessive edge lift. In these cases, a bicurve (base curve and one peripheral curve) or even reverse geometry (secondary curve steeper than base curve) may be necessary. Fortunately, many GP laboratories have the ability to fabricate nontraditional peripheral curve systems.

Lens Thickness: Consistent with our goals of maximizing oxygen transmission and minimizing lens mass, it is recommended to select the thinnest design possible. However, given the unusual topography and significant astigmatism associated with PK, clinicians must balance thinness with flexure and adherence resistance.

Fitting: Corneal topography systems can aid in lens fitting. The newer topographers have been shown to evaluate a large enough area of the cornea for better visualization of the corneal shape.[16] By analyzing the topography results, initial lens selection can be limited to only those designs that will seem most compatible with the corneal shape.

If the steepest area of the graft is inferior, a minus carrier lenticular or flatter posterior lens curvature may need to be incorporated into the lens design to aid in a lid attachment fit, as well as alignment in the flatter superior cornea. If the steep area of the graft is either nasal or temporal, a relatively successful option for lens stability is a larger overall diameter. A large overall diameter will aid in lens centration and pupillary coverage. Finally, if the steepest part of the graft is superior, increasing the mass of the lens with a prism ballast, high specific gravity lens, and/or a nonlenticular design can improve lens centration.[17] The authors have had good success with an intralimbal design in PK fitting (Fig. 19.2).

Although GPs provide excellent astigmatism correction and physiologic response, occasionally, lens instability or intolerance will prevail. In this situation, the patient might be best served with a soft or hybrid contact lens.

Soft Contact Lenses

Although used less frequently, soft contact lenses (SCLs) offer certain distinct advantages. In those situations in which the patient manifests an atypical corneal topography or graft tilt, an SCL often provides much improved contact lens stability and comfort. Unfortunately, these patients can also manifest a significant amount of astigmatism, thereby necessitating spectacle overcorrection. Additionally, PK patients wearing SCLs must be more carefully monitored for corneal edema, neovascularization, infiltrates, and papillary conjunctivitis.

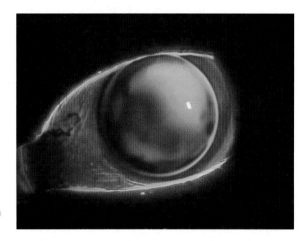

■ **FIGURE 19.2** An intralimbal lens design on a postpenetrating keratoplasty patient.

Lens Materials: As is often the case in postsurgical contact lens endeavors, the clinician must balance oxygen transmission with acceptable surface characteristics. Over the past several years, silicone hydrogel lenses have shown good efficacy and safety as therapeutic lenses,[18–20] and several have Food and Drug Administration (FDA) therapeutic approval. Bandage contact lenses are frequently used to splint compromised corneas. Oxygen is required to create the energy necessary for cellular division, synthesis of proteins and lipids, maintenance of pH/osmotic balance, and general repair. Irregular corneas can be extremely difficult to fit with silicone hydrogel lenses because of extreme curvature changes. Excessive movement, edge standoff, and fluting are common. Low oxygen transmission may stress an already compromised endothelium, whereas excessive movement may insult fragile or damaged epithelium. Silicone hydrogel made-to-order (MTO) lenses are customizable to both the fit and power needs of the patient, as well as maintaining a higher level of oxygen transmission.

Bandage contact lenses are frequently worn overnight during the healing process (see Chapter 11). Silicone hydrogel MTO lenses are currently only FDA approved for daily wear; prescribing overnight wear would be considered an off-label use. In some cases, overnight wear is unavoidable, such as in bullous keratopathy and other critical/sight-threatening diseases.[18–20] Some corneas have a higher than average requirement for oxygen. In these patients, extended wear with silicone hydrogel lenses may have a potentially irreversible effect on corneal homeostasis. The doctor should consider the risks and benefits, and discuss the off-label use with the patient, before sending the patient out with extended wear silicone hydrogel MTO lenses.

Silicone hydrogel lenses have a stiffer modulus of rigidity. Unlike thin disposable hydrogel lenses, these stiffer lenses are more significantly affected by base curve, corneal diameter, peripheral asphericity, and overall sagittal height of the cornea. Surprisingly, however, many high plus or high minus patients switching from custom HEMA designs complain of increased floppiness with subsequent difficulty in handling the custom silicone hydrogel lenses.

While stock silicone hydrogel lenses are designed to fit the majority of patients, similar to the empirical fitting of disposable hydrogel lenses, silicone hydrogel MTO lenses are best fit through trial lenses to achieve optimal fitting characteristics and power determination. Complications, ranging from discomfort to superior arcuate lesion and giant papillary conjunctivitis, may be related to less than ideal fits.[21] It is critical to select the appropriate diameter and base curve to ensure alignment to the cornea, especially in higher-power lenses, which tend to have even less flexibility. The base curve is selected after the diameter, since diameter will affect the overall sagittal depth of the contact lens. Flat lenses may not drape well on the cornea and can result in edge standoff and edge fluting. A steeper lens will typically be more comfortable; however, it may result in fluctuating vision if there is too much vault.

The lens should settle for a minimum of 10 minutes on the cornea to allow for osmotic equilibrium. Some patients may report mild lens awareness because of the stiff modulus of the lens.

This awareness is normal and generally quickly recedes. If the discomfort persists, it is important to check to make sure the lens is not inverted. The patient will also complain of discomfort if the lens is too flat and moves excessively; consider a larger, steeper lens in this case.

The lens is evaluated for corneal coverage and lens movement. The lens should exhibit 0.2- to 0.3-mm movement and have good limbal coverage in all gazes. A silicone hydrogel lens should be fit slightly loose, compared to some HEMA-based lenses, to allow for tear exchange behind the lens. A tight lens will exhibit decreased tear exchange. Retention of debris, cells, and microorganisms has been implicated in the development of inflammatory and infectious adverse events.[22]

If the sagittal depth of the cornea (caused by either an unusual corneal diameter, large or small or a steep or flat base curve) does not match the sagittal depth of the lens, the edge of the lens will produce a gap. If a gap, or "fluting," is present, the lens should not be dispensed since the lens will be uncomfortable because of lens edge awareness. In higher powers, a gap may induce cylinder across the entire lens, which will result in inadequate vision and challenging overrefractions.

Initial powers may be based on the patient's vertexed spectacle prescription or the current HEMA contact lens. A slight modification in prescription after the patient wears the lens is expected. Silicone hydrogel MTO lenses have aspheric optics and are also affected by a lacrimal lens power; therefore, do not assume the patient's current contact lens power will be optimal for a silicone hydrogel MTO lens. The power requirement for a silicone hydrogel MTO lens may be −0.25 to −0.50 D higher for myopic prescriptions and +0.25 to +0.50 D less for hyperopic prescriptions than the patient's current contact lens power.

Lens Design: Although clinicians have previously embraced the concept of prescribing standard thickness lenses to mask corneal astigmatism, there is very little evidence of this being practiced today with the advent of disposable lenses with high oxygen permeability (silicone hydrogels). Therefore, a thinner, more oxygen permeable design with adjunct spectacle overcorrection is preferable.

Certain PK patients may benefit from a toric SCL. This is acceptable if the patient achieves reasonable vision with a standard refraction, and does not manifest irregular astigmatism. A diagnostic lens fitting, overretinoscopy, and subjective overrefraction are mandatory to identify those patients who are destined to fail with this option. There are several silicone hydrogel toric lenses available today, including silicone hydrogel MTO lenses, with MTO toric lenses to be introduced in the very near future.

Piggyback Lenses

When a GP or SCL lens alone does not suffice, a combination of the two may be indicated. The concept of "piggybacking" a GP over an SCL has long been recognized as a niche application in specialty contact lens fitting. In this approach, an SCL is used for surface smoothing while the GP provides visual restoration.

Lens Materials: The potential for hypoxia is significant when one considers the oxygen transmissibility limitations of each material as well as the barrier effect. Therefore, high Dk materials should be routinely prescribed. This would include a silicone hydrogel soft lens and a hyper Dk GP lens material. During lens adaptation, the clinician must monitor corneal health and adjust wearing time accordingly.

Lens Design: SCL selection should be governed by each patient's prescription and topography. Piggybacking is an area where silicone hydrogels have substantial benefits, since a double lens system further reduces the oxygen flux to the cornea. However, daily disposable lenses offer substantial convenience and cleanliness. The power of the piggyback contact lens can be used to alter the fit of the GP lens. A plus lens will "steepen" the base curve of the eye. This creates a more prolate surface and is beneficial for a postsurgical/oblate cornea where centration of a GP lens may be difficult. Patients who manifest a "sunken" or plateau graft are best served by a moderate plus lens, thus addressing the anticipated need for hyperopic correction and providing an apex on which to center the GP. It can also be used with an existing GP fit to create a flatter lens-to-surface relationship, thereby "loosening" the GP lens. This is particularly beneficial in cases of a "proud" or steep graft. A myopic prescription will create a less prolate surface, useful, for example, on keratoconic patients, who are highly prolate. It will also "steepen" the lens-to-cornea relationship, effectively creating a "tighter" fit. In either of these situations, the value of incorporating a portion of the refractive power into the SCL lessens the thickness of the overlying GP.

The underlying SCL should be fit to center well and demonstrate optimal to excessive movement. Excessive movement is critical, as the GP will inevitably lessen SCL movement. Once a satisfactory SCL fit is obtained, over-keratometry is performed and serves as a starting point for GP selection. Averaging flat and steep keratometry is a good starting point for base curve radius selection or using the best fit sphere from the topographer. Final base curve radius, overall diameter, optical zone diameter, peripheral curve radii and widths, and power are determined by diagnostic fitting. High molecular weight sodium fluoride can be used to assess the GP–SCL relationship. The clinician should be careful to avoid a tightly fit GP, as this often traps interfacial debris. In the case where the GP is fit before piggybacking, an SCL can be added to increase lens comfort and wearing time or incorporate small refractive changes. It is imperative that the GP–SCL relationship remain as described above in both fitting scenarios.

It is generally accepted that any complication that occurs with either an SCL or a GP can develop with a piggyback combination. This is not entirely true, as GP peripheral corneal staining does not occur with piggyback combinations. However, papillary conjunctivitis, corneal edema, neovascularization, lens adherence, acute red eye, infiltrates, infection, and graft rejection can result from piggyback lens applications.

An SCL specifically designed for piggyback applications has been available for several years. Marketed as Flexlens Piggyback Lens (X-Cel Contacts), this midwater SCL lens has a partial thickness insert cut out of the center. The Flexlens concept allows for the GP to be fit within the "cut-out," thereby facilitating centration. However, this lens has a low oxygen permeability, increasing the likelihood for corneal edema to occur, which should be taken into consideration before fitting.

Hybrid Lenses

A relatively new entry in PK management involves the use of a hybrid design. This design fuses a GP center with an SCL skirt in an effort to provide good comfort and vision. Because of performance limitations (i.e., poor fitting characteristics, limited oxygen transmission, tearing at rigid–soft lens junction), the previous hybrid lens SoftPerm (Ciba Vision) is not regularly utilized. However, a new hybrid lens, SynergEyes, has recently entered the market. SynergEyes has an F-S/A center with a Dk of 100 (i.e., Paragon HDS100, Paragon Vision Sciences) and a poly-HEMA hydrophilic skirt (Fig. 19.3).

The SynergEyes lens has been found to allow significantly more oxygen to reach the cornea during wear than the SoftPerm lens at the central cornea, as well as 2.0 mm and 4.5 mm temporal to the central cornea.[23] The larger overall diameter, larger central optical zone, and GP peripheral curve provide a wider range of applications for the hybrid lens. Most recently, the SynergEyes PS lens has been introduced. This specific design is recommended for oblate corneas resulting from postrefractive surgery, ocular trauma, and postpenetrating keratoplasty.

Considerable debate exists regarding the risks and benefits of hybrid lenses in PK management. Lens adherence is relatively common and can result in corneal edema, neovascularization, epithelial erosion, acute red eye, infiltrative keratitis, and graft rejection. In addition, this lens can be difficult to handle; therefore, it is best inserted using the forefinger and the middle finger to cradle the lens. Likewise, although tearing at the GP–SCL junction is not as common as it is with

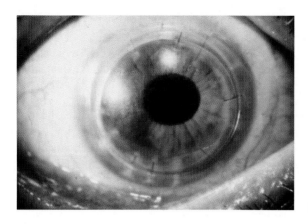

■ FIGURE 19.3 The SynergEyes lens (SynergEyes).

the SoftPerm lens, it is still recommended to push the lens onto the conjunctiva (where it is less adherent) before pinching it off of the eye. However, hybrid lenses offer excellent centration and stability as well as moderate astigmatism correction and provide an option for patients who experience discomfort or a poor lens-to-cornea fitting relationship with a GP lens. Our experiences with SynergEyes have been generally favorable; however, peripheral corneal/limbal compression accompanied by trapped debris can result in inflammatory events if the lens tightens over time. Therefore, certain precautions must be taken. The proper base curve selection is determined by diagnostic fitting, with each trial lens allowed to equilibrate for at least 15 minutes. Regardless of a good visual response and positive patient acceptance, adequate lens movement is essential.

■ RADIAL KERATOTOMY

Once the predominant mode of refractive surgery, RK has been relegated to a secondary status because of the widespread popularity of excimer laser-based procedures. At its height, RK was performed on approximately 250,000 Americans annually.[24] Although deemed relatively safe and effective by the Prospective Evaluation of Radial Keratotomy (PERK) study, RK has nonetheless been recognized for significant shortcomings.[25] Of primary concern is the incidence of residual refractive error, irregular astigmatism, diurnal fluctuations, progressive hyperopia, and glare.

Contact Lens Rationale

Although some patient symptoms are effectively managed by intermittent spectacle lens wear, many are best suited for contact lens wear. Once used regularly to address procedure-related micro- and macroperforations as well as persistent epithelial defects, bandage contact lenses are rarely used today. Refinement in surgical techniques, improved instrumentation, and the use of nonsteroidal anti-inflammatory drugs (NSAIDs) postoperatively have significantly lessened the need for bandage lenses. Occasionally, however, bandage lenses are employed to modulate refractive outcome. In those patients who are initially undercorrected, a bandage lens may be beneficial.[26] When worn on an extended wear basis, a bandage lens can increase peripheral corneal edema, spread the RK incisions, and possibly enhance the myopic effect. This strategy, however, is not without risk. The patient must be closely monitored for neovascularization, epithelial erosion, and signs of infiltrative keratitis.

Special Considerations

As is true of any corneal surgical procedure, RK can profoundly alter structure and function. Certainly, the topographic changes can provide a compelling argument for prescribing contact lenses. Conversely, the anatomic and physiologic alterations make contact lenses a riskier

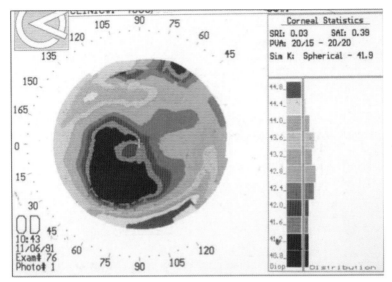

FIGURE 19.4 Optical zone decentration after radial keratotomy with associated visual fluctuation.

endeavor. The topographic changes can both support clinical suspicion as well as provide insight into contact lens fitting. Indeed, the idea of RK is to surgically induce a central corneal flattening accompanied by myopia reduction. Unfortunately, the degree of flattening is sometimes unpredictable and radially asymmetric. The net effect is residual myopia, unanticipated hyperopia, or induced astigmatism. Additionally, the post-RK topography can be complicated by an optical zone decentration (Fig. 19.4). Optical zone decentration has been associated with diurnal visual fluctuation and can complicate contact lens fitting, as the corneal apex is no longer centered.

The anatomic and physiologic changes associated with RK can be as challenging as the topographic alterations. The success of RK is, at minimum, partially because of the way in which the cornea heals. Initially, epithelial swelling is followed by hyperplasia into the wound margin. This epithelial "plug" interferes with normal stromal architecture, resulting in the desired flattening. Unfortunately, it is this epithelial "plug" that places the RK patient at greater risk while wearing contact lenses. Indeed, even after the RK incision has healed, it is more susceptible to neovascularization, epithelial erosion, and infiltrative keratitis. Finally, the RK incision often violates endothelial integrity. Fortunately, endothelial cell loss secondary to RK is often limited to the incision sight and is not widespread. However, the potential for endothelial cell loss underscores the importance of optimizing oxygen transmission.

Contact Lens Options

Although there are no time restraints on fitting contact lenses after RK, it is advisable to wait until both the corneal topography and refraction stabilize. For most RK patients, this occurs during the first 3 months after surgery.[27]

The goals in prescribing contact lenses after RK are correction of residual refractive error and stabilization of visual fluctuation. Much like in other postoperative contact lens fitting endeavors, the RK fit is as much an art as a science. Complicating this endeavor is the fact that many RK patients have a history of contact lens intolerance or have limited interest in returning to this modality.

Rigid Gas Permeable Lenses

Rigid GP lenses are the most frequently prescribed post-RK lenses for a variety of reasons. First, their ability to correct residual refractive error, mask irregular astigmatism, and stabilize diurnal variations is well recognized. Additionally, GP lenses provide a sound physiologic response by virtue of their excellent oxygen transmission, tear pump, and deposit resistance.

Lens Materials: The fluoro-silicone/acrylate lenses afford the RK patient a reasonable balance of oxygen transmission, stable surface characteristics, and flexural resistance. Hyper Dk (Dk >100) lenses are also a good choice for the RK patient; however, flexure can be an issue. Earlier generation gas permeable lenses should be relegated to a secondary status, and polymethylmethacrylate (PMMA) lenses are contraindicated. By adopting this strategy, the clinician minimizes the likelihood of corneal edema and warpage in this susceptible population.

Overall Diameter: Given the central flattening and apical displacement of the RK cornea, larger diameter GP lenses are imperative for adequate centration. Generally, overall diameters of 9.5 to 13.5 mm are used. In this fashion, the clinician can achieve centration through midperipheral corneal fitting or achieve lens control through lid attachment.

Optical Zone Diameter: As the RK cornea is flattened and plateaued, a relatively small optical zone diameter is necessary to avoid excessive tear pooling, bubble entrapment, and hypoxia. Therefore, a 9.5-mm overall diameter may require a 7.0-mm optical zone, considerably smaller than conventional designs.

Base Curve Radius: Both preoperative and postoperative keratometry readings are of limited value in fitting the RK eye, with the final base curve radius being somewhere in between. We have found that subtracting one-third of the refractive error reduction from the preoperative flat keratometry is a reasonable starting point for base curve radius selection. For example, if the patient's preoperative keratometry readings were 45.00 × 46.00 and the RK myopic reduction was 4.5 D, then a reasonable initial base curve radius would be = [45.00 − 1/3 (4.5)] = 43.50. This diagnostic lens is then assessed for fluorescein alignment, stability, and visual performance (Fig. 19.5). Additionally, base curve radius selection can be predicted with corneal topography. In this approach, the clinician often makes the initial base curve radius selection based on the flattest dioptric meridian at the bend of the transition zone (approximately 3-mm radius).[28]

Back surface aspheric designs have long been considered a viable option for post-RK fitting, presumably because of their junctionless nature and ability to accommodate unusual topographies. However, clinicians must be mindful of the fact that back surface aspheric lenses often

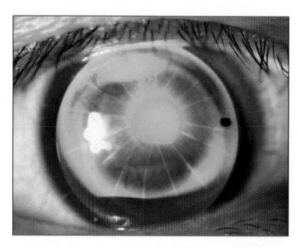

■ **FIGURE 19.5** Well-fitting gas permeable lens after radial keratotomy.

flatten more rapidly than do their spherical counterparts, a feature that may make centration more difficult.

Peripheral Curve Systems: Peripheral curve systems can be of paramount importance in post-RK fitting. Given the relative elevation of the midperiphery in comparison to the central cornea, it is understandable why peripheral curve radii are so important to proper lens fitting and centration. Often, the post-RK GP lens requires a peripheral curve system considerably steeper than in conventional lens designs. The secondary curve radius may need to be steeper than the base curve radius. Indeed, RK was considered the first application for reverse geometry lens designs.

Lens Thickness: The thinnest possible design lessens lens mass and should result in improved centration while optimizing oxygen transmission and facilitating comfort. However, thinner lens designs may also result in significant flexure with visual blur and lens adherence. Therefore, clinicians should balance these considerations when selecting a final lens thickness. Inevitably, certain patients are not successful with GP lenses. Whether because of discomfort, inadequate fit, or a previous GP intolerance, the clinician must be prepared to consider a soft contact lens.

Soft Contact Lenses

When indicated, SCLs are a reasonable option for the RK patient. Historically, SCLs were considered a relative contraindication in RK because of the increased likelihood of corneal neovascularization.[29] However, given the "mini-RK" techniques used in RK more recently, today it is rare for the clinician to encounter RK incisions to the limbus. Therefore, corneal neovascularization is less likely in RK today. Nevertheless, there is still a risk for corneal edema-related topographic changes, epithelial erosions along incision sites, and microbial keratitis. Therefore, certain clinical wisdoms should prevail when fitting the RK patient with an SCL.

Lens Materials: As in other postsurgical applications, the use of highly oxygen permeable lens materials, like a silicone hydrogel, are the rule. It is recommended to use extended wear materials on a daily wear basis. Additionally, as surface contamination issues are a concern, a frequently replaced modality is preferable. Fortunately, a variety of disposable and frequent replacement lenses meet these requirements. Regardless of the brand of silicone hydrogel lens selected, it is imperative for the patient to practice comprehensive lens hygiene.

Lens Design: Essential to a successful RK fit is the need for adequate lens centration and movement, a goal that is sometimes difficult to achieve. If lens centration is achieved through an excessively tight or steep design, a poor metabolic response and fluctuating vision may result. Conversely, if lens movement is obtained through an excessively loose or flat design, the patient may experience visual instability. In those patients requiring an inordinately flat base curve radius for optimal vision but a steep lens periphery for centration, the PRS (Post-Refractive Surgery Lens, X Cel Contacts) may be the most appropriate choice. When addressing residual astigmatism after RK, a low water standard thickness SCL might seem to be a logical choice, given the anecdotal evidence that these designs mask corneal astigmatism. In reality, this approach rarely compensates for the astigmatism and may actually exacerbate visual fluctuation by inducing peripheral corneal edema. In those cases in which residual astigmatism is consistent and regular, a toric SCL, in a silicone hydrogel material, is a logical choice. Fortunately, the proliferation of disposable and frequent replacement toric SCLs make this category of lenses much more efficacious. However, given the rather volatile nature of RK corneal topographies, the clinician must be mindful of the potential for "shifting" cylinder axis and power.

Considering the unusual structural and functional changes associated with RK, and given the success associated with GP and SCL options, there is limited need for combination or hybrid designs for this population. This is not to imply an absolute contraindication to these options, but to acknowledge the added risks of fitting combination or hybrid lenses to the RK patient.

■ EXCIMER PHOTOABLATIVE KERATECTOMY

Although the concept behind excimer laser medical applications dates back to 1981, it wasn't until 1995 that the FDA approved PRK. The elegance of 193-nm wavelength argon–fluoride excimer laser lies in its ability to excise the cornea in an optically smooth fashion with micron accuracy and with minimal collateral tissue damage. Since its inception, excimer laser keratectomy has been employed for both cosmetic refractive purposes (PRK) and therapeutic purposes (PTK). As a therapeutic device, the excimer laser has been effective in treating a variety of corneal pathologies, including superficial scarring, anterior corneal dystrophies, recurrent erosions, and band keratopathy. From a refractive perspective, the excimer laser has been particularly effective in managing myopia up to 9.00 D, astigmatism to 4.00 D, and hyperopia to 6.00 D.

Despite the attributes of excimer laser technology, surgeon skill and patient wound healing remain significant variables. Improper epithelial removal, ablation decentration, and inadequate/excessive lasering can result in residual refractive error, irregular astigmatism, or persistent corneal haze (Fig. 19.6).

Contact Lens Rationale

Although rare, contact lenses are prescribed for PRK patients manifesting residual ametropia, surgically induced astigmatism, and irregular astigmatism associated with persistent stromal haze or decentered ablations. Those patients undergoing PTK often require contact lens correction, as this procedure is directed toward eliminating corneal pathology or lessening corneal scarring. Fortunately, the topographic alterations associated with PRK and PTK are minimal, often requiring only standard rigid gas permeable and soft lens designs.

The use of bandage lenses after PRK, LASEK, and PTK has become standard procedure in recent years.[30] Their success has been largely because of the bandage lens' ability to lessen postoperative discomfort, in conjunction with topical NSAIDs. At the conclusion of each procedure, a bandage contact lens is placed on the eye and evaluated for proper fit. There are several disposable silicone hydrogel lenses approved for therapeutic bandage contact lens applications (see Chapter 11). Once the bandage lens has been deemed appropriate, the patient is prescribed an antibiotic-steroid drop and NSAID drop, each of which are used on a qid basis. The patient is evaluated for follow-up care in 24 hours. At the 24-hour visit, if the patient exhibits significant reepithelialization and minimal discomfort, the bandage lens and NSAID drop are discontinued. The patient continues the antibiotic-steroid drop qid for the balance of the week. If, at the 24-hour visit, there is minimal reepithelialization, the bandage lens and NSAID drop can be

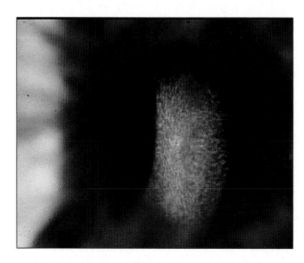

■ **FIGURE 19.6** Persistent stromal haze after surface photorefractive keratectomy.

continued for another 24 to 48 hours. In most all cases, bandage lens use is discontinued by the fifth postoperative day.

A postoperative technique that involves wearing an SCL in conjunction with a topical NSAID is termed *contact lens-assisted pharmacologically induced kerato-steepening* or CLAPIKS. This technique is implemented after refractive surgery (PRK, LASIK, LASEK, RK) in myopic patients who manifest overcorrection in the range of +0.50 to +3.00 D. The theory behind this process is to change the corneal contour with a steep contact lens, while the NSAID acts to thicken the anterior stroma. The procedure is usually initiated 1 week postoperatively. A tight-fitting (base curve radius 8.4 mm or steeper) disposable hydrophilic contact lens, in the patient's full hyperopic correction, is worn in an extended wear fashion while using Acular qid. Results are usually observed in 1 to 3 weeks.[31] Silicone hydrogel lenses are not used for CLAPIKS treatment.

Special Considerations

Corneal topography after excimer laser keratectomy can be quite varied from patient to patient. PTK patients often manifest unusual topographies to begin with and, therefore, exhibit the most unusual postoperative profiles. PRK patients manifest more predictable postoperative profiles. For example, a typical myopic PRK involves a 50- to 100-micron depth ablation over a 6-mm-diameter central zone while maintaining a normal midperipheral corneal topography. Conversely, in hyperopic PRK, the greatest ablation depth occurs in an annulus in the midperiphery, with the apex remaining centrally. In general, the topographic alterations associated with PRK are rarely extreme (Fig. 19.7).

The physiologic alterations associated with PRK, LASEK, and PTK are slightly more complex. Initially, the PRK cornea demonstrates epithelial closure by a sliding mechanism, with the basal cells secreting a basement membrane that behaves much like the Bowman membrane. This results in an epithelium–stroma interface with normal anchoring fibrils and hemidesmosome attachment. Although reepithelialization occurs within the first week, the epithelium remains poorly differentiated for up to 6 months, and can account for a certain amount of postoperative blur. At approximately 1 month, stromal keratocyte activity results in collagen production, stromal haze, and possible refractive error regression. In most patients, the haze fades and rarely interferes with vision beyond 6 months.

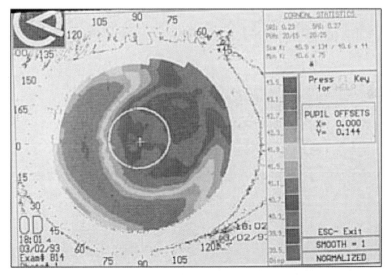

■ **FIGURE 19.7** Typical myopic photorefractive keratectomy topography with minimal decentration.

Contact Lens Options

Many questions remain with respect to contact lens wear following PRK, LASEK, or PTK. The short- and long-term sequelae of a contact lens on a poorly differentiated and thickened epithelium, in the absence of the Bowman layer or in the presence of stromal haze remains to be seen. It is uncertain whether contact lenses may adversely affect refractive outcome, although the experiences thus far have been generally favorable.[32]

Considerable debate exists regarding when it is appropriate to fit a contact lens after PRK, LASEK, or PTK. Most patients receive a bandage lens perioperatively, and some are prescribed soft lenses within the first month to modulate wound healing. However, for residual refractive errors, it is advisable to defer contact lenses for, at minimum, 3 months postoperatively, and preferably for 6 months.

Rigid Gas Permeable Lenses

The LASEK or PRK patient with residual ametropia rarely presents with an exceptionally altered topography or excessive irregular astigmatism and, therefore, GP lenses are not always mandatory. Nevertheless, the exceptional visual and physiologic response to GP lenses can be compelling.

Lens Materials: Because of their excellent oxygen transmission, stable surface characteristics, and flexural resistance, fluoro-silicone/acrylate lens materials remain the material of choice.

Overall Diameter: Most myopic patients manifest a central ablation zone of approximately 6 to 8 mm with a normal periphery. Contact lens centration or lid attachment is fairly easily attained with traditional designs, and an overall diameter of 9.0 to 10.5 mm often suffices.

Optical Zone Diameter: In myopic patients, where the ablation results in a central flat zone, a smaller than average optical zone diameter may be required to avoid excessive fluorescein pooling.

Base Curve Radius: For the post-PRK, -LASEK, or -PTK patient, the GP base curve radius often lies between the preoperative and postoperative flat keratometric reading. A reasonable initial base curve radius selection is approximately 0.50 D flatter than the flat preoperative keratometry reading. The base curve radius is then adjusted according to the fluorescein pattern, in an attempt to achieve light apical pooling and midperipheral alignment (Fig. 19.8).

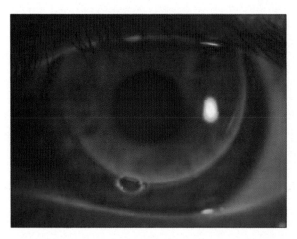

■ **FIGURE 19.8** Gas permeable fluorescein pattern after myopic photorefractive keratectomy, demonstrating light apical pooling and midperipheral alignment.

Peripheral Curves: The combination of more sophisticated ablation geometry and prompt epithelial healing accounts for the relatively smooth transition zone most often observed in these surface treatment procedures. For this reason, standard peripheral curve systems often suffice. Rarely is a reverse geometry design necessary.

Lens Thickness: Standard lens thickness profiles are sufficient for most patients as lens flexure and adherence are fairly rare. The thinnest profile consistent with enhanced comfort, vision, physiology, and patient handling is recommended.

Soft Contact Lenses

These patients do not seem particularly prone to chronic edema, neovascularization, or infiltrative keratitis and, as a result, SCLs are not contraindicated. Postmyopic patients require a fairly flat base curve radius and an average to larger diameter. Once proper lens centration and movement have been obtained, retinoscopy is used to validate an appropriate contact lens–cornea relationship. In those scenarios in which a toric SCL is indicated, a diagnostic fitting with spherocylindrical over-refraction is advisable. Therefore, the clinician can be certain that adequate rotational stability and visual acuity are obtainable. For optimal physiology, a disposable, silicone hydrogel lens, worn on a daily basis, is advisable. As is true in any contact lens endeavor, and in hydrogel wear in particular, compliance with a comprehensive lens care regimen is essential.

■ LASER-ASSISTED IN SITU KERATOMILEUSIS

In an effort to further advance the discipline of excimer laser photoablation, LASIK has become the procedure of choice for virtually every refractive surgeon. Relative to surface excimer laser procedures, LASIK results in less perioperative pain and inflammation and more rapid visual restoration, and requires fewer postoperative eyedrops. Additionally, with the advent of femtosecond laser flap technology, flap creation complications have become exceedingly rare.

Contact Lens Rationale

Although LASIK offers several advantages relative to its predecessors, it is nevertheless a more challenging procedure to perform. Aborted microkeratome passes, excessively thin or thick flaps, and inaccurate stromal bed ablations can lead to significant residual refractive error or irregular astigmatism. As adjustability is a significant advantage of LASIK, enhancements are performed in an effort to improve refractive outcomes. However, certain patients, especially presbyopes, are wary of undergoing additional surgery and prefer to address residual refractive error through more traditional means such as contact lenses.

Whereas bandage contact lenses are the standard in perioperative PRK management, they are less commonly used after LASIK. Certain surgeons prescribe bandage contact lenses after lifting the corneal flap for enhancement, in the presence of an epithelial defect, or to facilitate the flap settling in a thin or wrinkled flap. In these cases, the bandage lens is left in place for 1 to 3 days and the patient concomitantly receives antibiotic eyedrops. Much like in PRK, silicone hydrogel disposable lenses are often used as bandages.

Special Considerations

Topographically, myopic LASIK patients demonstrate the same general flattening experienced after myopic RK and PRK. However, as LASIK is an ablative procedure, the topographic alterations are often less dramatic than observed in RK. However, as LASIK is more frequently performed for higher degrees of myopia, the alterations can be more dramatic than in PRK. In considering the LASIK patient for contact lens fitting, clinicians must evaluate two features of the topography: the diameter of the flat zone and the midperipheral corneal curvature. In evaluating the flat zone diameter, one must be careful in interpreting sagittal topographic maps,

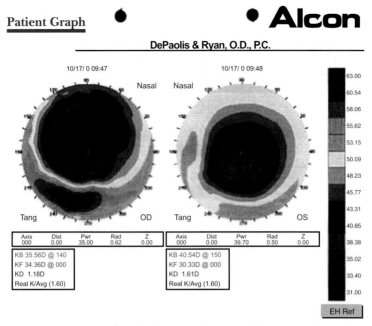

■ FIGURE 19.9 Sagittal corneal topography map after myopic laser in situ keratomileusis.

as the data-smoothing features make this dimension more difficult to delineate. Conversely, when evaluating midperipheral corneal curvature, tangential maps often provide widely variable dioptric values for a given annular area. As this region is critical in initial base curve radius selection, the data averaging of a sagittal map is more easily interpreted for initial base curve radius selection (Fig. 19.9). Of course, central flat zone diameter and midperipheral curvature measurements are only starting points for lens design, and their accuracy should be validated by fluorescein pattern evaluation.

Theoretically, the LASIK patient presents fewer physiologic problems than does the RK or PRK patient. Whereas RK, LASEK, and PRK significantly alter the corneal surface, LASIK results in minimal epithelial involvement. Nevertheless, LASIK presents with physiologic challenges of its own, including flap integrity. Every effort should be made to preserve flap edge integrity, so as to avoid epithelial defects or ingrowth. It is also important to avoid contact lens-related transient corneal thickness, curvature, or refractive changes. Additionally, the contact lens clinician must be cognizant of flap hypoesthesia, although this generally returns to normal by 3 to 6 months. A more lingering physiologic concern involves LASIK's proximity to the endothelium, although early studies have not associated LASIK with endothelial damage.[33] A frequent physiologic challenge involves ocular surface drying. The combination of corneal hypoesthesia and significant topographic alterations adversely affects tear production and distribution, often for up to 6 months and, in some cases, longer.

Contact Lens Options

As the corneal flap behaves much like a bandage, contact lenses are rarely used in the perioperative management of LASIK patients. There are two exceptions to this rule: (a) epithelial defects involving the flap and (b) wrinkles (irregularity) within the flap. In the former, a bandage lens may be beneficial in facilitating reepithelialization and mitigating against epithelial ingrowth. In the latter application, bandage lenses facilitate flap smoothing and may eliminate the need for flap lifting, cleaning, and repositioning. In either application, the bandage lens is used for no more than 1 week.

Given the physiologic and topographic alterations associated with LASIK, it is advisable to delay refractive contact lens fitting for at least 3 months. This approach provides the clinician with a more stable cornea and affords the patient a greater likelihood for successful contact lens wear.

A recent retrospective review, composed of 74 eyes of 45 patients with corneal ectasia after LASIK (72 eyes) or PRK (2 eyes), concluded that most of these patients could be corrected with contact lenses.[34] Specifically, final visual correction was achieved with GP lenses in 77% of eyes, spectacles in 9%, a corneal transplant in 8%, collagen cross-linking in 3%, and intra-corneal ring segments in 1%. Therefore, the majority of eyes avoided surgical intervention while achieving functional visual acuity with GP lenses.

Rigid Gas Permeable Lenses

Lens Materials: As is true in other postoperative GP lens applications, materials with high oxygen transmission, stable surface characteristics, and flexure resistance are desirable. For this reason, moderately transmissible fluoro-silicone/acrylates remain the lens material category of choice.

Overall Diameter: As the post-LASIK corneal topography is often less prolate in nature, fairly large overall diameters are indicated. This strategy facilitates lens centration, and where lens centration is unattainable, promotes a lid attachment fitting relationship. A larger diameter GP lens also vaults the flap, thereby lessening contact lens bearing. In general, overall diameters of 9.5 to 11.5 mm are indicated.

Optical Zone Diameter: In employing a large overall diameter, clinicians must not arbitrarily incorporate an excessively large optical zone diameter. Given the central flattening associated with myopic LASIK, a large optical zone diameter can cause lens adherence or excessive tear pooling, the latter resulting in poor vision, bubble entrapment, and/or hypoxia. To avoid these sequelae, it is reasonable to start with an optical zone diameter approximately 2.5 mm smaller than the overall diameter, considerably smaller than in a standard GP design. Of course, optical zone diameter is adjusted according to the fluorescein pattern and patient response.

Base Curve Radius: In selecting a GP base curve radius for the LASIK patient, clinicians should not rely on postoperative keratometry readings. In most cases, postoperative central keratometric readings will result in a lens design that is excessively flat. A more reasonable approach involves a base curve radius between preoperative and postoperative central keratometric readings. Similar to our recommendations for RK, we suggest an initial base curve radius that is flatter than the preoperative flat keratometry reading by one-fourth of the total LASIK dioptric reduction. Final base curve radius determination is then based on fluorescein assessment, contact lens stability, and visual outcome (Fig. 19.10). Those patients manifesting abrupt

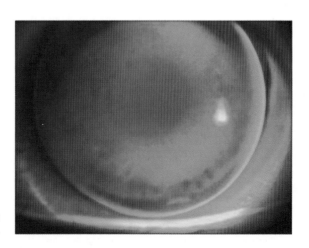

■ **FIGURE 19.10** Well-fitting gas permeable lens after myopic laser assisted in situ keratomileusis.

fluorescein pattern transitions between base curve radius and peripheral curves may benefit from a low eccentricity back surface aspheric geometry. If this strategy is adopted, however, a lid attachment fit might be necessary to facilitate centration.

Peripheral Curve System: The transition from central to midperipheral cornea in LASIK is often less dramatic than in RK, but more so than in surface PRK. It is prudent to start with a standard GP peripheral curve system and to modify accordingly. When evaluating fluorescein patterns, clinicians should be aware of the potential for excessive bearing in the transition zone and edge lift associated with standard designs. In either scenario, a steeper peripheral curve system is warranted. If the peripheral curve system necessary for alignment in the midperipheral transition zone results in inadequate edge clearance, a reverse geometry lens design may be necessary. In selecting the secondary curve for a reverse geometry lens, it is reasonable to start with a curvature that approximates the average dioptric value of the transition zone itself. This can be approximated by averaging four data points (0, 90, 180, and 270 meridians) along the transition zone from sagittal topography maps.

Lens Thickness: Whenever possible, the thinnest GP consistent with optimal comfort, centration, and oxygen permeability should be prescribed. Thicker designs are reserved for patients who experience lens flexure or warpage, lens adherence, or frequent lens damage.

Soft Contact Lenses

As LASIK patients are not at high risk for corneal neovascularization and rarely manifest significant irregular astigmatism, SCLs are often successful. As anticipated, myopic LASIK patients often require a fairly flat base curve radius. This mandate is not so much to ensure centration, but rather to optimize visual performance. Once SCL centration and movement is validated by biomicroscopy, retinoscopy is performed to substantiate an appropriate contact lens–cornea interface. If residual astigmatism necessitates a toric SCL, a diagnostic fitting with sphero-cylindrical over-refraction is advisable. Therefore, the clinician can be assured that rotational stability and consistent vision are attainable with this design.

Occasionally, the SCL diameter and base curve necessary for optimal centration and movement results in inadequate vision. In this scenario, a Post Refractive Surgery Hydrogel Lens (X-Cel) may be indicated. This lens features a mid-water-content material that fits like a reverse geometry design.

In light of the physiologic alterations associated with LASIK, we advocate a disposable silicone hydrogel design worn on a daily basis. As is true in any contact lens endeavor, compliance with a comprehensive care regimen is essential.

Alternate Design Lenses

As LASIK patients rarely present with inordinately abnormal topographies or excessive irregular astigmatism, nontraditional designs are rarely necessary. As a rule, hybrid, piggyback, and scleral lenses are not indicated. This is not to imply an absolute contraindication, but rather to relegate these designs to a special application status.

■ OCULAR TRAUMA

Generally, these patients are young to middle age with one eye that is correctable to 20/20. Trauma to the anterior segment may be limited to the cornea or penetrate to the crystalline lens. The trauma is often the result of an automobile accident, hunting or fishing accident, chemical burns, physical fighting/abuse, or penetration of a stick, rock, or toy. Contact lenses may be necessary to correct monocular aphakia or irregular astigmatism or to cosmetically improve their appearance. The patient's motivation may be high if contact lenses will improve cosmetic appearance or may be low if the other eye is correctable to 20/20. In lieu of the absence of motivation, it is important to educate the patient on the importance of correcting the traumatized eye for two reasons: (a) the traumatized eye may become amblyopic (depending on the patient's age) if it is not corrected and (b) there is the danger of an accident or disease affecting the opposite eye. Safety glasses should be worn, at minimum, during hazardous activities to reduce this risk.

Lenses for Visual Correction

In ocular trauma, contact lenses may aid in correcting irregular astigmatism or monocular aphakia. An intraocular implant may not be feasible, as the iris may have been destroyed as a result of the trauma. The fit is complicated by a flat, irregular cornea with possibly a high plus prescription.

The lens of choice is a GP fluoro-silicone/acrylate material in a low to moderate Dk (i.e., Dk 30–65) worn as daily wear. The first lens selected should be >9.0 mm in diameter with a base curve radius that is slightly flatter than the average keratometry reading. If a spherical lens is not adequate, a bitoric or aspheric GP may improve the fit.

If the lens decenters, a piggyback lens or the SynergEyes hybrid (SynergEyes, Inc.) lens may improve centration. The limitation of the SynergEyes A lens is that it is only available in flat base curve radius to 8.0 (42.25 D), which may be insufficiently flat for the traumatized cornea (i.e., flatter than 40 D). In these cases, a SynergEyes PS design may be more appropriate. It is, however, available in high plus powers up to +20.00 D. If the aforementioned options are not successful, a hydrogel or silicone hydrogel toric lens can be considered.

Lenses for Cosmesis

Some ocular trauma patients need a contact lens to improve the appearance of the eye, either via providing an iris, covering a disfigured cornea, or altering the pupil shape or size. The eye may also need a visual correction or may have no functional vision. GP lenses are generally too small in diameter and not available in the appropriate tints to be used for cosmetic purposes. The lens of choice in this case is a soft (not hydrogel) lens (SCL). These contact lenses are available in several iris tints and with clear or black pupils. Companies that provide custom, prosthetic tinted SCLs are listed in Table 19.1. Typically, the color-enhancing SCLs do not provide a sufficiently dark tint to be used in these patients. Successful fits have been achieved with the opaque tinted SCLs. Many times it is difficult to match the other eye; however, both eyes may be fitted with the tinted lenses to provide a good result.

TABLE 19.1 CUSTOM, PROSTHETIC, TINTED HYDROGEL LENS COMPANIES

Adventure in Colors	1-800-537-2845
Ciba Vision Corp.	1-800-488-6859
CooperVision	1-800-341-2020
Crystal Reflections Int'l., Inc.	1-800-807-8722
Custom Color Contacts	1-800-598-2020
Marietta Contact Lens Service	1-770-792-0208
Medlens, Inc.	1-877-533-1509
Ocu-Ease Optical	1-800-521-8984
Specialty Tint	1-800-748-5500

TABLE 19.2 GP SCLERAL LENS CATEGORIES

Corneoscleral: 12.9–13.5 mm
Semi-scleral: 13.6–14.9 mm
Mini-scleral: 15.0–18.0 mm
Full scleral: 18.1–24+ mm

From 37. Sindt C. Classifying and applications of large diameter GP lenses. Contact Lens Spectrum In press (to be published in October 2008 issue).

■ SCLERAL LENS APPLICATIONS IN POSTSURGICAL/IRREGULAR CORNEA PATIENTS

History and Classification

Scleral lenses have been used since 1888, when glass scleral lenses were first applied to the eye for the correction of optical and corneal irregularities. Many of the concepts and designs are still being used today. Glass, however, proved not to be a viable lens material and a switch was made to PMMA around 1934. Continued hypoxia with PMMA scleral lenses fostered the way for the first corneal lens designs in 1948.[35] Corneal GP lenses have become quite sophisticated through the use of complex computer-driven lathing systems, yet contact lens fitters have continued to look for easier, more comfortable contact lens designs. In recent years, there has been renewed interest in scleral lens designs with the advent of improved oxygen transmission materials.[36] Sclerals and other large lens designs have been categorized based on diameter.[37] This is provided in Table 19.2.

Benefits and Applications

For many experienced contact lens fitters, scleral lenses are becoming the lens of choice for PK, keratoconus, and other irregular corneal surfaces. Scleral lenses primarily align with the sclera and vault the irregularity of the cornea. These lenses offer superior comfort and handling and reduced chair time compared to other lens types. New lens materials, including Boston XO and Boston XO 2 (Bausch & Lomb) and HDS 100 (Paragon Vision Sciences) supply adequate oxygen transmission. In one author's experience (CS), scleral lenses should not be fitted on eyes with endothelial cells counts of <1,000 to avoid edema. Around 800 cells seem to be where problems arise, so a count of 1,000 leaves a margin of safety.

Fitting Principles

Scleral lenses are fitted based on sagittal depth as opposed to keratometric readings. While there are formulas to calculate the sagittal depth of the eye, a fitting set is the easiest way to determine necessary vault. The amount of sagittal depth of the eye is determined by the horizontal visible iris diameter, the corneal curvature, and the eccentricity value of the peripheral cornea. Therefore, two eyes with the same keratometry values could have vastly different sagittal depths. The diameter of the scleral lens will determine the fitting technique, and the manufacturer should be consulted on the subtleties of a particular lens. Sizes range from 13 to 24 mm. In general, the lens should exhibit alignment with the sclera, without impingement of blood vessel. Larger lenses will be less likely to cause a broad area of focal impingement. A large lens is similar to snowshoes, distributing weight over a broad area, and will allow the weight of the lens to be maintained above the sclera (Fig. 19.11). Small lenses are like stiletto heals, applying greater pressure over a small area, potentially causing scleral indentation and vascular impingement.

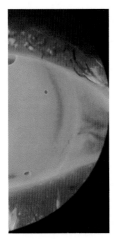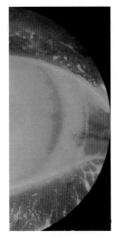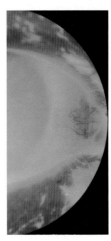

■ **FIGURE 19.11** Larger diameter lenses allow for broader distribution of weight and pressure.

There should be pooling in the limbal area and either complete vaulting or gracing touch over the central cornea. Smaller designs, generally <15 mm, will have greater interaction with the limbus and cornea and are frequently referred to as corneoscleral or mini-scleral. The 15- to 18-mm-diameter lenses are referred to as semi-scleral (Fig. 19.12). Larger lenses, considered to be >18 mm by many fitters, are easier to vault the entire cornea and are typically called full or true scleral lenses. A good fitting relationship is shown in Figure 19.13.

Limbal pooling is required to bath the fragile limbal stem cells, which are responsible for epithelial cell formation. Bearing over the cornea will cause erosions. In these cases, it is necessary to increase sagittal depth over the affected area through either curvature changes or diameter.

Bubbles should be avoided under the lens. Insertion bubbles can be avoided by filling the bowl with preservative-free saline before insertion. If the sagittal depth is too great in either the center or limbal area, steps will need to be taken to decrease the sagittal depth according the manufacturer's instructions. Preservative-free saline is preferred for insertion to avoid trapped preservative toxicity to the cornea. A thick fluid, such as GP solution or rewetting drops, will exacerbate mucin formation under the lens. Mucin can adhere to the posterior lens surface, causing discomfort upon insertion. Care should be taken to evaluate the lens for deposits.

Fluid is exchanged through a diaphragm movement during the blink. Unlike corneal lenses, vertical movement does not increase tear circulation. Vertical movement causes patient discomfort and should be avoided.

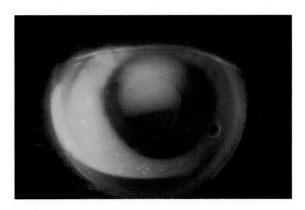

■ **FIGURE 19.12** The semi-scleral Macro lens. (Courtesy of Dr. Loretta Szczotka-Flynn.)

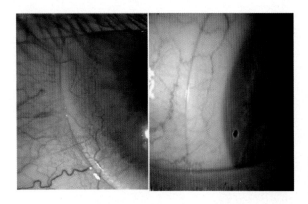

■ FIGURE 19.13 A good peripheral fit will demonstrate alignment of the sclera without impingement of blood vessels.

Excessive flexure will disrupt this fluid exchange. In this case, flexure causes suction of the lens to the eye, resulting in negative pressure build-up under the lens. In extreme cases, the limbal tissue will swell and become hyperemic (Fig. 19.14).

Although tight lenses will be comfortable at first, patients with scleral indentation, vascular impingement, and negative pressure build-up will complain of discomfort after lens removal and frequently an inability to wear the lens the next day.

In corneoscleral designs, a fenestration hole may be beneficial in relieving the negative pressure. This will aid in removal of the lens from the eye. A fenestration hole does not aid in fluid exchange under the lens. If a fenestration hole is desired, it should be approximately 1 mm in diameter and placed in the deepest pooling area over the limbus. If the fenestration hole is obstructed by the cornea or placed over the conjunctiva, the fenestration will not be effective. In cases of conjunctival chalasis, negative pressure can suck the conjunctiva up under the lens and herniate the conjunctiva through the hole. Fenestration holes are not advised in larger lenses because air will be sucked through the hole and obscure the optics (Fig. 19.15). It is necessary to break the suction before removal. This is easily performed by pressing on the sclera adjacent to the lens. Lens removal can be accomplished using the two-finger removal approach or by using a plunger.

■ SUMMARY

A central theme in addressing the postoperative cornea involves careful consideration of the physiologic and topographic alterations. Only in recognizing these structural and functional changes does the clinician better understand the indications and contraindications for various lens designs. Given the potential benefits as well as complications, the opportunities and challenges for the contact lens specialist are indeed significant.

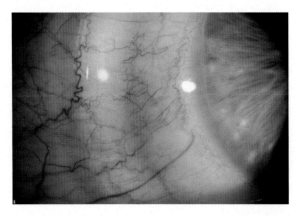

■ FIGURE 19.14 Excessive negative pressure under a scleral lens will cause limbal swelling.

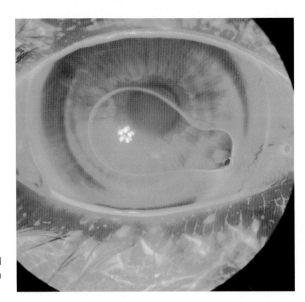

■ **FIGURE 19.15** Bubble under a fenestrated scleral lens coming in through the fenestration hole.

■ CLINICAL CASES

CASE 1

RB is a 53-year-old white man with a history of congenital cataract OS, exotropia, and amblyopia OS. He also manifests moderately advanced Fuch corneal dystrophy OU and is developing a significant cataract OD. With a best corrected visual acuity of OD 20/40− and OS CF (count fingers), RB's vision is reduced to OD 20/100 with glare source. RB elects to undergo cataract extraction, posterior chamber intraocular lens (IOL) implantation, and PK OD. Approximately 16 months after surgery, RB's continuous corneal suture is removed, a relaxing incision is performed, and wound prolapse ensues, requiring resuturing. Despite a clear corneal transplant and well-positioned IOL, his OD keratometry is 41.50 × 52.00 @ 157 and manifest refraction is OD −5.75 − 5.00 × 75 = 20/80. As RB manifests a highly irregular topography OD, a variety of GP lenses fail because of instability.

SOLUTION: A Ciba Vision Focus Night and Day (lotrafilcon A) 8.6 mm/13.8 mm/−0.25 D Rx contact lens was prescribed as the foundation for a piggyback combination. A Boston XO (Bausch & Lomb/Boston) 7.00 mm base curve radius (BCR)/9.5 mm overall diameter (OAD)/8.1 mm optical zone diameter (OZD)/−9.50 D Rx contact lens was prescribed for visual restoration. This combination provided RB visual acuity of 20/20, good comfort, and wearing time of 14 hours daily while maintaining a good physiologic response. RB maintains his lenses with Aquify Multi-purpose Solution (Ciba Vision) and Boston Daily Cleaner and Conditioner (Bausch & Lomb).

CASE 2

GT is a 77-year-old man with bilateral PK and IOL implantation. A manifest refraction yields best corrected visual acuity of OD +2.50 − 3.75 × 116/+2.50 = 20/200 and OS +3.50 − 5.50 × 23/+2.50 = 20/40. As GT's irregular astigmatism limits visual acuity OD, he is interested in additional surgery or contact lens correction. His surgeon has recommended against additional surgery for the OD, given GT's irregular astigmatism, secondary glaucoma, and mild background diabetic retinopathy. GT does articulate a history of previous GP failure because of frequent lens dislocation and loss. An initial diagnostic fitting visit confirms keratometry of OD 45.00 × 52.00 @ 90 with grade 4 distortion. Corneal topography reveals irregular astigmatism and PK "tilt" OD. Several standard-design GP lenses demonstrate variable fluorescein patterns and instability.

SOLUTION: A DYNA Intra-Limbal (Lens Dynamics, Inc) GP lens was ordered with Menicon Z material, 6.50 mm BCR/11.2 mm OAD/−10.00 D Rx. This lens provided exceptional centration, good stability, adequate movement, and a fluorescein pattern of slight apical clearance. Biomicroscopy confirmed an acceptable physiologic response. An over-refraction of OD +1.25 sph/+2.50 = 20/25 provided reasonable balance with the OS. GT uses Optimum Solutions (Lobob) for lens care.

CASE 3

JL is a 69-year-old woman who has developed pseudophakic bullous keratopathy OU. She previously underwent a PK with IOL exchange OD, and is currently having difficulty with her GP lens. The OS is increasingly symptomatic and JL is interested in resolving her contact lens problems OD before undergoing PK/IOL exchange surgery OS. Best corrected visual acuity with contact lens and overcorrection is OD 20/40, and with spectacle correction only, OS 20/400. Biomicroscopy demonstrates a nasally displaced and excessively mobile GP, healthy PK, and well-positioned IOL OD. The OS manifests grade 4 bullous keratopathy and an anterior chamber IOL. JL's history is complicated by secondary glaucoma OD. Keratometry is OD 46.25 × 47.75 @ 130 with slight distortion. Topography reveals a fairly central, symmetric, but steep PK OD.

SOLUTION: Given the fairly centered but steep PK OD, a Rose K contact lens (Blanchard Contact Lens, Inc.) 7.13 mm BCR/9.0 mm OAD/−5.75 D Rx/reduced edge lift profile was ordered. This lens offers slightly superior positioning, moderate fluorescein clearance, and reasonable edge clearance. Visual acuity with over-refraction is OD −0.50 − 0.75 × 80/+2.50 = 20/25. The PK remains clear, IOL well positioned, and glaucoma well controlled OD. JL has now undergone PK and IOL exchange OS, and is currently corrected with manifest refraction to +1.50 − 2.00 × 55/+2.50 = 20/40. JL uses Boston Daily Cleaner and Conditioner (Bausch & Lomb/Boston) for lens care.

CASE 4

WF is a 56-year-old man with a 35-year history of keratoconus OU and bilateral PK performed approximately 25 years ago. Additionally, WF is a bilateral pseudophake. He wears PureVision (Bausch & Lomb, Inc) 8.6 mm BCR/14.0 mm OAD/−9.00 D OD and 8.6 mm BCR/14.0 mm OAD/−1.25 D OS and spectacle overcorrection on a daily wear basis. WF ultimately developed graft failure OS, unrelated to contact lens wear. WF's visual acuity with contact lens and spectacle overcorrection was OD 20/40− and OS 20/150. A biomicroscopic examination of the involved OS revealed grade 3 full thickness corneal edema and a well-positioned posterior chamber IOL. Preferring to avoid the prolonged convalescence associated with full-thickness PK, WF elected to undergo a deep lamellar endothelial keratoplasty (DLEK). Approximately 1 month after the procedure, WF's biomicroscopy revealed a dramatic reduction in corneal edema. Figure 19.16A,B demonstrates the pre- and postsurgical corneal appearance.

SOLUTION: WF now wears a PureVision 8.6 mm BCR/14.0 mm OAD/−0.50D OS with a spectacle overrefraction of +0.50 − 2.75 × 082 = 20/30−. WF wears his contact lenses for 14 hours daily and uses Complete Easy Rub MPS (AMO, Inc.) nightly.

CASE 5 (COURTESY OF ROBERT M. GROHE, OD)[38]

A 56-year-old communications executive presented with distorted vision consisting of halos, spoking, and reduced scotopic vision. He has undergone seven GP refittings in the last 10 years with ongoing GP intolerance. He has had radial keratotomy performed OU with three enhancements for each eye and bilateral cataracts. He had previously been a 21-year wearer of PMMA lenses followed by 3 years of extended soft lenses wear and 3 years of daily wear of GP lenses. He has been fitted with four pairs of progression addition spectacle lenses, all which have failed because of poor vision. He spends 8 to 10 hours per day at a computer.

Keratometry (with −1.00 D extended range):

OD: 33.98 @ 26 × 32.69 @ 112 1+ distortion
OS: 37.62 @ 33 × 37.00 @ 115 Tr distortion

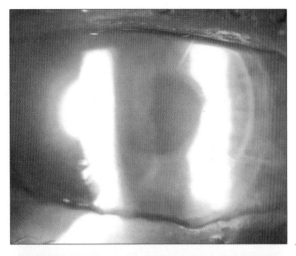

A

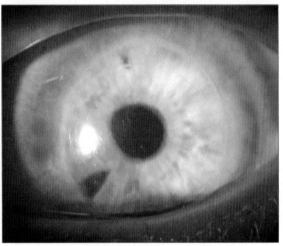

■ **FIGURE 19.16** Failed penetrating keratoplasty in patient with keratoconus who underwent deep lamellar endothelial keratoplasty. **(A)** Before surgery. **(B)** One month postoperative.

B

Manifest refraction:

OD: +2.75 − 1.25 × 115 = 20/40 with monocular diplopia
OS: +0.75 − 1.00 × 80 = 20/60 with monocular oblique triplopia

Slit lamp:
OD: Eight-incision RK with fibrotic recut channels and Tr anterior supcapsular cataract (ASC) and 1+ posterior subcapsular cataract (PSC)
OS: Eight-incision RK with fibrotic recut channels and 1+ ASC and 1+ PSC cataracts

Topography (Fig. 19.17A,B):

OD: Keratometry = 34.80 × 33.00
     Eccentricity = −1.51
     Central corneal thickness (CCT) = 426 microns
OS: Keratometry = 37.30 × 36.70
     Eccentricity = −1.07
     CCT = 453 microns

Diagnostic fitting:
Several different lens designs were attempted, including the following:
 1. Mini-scleral Jupiter 15.0-mm lens (unsuccessful because of intolerance)
 2. SynergEyes (unsuccessful because of severe residual monocular diplopia)
 3. Piggyback of Ciba Night & Day with Envision 10.2 mm (unsuccessful: similar to no. 2)

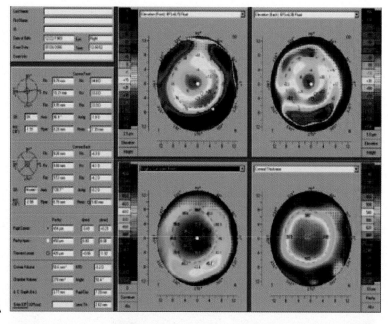

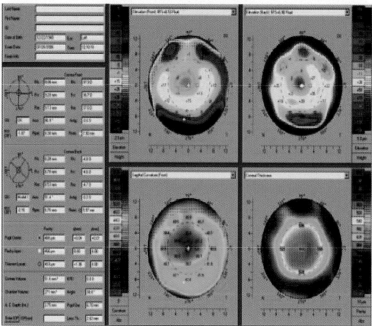

■ FIGURE 19.17 **(A)** OD topography in Case 5. **(B)** OS topography.

SOLUTION: He was successfully fitted into the Rose K2 IC lens OU (Blanchard):

OD: BCR: 9.20 mm (36.62 D)
Power: −0.75D
OAD: 11.2 mm
Peripheral curve (PC): standard flat
Visual acuity (VA): 20/40 + 2 (trace monocular vertical diplopia)
Lens position: central to temporal with 2-mm movement

OS: BCR: 9.25 mm (36.62 D)
Power: −1.00
OAD: 11.2 mm
PC: double flat
VA: 20/50 + 1 (1 + monocular vertical diplopia)
Lens position: central with 1- to 2-mm movement (Fig. 19.18A,B)

Before the refitting, a long discussion outlined the benefits and lingering compromises that would be experienced with any contact lens. Given the past history of unsuccessful spectacle and contact lens fittings and the presence of cataracts, it was necessary to reemphasize the need to compromise and that no contact lens could provide "perfect" vision. It was also stated that all-day wearing time may be unrealistic given the heavy computer use and anti-depressant medications, which together would enhance a dry-eye-like state. The patient begrudgingly agreed.

Success in this case was enhanced by the temporary use of Acular LS dosed as follows:

qid × 1 week
bid × 1 week
qd × 2 weeks
Now: prn

Vision was acceptable and bilaterally resulted in 20/40 − 1 with intermittent but tolerable ghosting and residual diplopia, especially under scotopic lighting. The patient wears his GP lenses 6 to 12 hours per day, depending on his computer use. He also alternates between two pairs of over-the-counter readers (+1.25 or +2.25) for near vision needs.

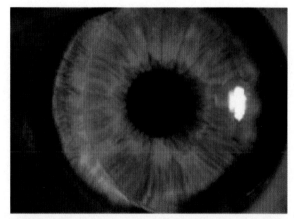

A

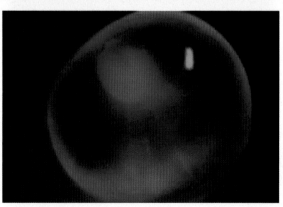

■ FIGURE 19.18 Lens position for patient in Case 5. **(A)** With white light. **(B)** Fluorescein application.

B

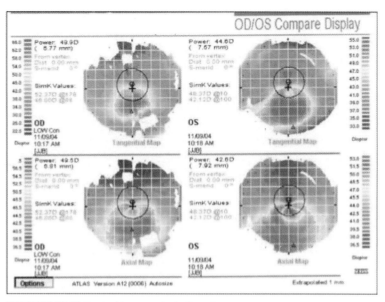

■ FIGURE 19.19 Corneal topography in Case 6.

CASE 6

KC is a 47-year-old woman who has undergone bilateral LASIK with two enhancements in each eye, resulting in ectasia. Her chief complaint is one of blurry vision and dryness OU. KC's spectacle best corrected visual acuity is OD 20/100 and OS 20/60, with ghosting OU. Biomicroscopy reveals well-healed LASIK with inferior apical thinning OU. Corneal topography confirms keratoectasia with a Pellucid morphology OU (Fig. 19.19). Simulated keratometry is OD 48.00 × 56.00 and OS 42.50 × 49.75. A manifest refraction yields OD +2.00 − 7.50 × 092 = 20/100 and OS +2.00 − 6.50 × 088 = 20/60.

SOLUTION: KC achieved excellent vision with a GP contact lens; however, she was intolerant because of her keratoconjunctivitis sicca. KC was subsequently fit with a SynergEyes KC (SynergEyes, Inc.) 6.90 mm BCR/14.5 mm OAD/−8.50 D OD and SynergEyes A 7.60 mm BCR/14.5 mm OAD/−3.50 D/8.6 sc OS, yielding an optimal fit and visual acuity of 20/30+ OD and 20/25 OS. We have performed bilateral lower lid punctal occlusion and KC uses OptiFree Express (Alcon Labs, Inc) nightly and Blink Contact Lens lubricating drops (AMO, Inc) prn.

CASE 7 (COURTESY OF ROBERT MAYNARD, OD)[38]

A 36-year-old computer sales executive presented in January 2003. He had radial keratotomy performed OU in 1995 and post-LASIK in 1998 OU.

Visual acuities (with spectacles):

OD: 20/80 − 1
OS: 20/100

Manifest refraction:

OD: −2.00 − 0.75 × 013   20/25 − 1 ghosting and doubling
OS: +3.00 − 5.00 × 098   20/25 − 1 ghosting and doubling

Keratometry:

OD: 41.37 @ 018; 45.37 @ 108
OS: 34.50 @ 109; 43.12 @ 019

SOLUTION:

INITIAL FIT

Lens parameters:

Power (D)	BCR (mm)	OAD/OZD (mm)	SCR/W (mm)	PCR/W (mm)
OD: −6.50	7.67	11.2/8.8	9.00/.5	11.75/.5
OS: −7.25	7.50	11.2/8.8	9.00/.5	11.75/.5

Overrefraction:

OD: +0.75 DS   20/30
OS: +0.75 DS   20/25

Slit-lamp examination:

OD: the lens is well centered and moved well with the blink. There was good fluorescein pooling centrally as well as superior and inferior.

OS: the lens is well centered and moved well with the blink. There was central pooling with slight touch superiorly-temporally, slight touch nasally, and slight touch inferiorly/temporally.

Two-week follow-up visit

Visual acuities (with lenses):

OD: 20/100 (foggy vision)
OS: 20/200 (foggy vision)

Slit-lamp examination:

OD: the lens is centered over the superior limbus with dimple veiling present over the papillary zone; the lens appears to be tilting backward over the superior limbus.

OS: identical fitting relationship as present OD

SECOND FIT

Lens parameters:

Power (D)	BCR (mm)	OAD/OZD (mm)	Cap Size (mm)	SCR/W(mm)	PCR/W(mm)
OD: −5.75	7.80	11.2/8.4	8.40	8.80/.7	10.00/.5
OS: −6.75	7.58	11.2/8.4	8.40	8.60/.7	10.00/.5

Overrefraction:

OD: +1.50 DS   20/30
OS: +1.75 DS   20/25 − 2

Slit-lamp examination:

OD: the lens is well centered and exhibits good movement with the blink. A bubble is present at 12 o'clock superior to the pupil.

OS: similar fitting relationship as present OD with the additional presence of mild dimple veiling.

Visual acuities:

OD: 20/30 + 2
OS: 20/40 − 1

Over-refraction:

OD: +0.50 DS   20/30 + 2
OS: +1.75 DS   20/25 − 2

Slit-lamp examination:

OD: the lens is well centered with apical clearance and good peripheral edge clearance.

OS: identical fitting relationship as present OD with the exception of mild dimple veiling superiorly.

THIRD FIT (NEW LENS OS ONLY)

Lens parameters:

Power (D)	BCR (mm)	OAD/OZD (mm)	SCR/W (mm)	PCR/W (mm)
OS: −6.75	7.58	11.2/8.4 × 9.0(oval)	8.60/.7	10.00/.5

Over-refraction:

OS: plano 20/25 − 2 (fluctuates)

Slit-lamp examination:

OS: good centration and movement, although dimple veiling was still present in various regions underneath the lens.

FINAL FIT

Essentially, the right contact lens was not changed, and continued to provide excellent vision as well as comfort. The left lens was modified several more times, including fenestrations to reduce the dimple veil problem. The final lens parameters were:

Power (D)	BCR (mm)	OAD/OZD (mm)	Cap Size (mm)	SCR/W(mm)	PCR/W(mm)
OD: −5.75	7.80	11.2/8.4	8.20	8.80/.7	10.00/.5
OS: −6.00	7.50	10.6/6.8 × 7.8(oval)	6.80	8.50/.85	10.50/.85

Five fenestrations (OS only)

Over-refraction:

OD: +0.50 DS 20/25 − 2
OS: −0.75 DS 20/20 − 2

Slit-lamp examination:

OD: the lens is decentered slightly superiorly with mild dimple veiling paracentrally at 4 o'-clock and just inside the superior limbus from 11:30 to 12:30.

OS: similar fitting relationship as present OD with good lid attachment. Fenestrations appear to be successful. There is a minor punctate stain at 4 o'clock, very minor scattered dimple veiling, and some inferior edge standoff. The fluorescein patterns of the lens-to-cornea fitting relationship of both lenses are provided in Figure 19.20A,B.

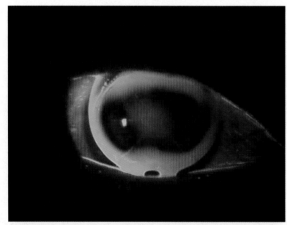

A

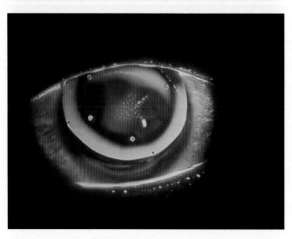

B

■ FIGURE 19.20 Fitting relationship of lenses fitted in Case 7. **(A)** Right lens. **(B)** Left lens.

Overall, the patient was "delighted" with his vision and comfort. We decided not to correct the prescription on the left eye, since he would not gain that much improvement. We sent him away to return for another complete primary care examination in 3 months. It took 10 months for him to be successfully fitted with a lens for his left eye, but it was well worth the effort. At the next eye examination visit, his vision was holding steady, the fitting relationship was still good, and he had no complaints; therefore, he was scheduled to return for a routine 6-month contact lens evaluation.

CASE 8

AB is a 36-year-old man who elected to undergo surface LASEK for myopia and astigmatism. His preoperative manifest refraction was OD $-4.00 - 1.25 \times 179 = 20/20$ and OS -4.50 sph $= 20/20$. Keratometry was OD 44.00×44.75 @ 102 and OS 43.75×44.25 @ 85. The surgery was performed with an excimer laser capable of spherical ablation only, and the procedure and postoperative course were uneventful in each eye. Postoperatively, the OS is 20/20 with a manifest refraction of plano. However, the OD is 20/30− with a manifest refraction of $-0.50 - 1.50 \times 15 = 20/20$. Postoperative keratometry OD is 41.25×43.25 @ 115.

SOLUTION: As AB previously wore GP lenses, he desired a contact lens OD rather than additional surgery. A Boston Envision lens (Bausch & Lomb/Boston) 8.10 mm BCR/9.6 mm OAD/−1.50 D Rx was prescribed. The contact lens positioned superiorly with lid attachment, demonstrated moderate apical clearance, moved well, and resulted in visual acuity of 20/20. AB uses Boston Daily Cleaner and Conditioning Solution (Bausch & Lomb) to care for his contact lenses.

CASE 9

HS is a 33-year-old man who became intolerant to contact lens wear and elected to undergo bilateral LASIK. His preoperative keratometry was OD 43.00×45.00 @ 90 and OS 43.25×45.00 @ 90. His preoperative manifest refraction was OD $-15.25 - 2.75 \times 165 = 20/30$ and OS $-13.50 - 3.00 \times 179 = 20/30$. HS underwent bilateral LASIK, bilateral enhancement, and a flap sweep OD. His final postoperative keratometry is OD 36.25×36.75 @ 63 and OS 36.50×36.75 @ 82, and his manifest refraction is OD -1.00 DS $= 20/25-$ and OS -0.25 DS $= 20/25-$. Despite an exceptional outcome, HS reports intermittent keratitis sicca symptoms and blurred vision.

SOLUTION: HS employs Restasis (Allergan) bid and Refresh (Allergan) artificial tears OU qid. Additionally, he wears a 1-Day Acuvue Moist contact lens (Vistakon) OD 9.0 mm BCR/14.2 mm OAD/−1.25 D Rx and OS 9.0 mm BCR/14.2 mm OAD/− 0.50 D Rx. These lenses provide visual acuity of OD 20/25+ and OS 20/25+, good centration and movement, and reasonable comfort. HS wears his lenses approximately 4 days each week.

CASE 10 (COURTESY OF MICHAEL WARD)[38]

A 46-year-old man complained of poor visual acuity and decreasing vision from his right eye and desires a contact lens for that eye only. Thirteen months before this visit he underwent hyperopic LASIK surgery for the right eye as a result of his emerging presbyopia. There was no record of his preoperative prescription. He reported that his vision was good immediately following the surgery. His contact lens history included successful wear of soft lenses before the surgery. He stated that he had attempted soft toric and GP lens wear without success during the past 6 months.

Visual acuity (without correction):

OD: 20/200
OS: 20/20 − 1

Manifest refraction:

OD: +3.00 − 3.00 × 085   20/80 − 1
OS: +0.75 − 0.25 × 138   20/20

Manual keratometry:

> OD: 46.7 @ 134; 43.0 @ 044 degrees 2+ mire distortion
> OS: 43.6 @ 156; 44.2 @ 066 degrees crisp mires

Corneal topography:
Indicates keratectasia (see map)

Slit-lamp examination:
OD: central and paracentral haze, vertical striae and thinned; nasal based flap with horseshoe-shaped microkeratome scar noted
OS: cornea clear

Contact lens diagnostic fitting:
Initial diagnostic lens
Design: Surgical C4
Base curve: 40.42 D
Diameter: 10.0 mm

Over-refraction: +2.50 DS 20/25 + 2

SOLUTION: Initial diagnostic lens selection was based on a combination of keratometry readings, topography maps, and fluorescein patterns. This type of lens fitting is similar to fitting keratoconus. It is not recommended in these cases to fit the apex of the ectatic protrusion. The base curve radius is often fit somewhat flatter than K, but not as flat as the superior corneal topography. The overall diameter is slightly larger than normal to increase centration; larger diameters may be beneficial. The fluorescein pattern should show complete tear exchange over the entire corneal surface with each blink.

Contact lens order:
Laboratory: ABBA
Material: Fluoroperm 60
BCR: 41.00 D
OAD/OZD: 10.0/9.0 mm
Power: +2.50D
Center thickness: 0.23 mm

At the 1-week follow-up visit, the patient's vision was unchanged and he was adjusting well to GP lens wear and enjoying both his vision and depth perception. He was ultimately successful with this design.

CASE 11

DA is a 37-year-old woman with a 20-year history of contact lens wear, who has developed mild ocular surface disease and a sporadic contact lens intolerance. Despite all efforts to alter DA's contact lenses and care regimen, she continues to experience intermittent episodes of related keratoconjunctivitis. After extensive consultation, DA elected to undergo bilateral LASIK. Preoperatively, DA's manifest refraction was OD −5.25 DS = 20/20 and OS −6.75 DS = 20/20. Postoperatively, DA has been successful with an uncorrected visual acuity of 20/25+ in each eye. Her keratometry readings are OD 41.00 × 41.25 @ 90 and OS 41.25 × 41.75 @ 83. Her refraction is OD −0.25 DS = 20/20 and OS −0.25 − 0.25 × 180 = 20/20. Biomicroscopy confirms a well-healed LASIK flap in each eye. Despite a nearly emmetropic outcome, DA would like to wear tinted contact lenses for cosmetic purposes on an intermittent basis.

SOLUTION: In light of DA's recent history of contact lens-related keratoconjunctivitis, we have advised against wearing contact lenses daily. She has been fit with Fresh Look One Day Colors (Ciba Vision) 8.6 mm BCR/13.8 mm OAD/−0.50 D Rx/blue in each eye. These lenses center well, move optimally, and provide visual acuity of 20/20− in each eye. DA currently wears the lenses approximately 2 nights each week for a wearing time of 4 to 6 hours per session, discarding the lenses after each wear. She uses no solutions regularly, as the lenses are daily disposable.

REFERENCES

1. EBAA Statistics.
2. Pahor D, Gracner B, Falez M, et al. Changing indications for penetrating keratoplasty over a 20-year period, 1985–2004. Klinische Monatsblatter fur Augenheilkunde 2007;224(2):110–114.
3. Fronterre A, Portesani G. Relaxing incisions for postkeratoplasty astigmatism. Cornea 1991;10:305–311.
4. Hjortdal J, Ehlers N. Treatment of post-keratoplasty astigmatism by topography supported customized laser ablation. Acta Ophthalmol Scand 2001;79:376–380.
5. Guell JL, Gris O, de Muller A, et al. LASIK for the correction of residual refractive errors from previous surgical procedures. Ophthalmic Surg Lasers 1999;30:341–349.
6. Bilgihan K, Ozdek SC, Akata F, et al. Photorefractive keratectomy for post-penetrating keratoplasty myopia and astigmatism. J Cataract Refract Surg 2000;26:1590–1595.
7. Geerards AJ, Vreugdenhil W, Khazen A. Incidence of rigid gas-permeable contact lens wear after keratoplasty of keratoconus. Eye Contact Lens 2006;32(4):207–210.
8. Afshari NA, Schirra F, Rapoza PA, et al. Laser in situ keratomileusis outcomes following radial keratotomy, astigmatic keratotomy, photorefractive keratectomy, and penetrating keratoplasty. J Cat Refract Surg 2005;31:2093–2100.
9. Lindahl KJ, Aquavella JV, DePaolis MD, et al. Applications of hydrophilic disposable contact lenses as therapeutic bandages. CLAO J 1991;17:241.
10. Szczotka, LB, Lindsay RG. Contact lens fitting following corneal graft surgery. Clin Exp Optom 2003;86(4):244–249.
11. Zadnik K, Mannis M. Use of the Saturn II lens in keratoconus and corneal transplant patients. Int Contact Lens Clin 1987;14:312.
12. Ward M. Contact lens management after refractive surgery. Contact Lens Spectrum 1996;11(10):23.
13. Weiner B. Contact lens correction of the post-keratoplasty patient. Contact Lens Update 1989;8:61.
14. Daniel R. Fitting contact lenses after keratoplasty. Br J Ophthalmol 1976;60:263.
15. Wicker D, Bleckinger P, Kowalski L, et al. Gaining efficiency in fitting the post-penetrating keratoplasty patient. Contact Lens Spectrum 1997;12:45.
16. Waring GO III, Hannush S, Bogan S, et al. Classification of corneal topography. In: Schanzlin DJ, Robin JB, eds. Corneal Topography: Measuring and Modifying the Cornea. New York: Springer-Verlag, 2992:70–71.
17. McMahon TT, Szczotka-Flynn LB. Contact lens applications for ocular trauma, disease, and surgery. In: Bennett ES, Weissman BA, eds. Clinical Contact Lens Practice. Philadelphia: Lippincott Williams & Wilkins, 2005:549–575.
18. Bendoriene J, Vogt U. Therapeutic use of silicone hydrogel contact lenses in children. Eye Contact Lens 2006;32(2):104–108.
19. Lim N, Vogt U. Comparison of conventional and silicone hydrogel contact lenses for bullous keratoplasty. Eye Contact Lens 2006;32(5):250–253.
20. Ozkurt Y, Rodop O, Oral R, et al. Therapeutic applications of lotrafilcon A silicone hydrogel soft contact lenses. Eye Contact Lens 2005;31(16):268–269.
21. Dumbleton KA, Chalmers RL, McNally J. Effect of lens base curve on/subjective comfort and assessment of fit with silicone hydrogel continuous wear contact lenses. Optom Vis Sci 2002;79(10):633–637.
22. Stapleton F, Stretton S, Papas E. Silicone hydrogel lenses and the ocular surface. Ocular Surface 2006;1:24–43.
23. Pilskalns B, Fink BA, Hill RM. Oxygen demands with hybrid contact lenses. Optom Vis Sci 2007;84(4):334–342.
24. Lindstrom RL, ed. Maximizing success in refractive surgery. Ocular Surg News 1997;Suppl 15(11):5.
25. Sanders DR, Hoffman RF, eds. Refractive Surgery: A Text of Radial Keratotomy. Thorofare, NJ: Slack Publishers, 1985.
26. Vickery JA. Post-RK and the soft lens. Contact Lens Forum 1988;13:34.
27. Salz JJ, Salz JM, Salz M, et al. Ten years' experience with a conservative approach to radial keratotomy. Refractive Corneal Surg 1991;7:12.
28. Szczotka LB. Contact lenses for the irregular cornea. Contact Lens Spectrum 1998;13(6):21.
29. Shivitz IA, Arrowsmith PN, Russell BM. Contact lenses in the treatment of patients with overcorrected radial keratotomy. Ophthalmol 1987;94:899.
30. Aquavella JV, Shovlin JP, Pascucci S, et al. How contact lenses fit into refractive surgery. Rev Ophthalmol 1994;1(12):36.
31. McDonald JE, Mertins A, Deitz D. Contact lens assisted pharmacologically induced keratoshaping. Eye Contact Lens 2004;30(3):122–126.
32. Shipper I, Businger U, Psarrer R. Fitting contact lenses after excimer laser photorefractive keratectomy for myopia. CLAO J 1995;21:281.
33. Kent DG, Solomon KD, Peng Q, et al. Effect of surface photorefractive and laser in situ keratomileusis on the corneal endothelium. J Cataract Refract Surg 1997;23:386.
34. Woodward MA, Randleman JB, Russell B, et al. Visual rehabilitation and outcomes for ectasia after corneal refractive surgery. J Cararact Refract Surg 2008;34:383–388.
35. Key JE. Development of contact lenses and their worldwide use. Eye Contact Lens 2007;33(6):343–345.
36. Pullum KW, Whiting MA, Buckley RJ. Scleral contact lenses: the expanding role. Cornea 2005;24(3):269–277.
37. Sindt C. Classifying and applications of large diameter GP lenses. Contact Lens Spectrum In press (to be published in October 2008 issue).
38. http://www.gpli.info. Accessed March 2008.

CHAPTER 20

Orthokeratology

Marjorie Rah and John Mark Jackson

$\mathbf{I}$t is clear from the success of refractive surgical procedures that patients are very interested in having good vision throughout the day without the need for optical devices such as glasses and contact lenses. Many patients may be wary of having surgery or making a permanent change to their eyes, however, and orthokeratology, the reshaping of the cornea using contact lenses, can be a successful option for many patients.

Orthokeratology (ortho-k) is a temporary correction of myopia and astigmatism using specially designed rigid contact lenses to flatten the central cornea. The effect is similar to that from refractive surgery: by flattening the cornea, the refractive power of the eye is reduced, which makes the eye less myopic. This procedure has also been known by a variety of terms, such as orthofocus, Precision Corneal Molding, Controlled Keratoreformation, Corneal Refractive Therapy, and Vision Shaping Treatment, among others. Ortho-k is still the most widely used term and will likely remain so.

■ ORTHOKERATOLOGY TECHNIQUES

Early Orthokeratology Techniques

Ortho-k has its origins from the early days of polymethylmethacrylate (PMMA) corneal contact lenses. Because the lenses did not allow any oxygen to pass through, clinicians often made their lenses flatter than the cornea to allow more tear exchange under the lens, increasing the available oxygen to the cornea. Clinicians observed that this caused a flattening of the corneal tissue and, usually, "spectacle blur" was the result. Patients noted that their vision was not correct when looking through their glasses for a period of time after removing their contact lenses. Some patients with low myopia reported they saw quite well without any correction at all for some time after removing their lenses.

The first literature reports of this effect were published in the 1950s.[1-3] In 1962, George Jessen published a paper on what he called "orthofocus."[4] This was the first report of a deliberate attempt to mold the cornea to reduce myopia. Jessen later called the technique "orthokeratology." Jessen's method was to use a standard PMMA lens that was flatter than the cornea by the amount of refractive error. If successful, this would flatten the cornea enough to eliminate the myopia. The lens itself had plano power, as the tear film provided all the visual correction. Unfortunately, lenses fitted this flat were very uncomfortable and likely would decenter, creating irregular astigmatism.

Although there were other techniques advocated in the early years of ortho-k, the technique of Grant and May was the most utilized by clinicians.[5] Their method was to use a series of gradually flatter and flatter large-diameter lenses, starting at about 0.12 D to 0.50 D flatter than K. As the cornea flattened, slightly flatter lenses were used until the myopia was reduced to the desired level. This process could take many months.

Proponents of ortho-k published many reports of success, but controlled studies using conventional lens designs were not published until the mid-1970s and early 1980s.[6-11] These studies varied in their design and results, but they all reached very similar conclusions: they found that (a) in general, ortho-k was as safe as standard contact lens fits with PMMA lenses;

(b) reduction in myopia was about 1.00 D on average, although significantly higher amounts were reported; (c) flat-fitting lenses may cause induced with-the-rule and irregular astigmatism; (d) no patient characteristics were found that allowed for prediction of success; (e) improvement in unaided visual acuity did not necessarily match the amount of corneal flattening or the amount of myopia reduced; and (f) the changes were not permanent and required wear of the lenses for some portion of each day to maintain the effect. After these studies were published, orthokeratology was mostly rejected by the eye care community.[12–14] Interest in the procedure did not evaporate completely, and a handful of proponents continued to advocate and refine the fitting techniques over the following years.

Modern Orthokeratology

A major advance in lens design resulted in a resurgence of interest in ortho-k. In contrast to early ortho-k using standard rigid lens designs, the modern procedure uses a completely different lens design known as a reverse geometry (RG) lens. Standard rigid lenses have curves that flatten from center to periphery. When fit flat for ortho-k, there is nothing to prevent the lens from decentering and causing poor results. In contrast, RG lenses are designed such that the secondary curve is *steeper* than the base curve. This secondary curve is often known as the *reverse curve*. The peripheral area of the lens then flattens out again to align with the peripheral cornea; this area is often called the *alignment curve*. These design changes allow the lens to maintain centration, even when the base curve is fit very flat to correct the myopia. RG lens designs also produce much faster results and can treat greater amounts of myopia, on average.

Although the first use of RG lenses was reported in 1972,[15] manufacturing technology at the time made them difficult to produce. Improvements in the RG design and the introduction of computer-driven lathes in the early 1990s led to better ortho-k outcomes.[16,17] The improvement in treatment with the new designs was remarkable enough to lead to the term *accelerated orthokeratology* to denote the use of these lenses and to differentiate it from the original ortho-k procedures. Results were achieved within weeks rather than months, as with the old procedure. There are now numerous contact lens laboratories that manufacture RG lenses and clinicians now have far more lens options for ortho-k (see section on lens designs).

The use of corneal topography also differentiates modern practice from old. Corneal topography is much more useful than keratometry because of the much greater area of the cornea measured. This allows for better lens designs, more accurate prediction of treatment success, and better monitoring of post-treatment effects. Although some RG ortho-k lenses could be fit without the use of a topographer, it would be very difficult to monitor progress of treatment and know how to change lens parameters if treatment is not optimal.

Rigid lens materials with high oxygen permeability (Dk) are now available that allow the ortho-k lenses to be worn during sleep (often referred to as "overnight orthokeratology"). This makes the procedure much more convenient for the patient, as there is no need to wear the ortho-k lens during waking hours. The lens is applied before bedtime and removed in the morning. When optimal results are achieved, the patient has good vision during all waking hours. Overnight wear of any contact lens can increase the risk of complications, and patients must be monitored carefully for any signs of problems related to lens wear.

Recent research supports the clinical observations that RG lenses lead to faster results and higher potential corrections than standard lens designs, particularly with overnight wear.[18–22] In general, these studies show an average treatment of about −2.50 D within 7 to 14 days of treatment, with corrections up to about −4.00 D possible. Preliminary studies of structural changes in the cornea that result from RG lens wear showed mostly central epithelial thinning and midperipheral epithelial thickening,[23] although more recent studies suggest stromal thickening may also play a role.[24,25] In a cat eye model, this change has been shown to be primarily compression rather than loss of cell layers.[26] Helen Swarbrick has conducted an extensive, excellent review of research on ortho-k effects on the cornea for the interested reader.[27]

TABLE 20.1 FDA APPROVAL CRITERIA FOR CRT AND VST

FDA approval for CRT
Up to −6.00 D of myopia
Up to −1.75 D of astigmatism
No age limitations
FDA approval for VST
−1.00 to −5.00 D of myopia
Up to −1.50 D of astigmatism
No age limitations

PATIENT EXPECTATIONS AND SELECTION

Overnight orthokeratology is not for every patient. It is important that the practitioner carefully screens potential candidates for this procedure. Although it is not possible to predict success completely, selecting patients carefully will help to eliminate frustration for both the patient and the doctor. Establishing a realistic goal is important for the success of the procedure. Because the lenses are worn overnight, it is especially important to select patients with no contraindications to overnight contact lens wear. The patient must understand that overnight orthokeratology does not change the cornea permanently and that if treatment is discontinued, myopia will return; however, some patients may be able to wear their ortho-k lenses less than 7 nights per week, whereas others may achieve functional unaided vision for only a few hours after lens removal.

The current Food and Drug Administration (FDA) approvals for overnight orthokeratology are provided in Table 20.1. Although the approvals are for patients with up to −5.00 to −6.00 D of myopia and up to −1.50 to −1.75 D of astigmatism at any axis orientation, the most success will be achieved by initially selecting patients with the lower baseline levels of myopia and with-the-rule astigmatism.

Two very important factors in myopia reduction are the corneal curvature and the asphericity of the cornea. The normal corneal curvature gradually becomes flatter from the center to the periphery and can be described as a prolate ellipsoidal surface. The rate of flattening from center to periphery is known as the corneal eccentricity (denoted by an *e*-value). Spherical surfaces have an *e*-value equal to zero, while *e*-values of elliptical surfaces are <1 but >0. The average eccentricity of the normal cornea is approximately $e = 0.5$. Corneal eccentricity is typically measured using corneal topography.

Efforts have been made to correlate corneal eccentricity to refractive changes or to use baseline corneal eccentricity values as a predictor of success with overnight orthokeratology. The studies have produced mixed results; some found no correlation between eccentricity and refractive changes,[28] whereas others found good correlation between change in apical corneal power and corneal eccentricity[29] or that shape factor (a measure of corneal shape similar to eccentricity) can be a good indicator of refractive changes.[30]

FITTING ORTHOKERATOLOGY LENSES

General Guidelines

Modern orthokeratology practice uses RG lenses almost exclusively. The focus of this section will be a description of basic techniques applicable to most RG lens designs.

To flatten the central cornea and reduce myopia, the base curve of an RG lens is made flatter than the corneal curvature. Exactly how flat is dependent on the lens design, but most make the base curve flatter than the cornea by the amount of treatment desired. This technique is sometimes called the Jessen method as this is how George Jessen chose the base curve for his standard lens "orthofocus" procedure.[4] For example, if the patient's spherical refractive error is −3.00 DS, the base curve radius is made 3.00 D flatter than the flat K reading. Most ortho-k lens design manufacturers will recommend selecting a base curve radius about 0.50 to 0.75 flatter than this value to slightly overcorrect the eye to a low amount of pseudohyperopia. This allows for a slight regression of the effect during the day so that the eye is close to plano by bedtime, allowing clear vision for all waking hours. A nice effect of this is that the tear film provides all the visual correction needed by the eye, and the lens power is close to plano. It should be noted that Mountford[31] argues that selecting the base curve radius in this manner has no scientific basis (see below).

To prevent the lens from decentering with such a flat base curve, the reverse curve steepens back toward the cornea. As the lens approaches the cornea, it then flattens into the alignment curve. The alignment curve aligns with the peripheral cornea, which "steers" the lens to center on the cornea. The lens must center over the pupil to prevent inducement of irregular astigmatism.

The designs of the reverse and alignment curves vary with each manufacturer, but they all work on the same principles. Some use more than one curve in the reverse and alignment areas, leading to so-called four- and five-zone lenses. Clinically, there is little difference in treatment outcome between lens designs.[22] In effect, the reverse and alignment curves control the overall sagittal depth of the lens to position the base curve radius close to the cornea without touching it, at least theoretically, while allowing the lens to center. While the base curve radius is important, the sag depth is more so. A lens with too little sag depth (shallow) will decenter, and a lens with excessive sag depth will provide little or no treatment. Typically, when altering an RG lens, the base curve radius should be left alone and the other parameters changed instead, as they have a greater effect on sag and the base curve radius was chosen to get the desired shape change (when fit with the Jessen method).

Most lenses have a diameter in the 10- to 11-mm range. This helps with centration but is also necessary to accommodate the zones of the lens. As most orthokeratology lenses are worn during sleep, high-Dk materials are used to maximize the oxygen available to the cornea.

A well-fitting RG lens will display a classic "bulls eye" appearance fluorescein pattern, where there is about 4 to 5 mm of central absence of fluorescein ("touch," see below), a ring of fluorescein about 1 mm wide in the midperiphery, alignment in the periphery, and a narrow ring of edge clearance (Fig. 20.1). Once an initial lens is chosen based on appearance, postwear topographic changes are a more useful guide regarding whether the lens parameters are correct to obtain the desired treatment centration and amount. The appearance of the lens in open-eye conditions may not correlate to how the lens performs with the lid closed during sleep.

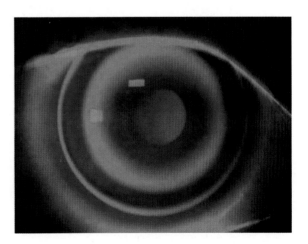

■ **FIGURE 20.1** Photo of reverse geometry lens with ideal fluorescein pattern.

Mountford[31] has written perhaps the most comprehensive mechanical description of how RG lenses achieve their effect. The tear reservoir that is formed under the reverse curve sets up a dramatic difference in tear film thickness between the center of the cornea and the edge of the optical zone of the lens. The tear film is much greater midperipherally than centrally. This creates a pressure gradient in the tear film. In effect, negative pressure is created near the edge of the optical zone that remodels the corneal epithelium. Mountford terms this the *squeeze film force*. This force, combined with lid pressure, creates the topographic shape change of ortho-k: central flattening and midperipheral steepening of the cornea.

Mountford also argues that, in order for ortho-k to work, there must actually be a very thin layer of tears at the corneal apex; the fluid force model provides little to no reshaping force if the lens touches the cornea centrally. A lens that touches centrally would also lose centration. The amount of central clearance is usually on the order of 10 μm (microns). Since fluorescein in the tear film is not visible at tear film thicknesses <20 μm, RG lenses will show an absence of fluorescein centrally, incorrectly interpreted as "touch" of the cornea. Also, within the tear reservoir under the reverse curve, small differences in tear film thickness, not discernible by observing the brightness of the fluorescein, make large differences in shaping forces. These observations have led Mountford and others to conclude that the fluorescein pattern of the lens is not a good indication of whether a lens will provide adequate treatment. An overnight trial and evaluation of postwear topography is a much better method to assess the performance of the lens. Nevertheless, fluorescein evaluation is helpful to evaluate lens centration and in making parameter changes in some lens designs.

Evaluation of postwear topography involves making a comparison of the pre- and postwear patterns. Most topography systems will produce a difference or subtractive map to show changes from one map to the next. The desired difference map pattern will show a circular area of central flattening well centered over the patient's pupil, with a circular area of steepening just beyond this (Fig. 20.2). This is similar to the appearance of a postrefractive surgery map, with the normally prolate corneal shape changed to an oblate shape. This result indicates that the lens has centered well during closed-eye conditions and is providing adequate shaping to continue lens wear. It is useful to compare the axial, tangential, and refractive maps when evaluating treatment centration and size. By moving the cursor of the topographer over the center of

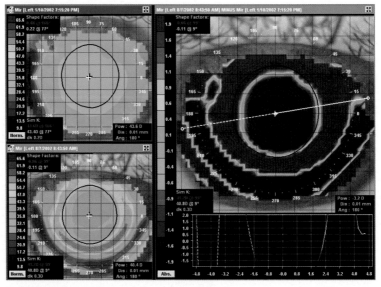

■ **FIGURE 20.2** Well-centered treatment following reverse geometry lens wear. (Courtesy Randy Kojima.)

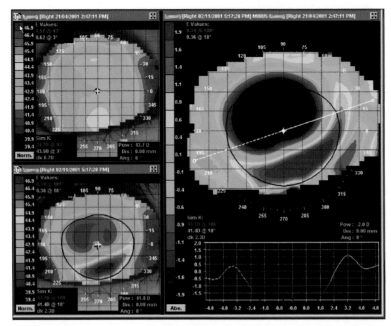

■ **FIGURE 20.3** Superior decentration pattern following wear of shallow sag depth reverse geometry lens. (Courtesy Randy Kojima.)

the treatment area on the difference map, an estimate of the amount of refractive change can be assessed.

Patterns other than centered flattening indicate that the lens fit is not optimal. A lens that has too little sagittal depth will tend to decenter superiorly, creating a flattened area on the topography map that is superior to the pupil, with an arc-shaped area of steepening below it (Fig. 20.3). This may still result in a decrease in the patient's myopia, but the treatment is suboptimal because this combination of treated/untreated pupil area may cause halos or diplopia. The fix for this is to increase the sag depth of the lens by altering the reverse curve(s), alignment curve(s), or both. The exact fix will depend on the lens design being used, and practitioners should refer to the fitting guide provided by the manufacturer.

A lens with excessive sagittal depth will tend to center well or may decenter slightly inferiorly. The classic topography pattern for a deep lens shows a central island, an area of central steepening surrounded by an area of flattening, surrounded again by a ring of steepening (Fig. 20.4). The patient may show no change in refraction or even an increase in myopia because of the central steepening. A slightly inferiorly decentered pattern usually means the sag depth was deep as well. To correct this would be to decrease the sag depth of the lens, again using the manufacturer's guidelines to do so. Other variations of topography patterns are possible, but the patterns presented here are the most common.

Lens Designs

Corneal Refractive Therapy

The Corneal Refractive Therapy (CRT) system (Paragon Vision Sciences, Mesa, AZ) was the first lens design FDA approved for overnight treatment. The fitting process uses a slide-rule-type guide to choose the initial lens and fluorescein analysis to refine the lens parameters.

The clinician finds the patient's flat K and spherical refractive error on the guide and a set of lens parameters is specified for the first lens. This lens is tried on and evaluated. A good lens fit will center well, have 4 to 5 mm of central "touch" (absence of fluorescein), and have edge

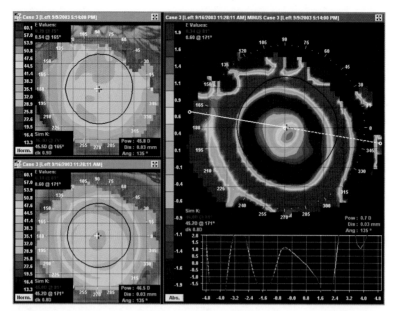

■ **FIGURE 20.4** Central island following wear of deep sag depth reverse geometry lens. (Courtesy Randy Kojima.)

clearance that is about 0.5 mm wide. The lens parameters are changed until an appropriate pattern is found.

The zones of the CRT lens are the treatment zone (base curve), the return zone (reverse curve), and the landing zone (alignment curve). The base curve is chosen by the Jessen method described above with 0.50 D regression factor. The CRT return zone uses a unique sigmoidal (S-shaped) curve. As it is not a simple spherical curve, the return zone is specified by its sag depth. Typical return zone depth (RZD) values are 500, 525, and 550 μm, although others are available in 25-μm steps. A lens with too little sag depth will tend to decenter superiorly, indicating the need to increase to the next deeper RZD (such as from 500 to 525 μm). Conversely, a lens that centers well but has <4 mm of central "touch" indicates the sag depth is too deep and the RZD should be decreased one step.

The landing zone is flat rather than curved and is specified by an angle. Typical landing zone angle (LZA) values are 32, 33, and 34 degrees, available in 1-degree steps. Increasing the LZA will decrease edge clearance, and decreasing it will increase edge clearance. For example, if the lens displays an edge clearance that is wider than 0.5 mm, the LZA should be increased by 1 degree (such as from 33 to 34 degrees). The standard overall diameter is 10.5 mm.

Practitioners have the choice of using a 110-lens fitting set or ordering lenses based on the slide-rule guide. The fitting set is valuable because the practitioner can make immediate changes in parameters to achieve an acceptable fit. Lenses can also be dispensed out of this inventory without having to wait for an ordered lens to arrive. For practitioners new to CRT, it may be more economical to order empirical lenses under warranty for the first few patients. Conversely, having the set on-hand makes the first fits easier to do.

Vision Shaping Treatment

The following lens designs all have FDA clearance for overnight wear under the Bausch & Lomb Vision Shaping Treatment approval.

BE Lens: The BE Retainer system (Precision Technology Services) uses corneal topography data to design the lens. Fluorescein analysis is not used.

The BE system is a lens-design software package and a 24-lens trial set. The patient's topography data and refractive error are entered into the software to design the lens. Necessary topography data include the corneal apical radius, sagittal height, and corneal diameter. The Medmont topographer is recommended for the BE system, in part because it generates a value for sag height, but other topographers can be used. The software also provides a predicted value for maximum possible treatment for the patient's eye; this is useful to determine whether the patient is a good candidate.

The software calculates lens parameters to provide an ideal tear film profile under the lens to obtain the necessary corneal change. This tear film shape provides what is referred to as the *squeeze-film force,* as discussed in the general fitting section. The BE system does not use the Jessen method of base curve calculation, unlike most other designs. Instead, the lens periphery is calculated to provide good lens centration, the alignment curve is chosen to provide the proper tear film thickness in this area, and the base curve is chosen to provide the correct apical tear film thickness. The lens periphery is flat rather than curved, and is designated by its cone angle.

A problem with using topography for lens design is that the corneal data may be incorrect. The trial lens set is used to overcome this problem. The software selects the trial lens that is closest in sag depth to the "ideal" lens based on topography. If the topographer calculated the corneal height correctly, wearing the trial lens overnight should result in the typical well-centered bull's eye of central flattening, although the amount of treatment will likely not be ideal. If this pattern is produced, the "custom" lens can be ordered for the patient. If not, then the topographer miscalculated the corneal sag. Depending on the type of pattern produced, the software adjusts the lens parameters and a new trial is selected. The process is repeated until a well-centered bull's eye is achieved. At this point, the custom lens can be ordered and should give predictable results.

Contex OK E-System: The Contex OK E-System is a reverse geometry lens design that utilizes the corneal eccentricity as a key fitting factor in lens design. The lens is composed of a back optical zone, a steeper reverse zone, one or more alignment curves, and a peripheral curve, which provides edge clearance and tear exchange. Each lens has a designated design code specific to the shape of the cornea and the refraction information of the eye. For example, the design code 44.00/−4.00 (.5 e) refers to a lens design for a cornea with a flat keratometry reading of 44.00 D, a targeted myopia reduction of 4 D, and a corneal eccentricity of 0.5. The base curve radius, overall lens diameter, and lens power are also specified on the lens packaging. The typical overall diameter of a Contex OK E-System lens is 10.6 mm with an optical zone diameter of 6.0 mm. When fitting a patient in the OK E-System lens design, the initial lens can be selected one of three ways:

1. By providing the laboratory with central keratometry readings and the manifest refraction
2. By providing the laboratory with central keratometry readings, the manifest refraction, and corneal topography maps
3. By trial fitting with an inventory fitting set

When a diagnostic fitting set is not used and information is provided to the laboratory for selection of an initial lens, the laboratory uses the average corneal eccentricity, or 0.5, to select the initial lens design. When corneal topography maps are available, the corneal eccentricity value from the map is used for the initial lens design. Fitting from the fitting set is the recommended method.

When troubleshooting the OK E-System design, the corneal eccentricity value is altered to loosen or tighten the lens fit. For instance, if the lens design code is 44.00/−4.00 (.5 e) and the lens is too tight, changing to a lens with a design code of 44.00/−4.00 (.55 e) will loosen the fit while maintaining the same targeted myopia reduction. When adjusting the eccentricity value to alter the fit of the lens, an adjustment of as least 0.05 e (equal to approximately 10 μm) is recommended. If an increase in myopia reduction is needed, the targeted myopia reduction in the design code should be changed. For example, if the patient in this example is undercorrected by 0.50 D, but the topography map and lens fit are ideal, a new lens with a design code of 44.00/−4.50 (.5 e) should be selected. A troubleshooting computer program and troubleshooting forms are available as an aid in clinical practice.

DreamLens: The DreamLens is also a reverse geometry design with a back optical zone, a steep reverse curve, one or more alignment curves, and a peripheral curve for edge clearance and tear exchange. The DreamLens is fitted using the proprietary DreamLens Software program. The program extracts the data from the corneal topography maps and combines the information with the spectacle prescription and the corneal diameter to design the initial lens for the eye. The corneal diameter is used to determine the overall diameter of the lens (10.0, 10.5, or 10.9 mm).

When troubleshooting a DreamLens fit, if the lens is centering inferior or superior to the pupil, changes in the alignment zone(s) are necessary to provide better lens centration. Changes of at least 0.50 D are recommended. Laboratory consultation is available as an aid in clinical practice.

Euclid Systems Corporation: Emerald Design: The Emerald lens is a reverse geometry lens with four zones: the back optic zone, the reverse curve, the alignment curve, and the peripheral curve. When fitting the Emerald lens, the parameters for the initial lens are determined by providing the patient refraction, keratometry measurements, and horizontal visible iris diameter to Euclid Systems. The laboratory will then use computer calculations to design the initial lens to best fit the patient. The standard lens diameters are 10.2, 10.6, and 11.0 mm and are selected based on the horizontal visible iris diameter. A diameter of 10.6 mm is typically recommended for the initial lens. The initial alignment curve is typically designed as equal to the flat keratometry measurement. The base curve radius is calculated based on the flat keratometry reading and the targeted myopia reduction (Jessen method described above) plus an additional 0.75 D. Once the alignment curve and base curve are determined, the reverse curve is calculated by Euclid.

Comment on Lens Designs

This is not an exhaustive list of lens designs for ortho-k. Rather, it is meant to give an overview of the different philosophies of the lens designers. Note that some require some decision making on the part of the practitioner, and some are very proprietary and the laboratory does all the lens design. The decision about which brand to try is up to the practitioner. As mentioned, all the designs can be successfully used and temporarily correct myopia. How easy it is for the practitioner to do so will vary with the brands. It is probably more important for the practitioner to select a method and learn as much as possible about it than to select the "right" brand.

It should also be noted that FDA approval for all these lenses requires that practitioners be "certified" to fit and order the lenses. This is to ensure that clinicians understand the unique fitting characteristics of RG lenses, the underlying concepts of treatment and follow-up, and troubleshooting that inevitably has to occur.

■ FOLLOW-UP CARE

Follow-Up Visits

It is typically recommended that the first follow-up visit occur on the morning following the first night of lens wear. Although not always possible, it is recommended that the patient ideally be examined within a few hours of lens removal. In addition to the 1-day visit, it is recommended that patients be evaluated again at 1 week, 1 month, 3 months, and 6 months following lens dispensing. The basic testing procedures to be conducted at each visit are provided in Table 20.2.

TABLE 20.2 RECOMMENDED TESTING PROCEDURES FOR FOLLOW-UP VISITS

- Entrance visual acuity
- Unaided visual acuity
- Refraction
- Slit-lamp examination
- Corneal topography
- Lens fit evaluation
- Over-refraction

The testing procedures are similar for each follow-up visit. Unaided visual acuity is recorded to monitor the vision and success of the treatment. Biomicroscopy is performed to monitor the ocular health. In addition to these basic procedures, corneal topography is critical for assessing the progress of treatment. If the patient's vision is unacceptable or slit-lamp signs are noted, corneal topography can be helpful in determining the cause. As mentioned previously, lenses with too little or excessive sagittal depth produce characteristic topography patterns, which can be used in addition to evaluating the lens fit on the eye to improve success. Lastly, an over-refraction will determine whether the base curve radius is appropriate. If minus power is detected in the over-refraction, the base curve radius should be flattened to fully correct the patient's distance refractive error.

Complications

As with any contact lens modality, complications are of concern with orthokeratology. There have been several reports of microbial keratitis associated with overnight orthokeratology.[32,33] The majority of reported cases were from Asian countries, predominantly China, Taiwan, and Hong Kong. Most of the cases were children between the ages of 9 and 15 years or young adults between the ages of 16 and 25 years. When interpreting these statistics, it is important to keep in mind that they do not necessarily indicate that patients in Asian countries or patients in the age ranges mentioned are more susceptible to infections. It could simply reflect the populations most likely to be fitted with overnight orthokeratology lenses.

The causative agent is also important in determining the appropriate treatment. In the cases mentioned above, *Pseudomonas aeruginosa* was the offending agent in most of the cases. The second most often noted was *Acanthamoeba*. Because there is a wide range of possible microorganisms that can be present, it is important to obtain a corneal culture before initiation of treatment.

The old adage, "an ounce of prevention is worth a pound of cure," is very appropriate when fitting any type of contact lenses, but especially with overnight orthokeratology. Education of patients regarding hygiene, proper cleaning techniques, and appropriate wearing times helps to reduce the risks of complications. In particular, given the number of cases of *Acanthamoeba* keratitis, patients should be firmly instructed to avoid any tap water coming in contact with the lenses and lens case.[34] Regular follow-up appointments that include similar education are also essential.

■ SUMMARY

A major advance in lens design, specifically the availability of custom-designed reverse geometry gas-permeable lenses, resulted in a resurgence of interest in ortho-k. The advanced manufacturing techniques in combination with corneal topography have improved the success of orthokeratology and brought it back into the mainstream of optometric practice. Higher amounts of myopia can be treated with the newer lens designs and materials available. Further research is still necessary to answer questions regarding topics such as the mechanism of action and the possibility of slowing myopia progression; however, orthokeratology is a viable option for many patients.

■ CLINICAL CASES

CASE 1

A 12-year-old Asian male presented to the New England Eye Institute interested in overnight contact lens corneal reshaping. A pretreatment manifest refraction of −4.25D sphere in the right eye and −4.25D − 0.50 × 150 in the left eye was obtained. Corrected Snellen visual acuity was 20/20 in each eye. Baseline keratometry readings were 44.00/44.75 @ 090 with clear and regular mires in the right eye and 43.50/44.75 @ 090 with clear and regular mires in the left eye. Baseline topography is observed in the top two maps of Figure 20.5.

SOLUTION: The patient was fitted with DreamLens design lenses with a 10.6-mm overall diameter.

At the 1-week follow-up appointment, the refraction was +0.25D sphere in the right eye and −0.25D sphere in the left eye, both corrected to 20/20. Unaided visual acuities were 20/20 in each eye; however, the treatment zone was decentered laterally (see Fig. 20.5, bottom images). At the 2-week follow-up appointment, the refraction was plano in the right eye and +0.50D sphere in the left eye, both corrected to 20/20. Unaided visual acuities in each eye were 20/20. Although the patient did not initially have visual complaints resulting from the decentered treatment zone, lenses with a larger diameter (11.0 mm) were ordered. This adjustment improved the centration of the treatment zone and the patient noticed an appreciable improvement in his vision. The final topography maps are provided in the bottom two maps of Figure 20.6.

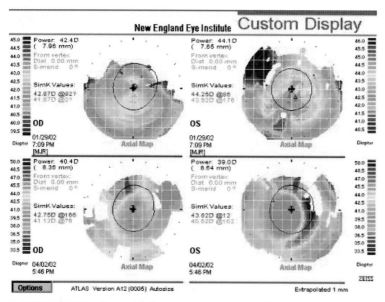

■ **FIGURE 20.5** Baseline and follow-up topography maps for the patient in Case 1 showing a decentered treatment zone. The top images represent the baseline corneal curvature and the lower images represent the corneal curvature after wearing the smaller-diameter lenses.

CASE 2

A 24-year-old Caucasian male presented for an annual contact lens examination. He complained that his eyes felt dry with his daily-wear disposable soft lenses.

SOLUTION: The option of contact lens corneal reshaping was discussed with the patient and he elected to try the procedure. Baseline manifest refraction was −2.50 DS corrected to 20/15 in each eye. Baseline simulated keratometry values were 44.62/44.50@090 OD and 44.62/44.00@122 OS. Baseline corneal topography maps are shown in the upper left of Figures 20.7 and 20.8.

The CRT lens design was chosen for this patient. The initial parameters from the slide rule were OD 8.2 mm base curve, 550 RZD, 34-degree LZA, 10.5 mm diameter; and OS 8.1 mm base curve, 550 RZD, 33-degree LZA, 10.5 mm diameter. The OD lens provided good centration over the pupil, 4-mm central "touch," and edge clearance of about 0.5 mm. The OS provided good centration, 4-mm central "touch," and excessive edge clearance. The parameters were left alone for the OD and the LZA was changed to 34 degrees for the OS to decrease the edge clearance. His visual acuity with the lenses was 20/20 in each eye. The patient was taught insertion, removal, and care of the lenses. He was instructed to wear them that night and return at 8 o'clock the following morning with the lenses in place.

When he returned, the patient reported no problems sleeping with the lenses in place. He used rewetting drops when he awoke and the lenses were moving freely when he arrived. After lens removal, corneal topography showed a well-centered treatment area in each eye and manifest refraction was −1.00 DS in each eye. Each cornea was quiet with no staining. He was given a pair of soft lenses of −1.25 DS power to wear for the first few days as needed until the full effect was obtained.

At his 1-week follow-up, unaided visual acuity was 20/20 in each eye. Topography maps again showed good treatment centration and he reported he could maintain the acuity for most waking hours. He noted it took about 4 days before he noticed his vision was stable most of the day. His 2-week topographies are shown in Figures 20.7 and 20.8. The patient was pleased with the results.

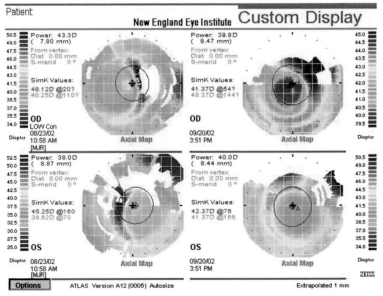

■ **FIGURE 20.6** Topography maps for the patient in Case 1 depicting the better-centered treatment zone after increasing the overall diameter of the reverse geometry lens. The right images depict the corneal curvature after wearing the smaller-diameter lenses. The left images depict the corneal curvature after wearing the larger-diameter lenses.

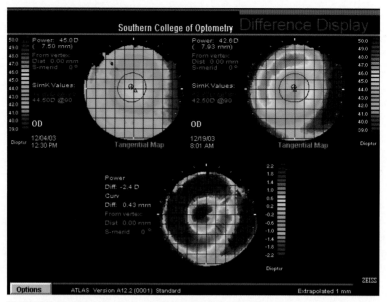

■ **FIGURE 20.7** Right eye 2-week CRT topography map for Case 2.

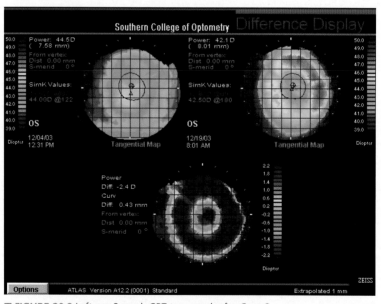

■ **FIGURE 20.8** Left eye 2-week CRT topography for Case 2.

CLINICAL PROFICIENCY CHECKLIST

■ Orthokeratology is a temporary correction of myopia and astigmatism using specially designed rigid contact lenses to flatten the central cornea.

■ Modern orthokeratology utilizes reverse geometry gas-permeable contact lenses, which have a secondary curve steeper than the base curve. This has resulted in greater refractive error reduction in a shorter period of time compared to earlier designs.

■ Corneal topography is much more useful than keratometry in evaluating the corneal changes because it enables the practitioner to measure a much greater area of the cornea.

■ The FDA-approved treatment range is up to −5.00 or −6.00 D of myopia and up to −1.50 or −1.75 D of astigmatism, depending on the lens design.

■ A well-fitting RG lens will display a classic "bull's eye" appearance fluorescein pattern, where there is about 4 to 5 mm of central absence of fluorescein ("touch"), a ring of fluorescein about 1 mm wide in the midperiphery, alignment in the periphery, and a narrow ring of edge clearance.

■ The performance of the lens on-eye after wearing overnight is more important than the fluorescein appearance of the lens, and must be assessed with a corneal topography difference map.

REFERENCES

1. Morrison RJ. Contact lenses and the progression of myopia. J Am Optom Assoc 1957;28:711–713.
2. Bier N. Myopia controlled by contact lenses. Optician 1958;135:427.
3. Carlson JJ. Basic factors in checking the progression of myopia. Opt J Rev Optom 1958;95(19):37–42.
4. Jessen GN. Orthofocus techniques. Contacto 1962;6(7):200–204.
5. Grant SC, May Ch. Orthokeratology control of refractive errors through contact lenses. J Am Optom Assoc 1971;42:345–359.
6. Kerns R. Research in orthokeratology. Part I: introduction and background. J Am Optom Assoc 1976;47: 1047–1051.
7. Kerns R. Research in orthokeratology. Part III: results and conclusions. J Am Optom Assoc 1976;47(8):1505–1515.
8. Binder PS, May CH, Grant SC. An evaluation of orthokeratology. Ophthalmology 1980;87(8):729–744.
9. Polse KA, Brand RJ, Schwalbe JS, et al. The Berkeley orthokeratology study, part II: efficacy and duration. Am J Optom Physiol Opt 1983;60(3):187–198.
10. Polse KA, Brand RJ, Keener RJ, et al. The Berkeley orthokeratology study, part III: safety. Am J Optom Physiol Opt 1983;60(4):321–328.
11. Coon LJ. Orthokeratology, part II: evaluating the Tabb method. J Am Optom Assoc 1984;55(6):409–418.
12. Polse KA. Orthokeratology as a clinical procedure (editorial). Am J Optom Physiol Opt 1977;54(6):345–346.
13. Eger MJ. Orthokeratology - fact or fiction (editorial). J Am Optom Assoc 1975;46(7):682–683.
14. Safir A. Orthokeratology, II. A risky and unpredictable "treatment" for a benign condition. Surv Ophthalmol 1980;24(5):291–302.
15. Fontana AA. Orthokeratology using the one piece bifocal. Contacto 1972;16(6):45–47.
16. Wlodyga RG, Bryla C. Corneal molding: the easy way. Contact Lens Spectrum 1989;4(8):58–65.
17. Harris HD, Stoyan N. A new approach to orthokeratology. Contact Lens Spectrum 1992;7(4):37–39.
18. Mountford J. An analysis of the changes in corneal shape and refractive error induced by accelerated orthokeratology. Int Contact Lens Clin 1997;24:128–143.
19. Lui WO, Edwards MH. Orthokeratology in low myopia. Part I: efficacy and predictability. Contact Lens Anterior Eye 2000;23(3):77–89.
20. Nichols JJ, Marsich MM, Nguyen M, et al. Overnight orthokeratology. Optom Vis Sci 2000;77:252–259.
21. Rah MJ, Jackson JM, Jones LA, et al. Overnight orthokeratology: preliminary results from the Lenses and Overnight Orthokeratology (LOOK) study. Optom Vis Sci 2002;79:598–605.
22. Tahhan N, Du Toit R, Papas E, et al. Comparison of reverse-geometry lens designs for overnight orthokeratology. Optom Vis Sci 2003;80:796–804.
23. Swarbrick HA, Wong G, O'Leary DJ. Corneal response to orthokeratology. Optom Vis Sci 1998;75:791–799.
24. Alharbi A, Swarbrick HA. The effects of overnight orthokeratology lens wear on corneal thickness. Invest Ophthalm Vis Sci 2003;44:2518–2523.

25. Alharbi A, La Hood D, Swarbrick HA. Overnight orthokeratology lens wear can inhibit the central stromal edema response. Invest Ophthalm Vis Sci 2005;46:2334–2340.

26. Choo JD, Caroline PJ, Harlin DD, et al. Morphological changes in cat epithelium following overnight lens wear with the Paragon CRT lens for corneal reshaping. ARVO abstract. Invest Ophthalm Vis Sci 2004;45:E-abstract 1552.

27. Swarbrick HA. Orthokeratology review and update. Clin Exp Optom 2006;89:124–143.

28. Joe JJ, Marsden HJ, Edrington TB. The relationship between corneal eccentricity and improvement in visual acuity with orthokeratology. J Am Optom Assoc 1996;67(2):87–97.

29. Mountford J. An analysis of the changes in corneal shape and refractive error induced by accelerated orthokeratology. Int Contact Lens Clin 1997;24:128–143.

30. El Hage SG, Leach NE, Colliac JP, et al. Controlled Kerato-Reformation (CKR): an alternative to refractive surgery. Presented at the American Academy of Optometry, New Orleans, LA, 1995.

31. Mountford J. Design variables and fitting philosophies of reverse geometry lenses. In: Mountford J, Ruston D, Dave T, eds. Orthokeratology—Principles and Practice. London: Butterworth-Heinemann, 2004.

32. Watt K, Swarbrick HA. Microbial keratitis in overnight orthokeratology: review of the first 50 cases. Eye Contact Lens 2005;31(5):201–208.

33. Watt KG, Boneham GC, Swarbrick HA. Microbial keratitis in orthokeratology: the Australian experience. Clin Exp Optom 2007;90(3):188–189.

34. Walline JJ, Holden BA, Bullimore MA, et al. The current state of corneal reshaping. Eye Contact Lens 2005; 31(5):209–214.

Management of Contact Lens-Associated or Lens-Induced Pathology

Ron Melton and Randall Thomas

▓ INTRODUCTION

Many contact lens wearers experience years of successful wear with no complications associated with or induced by contact lens wear. However, contact lens wearers can experience ocular complications that are related to the type of lens, the wearing schedule, the solutions they are using or not using, self-inoculation of bacteria from handling of the lens, the case or expired solution, deposits on the lens, hypoxia from the lens, a foreign body trapped by the lens, or something totally nonrelated to contact lens wear, such as lid disease, dry eyes, and nonrelated anterior segment disease. This chapter will address ophthalmic pharmaceuticals that can help restore afflicted tissues to normal.

▓ ANTIBIOTICS

Antibiotics can be overused with the contact lens patient. As red eyes are more likely to be inflammatory than infectious, prescribing an antibiotic only because the practitioner is unsure of the diagnosis of the red eye does not justify its use. The most common symptom/clinical sign to warrant antibiotic use is an acute mucopurulent discharge. However, there are conditions in contact lens wear that require antibiotic treatment. The most common contact lens-associated complications that require the use of antibiotics are infectious keratitis (corneal ulcers), corneal abrasion, bacterial conjunctivitis, blepharitis, and hordeola.

Sodium Sulfacetamide

Sulfa drugs are bacteriostatic, meaning they interfere with bacterial replication, in this case by inhibiting folic acid production. Sulfa drugs are broad spectrum; however, many staphylococcal and *Pseudomonas* species are resistant to them. In addition, many patients are allergic to sulfa drugs. Sulfa drugs are available in both solution (10%, 15%, and 30%) and ointment (10%) forms. These drugs are produced by various companies. Because of the bacterial resistance and allergic reactions, sulfa drugs are rarely used by eye care practitioners to treat contact lens patients.

Bacitracin

Bacitracin is bacteriocidal, meaning it kills the bacteria. It achieves this by destroying the cell wall of the bacteria. Primarily, it is most effective against gram-positive bacteria. Bacitracin is available only in ointment form. It is most effective in treating moderate to advanced staphylococcal blepharitis in combination with aggressive lid hygiene. The recommended treatment regimen for bacitracin would be to prescribe it 1 to 2 weeks to be used on the lid margins at bedtime.

Bacitracin and Polymyxin B

A combination of bacitracin and polymyxin B provides the excellent gram-positive effect of bacitracin with the potency of polymyxin B on gram-negative organisms (including *Pseudomonas*). Polymyxin B is bacteriocidal by destroying cell membranes. It is marketed under the name Polysporin (Monarch Pharmaceuticals) and is available in generic forms as an ointment in the United States. Adverse reactions, such as allergy, toxic reactions, and resistance, are uncommon. It is beneficial in treating staphylococcal blepharitis when used at bedtime for 2 weeks in combination with lid hygiene (i.e., lid scrubs before applying the ointment). In addition, Polysporin, in combination with another antibiotic drop during the day, could be used in hyperacute bacterial infections and bacterial keratitis.

Bacitracin, Polymyxin B, and Neomycin

The combination of bacitracin (or gramicidin), polymyxin B, and neomycin is marketed generically and under the name of Neosporin (Monarch Pharmaceuticals). Neomycin, an aminoglycoside, is a broad-spectrum antibiotic that inhibits protein synthesis. Neomycin is not effective against *Pseudomonas*, which is why the polymyxin B is included. Neomycin is prone to hypersensitivity reactions, which can occur within 5 to 10 days or 12 to 72 hours, depending on whether the patient has been previously sensitized. When a reaction occurs, the symptoms can consist of injection of the lids and conjunctiva, mild edema of the eyelids, and superficial punctate keratitis (SPK). The reaction is treated simply by discontinuing the drug. Neosporin is available in solution and ointment forms. Neosporin is rarely used as an ophthalmic drug because of the potential for a hypersensitivity reaction.

Trimethoprim with Polymyxin B

Trimethoprim with polymyxin B is marketed generically and as Polytrim (Allergan). Trimethoprim is bacteriostatic by interfering with folic acid production. It is active against common gram-positive and gram-negative organisms with the exception of *Pseudomonas*, which is why it is combined with polymyxin B. It is available as a solution and is effective for bacterial conjunctivitis, as adverse effects are rare. When treating a bacterial conjunctivitis, it is recommended that one drop be instilled every 2 hours for 2 days, then four times a day (q.i.d.) for 5 more days.

Chloramphenicol

Chloramphenicol is marketed generically by various manufacturers as a solution (0.5%) or as an ointment (1%). Its mechanism of action is bacteriostatic by inhibiting protein synthesis. It is broad spectrum in activity, but it is not effective against *Pseudomonas*. Although it is used in Europe and Australia, it is minimally used in the United States because of reports of aplastic anemia as an adverse effect. Even topical doses, in some individuals, might result in bone marrow aplasia, making it a legal liability to use when there are other alternatives.[1]

Erythromycin

Erythromycin is bacteriostatic by inhibiting bacterial protein synthesis. It is only available topically in ointment form (0.5%) and is available from various generic manufacturers. It is effective against many gram-positive and some gram-negative organisms; however, staphylococcal bacteria may develop resistance over a few days. This prohibits its use in long-term treatment; however, it is an effective drug for prophylactic use in the management of corneal abrasion or other forms of corneal compromise. It provides gentle lubrication and antibacterial cover for compromised epithelial tissues.

Azithromycin

Azithromycin is available as a 1% ophthalmic solution with the name AzaSite, manufactured by InSite Vision and licensed to Inspire Pharmaceuticals, Inc. Orally, azithromycin is known as Zithromax, which comes as Z-Pak, Tri-Pak, and Zmax, an extended-release, 2,000-mg oral suspension. Azithromycin is a macrolide, like erythromycin, and inhibits bacterial protein synthesis. Patients who have experienced an allergy to erythromycin should avoid using azithromycin. The benefits of this drug ophthalmically are yet to be determined via widespread clinical use, but initially it may be useful for bacterial conjunctivitis in pediatric patients and mild to moderate cases of bacterial conjunctivitis in adults.

Gentamicin and Tobramycin

Gentamicin and tobramycin are aminoglycosides that are bactericidal by inhibiting protein synthesis. They are effective against gram-negative and gram-positive organisms, although they are most effective against gram-negative organisms, including *Pseudomonas*. Both are available in solution (0.3%) and ointment (0.3%) forms by various manufacturers, including Genoptic (Allergan) and Tobrex (Alcon), and generic forms. Gentamicin and tobramycin are very effective drugs and carry a very minimal risk of toxicity or allergic reaction. The symptoms of this reaction would be similar to neomycin with conjunctival injection, edema of the lid, and SPK. Typically, any reaction occurs after use longer than 1 to 2 weeks. Both gentamicin and tobramycin are effective choices to treat bacterial infections when treatment is going to be brief and, because of the available generic forms, reduced patient cost is important. A typical treatment regimen for these antibiotics would be to use one drop q.i.d. for 7 days.

Fluoroquinolones

Since the introduction of fluoroquinolones, the effectiveness of these pharmaceuticals has led to a near dominance of use by practitioners for bacterial infections, especially when the cornea is involved. Ocular fluoroquinolones are Ciloxan (0.3% Alcon and generic), Ocuflox (0.3% Allergan and generic), Quixin (0.5% Vistakon Pharmaceuticals), Vigamox (0.5% Alcon), Zymar (0.3% Allergan), and Iquix (1.5% Vistakon Pharmaceuticals). There could be a debate pertaining to the overuse of fluoroquinolones, when other antibiotics like Polytrim and tobramycin might be equally effective. A fluoroquinolone is useful to provide rapid treatment with minimal risk of toxicity. Fluoroquinolones work by inhibiting DNA synthesis.[2] They are less toxic and more effective against gram-positive bacteria than aminoglycosides. Vigamox and Zymar perform more effectively against some gram-positive bacteria than the other fluoroquinolones. Vigamox is preservative free compared to Zymar, which is benzalkonium chloride (BAK) preserved and, along with enhanced penetration, results in often being the preferred drug.[3,4] The fluoroquinolones are all available in solution form, and Ciloxan is also available in an ointment. Use of fluoroquinolones is usually reserved for moderate to severe infections. Table 21.1 provides the dosing frequency. Antibiotics should never be tapered to less than four times a day, as this could result in resistance.

TABLE 21.1 DOSING FREQUENCY FOR FLUOROQUINOLONES

Bacterial conjunctivitis	Every 2 hr until controlled and then four times a day for 4–6 d
Bacterial keratitis	Every 15 min for the first several hours, then hourly until night for 2–4 d. Use Polysporin ointment at night until controlled, then discontinue the ointment and reduce the drops to every 2 hr for 4 d and then four times a day for 4–7 more d.

TABLE 21.2 TOPICAL ANTIBIOTICS AND ANTIBIOTIC/STEROID COMBINATIONS

GENERIC NAME	BRAND NAME	MANUFACTURER	FORM	SIZE
Topical antibiotics				
Sodium sulfacetamide	N/A	Generic	Solution	15 mL
Bacitracin		Generic	Unguent	3.5 g/3.75 g
Bacitracin/polymyxin B	Polysporin	Monarch/generic	Unguent	3.5 g
Bacitracin/polymyxin B/neomycin	Neosporin	Monarch/generic	Solution/unguent	10 mL/3.5 g
Trimethoprim/polymyxin B	Polytrim	Allergan/generic	Solution	10 mL
Chloramphenicol		Numerous	Solution/unguent	
Erythromycin 0.5%	Ilotycin	Dista/Generic	Unguent	3.5 g
Azithromycin 1%	AzaSite	Inspire Pharm.	Solution	2.5 mL
Gentamicin 0.3%	Genoptic	Allergan/Generic	Solution/unguent	5 mL/3.5 g
Tobramycin 0.3%	Tobrex	Alcon/Generic	Solution/unguent	5 mL/3.5 g
Ciprofloxacin 0.3%	Ciloxan	Alcon/Generic	Solution/unguent	2.5 mL/5 mL/10mL/3.5 g
Ofloxacin 0.3%	Ocuflox	Allergan/Generic	Solution	5 mL/10 mL
Levofloxacin 0.5%	Quixin	Vistakon Pharm.	Solution	2.5 mL/5 mL
Moxifloxacin 0.5%	Vigamox	Alcon	Solution	3 mL
Gatifloxacin 0.3%	Zymar	Allergan	Solution	2.5 mL/5 mL
Levofloxacin 1.5%	Iquix	Vistakon Pharm.	Solution	5 mL
Antibiotic/steroid combination				
Gentamicin/prednisolone	Pred-G	Allergan	Suspension/unguent	2.5 mL/5 mL/10 mL/3.5 g
Tobramycin/dexamethasone	TobraDex	Alcon	Suspension/unguent	2.5 mL/5 mL/10 mL/3.5 g
Tobramycin/loteprednol	Zylet	Bausch & Lomb	Suspension	2.5 mL/5 mL/10 mL

Combination Antibiotic/Steroid Preparations

Common aminoglycoside-steroid combination drugs include Zylet (tobramycin and loteprednol) and TobraDex (tobramycin and dexamethasone). These combination drugs can be useful when there is a bacterial infection or epithelial disruption combined with inflammation, such as rosacea, vascularized limbal keratitis (VLK), contact lens-induced acute red eye (CLARE), phlyctenular keratoconjunctivitis, noninfectious keratitis, herpes zoster with ocular involvement, and staphylococcal blepharitis.[5] These drugs should never be tapered below q.i.d. as this creates subtherapeutic levels of the antibiotic, which may cause antibiotic resistance. The section in this chapter pertaining to corticosteroids should be reviewed for a more complete understanding of this class of drugs. Table 21.2 provides a summary of the antibiotics covered in this section. Ocular conditions and the recommended antibiotic therapy are provided in Table 21.3.

■ ALLERGY MEDICATIONS

The incidence of allergies is on the rise; therefore, practitioners must be prepared to effectively treat ocular allergies.[6] Unfortunately, patients sometimes resort to over-the-counter drops that

TABLE 21.3 OCULAR CONDITIONS AND RECOMMENDED TREATMENT

OCULAR CONDITION	ANTIBIOTIC
Staphylococcal blepharitis	Bacitracin/Polysporin/TobraDex ointments
Acute eyelid infection	Bacitracin/tobramycin/erythromycin ($\pm$ oral medications)
Bacterial conjunctivitis	Aminoglycoside or fluoroquinolone
Corneal abrasion	Fluoroquinolone or aminoglycoside drops with ointment at night, nonsteroidal anti-inflammatory drug (NSAID) for pain, cycloplegic agent
Vascularized limbal keratitis, contact lens-induced acute red eye	Antibiotic/steroid combination such as Zylet or TobraDex
Corneal ulcer	Fluoroquinolone drops with ointment at night

"get the red out" without seeing an eye doctor. The symptoms of ocular allergy (redness and itching) should be evaluated to make sure that other forms of ocular disease, such as dry eyes or solution sensitivity, are not the cause. Patients manifesting dry eyes may experience itching and burning; therefore, tear film dysfunction should be ruled out initially. If patients are using a preserved contact lens care regimen, changing them to a nonpreserved system (i.e., hydrogen peroxide) to determine if that eliminates the symptoms should be attempted. Other helpful tips would include removing the offending source, frequent hand washing, use of cold compresses, refrigerating drops, and discouraging eye rubbing, which causes degranulation of mast cells, thus continuing the allergic cycle. Hair washing at night, before sleeping, has been found to help prevent irritants (pollutants, dirt, etc.) from being released onto the pillow, decreasing ocular allergies.[6]

If allergic conjunctivitis is the diagnosis, then antihistamine/mast cell stabilizers may be prescribed. There are four antihistamine/mast cell stabilizers: Elestat (Allergan), Optivar (MedPointe), and Patanol and Pataday (Alcon). Ketotifen 0.025% is available over the counter as Zaditor (Novartis), Alaway (Bausch & Lomb), and Refresh (Allergan). With the exception of Pataday, which is once-a-day (q.d.) dosage, the other medications are used twice a day (b.i.d.), morning and night. With the medications used twice a day, after the first 2 weeks, many patients can decrease to a maintenance dose of once a day.

Emadine (Alcon) is an antihistamine drop that can be used for ocular allergy; however, it may be more useful for lid myokymia (lid twitch). The dosage for this is q.i.d. for 2 weeks followed by b.i.d. for 1 to 2 weeks.

For patients experiencing ocular allergy with clinical inflammation, a topical steroid such as Alrex (Bausch & Lomb) or FML (Allergan) used every 2 hours for 2 days, then every 4 hours for a week, then once or twice a day for several more days to weeks, is beneficial. If the inflammation is more severe, Lotemax (Bausch & Lomb) can be used.

Mast cell stabilizers such as Alamast (Vistakon) and Alocril (Allergan) are best used as a maintenance drug than a treatment for acute allergy. First-generation mast cell stabilizers like Crolom, Opticrom, and Alomide have become relatively obsolete since the new formulations became available. When patients are aware of the trigger to their ocular allergy and realize that they will be exposed to the trigger, such as exposure to cats, use of a mast cell stabilizer used q.i.d. 1 week in advance can minimize or eliminate the allergic reaction. Mast cell stabilizers are safe to use for long periods of time, weeks to months. The various topical allergy drops are listed in Table 21.4.

For contact lens wearers, antihistamine/mast cell stabilizers can be used a few minutes before insertion and again after contact lens removal. If necessary, the drop can be instilled on top of the contact lens; however, preservative incompatibility may be an issue. For those contact lens wearers who experience seasonal ocular allergies, use of Lotemax with an antihistamine/mast cell stabilizer morning and evening, before and after contact lens wear, then decreasing the Lotemax to evening use only, will aid the patient in surviving the allergy season.

TABLE 21.4 TOPICAL ALLERGY DROPS

GENERIC NAME	BRAND NAME	MANUFACTURER	SIZE
Antihistamine/mast cell stabilizers			
Epinastine HCl 0.05%	Elestat	Allergan	5 mL
Azelastine hydrochloride 0.05%	Optivar	Med Pointe	6 mL
Olopatadine hydrochloride 0.1% and 0.2%	Patanol/Pataday	Alcon	2.5 mL/5 mL
Ketotifen fumarate 0.025%	Zaditor (OTC)	Novartis	5 mL
	Alaway (OTC)	Bausch & Lomb	
	Refresh (OTC)	Allergan	
Antihistamine			
Emedastine difumarate 0.05%	Emadine	Alcon	5 mL
Mast cell stabilizers			
Pemirolast potassium 0.1%	Alamast	Vistakon Pharmaceuticals	10 mL
Nedocromil sodium 4%	Alocril	Allergan	5 mL

OTC, over the counter.

See NSAIDs and Corticosteroids for Acular and Alrex.

Giant papillary conjunctivitis (GPC) is discussed in Chapter 13. Discontinuing contact lenses is warranted in severe cases; however, using nonpreserved solutions, new contact lenses (daily disposable contact lenses are very beneficial), and an antihistamine/mast cell stabilizer once or twice a day will benefit most patients. In very severe cases, where lenses are not discontinued, prescribing steroid use until the patient is stabilized and the tarsal conjunctiva has returned to a more normal looking appearance, followed by prescribing an antihistamine/mast cell stabilizer or mast cell stabilizer while tapering the steroid, is helpful.

Contact dermatitis may be caused by an environmental irritant or an allergic response. In either case, removal of the irritant, cold compresses, a topical steroid cream (such as 0.1% triamcinolone) applied around the lids (but not in the eye), and/or a systemic antihistamine will provide relief. In most cases, removing the irritant and use of cold compresses will be therapy enough. Severe cases may require the addition of the steroid cream (i.e., 0.1% triamcinolone) and/or the oral antihistamine (i.e., Benadryl). The allergic response with the recommended medications is provided in Table 21.5.

■ CORTICOSTEROIDS

General Information

The inflammatory process is the result of infectious, allergic, or traumatic factors, which cause the tissue to release prostaglandins as mediators of the response. Adverse effects of the inflammatory response may be mitigated by use of pharmaceutical agents, such as corticosteroids.

TABLE 21.5 SUMMARY OF ALLERGY TREATMENTS

ALLERGIC RESPONSE	MEDICATION
Allergic conjunctivitis	Antihistamine/mast cell stabilizer combination
Allergy with inflammation	Alrex/FML/Lotemax
Giant papillary conjunctivitis	Antihistamine/mast cell stabilizer combination

To better understand how anti-inflammatory agents are effective, it is useful to understand what occurs during the inflammatory process. When infections, allergy, or trauma affect the tissue, phospholipids are released from the cell membrane. These phospholipids convert to arachidonic acid. Arachidonic acid is converted to prostaglandins or leukotrienes via one of two enzymes, either cyclooxygenase or lipoxygenase. Corticosteroids inhibit phospholipid conversion to arachidonic acid; thus, corticosteroids work early in the inflammatory process. Nonsteroidal anti-inflammatory drugs (NSAIDs; which will be discussed in the next section) exhibit their effect further in the pathway to inhibit cyclooxygenase, which converts arachidonic acid to prostaglandins. NSAIDs do not affect the production of leukotrienes; thus, this limits their use in treating inflammatory processes.[2,7,8]

Corticosteroids' ability to suppress inflammation is based on their potency and bioavailability. The most commonly used ophthalmic corticosteroids are loteprednol, prednisolone, dexamethasone, fluorometholones and rimexolone. Loteprednol and prednisolone are most effective clinically. An important factor in treatment with corticosteroids is the frequency of instillation, which varies with the nature and the severity of the condition. High doses of topical steroids for brief periods of time (typically several days) are usually safe and effective. The treatment regimen should be customized for each case depending on the severity. A summary of corticosteroid medications in use today is found in Table 21.6.

The treatment regimen for corticosteroids almost always concludes with an interval of tapering. There are two reasons for the need to taper the patient off of this medication. First, the body produces natural steroids. When synthetic steroids are given, the body slows down production of natural steroids. By tapering the steroid, the body is given the opportunity to produce the appropriate amount of natural steroids again, without leaving the body momentarily with low levels of natural steroids. The second reason for tapering steroids is that a rebound effect can occur. The inflammatory process in the body is being inhibited by the synthetic steroids, and abrupt discontinuation of the steroid may allow the inflammation to rebound. Once the inflammation is controlled, the steroid use should be reduced by one-half for a few days, and then perhaps half again for a few more days. Such a tapering schedule will vary considerably from patient to patient.[9]

Regarding traumatic corneal abrasions, re-epithelialization should occur before steroid use in most cases. This is not the case when stromal inflammation is inhibiting re-epithelialization or the corneal epithelium is compromised by something other than an infectious agent (i.e., a welder's flash). In these cases, a combination antibiotic-steroid or a steroid in combination with a separate antibiotic may be prescribed.

Side effects from steroid use are less likely to occur with topical than with systemic steroids, but may include posterior subcapsular cataracts, increased intraocular pressure (IOP), retarding corneal wound healing, mydriasis, and ptosis.[2] Generally, these side effects are rare, and

TABLE 21.6 TOPICAL CORTICOSTEROID DRUGS

GENERIC NAME	BRAND NAME	MANUFACTURER	FORM	SIZE
Loteprednol etabonate	Alrex 0.2% Lotemax 0.5%	Bausch & Lomb	Suspension	5 mL/10 mL/ 15 mL
Prednisolone	Pred Forte	Allergan/Generic	Suspension	1 mL/5 mL/ 10 mL/15 mL
Dexamethasone	Maxidex/Decadron	Alcon/Merck	Suspension/ Solution	5 mL
Fluorometholone	FML/Flarex	Allergan/Alcon	Suspension/ (FML available as unguent)	2 mL/5 mL/ 10 mL/15 mL/ 3.5 g
Rimexolone	Vexol	Alcon	Suspension	5 mL/10 mL

TABLE 21.7 INDICATIONS AND CONTRAINDICATIONS OF CORTICOSTEROID USE

INDICATIONS	CONTRAINDICATIONS
Iritis	Herpes simplex infectious epithelial keratitis
Episcleritis	Acute bacterial infections
Chemical trauma	Significant epithelial compromise
Uveitic glaucoma	Fungal infections
Glaucomatocyclitic crisis	
Ocular trauma	
Postoperative care	
Phlyctenulosis	
Corneal microcystic edema	
Corneal infiltrates	
Ultraviolet keratitis	
Stromal keratitis	
Epidemic keratoconjunctivitis	
Peripheral corneal erosions	
Thygeson superficial punctate keratitis	
Vernal keratoconjunctivitis	
Inflammatory blepharitis	
Eczemoid blepharitis	
Angular blepharitis	
Contact blepharodermatitis	
Uveitis	
Herpes zoster (ocular involvement)	
Allergic conjunctivitis	
Rosacea	
Vascularized limbal keratitis	

From Krupin T, Mandell AI, Podos SM, et al. Topical corticosteroid therapy and pituitary adrenal function. Arch Ophthalmol 1976;94(6):919–920.

only occur after long-term use of a systemic or ocular steroid. If a patient uses a steroid for more than 1 to 2 weeks, it becomes important to monitor IOP. Loteprednol is less likely to increase IOP. Concomitant use of a beta blocker or brimonidine can be used for pressures of above 30 mm Hg. The indications and contraindications of steroid use are given in Table 21.7.

Loteprednol

Loteprednol is available in an ophthalmic suspension in two concentrations: 0.5% (Lotemax) and 0.2% (Alrex). Loteprednol differs from other corticosteroids in that it is ester based as opposed to ketone based. This is important as the ester-based corticosteroid has an anti-inflammatory effect and minimizes the potential for adverse side effects. This occurs because the body has enzymes to break down the ester, reducing the time it is in the body. The body does not have enzymes to break down ketones; therefore, ketone-based corticosteroids are more likely to cause side effects, especially with long-term use.

Alrex is approved for treating allergic conjunctivitis. Use of an antihistamine/mast cell stabilizer is preferred in most cases, but if there are clinical signs to accompany the symptoms of itching (i.e., conjunctival injection or chemosis), Alrex is beneficial in preventing the inflammatory response. Typical dosage is every 2 hours for 2 days, followed by q.i.d. for a week and b.i.d. or q.d. for several more days or weeks.

Lotemax is very popular today because of its clinical effectiveness. It is useful in treating ocular inflammation with little to no increase in intraocular pressure. Although the treatment regimen depends on the ocular condition, a typical treatment regimen would be one drop every 1 to 2 hours for a few days until control of the condition occurs; then the patient is tapered to q.i.d. for a few days, then b.i.d. for a few days; and then the use of the drops is discontinued. As a suspension drop, the patient should be instructed verbally and via written prescription to shake the bottle before use.

Prednisolone

Of all topical ophthalmic corticosteroids, prednisolone has the greatest anti-inflammatory efficacy. It is available as Pred Forte (Allergan) and in generic forms in 1% concentration, and as Pred Mild (Allergan) in 0.12% concentration. The 1% concentration is by far the more clinically useful form. Pred Forte has been demonstrated to be the most effective topical corticosteroid in the management of uveitis and corneal inflammation.[10] It can be used for severe ocular inflammations, such as iritis, episcleritis, and chemical or thermal burns of the cornea. The treatment regimen is similar to Lotemax, depending on the severity of the ocular condition.

Dexamethasone

Dexamethasone is available in a suspension (0.1%) manufactured by Alcon as Maxidex and a solution (0.1%) manufactured by Merck as Decadron. Dexamethasone is not as effective as prednisolone and has an increased risk of elevating IOP; therefore, it is not frequently used.

Fluorometholones

Fluorometholones exhibit good anti-inflammatory properties, in addition to being less likely to increase IOP. They are available in two forms: alcohol and acetate. An example of fluorometholone alcohol is FML (Allergan). It is available in 0.1% and 0.25% suspensions and 0.1% ointment. FML suspension is available generically. The 0.25% concentration is no more effective than the 0.1% and therefore is rarely used. This is a good choice when long-term therapy (>3–4 weeks) is necessary as it has a reduced risk of elevating IOP. Individuals exhibiting a chronic iridocyclitis or a long-term ocular allergy would benefit from use of FML or Lotemax.

Fluorometholone acetate is available in 0.1% generically and as Flarex (Alcon), both of which are ophthalmic suspensions. The acetate formulation is slightly more effective that the alcohol form, but less than loteprednol 0.5% (Lotemax) or prednisolone acetate. Fluorometholone acetate, like the alcohol form, has the benefit of reduced tendency to increase IOP.

Rimexolone

Rimexolone is available as a suspension [Vexol 1% (Alcon)]. It is the first steroid to be approved by the Food and Drug Administration (FDA) for use in postoperative inflammation, such as anterior chamber inflammation following cataract surgery. Pred Forte has also been used for postoperative inflammation; however, it has not been FDA approved for this use. Rimexolone has an efficacy almost but not quite as high as prednisolone acetate 1% and, like fluorometholones, has a reduced risk of increasing IOP. It is also used in the treatment of anterior uveitis.

Eye doctors have not utilized corticosteroids as often as indicated, most likely because of a fear of the potential side effects. However, when an accurate diagnosis is made of ocular

TABLE 21.8 CORTICOSTEROID USE FOR OCULAR CONDITIONS

Allergic conjunctivitis	Loteprednol 0.2%/fluorometholone 0.1%
Episcleritis/iritis	Prednisolone 1%/loteprednol 0.5%
Uveitis/corneal Inflammation	Prednisolone 1%/loteprednol 0.5%
Chemical/thermal burns	Prednisolone 1%/loteprednol 0.5%
Contact lens-induced acute red eye (CLARE)	Prednisolone 1%/loteprednol 0.5%/ fluorometholone 0.1%
Chronic iridocyclitis	Loteprednol 0.5%
Postoperative inflammation	Rimexolone
CLARE/vascularized limbal keratitis/ staphylococcal blepharitis	Combination antibiotic/steroid

inflammation and the drugs are used as intended for short periods of time, these agents are extremely successful in treating the inflammation. Steroids should not be used in herpes simplex keratitis, in acute bacterial or fungal infections, or when the epithelium is compromised, as they may exacerbate the condition and retard healing. Steroids are very beneficial in reducing the inflammation and the results of inflammation—scarring and neovascularization. The most important factors to consider when using steroids include an accurate diagnosis, selecting the appropriate steroid based on the severity of the condition, and aggressive treatment of the inflammation initially (i.e., every 1–2 hours until the condition is controlled). Tapering the drug and monitoring IOP is wise if the drug is used for more than 1 week. Ocular conditions treated with corticosteroids can be found in Table 21.8.

■ NONSTEROIDAL ANTI-INFLAMMATORY DRUGS

The use of topical NSAIDs for contact lens-related complications is rare. Systemic NSAIDs do have an anti-inflammatory effect, but topical NSAIDs provide only a minimal direct anti-inflammatory property, thus limiting their use in primary eye care. As discussed in the previous section, NSAIDs inhibit cyclooxygenase, one of two enzymes that convert arachidonic acid to prostaglandins. The other enzyme, lipoxygenase, which converts arachidonic acid to leukotrienes, is not affected by NSAIDs. Therefore, a patient with corneal inflammation and NSAID use may have reduced pain, but may also develop corneal infiltrates. The infiltrates are the result of leukocytes, which, in turn, are the result of the lack of inhibition of leukotriene.

The use of topical NSAIDs is primarily to treat ocular surface pain. Ocular treatment options with topical NSAIDs can be found in Table 21.9.

TABLE 21.9 USES OF TOPICAL NONSTEROIDAL ANTI-INFLAMMATORY DRUGS

Corneal abrasions
Postoperative care (i.e., penetrating keratoplasty, cataract surgery)
Treating inflamed pterygia and pinguecula
After foreign body removal
After laser surgery
Allergic conjunctivitis
Cystoid macular edema

TABLE 21.10 TOPICAL NONSTEROIDAL ANTI-INFLAMMATORY DRUGS

GENERIC NAME	BRAND NAME	MANUFACTURER	SIZE
Diclofenac sodium 0.1%	Voltaren	Novartis	2.5 mL/5 mL
Ketorolac tromethamine 0.4%	Acular LS	Allergan	5 mL
Bromfenac 0.09%	Xibrom	ISTA Pharmaceuticals	5 mL
Nepafenac 0.1%	Nevanac	Alcon	3 mL

There are four primary topical NSAIDs: Voltaren (Novartis), Acular LS (Allergan), Xibrom (ISTA Pharmaceuticals), and Nevanac (Alcon). The generic name of Voltaren is diclofenac sodium 0.1% and Acular LS is ketorolac tromethamine 0.4%. Both of these NSAIDs are prescribed q.i.d. and have similar responses; however, Voltaren may have a more pronounced effect and longer activity.[11] Acular LS is FDA approved to treat ocular allergy. Xibrom is used b.i.d. and Nevanac is used three times a day (t.i.d.). All of these NSAIDs are FDA approved to treat postoperative inflammation. It is important for the patient to not increase the frequency of administration over the FDA-recommended daily dosage and, with the exception of cystoid macular edema (CME), these drugs should not be used for more than 1 week. The drugs may need to be used for a month to treat CME. A summary table of topical NSAIDs in use today can be found in Table 21.10.

■ ANTIVIRAL MEDICATIONS

Contact lens wear does not cause viral infections, but contact lens wearers can still be affected by viral infections. The three primary viral diseases that eye doctors will encounter are herpes simplex virus, herpes zoster (varicella zoster) disease, and adenoviral infections [i.e., epidemic keratoconjunctivitis (EKC) and pharyngoconjunctival fever (PCF)]. The clinical sign of herpes simplex virus (HSV) is dendritiform or geographic epithelial keratitis. The herpes simplex virus is killed by an FDA-approved drug, Viroptic (trifluridine, Monarch Pharmaceuticals) or trifluridine 0.1% ophthalmic solution generically. The treatment regimen in the affected eye is one drop every 2 hours during waking hours for 4 to 5 days and then q.i.d. for 4 to 5 days. If the patient becomes intolerant or allergic to trifluridine, oral acyclovir (Zovirax) in the dosage of 400 mg taken five times a day for 1 week can be used. Other oral antivirals that may be used are Valtrex (valacyclovir), prescribed 500 mg t.i.d. for 1 week, or Famvir (famciclovir), prescribed 250 mg t.i.d. for 1 week. In addition, it is recommended that the patient use an artificial tear every 2 to 4 hours. HSV tends to have recurrent episodes.

A few cases of HSV occur as stromal immune keratitis or herpetic uveitis. The epithelial form must be treated with antiviral drugs, but these other immune-related forms benefit from treatment with Lotemax or Pred Forte. The recommended treatment would be to use one of these corticosteroids along with trifluridine q.i.d. or oral acyclovir 400 mg three to four times a day. This antiviral cover should be used until the steroid drops are decreased to b.i.d., which will take about 1 month. It will take another month or two before the steroid is tapered to once a day or every other day depending on the patient's response.

Herpes zoster most commonly affects the trunk, but the second most common location is the trigeminal nerve, specifically the first, or ophthalmic, division of the nerve on the head and/or face. When there is ocular involvement with herpes zoster, patients may present to eye doctors or be referred to eye doctors by their primary care physician. Herpes zoster is caused by the latent varicella zoster virus in the body of persons who have had chickenpox. Treatment of herpes zoster is 800 mg of Zovirax (acyclovir, GlaxoSmithKline) orally five times a day for 1 week. Valtrex (valacyclovir, GlaxoSmithKline) 1,000 mg and Famvir (famciclovir, Novartis) 500 mg dosages are taken three times a day for a week. When the eye is involved (this occurs in about 50% of the ophthalmic division cases), it is expressed predominantly as either iritis, keratitis, or both.[12] In these cases, aggressive use of Lotemax or Pred Forte is the standard of care.

Oral antiviral drugs are activated by viral thymidine kinase phosphorylation, which makes them biologically active. This characteristic makes them potent, but safe. Maximum effect occurs when the virus is treated during the first 3 days of the symptoms. Patients with poor kidney function should be treated in conjunction with their nephrologist or primary care physician, so as to calculate the proper dosage.

PCF is found primarily in children. Besides cool compresses, artificial tears, occasionally vasoconstrictors, and perhaps Alrex q.i.d. for 4 to 6 days, these children do not need more aggressive treatment. EKC is found primarily in adults and is much more virulent. Symptoms include acute red eye, watery discharge, clear cornea, petechial hemorrhages on bulbar conjunctiva, palpable ipsilateral lymphadenopathy, and, if left untreated, subepithelial infiltrates and pseudomembranes. One eye is typically affected first, with the second eye exhibiting clinical signs about 2 to 3 days later. There is an excellent therapy that is of yet an off-label application. The use of Betadine 5% Sterile Ophthalmic Prep Solution (Alcon), which is povidone-iodine, reduces the probability of spreading the virus by its excellent virucidal action, thus decreasing the length of the condition. The authors recommend the following use of Betadine for EKC:

- Rule out allergy to iodine.
- Anesthetize the eye with proparacaine as Betadine stings.
- Instill one to two drops of an NSAID as Betadine can cause corneal stippling.
- Instill four to five drops of Betadine 5% Ophthalmic Prep Solution and have the patient close the eye and roll the eye around to ensure contact with all the ocular surfaces.
- While the eye is closed, a swab moistened with Betadine should be used to wipe across the lid margins to eliminate the virus in that region.
- After 60 seconds, the eye should be thoroughly rinsed with sterile saline irrigation solution. The eye will still be inflamed from the adenovirus. Use Lotemax q.i.d. for 4 to 5 days to reduce inflammation and provide patient comfort.
- Instill one to two drops of an NSAID in the office to maximize patient comfort.

This recommended procedure will reduce the time period of EKC, maintain corneal clarity, and decrease the risk of subepithelial infiltrates and pseudomembranes by reducing the time period of the exposure to the virus. If the virus has already been present in the eye for 5 to 6 days, the authors do not use the Betadine therapy since EKC usually resolves in 7 to 8 days. In this case, use of Lotemax q.i.d. for a few days will aid in providing comfort to the patient. A listing of antiviral drugs is provided in Table. 21.11.

TABLE 21.11 ANTIVIRAL DRUGS

GENERIC NAME	BRAND NAME	MANUFACTURER	ROUTE OF ADMINISTRATION
Trifluridine 0.1%	Viroptic	Monarch	Topical
Acyclovir	Zovirax	GlaxoSmithKline	Oral
Valacyclovir	Valtrex	GlaxoSmithKline	Oral
Famciclovir	Famvir	Novartis	Oral
Povidone-iodine	Betadine 5% Sterile Ophthalmic Prep Solution	Alcon	Topical

◼ DRY EYES

Management

A large percentage of the population experiences "dry" eyes, and many contact lens "dropouts" attribute their discontinuation of lens wear to "dry" eyes.[13] There are many causes of dry-eye symptoms. Some of these symptoms have been discussed in other chapters, such as solution sensitivity (Chapter 12) and contact lens troubleshooting (Chapters 8 and 13). If the contact lens wearer complains of dry eyes, a thorough evaluation of the precorneal tear film should be performed (Chapter 1). Contact lens wearers should be carefully monitored if they have <10 seconds of tear breakup time (TBUT). Infrequent (<12 blinks per minute) and incomplete blinks may also contribute to dryness symptoms. Observation of the lacrimal lake height/volume should be noted as well.

Many times a solution sensitivity mimics dry-eye symptoms; therefore, altering the solution to preferably a nonpreserved solution, such as a hydrogen peroxide disinfection system; using one of the solutions that is formulated to improve dry-eye symptoms [i.e., Aquify (Ciba Vision), Opti-Free Replenish (Alcon)]; or using a daily disposable lens with no solutions should be beneficial. In gas-permeable (GP) wearers, using a different care regimen or using a daily cleaner and weekly enzyme may make lens wear more comfortable. Plasma-coated GP lenses may increase the lens comfort and decrease the dryness symptoms.[14–16] Another alternative for soft lens wearers is to use one of the commercially available soft lenses that have claimed to be more comfortable for patients with dry eyes, such as Proclear (CooperVision), Extreme H_2O (Hydrogel Vision Corp.), Dailies AquaComfort Plus (Ciba Vision), 1 Day Acuvue Moist (Vistakon), and silicone hydrogel materials. Frequent use of a nonpreserved contact lens rewetting drop will hydrate and rinse the lens in the eye. Initiating lid scrubs, warm compresses, and lid massage for 2 weeks before lens wear can increase the TBUT. More severe cases of blepharitis or meibomian gland dysfunction may require topical and/or oral antibiotics for 4 to 6 weeks.[17] If these alternatives do not help and a dysfunctional tear film has been diagnosed, rewetting drops, artificial tears, punctal plugs, anti-inflammatory therapy, and nutritional supplements may be beneficial.

Severe dry eyes are contraindicated for contact lens wear; however, therapy before instituting contact lens wear or concurrent therapy may improve the success of the dry-eye patient. This is especially important in patients who exhibit keratoconus, who need contact lenses to meet their visual needs but suffer from a dysfunctional tear film. In treating dry-eye patients, the practitioner and the patient need to be flexible to determine what will be most successful for each patient. Sometimes combining various therapies may increase success and sometimes a new therapy may eliminate an old one. For example, a particular lens type with a specific lens care regimen (or solution) used in conjunction with punctal plugs and rewetting drops may be most successful for one patient. Another patient may be able to eliminate rewetting drops after insertion of punctal plugs. Trial and error combined with patience is required to determine what will be most effective for each patient. Some other options to improve dryness symptoms are given in Table 21.12, after contact lens materials, solutions, and rewetting drops have been used to no avail. These therapy options may be successful alone or may require two or more options used concurrently for the patient's relief of symptoms. For contact lens wearers, it is hoped that this therapy would improve their likelihood of success and that, after an initial treatment period, these patients would be able to successfully wear lenses with rewetting drops, artificial tear use before and after lens wear, nutritional supplements, and/or punctal plugs.

Artificial Tears

When recommending artificial tears, the practitioner must decide on viscosity (low, medium, or high), preservatives (preserved, nonpreserved, or transiently preserved), container (bottled or unit dosage), and preparation (solution, emulsion, gel, or ointment). Probably the most

TABLE 21.12 OPTIONS TO IMPROVE DRYNESS SYMPTOMS

CONDITION	THERAPY
Mild dry eyes	Artificial tears
	Punctal plugs
	Omega-3 fatty acid supplementation
Moderate dry eyes	Artificial tears with gel use at bedtime
	Punctal plugs
	Omega-3 fatty acid supplementation
	Restasis trial for 3–6 mo
Severe dry eyes	Viscous preservative-free artificial tears
	Lotemax q.i.d. for 2 wk, then observe anti-inflammatory response
	Long-term Restasis if Lotemax response was positive
	Oral doxycycline (100 mg/d for 2 wk, then 50 mg/d for 6 mo)
	Omega-3 fatty acid supplementation for 3–6 mo
	Punctal plugs after the above measures have been in effect for 1–2 mo

From Krupin T, Mandell AI, Podos SM, et al. Topical corticosteroid therapy and pituitary adrenal function. Arch Ophthalmol 1976;94(6):919–920.

important factor is the patient usage. Patients tend to be negligent about frequency of instillation of the artificial tears. Instilling the drops as directed is the first hurdle in combating the dry-eye symptoms. Use of artificial tears every 4 hours is recommended. Use of a gel-type artificial tear, just before contact lens instillation, with rewetting drops during lens wear has been found to be beneficial.[18] Newer oil emulsion formulations, such as Soothe®XP, (Baush & Lamb), have been particularly helpful, especially with GP lenses.

Punctal Plugs

Punctal occlusion is underutilized. Possible reasons for this underutilization include the cost, lack of effectiveness of trial occlusion with collagen plugs, and loss of plugs. If punctal occlusion is indicated, it is best to directly proceed with "permanent" silicone plugs. Punctal plugs may be beneficial in patients with moderate tear film volume and those with markedly reduced tear film volume if they use artificial tears concurrently. Infrequent use of artificial tears with punctal occlusion and a small lacrimal lake results in a stagnant tear film, which may increase symptoms of dryness and increase inflammatory agents. Lotemax q.i.d. for 2 weeks, followed by b.i.d. for 2 weeks, and artificial tears should be used before punctal occlusion. To prevent loss of the punctal plug, it is suggested that the largest plug size that can be placed in the puncta should be used. Punctal gauges aid in determination of the optimal size. It is optional whether the doctor should administer a trial by occluding only one eye or occluding both eyes at the same time.

Anti-Inflammatory Therapy

Patients with tear dysfunction may have a significant inflammatory component. Use of a topical corticosteroid (Lotemax) or topical cyclosporine (Restasis) may benefit those patients with more severe clinical signs and symptoms. Typically, before Restasis therapy, a practitioner should perform a trial on the eye with Lotemax to determine if the patient will respond to anti-inflammatory therapy. The recommended procedure is to prescribe Lotemax q.i.d. for 1 month. If the results of this trial are beneficial for the patient, this patient's dry eye has an inflammatory component. At this time, the practitioner may continue with Lotemax b.i.d. for another month, then taper to once a day for 1 to 2 months accompanied by artificial tear use. Another option is to initiate Restasis therapy b.i.d. accompanied by b.i.d. Lotemax use if the patient shows benefits after the first month of Lotemax. The reason for this concurrent use is that it typically takes at least 1 month of Restasis therapy to render an effect. Utilization of the steroid first minimizes the inflammatory response and allows the Restasis time to achieve a therapeutic effect. Long-term therapy with Restasis is less of a risk for side effects, but if patients cannot afford the cost, Lotemax once or twice daily is more cost efficient. Although the potential side effects with Lotemax are remotely possible, using it once a day for several months is safe in most patients. Using the anti-inflammatory therapy for 6 to 12 months with concurrent use of artificial tears, punctal plugs, lid scrubs and massage, and nutritional supplements should increase patients' success and decrease their symptoms. Contact lens wear should be discontinued during the initial phases of this treatment (4–8 weeks minimum). After control of the condition has been obtained, the patient may occasionally experience acute symptoms, which can be treated by using Lotemax q.i.d. for 1 week, then b.i.d. for 1 to 2 weeks. The goal should be to use the minimum amount of medication; therefore, discontinuation of treatment will allow the doctor to see if the patient can now cease anti-inflammatory therapy.

Management of Meibomian Gland Dysfunction

Initially, aggressive treatment with lid scrubs, lid massage, and warm compresses (two to four times a day) may improve the appearance of the lid margins and the function of the meibomian glands in cases of meibomian gland dysfunction (MGD). However, patient compliance is a limiting factor, just as in artificial tear use. If bacterial blepharitis is observed, use of an antibiotic ointment in conjunction with lid scrubs, warm compresses, and lid massage will aid in improving this condition.[19] The use of oral doxycycline has been found to be beneficial in treating MGD.[20] The authors recommend using doxycycline 50 mg b.i.d. for 2 weeks and then 50 mg q.d. for 6 months. Side effects in adults are uncommon, but may include vaginal yeast infections and photosensitivity. The tetracyclines are contraindicated in pregnant women, nursing mothers, and children under the age of 8. After 6 months of therapy, transferring patients successfully treated with doxycycline to omega-3 supplements may be beneficial as patients may be more comfortable with using the nutritional supplement. Omega-3 supplementation usually takes 3 to 4 months for an effect to be observed. The recommended dosage is 2,000 mg of flaxseed oil a day. TheraTears Nutrition (Advanced Vision Research) capsules contain half fish oil and half flaxseed oil. The recommended dosage is three capsules taken in the morning. Patients should be aware that gastrointestinal upset can occur in some patients.

Dry-eye symptoms can be mild to severe. Treatment may include changing the contact lens material and altering the care regimen to anti-inflammatory therapy or oral antibiotics. It is recommended that after performing preliminary testing to determine the severity of the dry eye, the appropriate treatment interventions should then be initiated. It is important for the doctor and the patient to carefully consider which approaches are most successful for them. The goal should be to use the least amount of therapy that provides relief to the patient. Treatment should be initiated with less aggressive therapies and then progress to more aggressive treatment as indicated.

■ TREATMENT OF FUNGAL INFECTIONS

Up until recently, fungal infections were rare, usually more common in hot, humid climates. With the recent outbreak of *Fusarium* infections, primarily associated with patients who were using ReNu MoistureLoc and soft lens wear, an increase in the number of infections was observed. This solution was taken off the market.[21] Obviously, eye care practitioners must take seriously the risk of a fungal infection in their patients. *Candida, Aspergillus,* and *Curvularia* are other fungi that can commonly cause infection in the United States.[22] *Fusarium* is the most common cause of fungal keratitis in the United States, and *Aspergillus* is the most common cause in the world.[9] Fungi cause ocular damage by the presence of the organism, an infiltrative inflammatory response, and secondary damage caused by the fungal toxins and enzymes. Risk factors for infection include trauma, extended wear of contact lenses, poor care and hygiene of contact lenses, and diabetes. Presenting symptoms and clinical signs include foreign body sensation, decreased vision, tearing, redness, stromal infiltration with feathery borders, and a dry, whitish-gray, slightly elevated lesion on the cornea. The overlying epithelium may or may not be intact, and often satellite lesions, immune rings, and hypopyon may be observed.[23] Laboratory testing of corneal scrapings is cytologically diagnostic; however, deeper, more invasive biopsies may be required to obtain tissue samples. Because of the deep stromal infection, treatment may be difficult; therefore, partial debridement of the cornea may be necessary to enhance drug penetration. Several weeks of topical therapy is required to achieve clinical success.

The drug of choice is natamycin, manufactured by Alcon as Natacyn 5%, which is effective against a variety of fungi. Another drug is amphotericin B, which must be compounded by a pharmacist into an eyedrop formulation. Initially, one drop of natamycin should be used every 15 minutes for a few hours. In treating fungal infections, both natamycin and amphotericin B are used topically, alternating one drop every 30 minutes and a few times during the night until the epithelial defect has reduced in size. Typically, the eye would be cyclopleged during this treatment. Concurrent use of an oral antifungal like ketoconazole or voriconazole is rarely used. When the defect is decreased in size, drop administration can be decreased to alternating every hour. If the eye continues to improve after 2 weeks, amphotericin B can be discontinued as it tends to cause ocular irritation. Natamycin can be used every hour or two for another 10 to 14 days and then decreased to one drop every 2 to 4 hours until vision is improved and the lesion appears inactive. At this time, the patient should continue to be observed weekly. Natamycin can be used four times a day, decreasing to twice a day and then discontinuation if the eye continues to improve each week. Treatment with natamycin will typically take 4 to 8 weeks. In severe cases, a conjunctival flap, penetrating keratoplasty, or corneal graft may be required. Corticosteroids should not be used in these patients, except after several weeks of antifungal treatment; then they may be used with caution to quiet the eye and minimize scarring.

■ *ACANTHAMOEBA* KERATITIS

Acanthamoeba is a water-borne protozoan that exists as a cyst or in a trophozoite form. The cyst form is more difficult to eliminate. Fortunately, with increased knowledge and better patient education, this form of infection is rare, although recent outbreaks, which may be associated with changes in water purification, have been reported.[24,25] Thorough contact lens care, proper solution use, not using tap water on contact lenses, and not swimming in contact lenses are the best ways to prevent *Acanthamoeba* keratitis. Clinical signs and symptoms of this type of infection include a variably injected eye with pain, photophobia, and tearing. Generally, the symptoms will be more severe than the clinical signs. As the infection increases, epithelial lesions that may appear dendritic and a stromal ring or partial ring of infiltrates may be observed. Left untreated or misdiagnosed, this infection can lead to corneal perforation. As in most conditions, early diagnosis will enable the best results. Tissue biopsy can be helpful in diagnosing *Acanthamoeba*. When making a differential diagnosis with herpes simplex, whereas *Acanthamoeba* generally has severe pain and few associated clinical signs, generally herpes simplex will have more clinical signs and less discomfort.[26] Treatment of *Acanthamoeba* consists of medications including antifungals (fluconazole or clotrimazole), cationic antiseptics (polyhexamethylene biguanide or chlorhexidine), diamides (propamidine), and aminoglycosides (neomycin or paromomycin). A combination of two to three of the above medications is generally most effective, and treatment should continue for 3 to 6 months after all clinical signs have resolved. Successful treatment with cationic antiseptics and diamide, given every hour for

2 to 4 days, reducing to every 2 hours for 3 to 4 days, and then maintained on a maintenance dose of polyhexamethylene biguanide or chlorhexidine for 3 to 4 months, has shown effectiveness.[27] Epithelial debridement will sometimes improve the success of the treatment process. Another treatment regimen is to use a combination of polyhexamethylene biguanide or chlorhexidine, propamidine, and neomycin solution after debridement of the epithelium. Antibiotics prophylactically may be used in conjunction with these regimens.[28]

CLINICAL PROFICIENCY CHECKLIST

- Never taper antibiotics below the recommended dosage.
- Not knowing the diagnosis is not justification for prescribing an antibiotic.
- Bacterial eye infections in adults are uncommon events, whereas inflammatory conjunctivitis or keratoconjunctivitis is common.
- Monotherapy with corticosteroids is contraindicated in herpes simplex keratitis, acute bacterial infection, and fungal infections.
- For bacterial conjunctivitis or prophylaxis, select an aminoglycoside or fluoroquinolone. When treating an infectious keratitis, use a fourth-generation fluoroquinolone or fortified antibiotic.
- Prescribe a dosing frequency commensurate with the nature of the clinical presentation. The more severe the condition, the more frequent the dosage should be.
- Regarding steroid use, always gain good control of the inflammatory process before beginning the tapering process. The longer it takes to gain control, the longer the tapering process should be.
- Observation of any disease process at or near the limbus is almost always inflammatory in nature.
- Many inflamed eyes require a combination antibiotic/steroid as opposed to an antibiotic or steroid alone.
- Risk factors for ulcerative keratitis are overnight contact lens wear, poor tear film function, uncontrolled staphylococcal blepharitis, smoking, swimming with contact lenses, respiratory infection, and being under the age of 22.
- Perform a therapeutic trial with Lotemax q.i.d. for 2 weeks in the most symptomatic dry eye and if the patient finds this anti-inflammatory reduction beneficial, then consider a trial of Restasis, or continued b.i.d. or q.d. therapy with Lotemax.
- Drugs such as bacitracin, polymyxin B, and aminoglycosides are not used orally; therefore, resistance is exceedingly rare. These drugs remain excellent for topical ophthalmic use.

■ CLINICAL CASES

CASE 1

A GP patient presents with discomfort with his right eye for the last few weeks. Visual acuity is 20/20 OU. Upon slit-lamp examination, there is grade two, 3- and 9-o'clock staining OU, with increased staining on the right eye in the temporal area and a slightly elevated white lesion. The eyes are more injected in the temporal quadrant OU. Evaluation of the lens fit shows the lenses fit intrapalpebral and the lenses come to rest next to the area of the lesion.

DIAGNOSIS: Vascularized limbal keratitis (VLK)

TREATMENT: Lens wear is discontinued. An antibiotic/steroid combination drug like Zylet is prescribed to be used q.i.d. for 1 week and then tapered to b.i.d. The patient is to return for follow-up in 3 to 4 days. When it is determined that the patient can resume lens wear, the patient will be refitted in a lens that exhibits a tucked-under-the-upper-lid position and provides better tear exchange. Use of a contact lens rewetting drop or artificial tear, notably Soothe XP, will aid in lubricating the cornea.

CASE 2

A patient presents for a routine eye examination and contact lenses. She complains of itchy eyes in addition to decreased contact lens comfort toward the end of the day. She has a history of seasonal allergies and is taking Allegra q.d. She is currently wearing soft contact lenses that are replaced quarterly. Visual acuities are OD 20/30 and OS 20/25. Slit-lamp evaluation shows grade 3 papillae on the superior tarsal plates, mild injection, and deposited contact lenses.

DIAGNOSIS: Giant papillary conjunctivitis

TREATMENT: The patient is refitted into a daily disposable contact lens and is started on an antihistamine/mast cell stabilizer combination drug like Patanol, Elestat, Optivar, Zaditor, or Alaway (the latter two available over the counter) used b.i.d., or Pataday used q.d. The patient should return for a follow-up visit in 2 weeks. If an improvement is not observed, contact lens wear should be discontinued until symptoms have subsided.

CASE 3

A patient complains of an irritated, watery, and red left eye since awakening this morning. The patient reports sleeping in her hydrogel contact lenses the prior evening and had removed them upon awakening. Aided visual acuities are OD 20/20 and OS 20/30. Upon slit-lamp examination, four small infiltrates are present in the peripheral cornea OS. Diffuse SPK that stains lightly with fluorescein is also present in both eyes. The bulbar conjunctiva is grade 1+ injected in the right eye and grade 2 injected in the left eye.

DIAGNOSIS: Contact lens-induced acute red eye

TREATMENT: Discontinue contact lens wear until the condition fully resolves. Start an antibiotic/steroid combination drug like Zylet or TobraDex q.i.d. OS in addition to preservative-free artificial tears q.i.d. OU. The patient should be followed up in 2 or 3 days, sooner if there is any worsening. After resolution, the patient should be refitted into a silicone hydrogel contact lens material on a daily-wear regimen. The patient may be able to return to extended wear with silicone hydrogel lenses, but should be educated to wear lenses daily wear if suffering from a respiratory illness as this can provide an increased risk for infection.

CASE 4

A wearer of soft contact lenses with low oxygen permeability presents complaining of an irritated, red right eye for 2 days. The patient sleeps in lenses 3 to 4 days per week. Entering visual acuities are OD 20/25 and OS 20/20. Slit-lamp evaluation reveals three midperipheral subepithelial infiltrates located inferiorly on the right cornea. The bulbar conjunctiva is diffusely injected, grade 1+. There is grade 1 fluorescein staining of the epithelium over the infiltrates and the anterior chamber is deep and quiet.

DIAGNOSIS: Infiltrative keratitis

TREATMENT: Discontinue contact lens wear until the condition resolves. Start an antibiotic/steroid combination, like Zylet or TobraDex, every 2 hours OD for 2 days, then q.i.d. for 4 days. Preservative-free artificial tears may be used every 2 to 3 hours as palliative therapy. A follow-up visit should be scheduled in 2 to 3 days. When the condition is under control, refit the patient into a silicone hydrogel contact lens material and monitor him to determine whether he can return to extended-wear use.

CASE 5

A keratoconic patient complains of discomfort and dryness when wearing his contact lenses. As the patient's visual acuity through spectacles is reduced as compared to contact lens wear, the patient is highly motivated to continue contact lens wear.

DIAGNOSIS: Dry eyes

TREATMENT: The patient experiences better comfort with a piggyback design, and frequent use of rewetting drops improves the dryness symptoms. Punctal plugs are somewhat helpful. The patient is advised to take omega-3 fatty acid supplements. He finds that the supplements and lubricating drops in conjunction with the piggyback design lengthen his wearing time and increase his contact lens comfort.

REFERENCES

1. Rayner SA, Buckley RJ. Ocular chloramphenicol and aplastic anemia. Is there a link? Drug Saf 1996;14(5): 273–276, review.
2. Dewart MR, Elliott LJ. Management of contact lens-associated or lens-induced pathology. In: Bennett ES, Henry VA, eds. Clinical Manual of Contact Lenses, 2nd ed. Philadelphia: Lippincott Williams & Wilkins, 2000:582–610.
3. Solomon R, Donnenfield ED, Perry HD, et al. Penetration of topically applied gatifloxacin 0.3%, moxifloxacin 0.5%, and ciprofloxacin 0.3% into the aqueous humor. Ophthalmology 2005;112(3):466–469.
4. Kim DH, Stark WJ, O'Brien TP, et al. Aqueous penetration and biological activity of moxifloxacin 0.5% ophthalmic solution and gatifloxacin 0.3% solution in cataract surgery patients. Ophthalmology 2005;112(11):1992–1996.
5. Epstein AB, Quinn CJ. Diseases of the conjunctiva. In: Bartlett JD, Jaanus SD, eds. Clinical Ocular Pharmacology. Boston: Butterworth Heinemann, 2001:545–601.
6. Lanier B. Allergy-on the rise and in the news. Refractive Eyecare 2006;10(2):1, 32–34.
7. Silbert JA. Inflammatory responses in contact lens wear. In: Silbert JA, ed. Anterior Segment Complications of Contact Lens Wear, 2nd ed. Boston: Butterworth Heinemann, 2000:109–131.
8. Melton R, Thomas R. 2007 Clinical guide to ophthalmic drugs. Rev Optom 2007;144(6 Suppl.):1A–56A.
9. Krupin T, Mandell AI, Podos SM, et al. Topical corticosteroid therapy and pituitary adrenal function. Arch Ophthalmol 1976;94(6):919–920.
10. Leibowitz HM, Kuferman A. Antiinflammatory medications. Int Ophthalmol Clinics 1980;20(3):117–134.
11. Seitz B, Sorken K, LaBree LD, et al. Corneal sensitivity and burning sensation. Comparing topical ketorolac and diclofenac. Arch Ophthalmol 1996;114(8):921–924.
12. Pavan-Langston D. Herpes zoster ophthalmicus [Review]. Neurology 1995;45(12 Suppl 8):S50–51.
13. Begley C, Chalmers R, Mitchell L, et al. Characterization of ocular surface symptoms from optometric practices in North America. Cornea 2001;20:610–618.
14. Schafer J. Plasma treatment for GP contact lenses. Contact Lens Spectrum 2006;21(11):19.
15. Bennett ES. To plasma treat or not to plasma treat? Rev Cornea Contact Lenses 2006;Nov:9.
16. Rakow PL. Plasma treatments improve GP comfort. Vision Care Product News 2006;Oct:76–78.
17. Caffery B, Paugh JR. Tears, dry eye and management. In: Bennett ES, Weissman BA, eds. Clinical Contact Lens Practice, 2nd ed. Philadelphia: Lippincott Williams & Wilkins, 2005:457–474.
18. DeKinder JO. Maximizing soft lens comfort. Contact Lenses Today 2007;April.
19. Caroline PJ, Andre MP, Kame RT. Dermatologic complications of the lids and adnexa. In: Silbert JA, ed. Anterior Segment Complications of Contact Lens Wear, 2nd ed. Boston: Butterworth Heinemann, 2000:171–196.
20. Driver PJ, Lemp MA. Meibomian gland dysfunction. Surv Ophthalmol 1996;40(5):343–367.
21. Chang DC, Grant GB, O'Donnell K, et al. Fusarium Keratitis Investigation Team. Multistate outbreak of Fusarium keratitis associated with use of a contact lens solution. JAMA 2006;296(8):953–963.
22. Ward MA. Mycotic keratitis and lens care. Contact Lens Spectrum 2006;July.
23. Schornack MM. Clinical management of fungal keratitis. AOA News 2006;Apr 24:17–18.
24. Joslin CE, Tu EY, McMahon TT, et al. Epidemiological characteristics of a Chicago-area Acanthamoeba Keratitis outbreak. Am J Ophthalmol 2006;142(2):212–217.
25. Gutman C. Acanthamoeba Keratitis increasing at alarming rate. Ophthalmol Times 2006;Jan 1.
26. Townsend W. Beyond the branches: a closer look at ocular herpes, Part 1. Contact Lens Spectrum 2004;19(1):45.
27. Miller W. Acanthamoeba keratitis. Contact Lens Spectrum 2003;18(3):51.
28. Lingel N, Casser L. Diseases of the cornea. In: Bartlett JD, Jaanus SD, eds. Clinical Ocular Pharmacology, 4th ed. Boston: Butterworth Heinemann, 2001:603–672.

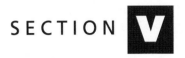

Practice Management

CHAPTER 22

Contact Lens Practice Management

Janice M. Jurkus, Brad Williams, Walter West, Peter G. Shaw-McMinn, Carmen Castellano, Jack Schaeffer, Walter Choate, N. Rex Ghormley, Stephanie Erker, and Jeff Harter

A successful contact lens practice must have an effective program for educating practitioners, staff, and patients. The fee system to be used must be well organized and factor in the amount of professional time to be devoted to a given type of patient. An effective system for follow-up care as well as patient retention is very important.

Of the 164.4 million ametropic patients in the United States, about 53 million people currently wear contact lenses. What about the remaining 68%? Many of these patients are good candidates, but the doctor needs to be proactive and offer contact lenses as an option. The doctor cannot wait for the patient to express interest.

Several studies have evaluated the importance of being proactive in recommending contact lenses. The Dillehay study[1] was a two-phase study looking at the ability of clinicians to offer contact lenses as a corrective option to good candidates. Ninety-five successful contact lens wearers were sent for eye examinations at 19 schools and colleges of optometry. Phase one consisted of the patients stating they did not wear contact lenses, nor did they ask for them. Even though all patients were successful lens wearers, none of the 95 patients were provided contact lenses as an option. In phase two of the study, the patients still stated that they were not current wearers but expressed interest in being fitted. In this round, 62 patients were scheduled for an evaluation. Of those patients, 47 were fitted into contact lenses. This study illustrates that if the practitioner waits for the patient to suggest fitting, a large percentage of good candidates will go unfitted. As indicated in Chapter 15, Jones et al[2] found that only 11.2% (9 of 80) of patients in their study were fitted into contact lenses if contact lenses were not proactively recommended to them, whereas 57.5% (46 of 80) were fitted into contact lenses if they were recommended as an option.

■ PREPARATION

Practitioner Education

It is the optometrist's skill and expertise that allow a patient to succeed with contact lens wear, not the result of any name-brand contact lens. Therefore, the emphasis should be placed on the service provided by the practitioner and not the material. The practitioner needs to stay informed about all technologic advances in the contact lens industry for lens materials, lens designs, and care systems to be updated frequently. To stay aware of the growing options, doctors can subscribe to various contact lens publications, such as *Contact Lens Spectrum*, *Review of Cornea and Contact Lenses*, *Eye and Contact Lens*, and *EyeWitness*, as well as the weekly e-mail newsletter *CL Today*.

Continuing education (CE) is another source of contemporary information. Some of the aforementioned journals offer CE credit if doctors read featured articles and then answer and submit questions based on the reading. Also, CE hours can be obtained by attending local, regional, or national conferences.

In addition, all optometrists have the opportunity to become involved in the Contact Lens and Cornea Section of the American Optometric Association (AOA) and the Cornea and Contact Lens Section of the American Academy of Optometry (AAO). Membership in the AOA Contact Lens and Cornea Section provides several benefits: free continuing education at the AOA's Optometry's Meeting, manufacturers' discount coupons, and a monthly e-newsletter supplying late-breaking clinical alerts. The Contact Lens and Cornea Section also affords optometrists the opportunity to work as liaisons with third-party programs, allowing optometrists to receive fair reimbursement for their clinical efforts.[3–5] For application and dues information, visit the AOA website (http://www.aoa.org). Optometrists can apply to be considered for fellowship in the American Academy of Optometry. Besides completing an application for candidacy, optometrists must also achieve 50 points by meeting several written requirements. After the written work is reviewed, candidates will be eligible for an oral examination held at the annual meeting. Successful completion of all stages grants the optometrist recognition as a Fellow. After achieving fellowship, one can also strive for the highly regarded status of Diplomate in the Cornea and Contact Lens Section, which requires completion of additional case studies as well as written, slide, oral, and practical examinations. Numerous symposia and educational position papers are available through membership in this Section.[6,7] For membership information, visit http://www.aaopt.org or write to the following address:

Membership Department
American Academy of Optometry
6110 Executive Boulevard, Suite 506
Rockville, MD 20852 USA

Finally, it is the doctor's responsibility to share his or her wealth of knowledge with the staff and patients. The optometrist should delegate and monitor tasks given to staff, ensuring that their knowledge level is adequate. Patient education is one of the most important factors in increasing patient compliance. The doctor should provide the tools necessary for the patient to succeed.

Staff Education

The best tool to educate your patients is to have an educated staff. Typically, a patient's original impression of a practice is not formed by direct communication with the optometrist, but rather by contact with a staff member. Therefore, staff personnel should be capable of answering patients' initial questions, providing sound advice, and making informed recommendations regarding general contact lens product information, care regimens, and basic ocular health. A well-educated staff member is then able to be a bridge between the patient and doctor, providing the best-quality care and instruction to the patient. Staff members can learn via several means: meetings, textbooks, journal articles, the Internet, workshops, and seminars.

Personnel can be educated by mandatory meetings scheduled on a regular basis (i.e., monthly, bimonthly). The primary focus of the meetings is to enhance communication and education, keeping staff members updated on recent contact lens issues. Some examples of topic ideas are new contact lens designs/materials, contact lens-related ocular diseases/conditions, lens wear complications, patient compliance, and proper lens care. To further review these subjects, the optometrist can provide the staff with textbooks, journal articles, and material from reputable online sources.

A few examples of textbooks available for use are the *Self-Study Course for Paraoptometric Certification*, 3rd ed., produced by the AOA (http://www.aoa.org) and Stein et al's *The Ophthalmic Assistant*, 8th ed., available at http://www.elsevier.com. Online sources include the following:

1. Gas Permeable Lens Institute: this website offers modules on care and handling instruction as well as educating presbyopic patients: http://www.gpli.info (Fig. 22.1).

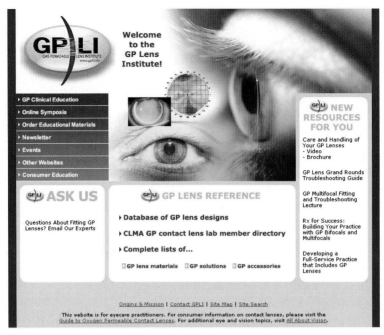

■ **FIGURE 22.1** Gas Permeable Lens Institute home page (www.gpli.info).

2. All About Vision: Guide to Eye Care and Vision Correction: this is a popular consumer site that provides good introduction information for new staff members: http://www. allaboutvision.com (Fig. 22.2).
3. Wink Productions: this company offers videos on telephone training and office etiquette as well as a book on professional medical staff training: http://www.winkproductions.com.
4. Contact Lens Society of America: this is a comprehensive source for online courses, contact lens fitting information, and staff guides: http://www.clsa.info.

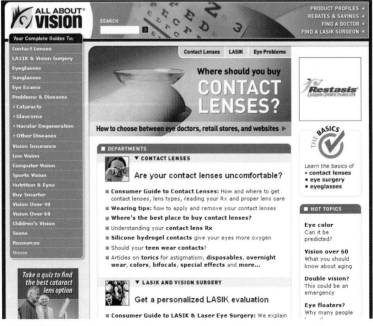

■ **FIGURE 22.2** All About Vision home page (www.allaboutvision.com).

Another method through which staff members can gain valuable information is by utilizing the knowledge available from pharmaceutical, lens care, and contact lens representatives. These representatives are experts of their particular product and are willing to share this information with practices. Some practitioners find it suitable to schedule seminars during lunch hour, for representatives often will provide refreshments.

In addition, companies may offer CDs/DVDs and printed information to be distributed to staff for further training. The American Optometric Association offers educational modules such as the "ABCs of Optical Dispensing," "Anatomy and Physiology," "Practice Management 101," etc. The modules are in a very easy-to-use PowerPoint format with accompanying audio. This information is available on the AOA website (http://www.aoa.org) under the Paraoptometric section.

Finally, staff can also attend state, regional, and national conferences. These conferences not only offer continuing education courses for optometrists, but also provide seminars for paraoptometric staff as well. A wide range of courses, from introductory to advanced, are provided to develop staff communication skills and general contact lens knowledge. An example of the array of courses provided at the 2008 Heart of America Contact Lens Society Conference begins with a fundamental course "The Essentials of Optometric Care: Facts, Terms and Anatomy" and extends to a more complex "Contemporary Contact Lens Correction for Presbyopia."[8] Workshops on technical skills are available as well as instruction on proper billing and coding. Enrollment fees for paraoptometrics are reduced and are typically paid for by the employing optometrist.

■ FEE ESTABLISHMENT

How to Establish the Fee

Setting fees for contact lenses falls into two areas, the professional service fee and the materials fee. Some practitioners will present a global fee that includes both the service and materials in a lump sum. Others will charge separate fees for each visit. A common approach to fees is to offer a service fee for the examination, fitting, and follow-up care and the fee for the products that includes the cost of the contact lenses. Some practitioners set their professional fees by staying within the "normal" range for a given area.

An option developed by the consulting firm The Williams Group recommends developing the retail fee in total. This fee is based on the amount of chair time with the patient in addition to the cost of the product. The basic formula for setting the fee is: Chair cost/hour × Clinic time + Material cost × % Mark-up needed = Your retail fee. First, your chair cost per hour should be determined. To accomplish this, the clinic/professional overhead per month should be determined. With knowledge of the office monthly gross income, operating costs are usually about 35% to 40% of this amount. The professional overhead is generally about 70% of the operating expenses and does not include the doctor's salary or cost of goods. Then, the professional overhead is divided by the number of practitioner hours per month. This will result in the dollar amount per hour. Table 22.1 provides an example of chair time determination.

The amount of time a specific contact lens-related examination requires is then used to determine the professional service fee. This should include the time involved for the initial examination, diagnostic fitting, dispensing, 2-week follow-up, 1-month follow-up, and any

TABLE 22.1 CHAIR TIME DETERMINATION

Monthly gross income	$40,000.00
Operating cost	$14,000.00 @ 35% gross income
Professional overhead	$9,800.00 @ 70%
Doctor hours/month	160 hours
Chair cost/hour	$9,800.00/160 = $61.25

TABLE 22.2 GUESS-ESTIMATING CLINIC TIME/YEAR/PATIENT TYPE

EXAM TYPES	INITIAL EXAM (MIN)	DIAGNOSTIC FITTING (MIN)	DISPENSING (MIN)	2-WEEK CHECK-UP (MIN)	1-MONTH CHECK-UP (MIN)	UNEXPECTED CHECK-UP (MIN)	TOTAL TIME (HR)	CHAIR COST/ HOUR ($61.25)
New spherical soft	20	20	30	15	10	15	1.8	$110
New toric soft	20	30	30	20	15	30	2.4	$147
New spherical gas permeable	20	35	30	20	15	30	2.5	$153
Refit	20	30	30	20	15	30	1.2	$73.50
Annual		30					0.5	$30

unexpected return visits. The complexity of a situation may greatly increase the amount of chair time with a patient and should be considered in the final determination of professional service fees. Some examples are provided in Table 22.2.

Each office should initiate their usual time-per-patient type. Following this example, the professional fees for a 3-month period varies depending on the type of service needed. The profit-goal percentage determined in the office forecasting may also be added to the fee. Once this initial fee determination is completed, many practitioners will develop a fee system that groups services. A sample grouping is in Table 22.3. The practitioner can insert his or her specific fees in each section.

The next step is to determine the cost of the product, the contact lenses. It is customary to mark up the cost of the product to pay for administrative costs involved in obtaining the lenses. A standard mark-up usually ranges from 20% to 30%. Lenses can be purchased directly from the manufacturer or through a buying group. Buying groups may offer a lower per unit cost but can charge an administrative fee (often approximately 5%). It is essential to be competitive in the material cost assessed to the patient. Some practitioners will determine the fees assessed by practitioners in the area via online or other alternative distributor sites and establish a fee

TABLE 22.3 GROUPING OF CONTACT LENS FEES

TYPE	NEW	REFIT	ANNUAL
Soft sphere DW	____	____	____
Soft sphere CW	____	____	____
Soft toric	____	____	____
Soft specialty	____	____	____
GP sphere	____	____	____
GP toric	____	____	____
GP specialty	____	____	____
Keratoconus	____	____	____

CW, continuous wear; DW, daily wear; GP, gas permeable.

similar to the average of the competition. A fee calculator for gas-permeable presbyopic patients is available as part of the "Rx for Success" program available at http://www.gpli.info.

The final part of the fee equation is to add the materials to the professional fees. If convenience is important to the patient, he or she should be encouraged to purchase a 1-year supply of lenses. For 2-week replacement lenses, this typically equates to eight boxes, although to reduce the initial purchase cost, patients may decide to initially order a 6-month supply. Many contact lens companies are now offering direct-to-patient rebates to help minimize the cost. These rebates are available from the corporate sales representative or the company websites.

To complete this example, the fees for a new patient wearing spherical soft lenses on a 2-week replacement schedule can be determined: Chair cost/hour × Clinic time + Material Cost × % Mark-up needed = Your retail fee: $61.25 × 1.8 + ($15 × 1.25) × 8 = $260.25.

Grouping professional fees by level of prescribing complexity and adding the material cost to professional fees is an easy way to present fees to the patient. The fees should normally be discussed with the patient by the administrative staff when the initial appointment is made. It is, however, important to inform the patient at this time that the exact fee cannot be determined until the conclusion of the contact lens examination. By evaluating the contact lens wearer's ocular physiology, eye health, visual problems, and goals, the doctor can more accurately recommend the course of treatment. Once in the office, both the doctor and the clinical assistants should present fees to the patient. The practitioner can educate the patient on the treatment plan and generally discuss the fee policy. The clinical assistant then discusses the exact fees, vision plan coverage, and any final costs to the patient. Forms that show the patient what the charges are, what is reimbursed by a third-party provider, and what the refund policy is should be developed and given to each patient before the services are provided. This will help that patient to make an informed decision regarding his or her potential management with contact lenses.

Third-Party Plans

Third-party plans may add a confusing element to the contact lens examination. This requires a well-educated staff that will be able to spend time explaining the reimbursement to the patient. Most healthcare providers only accept a patient's major medical health insurance. Optometry, however, is very different. Many patients have major medical insurance and a vision care plan. It is not uncommon for an office to submit to a major medical plan and vision care plan and for the patient to be responsible for the charges for all, or part of, the contact lens materials.

The popularity of third-party plans has increased in recent years. According to a recent national survey from the American Optometric Association, almost 50% of patients seeking the care of an optometrist have some form of vision care plan coverage. Approximately 30% of patients have coverage of vision services through their major medical health plan. According to the same survey, almost 40% of optometrists' total yearly revenue came from a vision care plan, while nearly 25% came from a major medical health plan. This survey helps to highlight the importance for practitioners to increase their participation in multiple vision care and major medical healthcare plans.[9]

Third-party plans can represent a double-edged sword. On one hand, they usually have limited coverage for contact lens-related expenses. Additionally, even a long-standing patient might choose another practitioner based on his or her insurance company's provider list, not based on the relationship with a practice or doctor's level of competence. One benefit of these third-party plans is that they do have the ability to bring patients into a practice on a more regular basis. Many times patients will seek an examination from an eye care professional so that they may receive all of the benefits provided by their third-party insurance plans.

Traditionally, third-party plans do not cover the cost of contact lens-related fees. However, this is beginning to change, especially with vision care insurance [i.e., Vision Service Plan

(VSP)]. A common trend with vision care insurance is to provide benefits for glasses or contact lenses. Usually, these companies provide the patient with either a set allowance amount that will apply to the cost of the contact lenses, examination fees, or both or require the patient to pay a certain percentage of their total costs.

Third-party insurance plans have changed the way a practitioner approaches a patient. The patient may attempt to persuade the doctor to choose a certain contact lens because it is covered by insurance. This requires the doctor to adapt to the situation by making sure not only that the patient is happy, but also that his or her ocular health remains uncompromised. The bottom line is that the doctor and staff must be well educated regarding third-party healthcare, and they must be prepared to explain any reimbursement policies to the patient.

Fairness to Contact Lens Consumers Act

The Fairness to Contact Lens Consumers Act was passed by the Federal Trade Commission (FTC) and enacted in December 2003. This act requires that any eye care professional prescribing contact lenses must supply their patients with a written copy of their contact lens prescription. The prescription must be given only after their eye care practitioner has finalized it for the patient. The act also allows for a third party to sell contact lenses to patients after a verification of the prescription by the doctor. The practitioner has up to 8 business hours to verify the patient's prescription to a third party. If the eye care professional does not respond to the third party within this time frame, the act allows for a "passive verification" and the third party may fill the prescription for contact lenses.[10]

It is critical, especially after the passing of this act, that there is a strong doctor–patient relationship. It is additionally important for the doctor to de-emphasize contact lens materials and emphasize the contact lens examination, patient education, and follow-up care. It must be relayed to patients that the practitioner's expertise is what will allow them to be successful contact lens wearers, not the purchasing of name-brand contact lenses from a third-party company. The doctor needs to inform patients of the benefits of the selected contact lens material and allow them to become part of the decision-making process. This interaction between the doctor and patient creates a bond and will help to ensure that the patient will return to the doctor for all of his or her contact lens needs, including the filling of the contact lens prescription.

Service Agreements

Service agreements are one efficient way to tie a patient to a practice. By having this bond, patients are less likely to seek care elsewhere, and it also increases the probability that they will return for an annual examination. This not only creates a cash flow into the practice, but also allows the practitioner to take control of the patient's healthcare. Once tied to the practice, the patient is more likely to seek the practitioner's assistance when a problem arises. In addition, this allows more of an opportunity for the practitioner to regularly assess the patient's ocular health. With this agreement, the patient is afforded the opportunity to pay a universal fee for services rendered. A printed brochure may offer an effective method to inform the contact lens patient of the service agreement. This brochure should be given to all new patients while they are completing their in-office forms. This strategy allows patients time to review the pamphlet before the examination begins. Presenting this information early allows them the time needed to make a well-informed decision. The brochure should include the pricing of the services provided during a normal contact lens examination, both with and without the service agreement. Additionally, what services are covered by the agreement should be present. An example of a service agreement is shown in Figure 22.3.

There are several different types of agreements, and they may be tailored to fit into the doctor's scope of practice. Two examples are supplemental and comprehensive service agreements. The supplemental plan is more beneficial for patients who have Medicare or other third-party insurance. Most third-party plans pay only for the health examination, but include neither the

Plan A – Supplemental

$　Annual Fee

Recommended for: those patients who have insurance that covers an annual eye health examination. This supplement covers services not included in your insurance.

Services Covered:

- **Unlimited** contact lens office visits
- **Unlimited** dispensing visits
- **Unlimited** cleaning visits
- **Complimentary** contact lens lab services
- **Unlimited** replacement lenses at a significant savings
- **15% discount on eyewear***

Lens Type	Price	Your cost
Type A		
Type B		
Type C		
Type D		
Type E		
Type F	Variable	Variable

Allows for online ordering of most soft contact lenses. You may establish an online account by visiting our website at www.koettingassoc.com

* 15% discount on eyewear not good with any other offer or third party plan and not applicable on all frames and sunwear.

Plan B – Comprehensive

Annual Fee

Recommended for: contact lens wearers whose annual eye health examination is not covered by third party insurance.

Services Covered:

- Annual eye health exam
- **Unlimited** contact lens office visits
- **Unlimited** dispensing visits
- **Unlimited** cleaning visits
- **Complimentary** contact lens lab services
- **Unlimited** replacement lenses at a significant savings
- **15% discount on eyewear***

Lens Type	Price	Your cost
Type A		
Type B		
Type C		
Type D		
Type E		
Type F	Variable	Variable

Allows for online ordering of most soft contact lenses. You may establish an online account by visiting our website at www.koettingassoc.com

* 15% discount on eyewear not good with any other offer or third party plan and not applicable on all frames and sunwear.

■ FIGURE 22.3 A representative contact lens service agreement.

cost of a contact lens fitting nor the price of materials. This plan allows patients to sign an agreement that will cover their contact lens-related material fees and any contact lens-related visits to the office for an entire year. As part of the agreement, the practitioner may also include a reduced fee for replacement of contact lenses as well as a reduced fee for eyewear. The comprehensive service agreement is similar to the supplemental plan, but additionally includes the cost of the yearly health examination. By signing these agreements, not only does the patient receive a discounted rate, but also the practitioner is able to bring a constant flow of patients into the practice.

Increasing Profitability

It is apparent that profitability can be optimized via consideration of the topics already discussed, including how to develop the fees, third-party plans, considering the Fairness to Contact Lens Consumers Act, and use of service agreements. There are several other important factors as well. Exhibiting a willingness to fit the patients deemed poor candidates by another practitioner can help build the practice. These can represent some individuals who can successfully be fitted quite easily including astigmatic, early presbyopic, and borderline dry-eye patients. Other individuals can represent a greater but far from insurmountable challenge, such as keratoconic, postsurgical, and some advanced presbyopic patients. However, the willingness to fit these patients provides the opportunity for practice growth, both via referrals and as a result of being able to charge higher professional fees for the chair time potentially involved with these individuals. The presbyopic patient market, in particular, has outstanding potential as only a relatively small percentage of presbyopic patients are fitted into contact lenses. This likely represents, in large part, practitioner apprehension in fitting multifocal contact lenses, which, as emphasized in Chapter 15, should not be perceived as overly complex. Offering corneal reshaping, particularly with young patients, can also help in building a practice. Selling solutions in the office, likewise, can represent an excellent source of practice revenue while ensuring that the patient continues to use the prescribed care regimen.

■ PATIENT ENCOUNTER

Pre-Examination Education: Media Impact

Public awareness of contact lenses has increased with widespread brand-name and alternative-source dispensing advertisements. Internet and news exposure has increased, especially after the *Fusarium* and *Acanthamoeba* outbreaks. Patients can enter the office with a wide variety of preconceived notions about contact lenses. Some will have a lack of knowledge but an interest in being fitted into lenses, while others may have been previously well informed. There are also patients who arrive misinformed on proper lens care, lens choice, etc. The optometrist and staff members should be aware of the patient's entering knowledge level and educate him or her appropriately.

Patient Education: Initial Contact

When a patient schedules an appointment, the staff member needs to ask about the patient's current correction status. If the patient is not in lenses, does he or she have interest in being fitted into contact lenses? If already prescribed lenses, the staff member should remind the patient to wear his or her current lenses to the examination and to bring his or her case and solutions.

Some offices believe that a pre-examination questionnaire is beneficial in determining a patient's interest level as well as potential candidacy for lens wear. Questions include inquiries about age, occupation and work environment, and medical/ocular history. Patients also can rate their level of desire to wear lenses and indicate their motivation toward lens wear. In addition, this questionnaire can be distributed to current lens wearers to monitor compliance and to test knowledge of contact lenses. Current lens wearers should be able to identify lens type, replacement schedule, average wear time, type of solution, and cleaning regimen. The form can be provided via the Internet or at the initial office visit. An example is provided in Appendix 1.

Staff employees should review basic fee information with the patient. These fees are merely estimates, because the patient's prescription will determine the final fee. At this time, any vision plan coverage by third-party or discount programs should be explained.

Patient Education: Reception Area

It is a good idea to have information available in the reception area for the patient to browse through while waiting. Some offices have a television in the reception room with videotapes or DVDs on the latest technologies as well as the new contact lens modalities available. Organizations such as the Gas Permeable Lens Institute (http://www.gpli.info) and the American Optometric Association (http://www.aoa.org/documents/Order-Dept-Catalog.pdf) provide information pieces and general brochures. These brochures and pamphlets about contact lens options and care products can be dispersed throughout the reception area or kept on a central bookcase. Other practices find it valuable to have a bulletin board with the latest news posted.

Although it is important to make written information available to the patient, it is imperative that the doctor recommend the use of contact lenses as a vision correction option. If the patient has any questions about eye health or contact lenses, the doctor can utilize acrylic drawing boards, models, diagrams, or even videotapes on examination room computers for further explanation.

Diagnostic Fitting Sets and Inventories

In-Office Fitting Set Recommendations

It is imperative to have a large and varied assortment of lens materials and design parameters with different replacement schedules, as shown in Table 22.4, to maximize options for fitting patients. Each patient will have different needs based on his or her personality, occupation, hobbies, desires, and motivations. With several available lens options, a more customized approach can be utilized.

Also, an extensive collection of designs is convenient for both the doctor and the patient. First, it allows multiple fittings at a single visit. The practitioner can easily assess the quality of the lens-to-cornea fitting relationship and, if need be, select an alternative lens from another diagnostic fitting set or inventory. Consequently, a patient could be dispensed lenses at the initial fitting visit, reducing the number of appointments needed to obtain a successful prescription. This can provide a sense of gratification for the patient, increasing his or her motivation and enthusiasm toward contact lens wear. Finally, if a patient is in need of a replacement lens, the lens can simply be pulled from the in-office supply.

TABLE 22.4 RECOMMENDED MINIMUM NUMBER OF DIAGNOSTIC FITTING SETS AND INVENTORIES FOR CONTACT LENS PRACTICE

1. Spherical soft lenses: two silicone hydrogel lens sets and one hydrogel set

2. Toric soft lenses: two silicone hydrogel lens sets and one hydrogel set

3. Soft bifocal/multifocal lenses: one silicone hydrogel lens set and one hydrogel set

4. Gas-permeable (GP) spherical sets (low minus, high minus, and plus sets as given in Chapter 5)

5. Bifocal/multifocal GP lenses: one aspheric multifocal and one segmented, translating set; a concentric set should also be considered

6. Bitoric GP lenses: either a 3-D SPE set from your laboratory or use an empirical method such as Mandell-Moore

7. Keratoconic GP lenses: at minimum, both a small-diameter and an intralimbal fitting set; if the practice specializes in contact lenses, both a semi-scleral set and a hybrid set should be considered

8. Postsurgical GP lenses: at minimum, one postsurgical fitting set, often an intralimbal diameter with a reverse geometry midperiphery, although multiple sets (i.e., non–reverse geometry, semi-scleral, and hybrid) should be available if the practice specializes in contact lenses

Sales representatives from the various contact lens companies are excellent resources for answering questions about different contact lenses and care systems. They should be encouraged to meet on a regular basis with both practitioners and staff members. They also represent the source for fitting sets and inventories of recently introduced lenses.

Lens Storage

Storage: Soft Lenses: Soft lenses are available in convenient disposable blister packing; thus, after fitting, the patient can either wear lenses home or the lenses can be disposed. If cleaning and reuse are necessary, disinfect with a surfactant cleaner or a two-step peroxide system (e.g., Clear Care) and store in a soft lens-compatible solution. If long-term storage is necessary, redisinfect every 90 days.

Storage: Gas-Permeable Lenses: Most gas-permeable lenses are typically stored dry. After each use, properly disinfect lenses with either a strong surfactant cleaner (e.g., Miraflow) or hydrogen peroxide for 10 minutes, blot clean, and store. Some gas-permeable lenses require storage in solution, such as Claris or Optimum. As both of these products are nonabrasive cleaners with benzyl alcohol, lenses should be rinsed before insertion.

Patient Education: Postexamination

After the examination, the practitioner or staff member needs to instruct the patient on several topics. The following items should be emphasized: insertion and removal techniques, lens type and replacement schedule, and lens care regimens. These are discussed in Chapters 6 and 12. Fee information should also be discussed. Many offices have a management agreement that breaks down the various charges associated with the examination, materials, and follow-up care. Figure 22.4 provides an example of a management agreement.

These agreements can also include information pertaining to refund policy and a listing of solutions, and reminding the patient that successful contact lens wear is not guaranteed. It is also advisable to have an agreement specifically for patients who will be wearing continuous-wear lenses (see Appendix 2) or for corneal reshaping.

■ PATIENT RETENTION

One of the most important factors in patient retention is to have a strong bond with the patient. One way to help solidify this bond is for the patient to be seen on a regular basis. After the initial contact lens examination and subsequent follow-up visits, the contact lens wearer should typically be scheduled to return to the office every 6 months. The office staff needs to make this appointment for the patient before he or she leaves the office. Seeing patients semi-annually not only allows the doctor to detect small visual and physiologic problems before they become an issue, but also allows for the monitoring of contact lens care and compliance. The bond with the patient may be strengthened during these visits as well. It is easier to retain a patient who is happy, successful, and compliant and knows the doctor and staff on a personal basis.

Another way to solidify the doctor–patient relationship is to know the patient by name. The patient will feel important if the office staff personally walks up and addresses him or her by name when it is time for the appointment to begin. One way to accomplish this task is to take photographs of all new patients and keep them in their permanent files. A public relations card kept within the patient's permanent file is another mechanism that allows the doctor and staff to have a relationship with the patient. This card contains personal notes about the patient such as hobbies or upcoming vacations. When the patient returns for a visit, the card helps the practitioner and staff relate to him or her on a more personal level, thus enhancing the in-office experience.

A follow-up call by the optometric staff to patients should be considered. These calls may be made to new patients or to established patients who have recently had changes in their

Figure 5 Prescription and management agreements

Cornea Center for Clinical Excellence
3241 S. Michigan Avenue
Chicago, IL 60616
(312) 949-7240

ILLINOIS EYE
INSTITUTE

Contact Lens Prescription and Management Agreement

At the Illinois Eye Institute, we are dedicated to providing the highest level of contact lens services to our patients. This agreement outlines our contact lens policies.

Professional Fees

Professional fees are due at the time of service and are for 90 days of contact lens related visits. In addition, they are non-refundable. Those fees not covered by insurance are the responsibility of the patient. When this agreement expires in 90 days, additional professional fees will apply.

Orders

All orders must be paid in full at the time they are placed. Disposable lens orders of four boxes or more will be direct shipped to you. Non-standard orders are subject to a $5 processing fee. If you request a non-standard order be shipped that fee is an additional $5. If a more advanced or different design is needed additional fees may arise. Material returns are only permitted within 60 days of the original order date. Only unopened boxes of multi-packaged lenses may be returned. There are no discounts on lost or damaged lenses. There are no returns or refunds on custom, donated, or colored lenses. Orders that are not picked up within 60 days will be returned and deposit forfeited.

Presciptions

Each year you will receive a copy of both your contact lens and spectacle prescriptions in accordance with federal law. You may re-order on a valid prescription up to the maximum number of refills listed by calling 312-949-7268.

Preliminary fee estimate   Recommended follow-up schedule
_____ Health Exam Fee   _____ 1 day
_____ 90 day professional fee for fit and follow-up   _____ 1-2 weeks
_____ One year supply of contact lenses   _____ 1 month
_____ Present total   _____ 3 months
_____ Discounts and/or co-pays   _____ 6 months
_____ Balance   _____ As needed

Important information about your eye health

Yearly eye examinations are necessary to ensure complete eye health. Therefore, we recommend yearly-dilated eye examinations at the Illinois Eye Institute.

Contact lens patients require special care because of the increased risk of eye infection that may lead to severe vision loss. If you experience any of the following symptoms, you should remove your contact lenses immediately and call the Illinois Eye Institute at (312) 225-6200 (24-hour urgent care service). **During normal business hours you should also contact the Cornea Center for Clinical Excellence at (312) 949-7240.**
Eye pain or unusual irritation   Cloudy or decreased vision
Watering of a discharge from the eye(s)   Sensitivity to light
Redness of the eye(s)   Any disturbance in vision or eye comfort
*Please note after-hours visits may be subject to additional fees.

I have been given the opportunity to ask questions about this agreement and my responsibilities associated with contact lens wear. With my signature below, I acknowledge having received a copy of this agreement and accept it as it is written.

_____   _____
Signature of patient or guardian   date

■ **FIGURE 22.4** A fee information agreement.

prescription. For example, an established patient who is attempting contact lenses for the first time would appreciate a telephone call from the office. The staff can use this time to not only obtain information about the patient's experience, but also ascertain whether or not any complications have arisen since the examination.

An effective approach to retaining established contact lens wearers is to send out regular mailings (i.e., office updates or a newsletter could be mailed or e-mailed) (Fig. 22.5). These may be sent out several times a year and can highlight the practitioners and the staff. They may be written by the staff or the practitioner (or, preferably, both), and should be used to make the patient feel like he or she is part of the practice family, not just another patient. Mailed or e-mailed materials may also be used to focus on new developments in contact lenses or to address any eye-related concerns that may have received recent media attention. For example, when the *Fusarium* outbreak was prevalent in the media, a mailing/e-mailing to current contact lens patients, including basic information about the disease as well as preventative measures, may have been greatly appreciated by the patients.

Some of the strategies that are used to help retain patients may also be used to attract new ones. Holding an open house is a great way to make patients aware of the different services the doctor provides. This may also provide an opportunity to show office renovations, feature new equipment, or inform the public about new innovations in contact lenses. Additionally, the open house is a useful occasion for informing patients of the office hours. Having extended office hours is an effective method for attracting new patients. Most patients work during

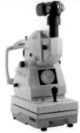

The newest in eye care technology has arrived at Vision Care Consultants. We now have the latest in digital cameras that allow us to photograph both the outside and the inside of the eye. Our new Biomicroscope camera can take high-resolution digital photographs of the exterior or front part of the eye while our digital retinal camera can take high-resolution photos of the interior portion of the eye called the retina. This new technology can greatly aid our doctor's ability to accurately diagnosis and document many diseases. High-resolution photographs can show early abnormalities of the eye that may threaten normal vision. It also provides a baseline for comparison with patient's previous and future visits, which aids in monitoring disease progression and response to therapy.

Our new digital retinal camera is the latest in eyecare technology.

Other advantages of Digital Ocular Photography:

✦ Your images are available immediately, allowing for quick diagnosis and an appropriate management for your individual case.

✦ The images can be enhanced using sophisticated software to highlight any problem areas. This helps our doctors with diagnostic decisions.

✦ Our doctors now can show you images of your eye on high resolution computer monitors in the privacy of your exam room so you can make the most informed decision on the health of your eyes.

continued on page 3

WE ARE PROVIDERS FOR MANY VISION & MEDICAL INSURANCE PLANS

Vision Care Consultants is a provider for many Vision & Medical insurance plans. You may have vision insurance or major medical insurance or you may have both. Check the list below or call (314) 843-5700 to see if we accept your plan.

A vision care plan may partially pay for your vision examination, glasses or contact lenses. Medical insurance may pay a portion of your charges for a medical emergency (eye infection, eye injury, retinal detachment, etc.) or for necessary medical testing needed to manage ocular disease (glaucoma, cataract, diabetes, etc.). Medical insurance usually has a co-payment that needs to be paid at the time that services are rendered in the office.

In order for us to help you get your full insurance benefits, it is very important that every patient present their insurance cards to our front desk before they see our doctors. If you send your son or daughter to our office without a patient, please give them your vision and/or medical insurance card so they can provide that information to our staff. We appreciate your cooperation.

Medical Insurance Plans:		Vision Plans:
✦ Aetna	✦ GHP & GHP Advantra	✦ EyeMed
✦ Blue Cross/Blue Shield -	✦ Health & Welfare Funds	✦ Great West
Many Plans	✦ HealthLink - All Plans	✦ Premier Benefits
✦ Cigna - Primary Eye Care	✦ Medicare	✦ Spectera
✦ EPOCH	✦ Mercy	✦ Vision Service Plan (VSP)
✦ GHP/CMR-Carpenters'/Coventry	✦ United Healthcare	✦ Vision Benefits of America (VBA)

Plus many more! When you make an appointment, please let us know if you have vision or medical insurance. Do not assume that you do not have any insurance coverage for vision or medical procedures. We are happy to assist with your insurance questions.

VisionCareConsultants™

■ FIGURE 22.5 A contact lens practice patient newsletter.

regular office hours. If the office is open later in the evening (e.g., until 8:00 p.m. one evening a week and until 3:00 p.m. on a Saturday), patients have more opportunities to make an appointment. This may be just what is needed to encourage new patients to seek eye care.

Another beneficial strategy is in-office seminars. For example, such a seminar could be designed for patients interested in multifocal contact lenses. During this time, the practitioner would provide a formal presentation and allow time for the participants to ask any questions about contact lenses. It is also recommended to have some of the office staff working during the event. These seminars allow the patients an opportunity to be fitted with some of the different types of contact lenses and determine if this is a worthwhile investment. If the opportunity exists for potential patients to schedule appointments, they will be more likely to return to the office for their contact lens examination and fitting. Orthokeratology, or corneal reshaping, represents another such opportunity to provide a seminar/workshop.

As a practitioner, it is crucial that one is not afraid to advertise. Most practitioners will utilize the phonebook yellow pages, but they should not be limited by them. The local media offers a great way to reach new patients. Contacting local radio stations, television stations, and newspapers and informing them of your expertise in contact lenses could result in opportunities that could both be enjoyable and help build the practice. A curriculum vitae complete with qualifications as well as potential topics for discussion or publication should be included. These opportunities again provide the doctor with name recognition.

The bottom line is that a happy patient will return. Patients must be able leave the office and feel like they have had a successful contact lens fit. Establishing a strong doctor–patient relationship through strategies such as public relations cards, mailings, and accessible educational materials will keep the contact lens wearer returning to the office again and again.

■ SUMMARY

It is evident that the key to a successful contact lens practice is a comprehensive education program for the practitioner, staff, and patients. The ideas presented in this chapter will not all apply to every practice, but the important outcome is the understanding that a large percentage of income generated in an eye care practice is from contact lenses. In particular, specialty lenses represent a great potential source of practice profitability and growth, not to mention personal satisfaction.

■ APPENDIX 1

Patient Visual Needs Assessment

Drs. Quinn, Quinn, and Associates

Your Name _____ Age _____ Today's Date _____

1. So we may best meet your visual needs, please list specific visual demands you have (work or recreation related):

   _____

2. What is your primary form of visual correction? (please circle)

   Glasses   Soft contact lenses   Gas-permeable contact lenses   No correction

3. How do you wear your current glasses? (please circle)

   All day   Distance tasks   Near tasks   As needed   Don't wear

4. Are you interested in considering contact lenses? (please circle one)

   To wear daily   To wear on occasion To wear continuously for up to 1 month

   Haven't considered I already wear   Not interested

5. Are you interested in contact lenses that will change or enhance eye color?   Yes   No

6. Have you worn contact lenses in the past? (please circle)

   Soft lenses   Gas-permeable lenses   Hard lenses   Haven't worn

7. Are you interested in considering corneal refractive therapy (wearing a gas-permeable lens overnight to reshape the eye, so when removed in the morning, uncorrected vision is clear)?

   Yes   No   Not sure

8. Are you interested in considering laser treatment to reduce your dependence on corrective lenses?

   Yes   No   Not sure

Thank you! Please return this form to the receptionist.

■ **APPENDIX TWO**

Your Continuous Wear Contact Lens Care Plan (Courtesy of Dr. Walter Choate)

Soft contact lenses have been prescribed for extended wear for up to 7 nights since 1981. Unfortunately, the early generations of extended-wear soft contact lenses have now been shown to not be as safe for many people as we once thought. In November 2001, the Food and Drug Administration (FDA) issued final approval for two new silicone hydrogel soft lens materials for continuous wear for up to 30 nights. The difference in these materials and the first-generation materials is significant in several areas: truly safe amounts of oxygen are able to flow through the lens to the cornea, adequate movement, greater comfort, less dryness, greater deposit resistance, and less chance for eye infection. We are, therefore, in a new era for overnight wear of contact lenses, providing you with new levels of comfort, safety, visual performance, and convenience.

Quality contact lens care begins with a medical eye examination and vision analysis. This will establish your suitability for wearing contact lenses, and will determine your prescription needs for spectacles. Following this evaluation, your contact lens evaluation will include special tests specific to contact lenses: computerized corneal mapping, tear chemistry evaluation, diagnostic fitting and evaluation of lenses on the eye, and finally a class to properly instruct you on the care and handling of your lenses. After your lenses have been dispensed, you will be asked to return to the office for progress evaluations. The duration of these visits should be brief, but please do not underestimate their importance. From these visits we will determine the following: quality of the contact lens fitting relationship to the cornea, reaction of the eye to overnight wear, suitability of the solution system, frequency of lens replacement, proper number of safe nights of continuous wear, and visual adaptation. The prescribed schedule of visits for a first-year patient is as follows: 2 weeks, 4 weeks, 6 weeks, 3 months, 6 months, and 9 months.

Our office stands for excellence in eye care. We only know how to do things one way—the right way! Our goals for you are higher than your own, in that we want your eyes to remain healthy, your vision better than 20/20, and for you to not even know that your lenses are in your eyes. These goals are lofty, but we achieve them most of the time.

For us to be successful, you have to be a dedicated partner in this process. That means the following: follow all of our instructions carefully, come in for all prescribed follow-up visits, use only prescribed contact lens care products, replace your lenses per our professional instructions, and never wear your lenses when your eyes are red or uncomfortable or your vision is blurry. Please realize that many of the potential risks you will face with contact lens wear are environmental in nature. That means if you find yourself in conditions that will normally irritate your eyes, you should never make matters worse by sleeping in your contacts. Always maintain the highest standards of personal hygiene, washing your hands with an antibacterial soap before handling your lenses. You should also inspect your eyes every night before considering overnight wear. They should be WHITE and COMFORTABLE (you can't feel them), and you should be SEEING CLEARLY (check both eyes individually). If any one of these issues is a problem, DO NOT SLEEP IN YOUR LENSES THAT NIGHT. You can then revisit your contact lens wear the following morning. Always report to us immediately if you have persistent redness, pain, light sensitivity, or blurry vision.

In constructing fees for your care, please remember that our fees are customized for each individual patient according to the complexity of the case and the predicted time necessary to take care of the individual patient. Below is a breakdown of your fees.

Medical Eye Examination and Visual Analysis... _____
Comprehensive evaluation of internal and external eye health, review of general health status and its impact on ocular health, and visual analysis resulting in a prescription for glasses (approximately 1 hour).

Contact Lens Evaluation .... _____
Includes computerized corneal mapping, tear chemistry evaluation, diagnostic fitting/dispensing of initial lenses, and a class to cover all appropriate aspects of the care and handling of your lenses (approximately 1½ hours).

Prescribed Follow-Up Care .... _____
Your number of follow-up visits will be greater if you are new to contact lenses and less if you are a return patient with no complications. Prescribed follow-up visits for new patients are approximately seven for the year and for return patients are approximately four for the year. Your fee covers all scheduled and unscheduled contact lens-related visits for the year. It is during these visits that refinements in your contact lens fit and care system are made to maximize your comfort, vision, and health (approximately 1½–2½ total hours).

Contact Lenses and Solutions .... _____
This fee is for a 1-year supply of your prescribed lenses. You may purchase a 3-month or a 6-month supply, but typically your cost is lower if an annual supply is purchased, because of manufacturer rebates. As a convenience to you, we are always happy to have your lenses direct shipped to you at your home or office at no additional charge. Please also note that we also replace all lenses that are lost, torn, or defective at no additional charge to you. When you come in for routine visits, we also give you complimentary cases and travel sizes of your solutions.

I have read and understand the care plan that has been developed for me by Dr. _____'s. Furthermore, I agree to follow Dr. _____'s recommendations regarding follow-up care visits, contact lens replacement, contact lens solutions, and frequency of lens removal. I furthermore agree to never sleep in my lenses if my eyes are red or uncomfortable or my vision is blurry. I will also contact Dr. _____'s office immediately if my eyes become persistently red, light sensitive, or painful, or if my vision becomes blurry. I am aware that my continuous-wear lenses can jeopardize my eye health and vision if I do not adhere to these instructions.

_____

Patient Signature   Date

REFERENCES

1. Dillehay SM. Recommendation rates of contact lenses at North American schools and colleges of optometry. Optom Vis Sci 1997;74(12s):77
2. Jones L, Jones D, Langley C, et al. Reactive or proactive contact lens fitting – does it make a difference? J Br Contact Lens Assoc 1996;19(2):41–43.
3. American Optometric Association Contact Lenses and Cornea Section. CLCS scope and function. Available at http://www.aoa.org/x5989.xml. Accessed March 20, 2008.
4. American Optometric Association Contact Lenses and Cornea Section. CLCS membership benefits. Available at http://www.aoa.org/x5992.xml. Accessed March 20, 2008.
5. American Optometric Association Contact Lenses and Cornea Section. CLCS membership information. Available at http://www.aoa.org/x5993.xml. Accessed March 20, 2008.
6. American Academy of Optometry Cornea & Contact Lens. Becoming a diplomate - history. Available at http://www.aaopt.org/section/cl/becoming/history/index.asp. Accessed March 20, 2008.
7. American Academy of Optometry Cornea & Contact Lens. Becoming a diplomate in the American Academy of Optometry's Section on Cornea and Contact Lenses. Available at http://www.aaopt.org/section/cl/becoming/index.asp. Accessed March 20, 2008.
8. Heart of America Contact Lens Society 2008 Conference Links. 2008 courses - paraoptometirc. Available at http://www.hoacls.com/registration/CLASSSCHEDr.ASP?rtc=p. Accessed March 20, 2008.
9. American Optometric Association. Third party/managed care surveys. Available at http://www.aoa.org/x4849.xml. Accessed March 20, 2008.
10. Federal Trade Commission: Protecting America's Consumers. FTC issues final rule implementing Fairness to Contact Lens Consumers Act. Released June 29, 2004. Available at http://www.ftc.gov/opa/2004/06/contactlens.shtm. Accessed March 20, 2008.

Appendices

CURVATURE (D)	CONVEX RADIUS (MM)	CURVATURE (D)	CONVEX RADIUS (MM)	CURVATURE (D)	CONVEX RADIUS (MM)
60.00	5.63	54.37	6.21	48.87	6.91
59.87	5.64	54.25	6.22	48.75	6.92
59.75	5.65	54.12	6.24	48.62	6.95
59.62	5.66	54.00	6.25	48.50	6.96
59.50	5.67	53.87	6.26	48.37	6.98
59.37	5.68	53.75	6.28	48.25	7.00
59.25	5.70	53.62	6.29	48.12	7.01
59.12	5.71	53.50	6.31	48.00	7.03
59.00	5.72	53.37	6.32	47.87	7.05
58.87	5.73	53.25	6.34	47.75	7.07
58.75	5.75	53.12	6.35	47.62	7.09
58.62	5.76	53.00	6.37	47.50	7.11
58.50	5.77	52.87	6.38	47.37	7.12
58.37	5.78	52.75	6.40	47.25	7.14
58.25	5.79	52.62	6.41	47.12	7.16
58.12	5.81	52.50	6.43	47.00	7.18
58.00	5.82	52.37	6.44	46.87	7.20
57.87	5.83	52.25	6.46	46.75	7.22
57.75	5.84	52.12	6.48	46.62	7.24
57.62	5.86	52.00	6.49	46.50	7.26
57.50	5.87	51.87	6.51	46.37	7.28
57.37	5.88	51.75	6.52	46.25	7.30
57.25	5.90	51.62	6.54	46.12	7.32
57.12	5.91	51.50	6.55	46.00	7.34
57.00	5.92	51.37	6.57	45.87	7.36
56.87	5.94	51.25	6.59	45.75	7.38
56.75	5.95	51.12	6.60	45.62	7.40
56.62	5.96	51.00	6.62	45.50	7.42
56.50	5.97	50.87	6.63	45.37	7.44
56.37	5.99	50.75	6.65	45.25	7.46
56.25	6.00	50.62	6.67	45.12	7.48
56.12	6.01	50.50	6.68	45.00	7.50
56.00	6.03	50.37	6.70	44.87	7.52
55.87	6.04	50.25	6.72	44.75	7.54

Continues

APPENDIX 1 *(Continued)* KERATOMETER DIOPTER CONVERSION TO MILLIMETERS

CURVATURE (D)	CONVEX RADIUS (MM)	CURVATURE (D)	CONVEX RADIUS (MM)	CURVATURE (D)	CONVEX RADIUS (MM)
55.75	6.05	50.12	6.73	44.62	7.56
55.62	6.07	50.00	6.75	44.50	7.58
55.50	6.08	49.87	6.77	44.37	7.61
55.37	6.10	49.75	6.78	44.25	7.63
55.25	6.11	49.62	6.80	44.12	7.65
55.12	6.12	49.50	6.82	44.00	7.67
55.00	6.14	49.37	6.84	43.87	7.69
54.87	6.15	49.25	6.85	43.75	7.72
54.75	6.16	49.12	6.87	43.62	7.74
54.62	6.18	49.00	6.89	43.50	7.76
54.50	6.19				
43.37	7.78	40.62	8.31		
43.25	7.80	40.50	8.33		
43.12	7.83	40.37	8.36		
43.00	7.85	40.25	8.39		
42.87	7.87	40.12	8.41		
42.75	7.90	40.00	8.44		
42.62	7.92	39.87	8.46		
42.50	7.94	39.75	8.49		
42.37	7.97	39.62	8.52		
42.25	7.99	39.50	8.55		
42.12	8.01	39.37	8.57		
42.00	8.04	39.25	8.60		
41.87	8.06	39.12	8.63		
41.75	8.08	39.00	8.65		
41.62	8.11	38.87	8.68		
41.50	8.13	38.75	8.71		
41.37	8.16	38.62	8.74		
41.25	8.18	38.50	8.77		
41.12	8.21	38.37	8.80		
41.00	8.23	38.25	8.82		
40.87	8.26	38.12	8.85		
40.75	8.28	38.00	8.88		

APPENDIX 2 EFFECTIVE SPECTACLE LENS POWER AT THE CORNEAL PLANE (12-MM VERTEX DISTANCE)

	MINUS LENSES (D)		
SPECTACLE LENS POWER	EFFECTIVE POWER	SPECTACLE LENS POWER	EFFECTIVE POWER
−4.00	−3.82	−11.25	−9.91
−4.25	−4.05	−11.50	−10.11
−4.50	−4.27	−11.75	−10.30
−4.75	−4.49	−12.00	−10.49
−5.00	−4.72	−12.25	−10.69
−5.25	−4.94	−12.50	−10.87
−5.50	−5.16	−12.75	−11.06
−5.75	−5.38	−13.00	−11.25
−6.00	−5.60	−13.25	−11.43
−6.25	−5.82	−13.50	−11.62
−6.50	−6.03	−13.75	−11.80
−6.75	−6.25	−14.00	−11.99
−7.00	−6.46	−14.25	−12.17
−7.25	−6.67	−14.50	−12.38
−7.50	−6.88	−14.75	−12.54
−7.75	−7.09	−15.00	−12.72
−8.00	−7.30	−15.25	−12.90
−8.25	−7.51	−15.50	−13.07
−8.50	−7.71	−15.75	−13.25
−8.75	−7.92	−16.00	−13.43
−9.00	−8.13	−16.25	−13.61
−9.25	−8.33	−16.50	−13.78
−9.50	−8.53	−16.75	−13.95
−9.75	−8.73	−17.00	−14.12
−10.00	−8.93	−17.25	−14.30
−10.25	−9.13	−17.50	−14.47
−10.50	−9.33	−17.75	−14.64
−10.75	−9.52	−18.00	−14.80
−11.00	−9.72		

	PLUS LENSES (D)		
SPECTACLE LENS POWER	EFFECTIVE POWER	SPECTACLE LENS POWER	EFFECTIVE POWER
+4.00	+4.20	+11.25	+13.01
+4.25	+4.48	+11.50	+13.30
+4.50	+4.76	+11.75	+13.68
+4.75	+5.04	+12.00	+14.02
+5.00	+5.32	+12.25	+14.37
+5.25	+5.60	+12.50	+14.71
+5.50	+5.89	+12.75	+15.06
+5.75	+6.18	+13.00	+15.41

Continues

APPENDIX 2 *(Continued)* EFFECTIVE SPECTACLE LENS POWER AT THE CORNEAL PLANE (12-MM VERTEX DISTANCE)

	PLUS LENSES (D)		
SPECTACLE LENS POWER	EFFECTIVE POWER	SPECTACLE LENS POWER	EFFECTIVE POWER
+6.00	+6.47	+13.25	+15.76
+6.25	+6.76	+13.50	+16.11
+6.50	+7.05	+13.75	+16.47
+6.75	+7.35	+14.00	+16.83
+7.00	+7.64	+14.25	+17.20
+7.25	+7.94	+14.50	+17.56
+7.50	+8.24	+14.75	+17.93
+7.75	+8.55	+15.00	+18.30
+8.00	+8.85	+15.25	+18.67
+8.25	+9.16	+15.50	+19.05
+8.50	+9.52	+15.75	+19.43
+8.75	+9.83	+16.00	+19.81
+9.00	+10.09	+16.25	+20.02
+9.25	+10.41	+16.50	+20.59
+9.50	+10.73	+16.75	+20.97
+9.75	+11.05	+17.00	+21.37
+10.00	+11.36	+17.50	+22.16
+10.50	+12.02	+17.75	+22.57
+10.75	+12.35	+18.00	+22.97
+11.00	+12.68		

APPENDIX 3 EXTENDED KERATOMETER RANGE WITH +1.25 D LENS

ACTUAL DRUM VALUE READING (D)	EXTENDED VALUE (D)	ACTUAL DRUM READING (D)	EXTENDED VALUE (D)
43.00	50.13	47.62	55.53
43.12	50.28	47.75	55.67
43.25	50.42	47.87	55.82
43.37	50.57	48.00	55.96
43.50	50.72	48.12	56.11
43.62	50.86	48.25	56.25
43.75	51.01	48.37	56.40
43.87	51.15	48.50	56.55
44.00	51.30	48.62	56.69
44.12	51.44	48.75	56.84
44.25	51.59	48.87	56.98
44.37	51.74	49.00	57.13
44.50	51.88	49.12	57.27
44.62	52.03	49.25	57.42
44.75	52.17	49.37	57.57
44.87	52.32	49.50	57.71
45.00	52.46	49.62	57.86
45.12	52.61	49.75	58.00
45.25	52.76	49.87	58.15
45.37	52.90	50.00	58.30
45.50	53.05	50.12	58.44
45.62	53.19	50.25	58.59
45.75	53.34	50.37	58.73
45.87	53.49	50.50	58.88
46.00	53.63	50.62	59.02
46.12	53.78	50.75	59.17
46.25	53.92	50.87	59.31
46.37	54.07	51.00	59.46
46.50	54.21	51.12	59.61
46.62	54.36	51.25	59.75
46.75	54.51	51.37	59.90
46.87	54.65	51.50	60.04
47.00	54.80	51.62	60.19
47.12	54.94	51.75	60.33
47.25	55.09	51.87	60.48
47.37	55.23	52.00	60.63
47.50	55.38		

Continues

APPENDIX 3 *(Continued)* EXTENDED KERATOMETER RANGE WITH −1.00 D LENS

ACTUAL DRUM VALUE READING (D)	EXTENDED VALUE (D)	ACTUAL DRUM READING (D)	EXTENDED VALUE (D)
36.00	30.87	39.12	33.55
36.12	30.98	39.25	33.66
36.25	31.09	39.37	33.77
36.37	31.20	39.50	33.88
36.50	31.30	39.62	33.98
36.62	31.41	39.75	34.09
36.75	31.51	39.87	34.20
36.87	31.62	40.00	34.30
37.00	31.73	40.12	34.41
37.12	31.84	40.25	34.52
37.25	31.95	40.37	34.63
37.37	32.05	40.50	34.73
37.50	32.16	40.62	34.84
37.62	32.27	40.75	34.95
37.75	32.37	40.87	35.05
37.87	32.48	41.00	35.16
38.00	32.59	41.12	35.27
38.12	32.70	41.25	35.38
38.25	32.80	41.37	35.48
38.37	32.91	41.50	35.59
38.50	33.02	41.62	35.70
38.62	33.13	41.75	35.81
38.75	33.23	41.87	35.91
38.87	33.34	42.00	36.02
39.00	33.45		

Index

Page numbers followed by *f* denote figures; those followed by *t* denote tables.

RE 977 .B43 2009 c.4

Clinical manual of contact
lenses

CCS1108